Thieme

The Brain, Spine and Nerves in Sports

Nicholas Theodore, MD
Professor
Department of Neurosurgery
Johns Hopkins University
Baltimore, Maryland, USA

Russell R. Lonser, MD
Chair
Department of Neurological Surgery
The Ohio State University
Columbus, Ohio, USA

124 illustrations

Thieme
New York • Stuttgart • Delhi • Rio de Janeiro

Library of Congress Cataloging-in-Publication Data is available with the publisher.

Important note: Medicine is an ever-changing science undergoing continual development. Research and clinical experience are continually expanding our knowledge, in particular our knowledge of proper treatment and drug therapy. Insofar as this book mentions any dosage or application, readers may rest assured that the authors, editors, and publishers have made every effort to ensure that such references are in accordance with **the state of knowledge at the time of production of the book.**

Nevertheless, this does not involve, imply, or express any guarantee or responsibility on the part of the publishers in respect to any dosage instructions and forms of applications stated in the book. **Every user is requested to examine carefully** the manufacturers' leaflets accompanying each drug and to check, if necessary, in consultation with a physician or specialist, whether the dosage schedules mentioned therein or the contraindications stated by the manufacturers differ from the statements made in the present book. Such examination is particularly important with drugs that are either rarely used or have been newly released on the market. Every dosage schedule or every form of application used is entirely at the user's own risk and responsibility. The authors and publishers request every user to report to the publishers any discrepancies or inaccuracies noticed. If errors in this work are found after publication, errata will be posted at www.thieme.com on the product description page.

Some of the product names, patents, and registered designs referred to in this book are in fact registered trademarks or proprietary names even though specific reference to this fact is not always made in the text. Therefore, the appearance of a name without designation as proprietary is not to be construed as a representation by the publisher that it is in the public domain.

Thieme addresses people of all gender identities equally. We encourage our authors to use gender-neutral or gender-equal expressions wherever the context allows.

Thieme Publishers New York
333 Seventh Avenue, 18th Floor
New York, NY 10001, USA
www.thieme.com
+1 800 782 3488, customerservice@thieme.com

Cover design: © Thieme
Cover image source: © Laura Roy
Typesetting by TNQ Tech Private Limited, India

Printed in India by Replika Press Pvt. Ltd. 5 4 3 2 1

MIX
Paper | Supporting responsible forestry
FSC™ C016779

DOI: 10.1055/b-006-164736

ISBN: 978-1-68420-114-3

Also available as an e-book:
eISBN (PDF): 978-1-68420-115-0
eISBN (epub): 978-1-63853-663-5

Contents

Part II: Spine

Videos

Video 9.1: Maximum principal strain in the brain (warmer colors represent higher brain strains) from a pulse with a peak linear acceleration of 35 *g* with low rotational kinematics (top) and high rotational kinematics (bottom). Results generated using the Global Human Body Models Consortium (GHBMC)-owned, 50th percentile male, detailed, seated occupant (v4.3) head. (No audio.)

Video 9.2: Maximum principal strain in the brain (warmer colors represent higher brain strains) from rotational impacts with peak kinematics of 40 rad/s and 4 krad/s^2 applied in difference planes: sagittal (left), coronal (center), and transverse (right). Results generated using the Global Human Body Models Consortium (GHBMC)-owned, 50th percentile male, detailed, seated occupant (v4.3) head. (No audio.)

Video 9.3: Test setup for the Virginia Tech helmet test program. In this example, a hockey helmet is mounted on the head and neck of an anthropometric surrogate (head: NOCSAE headform; neck: 50th percentile Hybrid III). A pendulum impactor with a flat, rigid impactor face impacts the helmeted head at multiple impact locations and velocities to mimic relevant hockey impacts. The head–neck assembly is mounted on a sliding table to allow for linear and rotational motions to be measured. (No audio.)

Video 19.1: Case presentation of a 16-year-old girl with spondylolysis treated with direct pars repair via the Buck procedure. (Used with permissions from Barrow Neurological Institute, Phoenix, Arizona.)

Foreword

The first responsibility of a physician is to prevent disease.
If that be impossible, to cure it.
If that too be impossible, to relieve pain.

These words summarize an approach to care set forth by the famous Greek Hippocrates over 2,000 years ago. And for the last 50 years, I have been committed to this approach when treating athletes "on the fields of friendly strife." From youth sports to the NFL and beyond, I have prioritized prevention of sports-related brain and spinal injuries, performed surgeries in an attempt to cure, and offered methods for pain reduction and rehabilitation.

As someone who has always sought new and better ways to prevent, cure, and relieve pain, I was honored when Dr. Nick Theodore and Dr. Russell Lonser asked me to write this foreword for *The Brain, Spine and Nerves in Sports*. Russell and I are both past presidents of the Congress of Neurological Surgeons, and I have worked closely with both Nick and Russell on the NFL Head, Neck and Spine Committee. These fine physicians have collaborated to create a superb compendium that blends their own experiences with many of the world's most informed professionals in brain and spinal injuries in sports medicine.

While this book addresses the goals set forth by Hippocrates, it also deftly embraces Sir William Osler's notion that medicine is both a science and an art. Readers will benefit from meticulous scientific research on everything, from the epidemiology of concussions to novel surgical approaches for the repair of spondolytic defects. The book contains detailed and critical overviews of unique sports-related injuries in soccer, cycling, skiing, hockey, rugby, and more. But readers will also learn the more subtle art of medicine, including advice on how to navigate through challenging—often time-sensitive—options, and how to handle the complex decisions concerning a return to play.

What Nick and Russell have created is a profound and definitive text on the diagnosis and treatment of the most important neurological and neurosurgical conditions pertinent to all sports. It is a timely, well-referenced, and succinctly written resource and will no doubt contribute to the ultimate goals of sports medicine: prevention, cure, and treatment. Hippocrates would be proud.

Joseph C. Maroon, MD, FACS
Clinical Professor
Department of Neurological Surgery
Heindl Scholar in Neuroscience
University of Pittsburgh Medical Center
Pittsburgh, Pennsylvania, USA

Preface

Homer's the *Iliad* brings us what is likely the first description of a sports-related neurological injury, with the epic poet describing a vicious boxing match between Epeus and Euryalus. Homer recounts a blow Epeus delivers to Euryalus' cheek that knocked him off his feet—Epeus' movements were so fast that they were likened to that of a fish. Since the early period in history, athletic endeavors have thankfully become much safer. Sports medicine as a discipline has evolved through an understanding of the complex interplay between the physiology of the human body and the demands of athletic performance.

Although musculoskeletal injuries are by far the most common injuries seen in sports, neurological injuries are often the most serious and potentially devastating. As athletes push the boundaries of physical achievement, they inevitably encounter challenges and trauma that require specialized medical attention, particularly in critical structures such as the brain, spinal cord, and peripheral nerves.

The Brain, Spine and Nerves in Sports is a comprehensive textbook that delves into the intricacies associated with the diagnosis and treatment of sports-related neurological injuries. This book is a collaborative effort by leading experts in the fields of neurosurgery, spine surgery, sports medicine, and rehabilitation, and aims to provide a thorough exploration of the latest advancements, techniques, and best practices in managing neurological conditions in athletes.

The chapters within this textbook are thoughtfully curated and cover a wide range of topics, including traumatic brain injuries, spinal cord injuries, peripheral nerve injuries, concussions, neurovascular disorders, and neurological considerations in sports-related spine pathology. Each chapter is structured to offer a blend of theoretical knowledge, evidence-based practices, case studies, and practical insights derived from the authors' years of clinical experience.

Furthermore, this textbook acknowledges the multidisciplinary nature of sports medicine, emphasizing the importance of collaboration between neurosurgeons, orthopedic surgeons, sports physicians, physical therapists, and other healthcare professionals. Through this collaborative approach, we aim to optimize patient outcomes, enhance performance, and promote the overall well-being of athletes at all levels of competition.

We extend our sincere gratitude to all the contributors, editors, reviewers, and medical illustrators who have dedicated their expertise and passion to bring this volume to fruition. It is our sincere hope that this book will serve as a beacon of knowledge and inspiration in the dynamic and ever-evolving field of neurological injuries in sports.

Nicholas Theodore, MD
Russell R. Lonser, MD

Acknowledgments

"Upon the fields of friendly strife are sown the seeds that, upon other fields, on other days, will bear the fruits of victory."

General Douglas MacArthur, General of the US Army

"By failing to prepare you are preparing to fail."

Benjamin Franklin

"He who is only an athlete is too crude, too vulgar, too much a savage. He who is a scholar only is too soft, to effeminate. The ideal citizen is the scholar athlete, the man of thought and the man of action."

Plato

In life, as in sports, a unified team is everything.

To my home team, including my wonderful wife Effie and my sons Costa and John, you are a constant source of love, encouragement, and inspiration and make it possible for me to keep playing.

To my work team, including Andrew Hersh, Carly Weber-Levine, and Kelly Jiang, you are a collective tour de force and bring me great solace in knowing that the future generation is in great hands.

To my editorial team, Clare Sonntag, and Deepanshu Manral from Thieme, you have helped referee this book to a finish. And finally, to the authors of this book, your wisdom, time, and skill have made this effort a winner!

Nicholas Theodore, MD

I want to express my deepest gratitude to my family—my wife Carolyn, and my daughters, Hannah, Sarah, and Alicia—for their endless support and inspiration. Their patience and encouragement have been pivotal throughout this process.

I am equally thankful to my colleagues at the Department of Neurological Surgery at The Ohio State University for their invaluable support and contributions. Critically, I want to acknowledge Clare Sonntag, and Deepanshu Manral from Thieme, who were instrumental in shaping this textbook.

This work reflects a shared commitment to advancing the understanding and treatment of head injuries in sports. My heartfelt thanks go out to all of the authors involved.

Russell R. Lonser, MD

Contributors

Hussam Abou-Al-Shaar, MD
Neurosurgery Resident
Department of Neurological Surgery
University of Pittsburgh Medical Center
Pittsburgh, Pennsylvania, USA

A. Karim Ahmed, MD
Resident
Department of Neurosurgery
Johns Hopkins School of Medicine
Baltimore, Maryland, USA

Adam Ammar, MD
Pediatric Neurosurgeon
Department of Neurosurgery
New Jersey Pediatric Neuroscience Institute
Morristown, New Jersey, USA

Kristy B. Arbogast, PhD
Scientific Director
Center for Injury Research and Prevention
Children's Hospital of Philadelphia
Professor
R. Anderson Pew Endowed Chair
Department of Pediatrics
University of Pennsylvania
Philadelphia, Pennsylvania, USA

Kimberly Ashayeri, MD
Spine Fellow
Department of Neurosurgery
Johns Hopkins School of Medicine
Baltimore, Maryland, USA

Allan J. Belzberg, MD, FRCSC
Professor
Department of Neurosurgery and Plastic & Reconstructive Surgery
Johns Hopkins School of Medicine
Baltimore, Maryland, USA

Victoria Bergstein, BA
Medical Student
School of Medicine
Johns Hopkins School of Medicine
Baltimore, Maryland, USA

Meghana Bhimreddy, BA
Medical Student
Department of Neurosurgery
Johns Hopkins School of Medicine
Baltimore, Maryland, USA

James R. Borchers, MD, MPH
Professor
Family Medicine/Sports Medicine
The Ohio State University
Columbus, Ohio, USA

Benjamin L. Brett, PhD
Assistant Professor
Department of Neurosurgery
Medical College of Wisconsin
Milwaukee, Wisconsin, USA

Javier Cardenas, MD
Professor
Barrow Concussion and Brain Injury Center
Department of Neurology
Barrow Neurological Institute, St. Joseph's Hospital and Medical Center
Phoenix, Arizona, USA

Nicholas D. Cassimatis, BS
Medical Student
Department of Neurosurgery
Hackensack Meridian School of Medicine
Cornwall, New York, USA

Andrew K. Chan, MD
Co-Director, Minimally Invasive Scoliosis Surgery
Director, Neurosurgical Spine Research
Assistant Professor of Neurological Surgery
Department of Neurological Surgery
Columbia University
Och Spine at NewYork-Presbyterian Hospital
New York, New York, USA

Mitchell J. Christiansen, BA
Medical Student
Department of Neurosurgery
Barrow Neurological Institute, St. Joseph's Hospital and Medical Center
Phoenix, Arizona, USA

Alan R. Cohen, MD
Professor
Department of Neurosurgery
Johns Hopkins School of Medicine
Baltimore, Maryland, USA

Alexis M. Coslick, DO, MS
Assistant Professor
Department of Physical Medicine and Rehabilitation and Orthopaedics
Johns Hopkins University School of Medicine
Baltimore, Maryland, USA

A. Daniel Davidar, MBBS
Post-doctoral Research Fellow
Department of Neurosurgery
Johns Hopkins University School of Medicine
Baltimore, Maryland, USA

Joseph D. DiDomenico, MD
Neurosurgery Resident
Department of Neurosurgery
Barrow Neurological Institute, St. Joseph's Hospital and Medical Center
Phoenix, Arizona, USA

Ryan G. Eaton, MD
Clinical Instructor House Staff
Department of Neurological Surgery
The Ohio State University
Columbus, Ohio, USA

Jeff Ehresman, MD
Neurosurgery Resident
Department of Neurosurgery
Barrow Neurological Institute, St. Joseph's Hospital and Medical Center
Phoenix, Arizona, USA

James Bradley Elder, MD
Professor
Department of Neurological Surgery
The Ohio State University
Columbus, Ohio, USA

Mark I. Ellen, MD
Medical Director
Anthem Federal Health Care
Ocala, Florida, USA

Mohammed Emam, MD
Assistant Professor
Department of Physical Medicine and Rehabilitation
Johns Hopkins University
Baltimore, Maryland, USA

S. Harrison Farber, MD
Neurosurgery Resident
Department of Neurosurgery
Barrow Neurological Institute, St. Joseph's Hospital and Medical Center
Phoenix, Arizona, USA

Gerard A. Gioia, PhD
Pediatric Neuropsychologist/Director
Safe Concussion Outcome, Recovery & Education (SCORE) Program
Division of Pediatric Neuropsychology
Children's National Hospital/George Washington University School of Medicine & Health Sciences
Rockville, Maryland, USA

Jakub Godzik, MD
Assistant Professor
Department of Neurosurgery
University of Alabama at Birmingham
Birmingham, Alabama, USA

Danielle Golub, MD, MSCI
Resident Physician
Department of Neurosurgery
Northwell Health
Manhasset, New York, USA

Andrew M. Hersh, MD
Resident
Department of Neurosurgery
Johns Hopkins School of Medicine
Baltimore, Maryland, USA

Mackenzie M. Herzog, PhD, MPH
Director, Epidemiology, Injury Surveillance and Analytics
Real World Solutions
IQVIA
Durham, North Carolina, USA

Melanie Alfonzo Horowitz, BA
Medical Student
Department of Neurosurgery
Johns Hopkins School of Medicine
Baltimore, Maryland, USA

Kelly Jiang, MS
Medical Student
Department of Neurosurgery
Johns Hopkins School of Medicine
Baltimore, Maryland, USA

Soren Jonzzon, MD
Resident Physician
Department of Neurological Surgery
Vanderbilt University Medical Center
Nashville, Tennessee, USA

U. Kumar Kakarla, MD
Professor
Department of Neurosurgery
Barrow Neurological Institute, St. Joseph's Hospital and Medical Center
Phoenix, Arizona, USA

Nicholas Kats, BS
Undergraduate Student
Department of Biomedical Engineering
The Johns Hopkins University School of Medicine
Baltimore, Maryland, USA

Max J. Kerensky, BSE
PhD Candidate
Department of Biomedical Engineering
The Johns Hopkins University School of Medicine
Baltimore, Maryland, USA

John Knightly, MD
Neurosurgeon
Department of Neurosurgery
Atlantic Neurosurgical Specialists
Cedar Knolls, New Jersey, USA

Daniel Krasna, MD
Assistant Professor
Department of Physical Medicine and Rehabilitation
Johns Hopkins School of Medicine
Baltimore, Maryland, USA

D. Scott Kreiner, MD
Director
Interventional Spine and Musculoskeletal Medicine
Barrow Brain and Spine
Department of Neurosurgery
Barrow Neurological Institute, St. Joseph's Hospital and Medical Center
Phoenix, Arizona, USA

Wayne Kuhl, MD
Head Team Physician
Arizona Cardinals
Phoenix, Arizona, USA

Minh Quan Le, MD
Attending Physician
Department of Physical Medicine and Rehabilitation
Broward Health System
Deerfield Beach, Florida, USA

Russell R. Lonser, MD
Chair
Department of Neurological Surgery
The Ohio State University
Columbus, Ohio, USA

Noah Lu, BS (Biomedical Engineering and Neuroscience)
Master of Science in Engineering (MSE) Candidate;
Founder of Johns Hopkins Undergrad Brain-Computer Interface Society;
Research Assistant
Department of Biomedical Engineering
Johns Hopkins School of Medicine
Baltimore, Maryland, USA

Christina Mack, PhD
Chief Scientific Officer and Head, Agile Analytics
Real World Solutions
IQVIA
Durham, North Carolina, USA

Mark A. Mahan, MD
Associate Professor
Department of Neurosurgery
University of Utah
Salt Lake City, Utah, USA

Michael A. McCrea, PhD
Endowed Professor of Neurosurgery
Department of Neurosurgery
Medical College of Wisconsin
Milwaukee, Wisconsin, USA

Arjun K. Menta, BBA, BSA
Medical Student
Department of Neurosurgery
Johns Hopkins School of Medicine
Baltimore, Maryland, USA

Michael A. Miller, DC, CCSP
Certified Chiropractic Sports Physician
Professional Football Chiropractic Society Hall of Fame Inductee
Palmer College of Chiropractic
Norwood, Massachusetts, USA

Lindsay D. Nelson, PhD
Professor of Neurosurgery and Neurology;
Director of Translational Research for Neurosurgery
Departments of Neurosurgery and Neurology
Medical College of Wisconsin
Milwaukee, Wisconsin, USA

Annie Pan
Student
Department of Applied Mathematics and Statistics
Johns Hopkins School of Medicine
Baltimore, Maryland, USA

Declan A. Patton, PhD
Senior Research Scientist
Center for Injury Research and Prevention
Children's Hospital of Philadelphia
Philadelphia, Pennsylvania, USA

Randall W. Porter, MD
Director
Interdisciplinary Skull Base Program;
Co-Director
Acoustic Neuroma Center;
Team Neurosurgeon
Arizona Cardinals
Department of Neurosurgery
Barrow Neurological Institute, St. Joseph's Hospital and Medical Center
Phoenix, Arizona, USA

Margot Putukian, MD, FACSM, FAMSSM
Consultant;
Chief Medical Officer
Major League Soccer;
Former Director of Athletic Medicine;
Head Team Physician
Princeton University
Princeton, New Jersey, USA

Nicholas M. Rabah, MD
Neurosurgery Resident
Department of Neurosurgery
Barrow Neurological Institute, St. Joseph's Hospital and Medical Center
Phoenix, Arizona, USA

Patricia Roby, PhD, ATC
Epidemiologist
Real World Solutions
IQVIA
Durham, North Carolina, USA

Denis Routkevitch, BS (Biomedical Engineering)
MD/PhD Student
Department of Biomedical Engineering/Neurosurgery
Johns Hopkins School of Medicine
Baltimore, Maryland, USA

Christina Sarris, MD
Assistant Professor
Department of Neurosurgery
New York University Grossman School of Medicine
New York, New York, USA

Allen Sills, MD
Professor
Department of Neurosurgery
Vanderbilt University Medical Center
Franklin, Tennessee;
Chief Medical Officer
National Football League, USA

Laura A. Snyder, MD
Professor of Neurosurgery;
Director of Neurotrauma;
Associate Residency Program Director
Department of Neurosurgery
Barrow Neurological Institute, St. Joseph's Hospital and Medical Center
Phoenix, Arizona, USA

Gary S. Solomon, PhD
Senior Medical Advisor
Player Health and Safety
National Football League
Colchester, Vermont, USA

Zoe Soulé, BS (Neuroscience)
Research Assistant
Department of Neurosurgery
Johns Hopkins Hospital
Baltimore, Maryland, USA

Jesse Stokum, MD, PhD
Resident
Department of Neurosurgery
University of Maryland School of Medicine
Baltimore, Maryland, USA

John Theodore, BA
Student
Department of Neurosurgery
Johns Hopkins School of Medicine
Baltimore, Maryland, USA

Nicholas Theodore, MD
Professor
Department of Neurosurgery
Johns Hopkins University
Baltimore, Maryland, USA

Luis M. Tumialán, MD
Professor
Department of Neurosurgery
Barrow Neurological Institute, St. Joseph's Hospital and Medical Center
Phoenix, Arizona, USA

Stephanie Van, MD
Assistant Professor
Department of Physical Medicine & Rehabilitation
Johns Hopkins University School of Medicine
Baltimore, Maryland, USA

Vikas Vattipally, BS
Medical Student
School of Medicine/Neurosurgery
Johns Hopkins University School of Medicine
Baltimore, Maryland, USA

Corey T. Walker, MD
Assistant Professor
Department of Neurosurgery
Cedars-Sinai Medical Center
Los Angeles, California, USA

Joshua L. Wang, MD
Resident
Department of Neurological Surgery
The Ohio State University
Columbus, Ohio, USA

Erin B. Wasserman, PhD
Associate Director, Epidemiology, Injury Surveillance and Analytics
Real World Solutions
IQVIA
Durham, North Carolina, USA

Carly Weber-Levine, MS
Medical Student
Department of Neurosurgery
Johns Hopkins University School of Medicine
Baltimore, Maryland, USA

Michael D. White, MD
Neurosurgery Resident
Department of Neurosurgery
Barrow Neurological Institute, St. Joseph's Hospital and Medical Center
Phoenix, Arizona, USA

Timothy G. White, MD
Resident
Department of Neurosurgery
Zucker School of Medicine at Hofstra Northwell
Manhasset, New York, USA

Faisel M. Zaman, MD
Medical Director
Encompass Health
Prosper, Texas, USA

Scott L. Zuckerman, MD, MPH
Assistant Professor
Department of Neurological Surgery and Orthopaedic Surgery
Vanderbilt University Medical Center
Nashville, Tennessee, USA

Part I

Brain

I

1 Sports-Related Head Injury

Minh Quan Le, Mohammed Emam, Alexis M. Coslick, and Daniel Krasna

Summary

Traumatic Brain Injury (TBI) is a significant public health concern. There are various classification systems used to describe injury severity. The majority of TBI are mild both in the general population as well as in athletes. Injuries occur more commonly in contact sports. In this chapter we describe the classification and pathophysiology of TBI and review complications and rehabilitation strategies to manage patients with an emphasis on mild, sports-related injuries.

Keywords: brain injury, sports, concussion

1.1 Traumatic Brain Injury Overview

1.1.1 Classification

Traumatic brain injury (TBI) is defined as an "alteration in brain function, or other evidence of brain pathology, caused by an external force."[1] Clinically, TBI severity is often based on the Glasgow Coma Scale (GCS). Mild injuries make up the overwhelming majority of sports-related injuries both in the general population engaging in recreational sports and professional athletes.[2] There are numerous scales to classify severity of brain injury, many of which incorporate some combination of the GCS level, duration of post-traumatic amnesia (PTA), duration of loss of consciousness (LOC), alteration of consciousness (AOC), and focal neurologic deficits.[3,4,5] Based on these scales, patients can be classified as having mild, moderate, or severe brain injury (▶ Table 1.1). Given the inconsistency of accurate reporting for both PTA and LOC, GCS scores are most commonly used clinically for assessing severity.[6] However, it is important to recognize that GCS alone provides insufficient information for capturing both extremes of severity and does not correlate well to outcomes.[7,8] Even with additional demographic information and examination findings, the accuracy of predicting outcomes is below 40%.[6]

Table 1.1 Classification of injury severity

	Mild	Moderate	Severe
GCS	13–15	9–12	< 8
PTA	< 24 hours	24 hours–7 days	> 7 days
LOC	< 30 min	30 min–24 hours	> 24 hours

Abbreviations: GCS, Glasgow Coma Scale; PTA, post-traumatic amnesia; LOC, loss of consciousness.

Source: Adapted from Appendix C, Definition of mTBI from the VA/DOD Clinical Practice Guideline for Management of Concussion/Mild Traumatic Brain Injury (2009). In: O'Neil ME, Carlson K, Storzbach D, et al. Complications of Mild Traumatic Brain Injury in Veterans and Military Personnel: A Systematic Review [Internet]. Washington (DC): Department of Veterans Affairs (US); 2013. Available from: https://www.ncbi.nlm.nih.gov/books/NBK189784/

The diagnostic criteria for mild TBI vary among different guidelines.[5,9,10] Within the world of sports, mild TBI is often used interchangeably with concussion. The consensus statement from the international Concussion in Sport Group (CISG) defines sports-related concussion (SRC) as an alteration of brain function caused by an external force that usually has "rapid onset of short-lived impairment of neurological function that resolves spontaneously," though signs and symptoms may "evolve over a number of minutes to hours." LOC is not required but possible.[11]

1.1.2 Epidemiology

Global estimates of TBI show an annual incidence of 69 million of which over 80% are mild.[12] Sports and recreational activities may be responsible for over 1.6 million TBIs with a similar predominance of mild injuries.[2] Severe brain injuries in sport are more often related to cycling and equestrian sports. In both groups, more severe injuries are seen in unhelmeted riders.[13] A study by Winkler et al further illustrates the importance of proper helmet use. They noted that winter board sports such as skiing and snowboarding where helmet use is high had lower mortality than roller sports such as skateboarding where helmet use is very low.[14]

Given that the majority of TBIs in sports are mild, databases have been set up looking at SRC across various sports associations. During the National Collegiate Athletic Association (NCAA) seasons 2014/15 to 2018/19, there were 4.13 mild TBIs per 10,000 athlete-exposures (AEs) reported for 23 sports, showing a decrease from 4.47 per 10,000 AEs in 2009/10 to 2013/14 reported for 25 sports.[15,16] Across both men's and women's collegiate sports, men's ice hockey had the highest rate of SRC at approximately 7.35 per 10,000 AEs, followed by women's soccer with 7.15 per 10,000 AEs. Men's track and field had 0.33 per 10,000 AEs and women's track and field reported 0.17 in 1,000 AEs.[15] An analysis of high school sports during the 2013/14 to 2017/18 school years found 4.17 concussions per 10,000 AEs across 20 sports.[17] American football had the most reported concussion at 10.40 per 10,000 AEs and girls' soccer registered 8.19 per 10,000 AEs.[17]

The highest reported mechanism of injury was player contact, which accounted for approximately 85.1% of concussions in collegiate men's American football and 83.8% in men's basketball.[15] Most SRC in women's sports was attributed to equipment/apparatus contact in collegiate and high school sports, although collegiate women's ice hockey (45.9%), women's soccer (42.5%), and women's basketball (64.1%) had a greater incidence of player contact.[15] Across both sexes, and disciplines, the majority of SRC occurred during competition, with 54.5% of concussions happening in the second half or third or fourth quarter.[15,17,18]

Partitioning for sex, there was a higher incidence of SRC in collegiate soccer, basketball, and softball/baseball in women relative to men.[15,19] A similar trend was demonstrated in high school, with higher SRCs in girls than boys at 3.35 versus 1.51 per 10,000 AEs, respectively. High school boys and collegiate men's ice hockey had the highest prevalence of recurrent concussion at 14.4 and 10.6%, respectively.[15,17]

1.1.3 Pathophysiology

Injuries to the brain can be described both by timing as well as by location. Patients can have injuries focally at the site of impact as well as diffusely due to global force from acceleration and deceleration. Examples of focal injuries include skull fractures, contusions, and hemorrhage.[20] Focal injuries cause specific functional deficits depending on laterality and lobe. The structure of the skull puts the temporal and frontal lobes at higher risk of injury. Damage to these areas is responsible for the neurobehavioral profile often associated with more severe TBI.[21]

Diffuse injuries include axonal injury. The different tissue densities within the brain makes the axons in white matter particularly susceptible to damage from rotational acceleration. Damage initially affects the axon membranes at nodes of Ranvier, causing disruption of ion transport, subsequent swelling, and potential retraction of the axon. More severe injuries can cause structural damage. Given the role of axons in connecting various regions of the brain, diffuse axonal injury (DAI) can cause a wide range of impairments, and the severity of DAI correlates with the duration of LOC.[22]

Diffuse and focal injuries present at the time of impact are referred to as primary injury and these trigger cascades in the following minutes to days causing secondary injury.[20] TBI initially causes disruption of cell membranes leading to glutamate and potassium release as well as accumulation of intracellular calcium. This is followed by energy consumption and a drop in glucose levels. The degree of ionic disruption and glucose depletion correlates with injury severity.[23] These changes occur in the immediate minutes to hours following injury but can lead to further downstream dysfunction in the following days from edema and oxidative stress.[20] Focal injuries such as ischemia and edema can also trigger these secondary cascades in a more localized fashion.[24]

Mild Injury

Mild TBI involves a less severe injury to the brain but as per the definition of TBI above, the force incurred needs to be of sufficient strength to alter brain activity.[25] Although many of the aforementioned diffuse processes occur to a degree, mild TBIs are usually without focal injuries. Some classification systems identify the presence of focal injury as consistent with moderate TBI whereas others label these cases complicated mild TBI.[25,26] Axonal injury is hypothesized to be the main mechanism of initial symptoms[27]; however, ion dysregulation is usually not severe enough to progress to secondary injuries. Therefore, recovery is possible before structural damage occurs.[22,24] This pathophysiology informed the CISG definitions and expected clinical course of SRC as already mentioned.[11]

1.2 Management Principles

The principles of management for TBI are different for mild injuries compared to moderate and severe injuries. In general, all patients require an initial neurologic examination to determine the level of severity and assess the need for further immediate care and stabilization. Additionally, depending on the mechanism of injury a full body trauma examination is often indicated to find concurrent injuries, especially in more severe cases.

1.2.1 Workup and Treatment

Moderate and Severe

Patients with more severe injuries will need prolonged observation or admission to an acute hospital to continue stabilization started in the outpatient setting. For patients with a GCS of < 15, a computed tomography (CT) scan is recommended. A major concern during the acute period is control of edema and ischemia by monitoring cerebral perfusion pressure (CPP) through the surrogate of intracranial pressure (ICP). Patients with GCS below 9 or significant vital sign or neurologic abnormalities are at the highest risk and should be monitored by invasive means.[6]

Moderate and severe TBI patients have a risk of seizure between 2 and 17% in the first week after TBI.[28] It is recommended that patients be given 7 days of seizure prophylaxis to reduce complications from seizure during this often critical time of medical instability. Prophylaxis is meant to address early seizures but does not prevent the development of late seizures after the first week. Early studies were done using older antiepileptics which have fallen out of favor due to their side effect profile.[29] Many practitioners now utilize levetiracetam, though higher quality studies are still needed.[30]

Once a patient is medically and surgically stable, assessment of the functional status is important to guide the next level of care. This is best done via a multidisciplinary rehabilitation team, even in the acute hospital, consisting of a physiatrist, physical and occupational therapists, and speech-language pathologists. Depending on the deficits, this team can work on medications and therapies to improve function and recommend the next level of care including acute inpatient rehabilitation where specialized teams can continue this work.

Given the heterogeneous population, there are not many medical interventions that are recommended for all TBI patients. Some randomized controlled trials have demonstrated efficacy for specific medications in specific instances including amantadine for disorders of consciousness.[31] Beyond this, the main guidance for medications in brain injury medicine is the adage "start low and go slow," in that medications of various drug classes can be used for cognitive and behavioral sequelae of injury but are started at lower doses and gradually increased.[32] Providers need to be aware that certain classes of medications can lead to delayed neurorecovery including benzodiazepines, drugs with anticholinergic effects, and antipsychotics with typicals often having greater impairment than atypicals.[33]

Mild

Baseline Assessment

A baseline assessment can aid in recognition of comorbid conditions and assist in diagnosis and return to play decisions.[11,34] One such validated tool is the Sports Concussion Assessment Tool (SCAT), which was originally developed in 2004 by the

CISG for medical professionals to evaluate SRC for individuals 13 years or older.[35] Participants between the age of 5 and 12 years old utilize the Child SCAT5. Additionally, computerized neuropsychological testing can be performed preseason and can aid health care providers in tracking SRC and recovery.[34]

On-Field Assessment

Since its early conception, the SCAT underwent multiple revisions with the latest edition updated in 2016 as SCAT5. The test comprises immediate on-field assessments of red flag symptoms, observable signs, memory assessment questions, GCS, and cervical spine assessment. Athletes with signs of LOC, impact seizure, tonic posturing, gross motor instability, confusion, or amnesia should be removed from play.[34] Given the heterogeneity of concussive injury, combined with low sensitivity and specificity of assessment tests, close attention should be given to the athlete's symptoms.[36] For laypersons, the Concussion Recognition Tool 5 (CRT5) can be used to detect signs and symptoms of possible concussion.[37] Ultimately, if there are any concerns for SRC, the athlete should be removed from play for further evaluation. If the athlete is diagnosed with concussion, he or she must be excluded from play that day.

Off-Field Assessment

Additional tests off the field in a quiet, controlled environment consists of modified balance error scoring system (mBESS) to assess for postural stability, vestibular/ocular motor screening (VOMS) to evaluate oculomotor functions, neurocognitive function questions, and post-concussion symptoms scale from the SCAT5.[38] Clinicians should be mindful of an attenuation effect to detect SRC after 3 days following an inciting event.[35] During the off-field assessment, athletes should be evaluated for comorbid conditions such as attention deficit disorders, prior concussion, migraines, depression, and anxiety which may prolong recovery as detailed in the following.[39]

Routine use of CT, magnetic resonance imaging (MRI), or skull radiograph are not recommended without high clinical suspicion for intracranial structural injuries.[34] Clinical decision rules such as the Canadian CT Head Rule for patients older than 16 and the Pediatric Emergency Care Applied Research Network algorithm can help guide imaging decisions.[40,41]

Given the initial ion exchange and glutamate excitotoxicity following head injury, research is being done on the role of utilizing fluid biomarkers to aid in the diagnosis of concussion and prognosis.[38] Currently, there is no scientific consensus to recommend the use of biomarkers for management or diagnosis.[42] Recently, use of glial fibrillary acidic protein (GFAP) and ubiquitin C-terminal hydrolase L1 (UCH-L1) has been shown to aid prognosis in patients presenting with same-day injury with GCS of 3 to 12 and may be able to predict imaging findings.[43,44]

At this time, since there are no imaging or laboratory tests that can confirm the occurrence of concussion, clinicians need to use their judgment to assess the likelihood a concussion occurred. If LOC or posturing following trauma to the head or rapid deceleration with subsequent return to normal neurologic functioning is witnessed, one can be reasonably diagnose a concussion with certainty. In cases without such findings, the degree of force and chance of other diagnoses needs to be carefully considered to ensure the correct diagnosis, though it is always safer to manage acutely as if the patient did indeed suffer a mild TBI.[45] Allowing athletes to continue playing increases the risk of a feared complication of second impact syndrome. Second impact syndrome occurs when patients sustain a second concussion prior to the resolution of the first one, resulting in disruption of the brain's autoregulatory mechanism which can lead to severe brain injury, disability, or death.[46] Previous studies have identified young athletes (13 to 24 years old) and male gender to be associated with second impact syndrome.[46] This issue rose to prominence with the passing of a law in Washington state after the injury of a middle school student who suffered severe sequalae after returning to play with a concussion. The Washington state's Lystedt law which went into effect in 2009 requires athletes with suspected head injury or concussion to be removed from play and not return to practice or competition until evaluated by a medical provider.[47]

Rest

Relative cognitive and physical rest after initial injury has been the mainstay treatment for SRC to allow for optimal recovery.[11] Following the first 24 to 48 hours after the event, patients are encouraged to participate in light aerobic activities as symptoms permit to decrease delayed recovery (greater than 30 days of symptoms).[48] Any aerobic activities which exacerbate post-concussive symptoms scores by two or more points on the post-concussive symptom scale, a 22-question Likert scale with higher scores indicating greater severity, should be halted. Exercise tolerance testing, such as the Buffalo Concussion Treadmill Test, can be used to gradually promote athletes' return to activity.[48]

Rehabilitation

A multidisciplinary team approach is beneficial to identify deficits and address impairments. Common symptoms such as headache or dizziness may arise because of autonomic, cervicogenic, vestibular, or cognitive dysfunction.[49] Up to 81% of patients report dizziness within the first day following concussion.[50] Vestibular rehabilitation has been shown to be beneficial in patients with persistent impairments such as dizziness, gait abnormalities, and balance deficits.[50] Exercises consist of gaze stabilization, standing balance, walking with balance challenge, as well as canalith repositioning maneuver. Therapies aimed at addressing cervicogenic pain include manual treatment, cervical proprioception, and motor control.[49]

Given the transient nature of concussion pathophysiology, conservative symptom management is preferred for most symptoms. Headache can be managed with medications such as nonsteroidal anti-inflammatory drugs (NSAIDs) and acetaminophen. Athletes and parents should be educated on warning signs such as vomiting, changes in baseline mentation, and acutely worsening headaches, which should prompt immediate medical attention and consideration of advanced imaging.[51] Other pharmacological supplements have limited in vivo analysis with no FDA regulations, leading to their low recommendations for treatment.[34]

Return to School

Although students report improvement in their learning ability with slow integration back to academics, many report initial challenges with poor attention, fatigue, and difficulty understanding materials.[52] On average, students are absent for 3 to 5 days following a concussion, with older students missing for a longer period.[53] Earlier return to school has been associated with lower symptom burden at 2 weeks post injury likely due to socialization, maintaining sleep–wake cycle, lower stress from missed work, and physical activities.[53,54]

A customized learning plan in collaboration with health care providers, students and parents, and the school is important for students to reintegrate into their academic environment.[51] Accommodations include appropriate workloads, extended time for tests, quizzes, and assignments, along with adequate breaks and an environment which does not exacerbate symptoms. Symptoms should be monitored, and adjustments of learning activities should progress such that students are back to full academic workload without symptom exacerbation. In this way, although it is not as easily measured, return to school should mirror return to play with increasing difficulty as the student masters activities without symptom exacerbation.

Return to Play

The Consensus Statement on Concussion in Sports characterizes a stepwise gradual return to sports protocol in six stages. Athletes graduate through each stage if their symptoms are not exacerbated. These stages consist of starting with symptom limited activity, light aerobic exercise, sports-specific exercise, noncontact training drills, full contact practice, and subsequent return to sport. If athletes experience exacerbation of their concussive symptoms in any of the stages, they must stop physical activity, rest for 24 hours, and resume the previous stage.[11] Individualized time frame may vary depending on age, sports, and medical history. Furthermore, athletes must demonstrate psychological readiness with progression in return to play protocol for final clearance.[34]

1.2.2 Complications

Mild

Majority of individuals with mild TBI have resolutions of symptoms, but the time course of recovery is unclear. In a study by the World Health Organization, most patients seemed to recover over the span of 3 months to 1 year.[55] Clinical recovery from concussion often precedes physiological recovery, and there is no single test that can be used to definitively mark the time of full recovery from concussion.[56] Many children recover from concussion within 4 to 12 weeks, and adults generally recover in 2 months.[11,57,58,59] The median time for return to work for adults is 1 to 2 weeks.[60]

In contrast, McCrea and colleagues studied 570 athletes with concussion. Of these, only 10% had a prolonged recovery as measured by persistent elevation of Graded Symptom Checklist score at the 1-week mark; however, their cognitive and balance testing returned to normal limits. These individuals had higher symptom scores early on as well.[61] The faster return compared with the general adult population may be due to differences in responsibilities and life stressors, general health at the time of injury, as well as the potential for underreporting symptoms in order to return to play. Underreporting may also explain why female athletes have higher rates of delayed recovery than males.[62]

There are specific underlying comorbidities that predispose patients to a prolonged recovery. These include prior concussion, ADHD, anxiety, learning disorder, and migraines.[39,63,64] Additionally, a prior history of mental health diagnoses increases one's risk for persistent symptoms. Similarly, initial symptoms including headaches or depression are a risk factor for concussion symptoms to be present for greater than 1 month.[62]

For those patients with delayed or incomplete recovery, the term post-concussive syndrome (PCS) or post-concussional disorder (PCD) has been used. The terms are defined differently by the Diagnostic and Statistical Manual of Mental Disorders IV (DSM-IV) and the International Classification of Diseases 10 (ICD-10), the biggest difference being the DSM definition of PCD requiring cognitive impairment to be present.[65] Neither definition provides a mechanism for why the symptoms persist beyond the usual recovery period.

Further highlighting that these symptoms are not clearly linked to brain pathology are studies which have looked at the rates of occurrence of PCS symptoms in healthy controls.[66,67] Based on this, the clearest guidance from Silverberg et al in their Synthesis of Practice Guideline for managing symptoms that persist after an initial head injury is to utilize best practices for those symptoms from the general population and to prioritize sleep, headaches, and mood issues. They reserve referral to specialty treatment teams once symptoms last for a month despite appropriate management of these key symptoms.[60]

Moderate and Severe

The long-term management of more severe brain injuries is complex and relates to the various sequelae of injury these patients may deal with. One main guiding principle is that acute changes in mental status or neurologic function require a thorough workup as multiple complications can arise at variable times post injury. This can include lab work for metabolic or infectious etiologies, repeat imaging, and patient and family interviewing. Some of the most common complications are seizures, urinary tract infections, pneumonia, and central nervous system infections, particularly in patients with history of neurosurgical intervention or skull fractures, hydrocephalus, or intraventricular hemorrhage. Patients are also at risk of other neurologic sequelae of injury including movement disorders, spasticity, and paroxysmal sympathetic hyperactivity.[6,68] The specific workup and management of these issues are beyond the scope of this chapter and readers are referred to the citations and brain injury medicine textbooks.

Preventative screening is possible for some other sequelae of TBI. Around 30% of patients have injury to the pituitary which can cause reversible symptoms that overlap with impairment from TBI.[69] An endocrine panel should be obtained if symptoms are noted. For a preventative screen, there is some debate on the timing and what lab work to include, but a screen at 3 to 6 months is reasonable.[69,70,71]

Another common complication after TBI is sleep dysfunction. Some estimates suggest that every patient will experience sleep disturbance, at least initially after TBI.[72] Overall sleep disorder prevalence decreases over time after injury, but a large proportion of patients report it as a chronic issue.[72,73] Most commonly diagnosed are insomnia, obstructive sleep apnea, and circadian rhythm disorders. Sleep hygiene should be discussed to optimize recovery. Melatonin, an over-the-counter supplement, can be used to help facilitate sleep. If patients continue to have sleep disturbance, a referral to a sleep specialist is warranted.[51]

Lastly, depression is a common occurrence after TBI affecting 25 to 60% of patients. Screening can be done to allow for early intervention and prevent symptom progression.[33] This unfortunately is not always conducted and not always successful, and the rates of suicide in this population are 3 to 4 times higher than the general population.[74]

1.3 Clinical Pearls

- TBI is broadly defined as an alteration in brain function caused by force to the brain which can be a result of direct impact or significant acceleration and deceleration forces.
- Most injuries in the general population and in sports are mild TBI, which has a greater focus on outpatient management. SRC is defined as an alteration of brain function caused by an external force that usually resolves on its own.
- The most important aspect of SRC is identifying its occurrence to remove athletes from play and avoid potential further injury from subsequent impacts before the concussion has resolved.
- More severe brain injuries occur in fast sports with unhelmeted participants.

References

[1] Menon DK, Schwab K, Wright DW, Maas AI, Demographics and Clinical Assessment Working Group of the International and Interagency Initiative toward Common Data Elements for Research on Traumatic Brain Injury and Psychological Health. Position statement: definition of traumatic brain injury. Arch Phys Med Rehabil. 2010; 91(11):1637–1640

[2] Langlois JA, Rutland-Brown W, Wald MM. The epidemiology and impact of traumatic brain injury: a brief overview. J Head Trauma Rehabil. 2006; 21 (5):375–378

[3] Malec JF, Brown AW, Leibson CL, et al. The mayo classification system for traumatic brain injury severity. J Neurotrauma. 2007; 24(9):1417–1424

[4] O'Neil ME, Carlson K, Storzbach D, et al. Complications of Mild Traumatic Brain Injury in Veterans and Military Personnel: A Systematic Review. VA Evidence-based Synthesis Program Reports. Washington (DC): Department of Veterans Affairs (US); 2013

[5] National Academies of Sciences, Engineering, and Medicine; Health and Medicine Division; Board on Health Care Services; Committee on the Review of the Department of Veterans Affairs Examinations for Traumatic Brain Injury. Evaluation of the Disability Determination Process for Traumatic Brain Injury in Veterans. Washington, District of Columbia: The National Academies Press; 2019

[6] Robinson CP. Moderate and severe traumatic brain injury. Continuum (Minneap Minn). 2021; 27(5):1278–1300

[7] Bodien YG, Barra A, Temkin NR, et al. TRACK-TBI Investigators. Diagnosing level of consciousness: the limits of the Glasgow Coma Scale total score. J Neurotrauma. 2021; 38(23):3295–3305

[8] Maas AI, Harrison-Felix CL, Menon D, et al. Common data elements for traumatic brain injury: recommendations from the interagency working group on demographics and clinical assessment. Arch Phys Med Rehabil. 2010; 91(11):1641–1649

[9] Silverberg ND, Iverson GL, Cogan A, et al. The American Congress of Rehabilitation Medicine Diagnostic Criteria for Mild Traumatic Brain Injury. Arch Phys Med Rehabil. 2023; 104(8):1343–1355

[10] Powell D, Affuso O, Chen Y. Weight change after spinal cord injury. J Spinal Cord Med. 2017; 40(2):130–137

[11] McCrory P, Meeuwisse W, Dvořák J, et al. Consensus statement on concussion in sport—the 5th international conference on concussion in sport held in Berlin, October 2016. Br J Sports Med. 2017; 51(11):838–847

[12] Dewan MC, Rattani A, Gupta S, et al. Estimating the global incidence of traumatic brain injury. J Neurosurg. 2018; 130(4):1080–1097

[13] Coronado VG, Haileyesus T, Cheng TA, et al. Trends in sports- and recreation-related traumatic brain injuries treated in US emergency departments: The National Electronic Injury Surveillance System-All Injury Program (NEISS-AIP) 2001–2012. J Head Trauma Rehabil. 2015; 30(3):185–197

[14] Winkler EA, Yue JK, Burke JF, et al. Adult sports-related traumatic brain injury in United States trauma centers. Neurosurg Focus. 2016; 40(4):E4

[15] Chandran A, Boltz AJ, Morris SN, et al. Epidemiology of concussions in National Collegiate Athletic Association (NCAA) sports: 2014/15–2018/19. Am J Sports Med. 2022; 50(2):526–536

[16] Zuckerman SL, Kerr ZY, Yengo-Kahn A, Wasserman E, Covassin T, Solomon GS. Epidemiology of sports-related concussion in NCAA athletes from 2009–2010 to 2013–2014: incidence, recurrence, and mechanisms. Am J Sports Med. 2015; 43(11):2654–2662

[17] Kerr ZY, Chandran A, Nedimyer AK, Arakkal A, Pierpoint LA, Zuckerman SL. Concussion incidence and trends in 20 high school sports. Pediatrics. 2019; 144(5):e20192180

[18] Pierpoint LA, Collins C. Epidemiology of sport-related concussion. Clin Sports Med. 2021; 40(1):1–18

[19] Prien A, Grafe A, Rössler R, Junge A, Verhagen E. Epidemiology of head injuries focusing on concussions in team contact sports: a systematic review. Sports Med. 2018; 48(4):953–969

[20] Mckee AC, Daneshvar DH. The neuropathology of traumatic brain injury. Handb Clin Neurol. 2015; 127:45–66

[21] McAllister TW. Neurobiological consequences of traumatic brain injury. Dialogues Clin Neurosci. 2011; 13(3):287–300

[22] Smith DH, Hicks R, Povlishock JT. Therapy development for diffuse axonal injury. J Neurotrauma. 2013; 30(5):307–323

[23] Prins M, Greco T, Alexander D, Giza CC. The pathophysiology of traumatic brain injury at a glance. Dis Model Mech. 2013; 6(6):1307–1315

[24] Gaetz M. The neurophysiology of brain injury. Clin Neurophysiol. 2004; 115 (1):4–18

[25] Silverberg ND, Iverson GL, ACRM Mild TBI Definition Expert Consensus Group and the ACRM Brain Injury Special Interest Group Mild TBI Task Force. Expert panel survey to update the American Congress of Rehabilitation Medicine definition of mild traumatic brain injury. Arch Phys Med Rehabil. 2021; 102(1):76–86

[26] Williams DH, Levin HS, Eisenberg HM. Mild head injury classification. Neurosurgery. 1990; 27(3):422–428

[27] Barkhoudarian G, Hovda DA, Giza CC. The molecular pathophysiology of concussive brain injury. Clin Sports Med. 2011; 30(1):33–48, vii–iii

[28] Frey LC. Epidemiology of posttraumatic epilepsy: a critical review. Epilepsia. 2003; 44 s10:11–17

[29] Temkin NR, Dikmen SS, Wilensky AJ, Keihm J, Chabal S, Winn HR. A randomized, double-blind study of phenytoin for the prevention of post-traumatic seizures. N Engl J Med. 1990; 323(8):497–502

[30] Yang Y, Zheng F, Xu X, Wang X. Levetiracetam versus phenytoin for seizure prophylaxis following traumatic brain injury: a systematic review and meta-analysis. CNS Drugs. 2016; 30(8):677–688

[31] Giacino JT, Whyte J, Bagiella E, et al. Placebo-controlled trial of amantadine for severe traumatic brain injury. N Engl J Med. 2012; 366(9):819–826

[32] Arciniegas DB, Held K, Wagner P. Cognitive impairment following traumatic brain injury. Curr Treat Options Neurol. 2002; 4(1):43–57

[33] Polich G, Iaccarino MA, Zafonte R. Psychopharmacology of traumatic brain injury. Handb Clin Neurol. 2019; 165:253–267

[34] Harmon KG, Clugston JR, Dec K, et al. American Medical Society for Sports Medicine position statement on concussion in sport. Clin J Sport Med. 2019; 29(2):87–100

[35] Echemendia RJ, Meeuwisse W, McCrory P, et al. The Sport Concussion Assessment Tool 5th Edition (SCAT5): background and rationale. Br J Sports Med. 2017; 51(11):848–850

[36] Chin EY, Nelson LD, Barr WB, McCrory P, McCrea MA. Reliability and validity of the Sport Concussion Assessment Tool-3 (SCAT3) in high school and collegiate athletes. Am J Sports Med. 2016; 44(9):2276–2285

[37] Echemendia RJ, Meeuwisse W, McCrory P, et al. The Concussion Recognition Tool 5th Edition (CRT5): background and rationale. Br J Sports Med. 2017; 51(11):870–871

[38] McKeithan L, Hibshman N, Yengo-Kahn AM, Solomon GS, Zuckerman SL. Sport-related concussion: evaluation, treatment, and future directions. Med Sci (Basel). 2019; 7(3):44

[39] Cuff S, Maki A, Feiss R, et al. Risk factors for prolonged recovery from concussion in young patients. Br J Sports Med. 2022; 56(23):1345–1352

[40] Kuppermann N, Holmes JF, Dayan PS, et al. Pediatric Emergency Care Applied Research Network (PECARN). Identification of children at very low risk of clinically-important brain injuries after head trauma: a prospective cohort study. Lancet. 2009; 374(9696):1160–1170

[41] Stiell IG, Wells GA, Vandemheen K, et al. The Canadian CT Head Rule for patients with minor head injury. Lancet. 2001; 357(9266):1391–1396

[42] McCrea M, Meier T, Huber D, et al. Role of advanced neuroimaging, fluid biomarkers and genetic testing in the assessment of sport-related concussion: a systematic review. Br J Sports Med. 2017; 51(12):919–929

[43] Korley FK, Jain S, Sun X, et al. TRACK-TBI Study Investigators. Prognostic value of day-of-injury plasma GFAP and UCH-L1 concentrations for predicting functional recovery after traumatic brain injury in patients from the US TRACK-TBI cohort: an observational cohort study. Lancet Neurol. 2022; 21(9):803–813

[44] Papa L, Brophy GM, Welch RD, et al. Time course and diagnostic accuracy of glial and neuronal blood biomarkers GFAP and UCH-L1 in a large cohort of trauma patients with and without mild traumatic brain injury. JAMA Neurol. 2016; 73(5):551–560

[45] Kutcher JS, Giza CC. Sports concussion diagnosis and management. Continuum (Minneap Minn). 2014; 20(6 Sports Neurology):1552–1569

[46] McLendon LA, Kralik SF, Grayson PA, Golomb MR. The controversial second impact syndrome: a review of the literature. Pediatr Neurol. 2016; 62:9–17

[47] Bompadre V, Jinguji TM, Yanez ND, et al. Washington State's Lystedt law in concussion documentation in Seattle public high schools. J Athl Train. 2014; 49(4):486–492

[48] Leddy JJ, Haider MN, Ellis MJ, et al. Early subthreshold aerobic exercise for sport-related concussion: a randomized clinical trial. JAMA Pediatr. 2019; 173(4):319–325

[49] Brown L, Camarinos J. The role of physical therapy in concussion rehabilitation. Semin Pediatr Neurol. 2019; 30:68–78

[50] Alsalaheen BA, Mucha A, Morris LO, et al. Vestibular rehabilitation for dizziness and balance disorders after concussion. J Neurol Phys Ther. 2010; 34(2):87–93

[51] Lumba-Brown A, Yeates KO, Sarmiento K, et al. Centers for Disease Control and Prevention guideline on the diagnosis and management of mild traumatic brain injury among children. JAMA Pediatr. 2018; 172(11): e182853

[52] DeMatteo CA, Jakubowski J, Randall S, Stazyk K, Lin CY, Yakubov R. School performance in youth after a concussion. Front Sports Act Living. 2022; 4: 1008551

[53] Vaughan CG, Ledoux AA, Sady MD, et al. PERC 5P Concussion Team. Association between early return to school following acute concussion and symptom burden at 2 weeks postinjury. JAMA Netw Open. 2023; 6(1): e2251839

[54] Ledoux AA, Barrowman N, Bijelić V, et al. PERC PedCARE Concussion team. Is early activity resumption after paediatric concussion safe and does it reduce symptom burden at 2 weeks post injury? The Pediatric Concussion Assessment of Rest and Exertion (PedCARE) multicentre randomised clinical trial. Br J Sports Med. 2022; 56(5):271–278

[55] Carroll LJ, Cassidy JD, Peloso PM, et al. WHO Collaborating Centre Task Force on Mild Traumatic Brain Injury. Prognosis for mild traumatic brain injury: results of the WHO Collaborating Centre Task Force on Mild Traumatic Brain Injury. J Rehabil Med. 2004(43) Suppl:84–105

[56] Kamins J, Bigler E, Covassin T, et al. What is the physiological time to recovery after concussion? A systematic review. Br J Sports Med. 2017; 51 (12):935–940

[57] Meehan WP, III, Mannix R, Monuteaux MC, Stein CJ, Bachur RG. Early symptom burden predicts recovery after sport-related concussion. Neurology. 2014; 83(24):2204–2210

[58] Heyer GL, Schaffer CE, Rose SC, Young JA, McNally KA, Fischer AN. Specific factors influence postconcussion symptom duration among youth referred to a sports concussion clinic. J Pediatr. 2016; 174:33–38.e2

[59] Wäljas M, Iverson GL, Lange RT, et al. Return to work following mild traumatic brain injury. J Head Trauma Rehabil. 2014; 29(5):443–450

[60] Silverberg ND, Iaccarino MA, Panenka WJ, et al. American Congress of Rehabilitation Medicine Brain Injury Interdisciplinary Special Interest Group Mild TBI Task Force. Management of concussion and mild traumatic brain injury: a synthesis of practice guidelines. Arch Phys Med Rehabil. 2020; 101 (2):382–393

[61] McCrea M, Guskiewicz K, Randolph C, et al. Incidence, clinical course, and predictors of prolonged recovery time following sport-related concussion in high school and college athletes. J Int Neuropsychol Soc. 2013; 19(1):22–33

[62] Iverson GL, Gardner AJ, Terry DP, et al. Predictors of clinical recovery from concussion: a systematic review. Br J Sports Med. 2017; 51(12):941–948

[63] Wang EX, Hwang CE, Nguyen JN, Segovia NA, Abrams GD, Kussman A. Factors associated with a prolonged time to return to play after a concussion. Am J Sports Med. 2022; 50(6):1695–1701

[64] Martin AK, Petersen AJ, Sesma HW, et al. Learning and attention deficit/ hyperactivity disorders as risk factors for prolonged concussion recovery in children and adolescents. J Int Neuropsychol Soc. 2022; 28(2):109–122

[65] McCauley SR, Boake C, Pedroza C, et al. Postconcussional disorder: are the DSM-IV criteria an improvement over the ICD-10? J Nerv Ment Dis. 2005; 193(8):540–550

[66] Lange RT, Iverson GL, Brubacher JR, Mädler B, Heran MK. Diffusion tensor imaging findings are not strongly associated with postconcussional disorder 2 months following mild traumatic brain injury. J Head Trauma Rehabil. 2012; 27(3):188–198

[67] Iverson GL, Lange RT. Examination of "postconcussion-like" symptoms in a healthy sample. Appl Neuropsychol. 2003; 10(3):137–144

[68] Masel BE, DeWitt DS. Traumatic brain injury: a disease process, not an event. J Neurotrauma. 2010; 27(8):1529–1540

[69] Gasco V, Cambria V, Bioletto F, Ghigo E, Grottoli S. Traumatic brain injury as frequent cause of hypopituitarism and growth hormone deficiency: epidemiology, diagnosis, and treatment. Front Endocrinol (Lausanne). 2021; 12:634415

[70] Ghigo E, Masel B, Aimaretti G, et al. Consensus guidelines on screening for hypopituitarism following traumatic brain injury. Brain Inj. 2005; 19(9): 711–724

[71] Tan CL, Alavi SA, Baldeweg SE, et al. The screening and management of pituitary dysfunction following traumatic brain injury in adults: British Neurotrauma Group guidance. J Neurol Neurosurg Psychiatry. 2017; 88(11): 971–981

[72] Nakase-Richardson R, Sherer M, Barnett SD, et al. Prospective evaluation of the nature, course, and impact of acute sleep abnormality after traumatic brain injury. Arch Phys Med Rehabil. 2013; 94(5):875–882

[73] Barshikar S, Bell KR. Sleep disturbance after TBI. Curr Neurol Neurosci Rep. 2017; 17(11):87

[74] Simpson G, Tate R. Suicidality in people surviving a traumatic brain injury: prevalence, risk factors and implications for clinical management. Brain Inj. 2007; 21(13–14):1335–1351

2 Imaging of Sports-Related Neurological Injuries

Joshua L. Wang, Ryan G. Eaton, James R. Borchers, and James Bradley Elder

Summary

Advances in cross-sectional medical imaging have drastically improved the ability of clinicians to diagnose sports-related neurological injuries that are seen or suspected based on history, physical examination, and plain radiography. Several screening tools or scoring systems have been developed to indicate use of these modalities in assessing the acutely injured patient. This chapter will provide a brief overview of normal anatomy and physiology of the neuroaxis, scoring systems used for triaging further imaging for the injured athlete, and imaging findings in specific, common injuries.

Keywords: concussion, traumatic brain injury, spinal cord injury, spinal trauma

2.1 Basic Anatomy and Pathophysiology of the Spine

The spinal column is composed of 33 vertebrae, with the cervical spine beginning at the base of the skull and connecting to the thoracic vertebrae. The lumbar vertebrae connect the thoracic spine to the sacrum which is attached to the pelvic ring and the coccyx. The bony structures of the vertebrae surround and protect the spinal cord and nerves, which run in the spinal canal. Fibrous disks anteriorly and synovial facet joints posteriorly form the articulations between each vertebra from C2 to S1. A series of longitudinal continuous (i.e., anterior longitudinal and posterior longitudinal ligaments) and segmental (e.g., ligamentum flavum and interspinous ligaments) ligaments provide additional longitudinal stability to the vertebral column. At the craniocervical junction (base of skull through C2), a complex series of ligaments and synovial joints stabilize the skull on top of the spine while also allowing physiologic range of motion.

Damage to the neural elements within the spinal column can occur due to direct compression or transection by the surrounding structural elements, compressive hematomas, infarction, or traumatic shear injury of neural tissue. Careful neurologic examination can localize the neurologic deficit, but modern imaging techniques can identify causative lesions which may allow medical staff to prescribe treatment in cases when the patient is unable to participate adequately in the examination, when there may be an unstable injury without neurologic deficit, or when the examination does not correlate with the mechanism of trauma.

2.2 Specific Injuries

It is beyond the scope of this chapter to cover all possible injuries involving the spine, although we will review some special cases that are most relevant to athletes and must be kept in mind when treating these individuals.

2.2.1 Craniocervical Junction Injuries

Craniocervical junction injuries present quite rarely in sports due to the high forces required for such injuries to occur, but should still be considered. Atlantooccipital dissociation (AOD) is caused by disruption of the ligaments involved in stabilizing the occipital condyles in their articulation with C1 and is associated with a mortality rate of 50 to 80%.[1] The diagnosis of AOD can be made on computed tomography (CT) imaging alone if there is already distraction or subluxation, although magnetic resonance imaging (MRI) can be obtained to evaluate the ligaments directly. A common finding on CT that may indicate AOD in the absence of subluxation includes ventral epidural hematoma along the clivus or upper cervical spine due to rupture of the tectorial membrane.

Fractures of C1 (eponymously named Jefferson fractures) are similarly rare and usually arise from heavy axial loading, such as diving into a shallow body of water. Integrity of the transverse ligament may be inferred on open mouth radiograph or on CT scan but may also be directly assessed with MRI. C2 fractures primarily occur due to high-velocity hyperextension injuries in younger individuals and are less common in sports like football where axial loading, commonly caused by "helmet spearing," is the primary mechanism of injury. An example of a C2 injury is shown in ▶ Fig. 2.1.

2.2.2 Subaxial Cervical Spine

The cervical spine is particularly vulnerable to injury in contact sports, equestrian activities, gymnastics, and competitive diving given its mobility. The most flexible segments descend with increasing age, from C1–C3 at less than 8 years down to C5–C6 in adolescence, where it remains into adulthood.

Fractures and dislocations of the cervical spine can be observed on plain radiographs, which should be obtained in lateral and anteroposterior (AP) projections. An open mouth AP view should also be obtained to appropriately image the occipital condyles down to the C1–C2 articulations. CT images of the cervical spine have a higher sensitivity and specificity for identifying bony injuries to the spine compared to radiographs.

Common injuries of the cervical spine include fractures of nonstabilizing structures, fractures of the vertebral bodies, and fractures or dislocations of the facets (▶ Fig. 2.2). In patients with facet dislocations (e.g., "jumped" or "locked" facets), expedient reduction of the dislocation is associated with improved neurologic outcomes.[2] However, in the neurologically intact patient, if MRI is readily available in an emergent fashion, MRIs of the cervical spine may be obtained prior to attempting reduction to evaluate for possible epidural hematoma or traumatic disk herniation that may need to be addressed during open fixation.

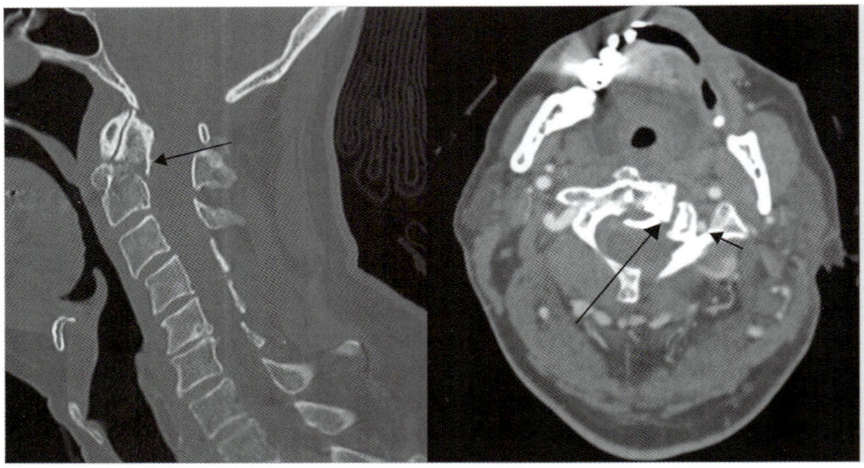

Fig. 2.1 Traumatic C2 injury. Sagittal computed tomography (CT) image (left) shows a fracture involving the base of the C2 dens resulting in posterior translation (*arrow*). Axial CT image (right) characterizes the degree of rotational subluxation and facet joint involvement. Contrast angiography is performed as well to rule out vessel dissection given the proximity of the patent vertebral artery (*short arrow*) to the fracture (*long arrow*).

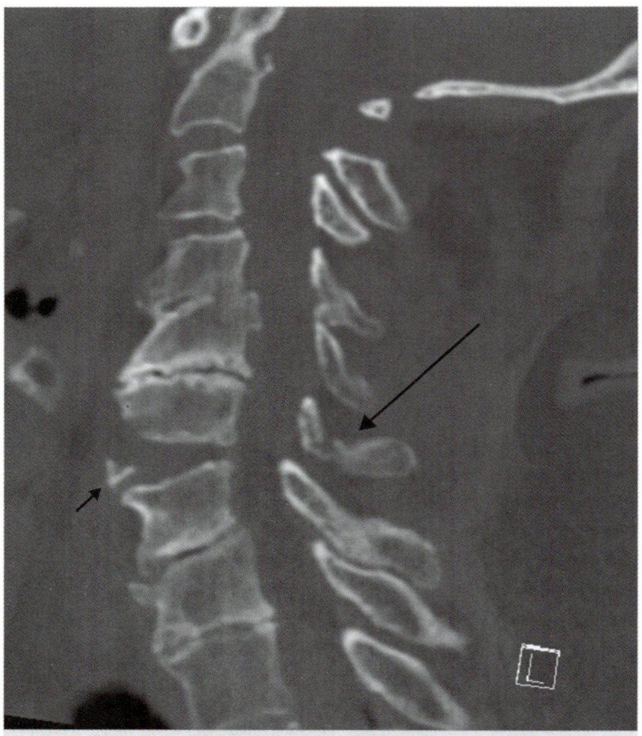

Fig. 2.2 Sagittal computed tomography (CT) images of a subaxial cervical fracture. The C6/C7 disk space widening, C6 teardrop fracture of anterior–inferior vertebral body (*short arrow*) as well as C6 spinous progress fracture (*long arrow*) are all suggestive of an extension-type injury.

2.2.3 Thoracolumbar Spine

Compression fractures are among the most common acute thoracolumbar spine sports injuries (▶ Fig. 2.3). Most thoracic spine sports injuries are mechanically stable as this region of the spine is additionally supported by the ribs and sternum. Repetitive stress on the low back in many sports puts the lumbar spine at high risk of injury. In sports with repeated axial loading such as football, basketball, equestrian, and gymnastics, disk degeneration and herniation are commonly reported.[3]

Repetitive hyperextension such as in dance, gymnastics, rowing, weightlifting, and football can result in spondylolysis, a stress fracture of the pars interarticularis which connects the superior and inferior facets of a given spinal vertebrae. Spondylolysis is often managed conservatively as demonstrated by an analysis by Choi et al who evaluated 201 cases of lumbar spondylolysis in adolescent athletes with all but one successfully undergoing conservative management.[4] Acute fractures and spondylolysis can both be seen on CT, or classically on oblique lumbar radiographs. MRIs are useful in identifying the degree of neural compression, particularly in cases of isthmic spondylolisthesis, disk herniations, or epidural hematomas.

2.3 Imaging of Spine Trauma

2.3.1 Radiographs and Computed Tomography (CT)

Two major cervical spine evaluation "rules" were created to guide clinicians on whether to obtain radiographs or CTs (NEXUS and Canadian C-spine Rule). These evaluations are within the scope of the sideline assessment and may be easily performed by any provider. These guidelines are tabulated in ▶ Table 2.1.

In pediatric patients, radiographs of the spine are often obtained first before CTs to minimize overall radiation exposure.[5] Additionally, bony spinal features and pathology are often easier to detect in a pediatric patient versus an adult patient due to decreased body size and improved penetration of X-rays. X-ray machines and qualified technologists are broadly available, even in some urgent care settings. Radiographs are thus often the first imaging modality obtained in the pediatric athlete presenting with spinal symptoms or pathology; however, padding serves as an impediment to radiographic visualization and should be removed prior to imaging.[6,7]

Bony injuries, fractures, and dislocations are best assessed using CT imaging, given the widespread availability and relative speed with which the images can be obtained. Although CT has largely supplanted plain radiography for initial diagnosis and screening, radiographs can be used adjunctively to assess stability and deformity in dynamic imaging and with weight-bearing. While CTs are used to identify bony injuries, certain findings on radiograph or CT may suggest ligamentous injuries, such as

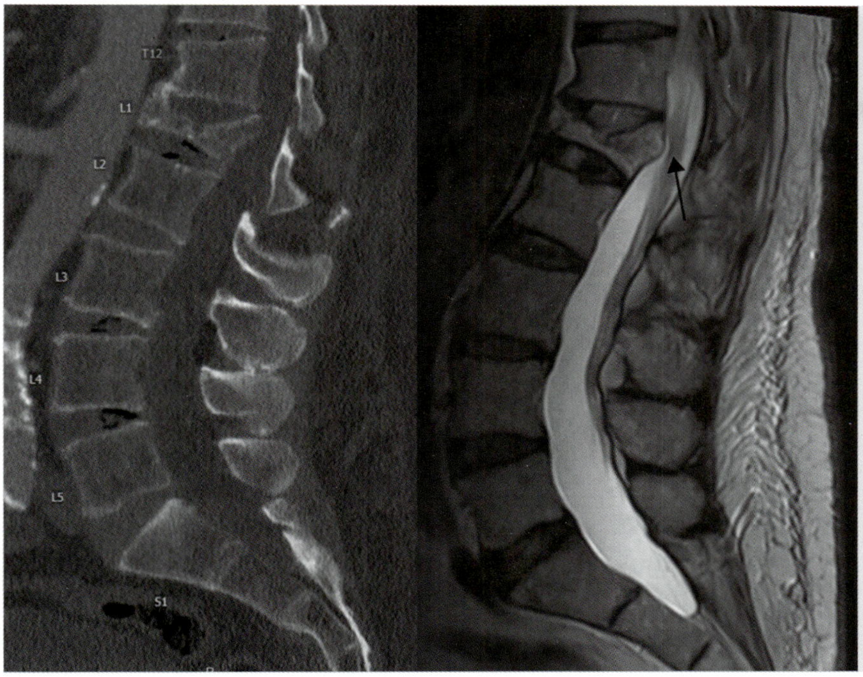

Fig. 2.3 Thoracolumbar fracture with burst morphology at L1. Sagittal computed tomography (CT) (left) shows nearly 80% vertebral body height loss at L1. T2-weighted magnetic resonance imaging (MRI) (right) better delineates the degree spinal canal narrowing and compression of neural structures from the retropulsed fragment (*arrow*).

Table 2.1 Cervical imaging guidelines

	NEXUS	Canadian C-spine rules
Require awake and reliable patient	Yes	Yes
Requires patient to be able to actively rotate neck by 45 degrees	No	Yes
Low-risk criteria (must have all present to forgo imaging)	• No posterior midline cervical spine tenderness • No evidence of intoxication • Normal level of alertness • No focal neurologic deficit • No painful distracting injury	• Simple rear-end motor vehicle accident • Sitting position in emergency department • Ambulatory at any time • Delayed (not acute) onset of neck pain • Absence of midline cervical spine tenderness
High-risk factors that mandate radiography	N/A	• Age at least 65 years • Dangerous mechanism • Paresthesia in extremities

prevertebral hematomas, spondylolisthesis, asymmetric disk space widening, facet joint widening or dislocations, or interspinous widening.

CT angiography (CTA) is a noninvasive technique using a bolus of intravenous contrast with CT image acquisition gated by a predefined Hounsfield unit threshold in the descending aorta, to minimize venous contamination of the acquired image stack. In the setting of trauma, these images are useful for assessing vascular injuries of the head and neck due to blunt or penetrating trauma (▶ Fig. 2.4). The Denver criteria provide indications for obtaining CT angiograms of the neck and head for trauma patients.

CTs and CT angiograms require more time and resources to obtain than plain radiographs, although most emergency departments in the United States are equipped with CT scanners. These studies are still expedient enough that they can be obtained safely and with good imaging quality even in a mildly uncooperative patient. CTA additionally requires bolus-timed acquisition following a contrast load given by a powered intravenous injector, which is not equipped with every CT scanner, so even though a particular emergency department may have CT capabilities, patients meeting clinical indications for CTAs may still need to be transferred to a secondary or tertiary center. Radiation exposure is vastly increased with CTs compared to radiographs, in exchange for three-dimensional data.

Iodinated contrast administration carries a risk of acute kidney injury, which can be exacerbated in patients experiencing rhabdomyolysis as a part of their overall athletic trauma. Use of contrast should be weighed carefully, and volume expansion with intravenous hydration may be used to decrease the risk of contrast-associated acute kidney injury in high-risk patients.

2.3.2 Magnetic Resonance Imaging (MRI)

MRIs provide superior imaging of soft tissue injuries, ligamentous disruptions, and spinal cord pathologies, including sources of extrinsic compression, such as hematoma or disk herniations, and intrinsic injury, such as infarct or shear injury, when compared to CTs and radiographs. However, they are the most time and resource intensive modality routinely used for imaging of

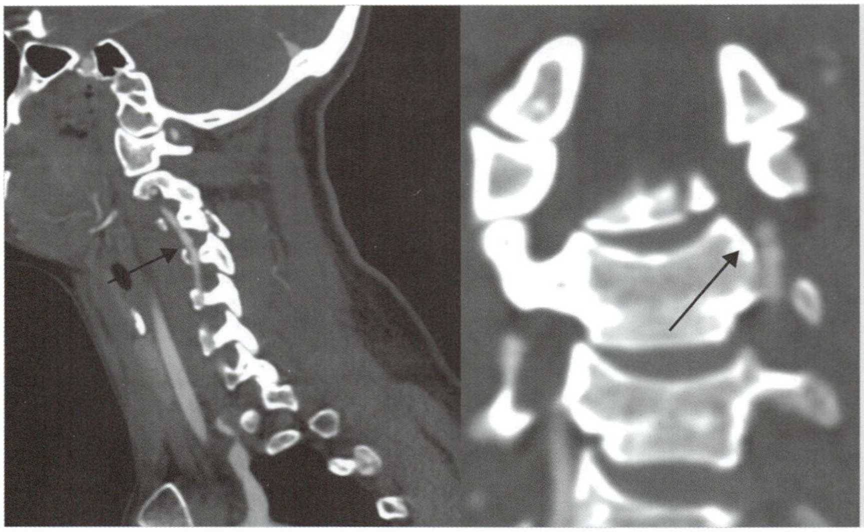

Fig. 2.4 Computed tomography (CT) angiography of a left vertebral artery dissection. The sagittal image (left) shows focal stenosis of the vertebral artery (*arrow*) while the magnified coronal image (right) shows the dissection flap in greater detail (*arrow*).

sports-related injuries and are less commonly available compared with CT and plain X-ray.

MRIs are indicated to evaluate radiographic or CT findings suggestive of ligamentous injury, epidural hematomas, disk herniations, patients with impaired neurologic status, and patients with suspected occult fractures or ligamentous injuries and to discern hemorrhagic and nonhemorrhagic spinal cord injuries for prognostication. The American College of Radiology appropriateness criteria indicate MRI of the spine following CT in the setting of acute spinal trauma if NEXUS or Canadian Cervical Spine criteria are met and if there is also clinical myelopathy, imaging findings suspicious for ligamentous injury, or suspected mechanical instability.[8]

MRIs for acute spinal injury have the highest sensitivity for identifying ligamentous injury within the first 72 hours, as the T2 hyperintensity produced by the injury edema improves the contrast of the ligaments, which are hypointense in the normal state. As edema and hemorrhage resolve over time, sensitivity of MRI to detect ligamentous injuries decreases.[9,10] For most sports-related indications for MRI, gadolinium-based intravenous contrast is not required.

High-resolution MRI also plays a role in sports-related injuries specifically in the workup of suspected ligamentous injury.[1,2,3] For instance, in patients with suspected craniocervical junction injuries, protocols using at least 1.5 T field strength scanners allow for adequate visualization of the structures in question.[11] These three-dimensional volumetric proton density sequences with variable flip angle, commercially called Cube (GE Healthcare, Chicago, Illinois, United States) or SPACE (Siemens, Berlin, Germany), require slightly longer scan times but produce high spatial resolution and isotropic voxels which allow for reconstruction in any plane.

2.4 Imaging of Cranial Trauma

2.4.1 Initial Evaluation

Sports-related head injuries may range from imaging negative concussions to severe traumatic brain injuries (TBIs) with concurrent bleeding. Several decision-making tools have been created to assist physicians in identifying which patients to evaluate for intracranial injury. These include the Canadian Head CT Rule,[12] the NEXUS Head CT Instrument,[13] and the PECARN Pediatric Head Injury/Trauma Algorithm.[14] These decision-making tools generally consider global mental status, focal neurologic deficits, and external signs of trauma to indicate further imaging.

Cranial trauma is common in certain athletic competitions such as football, soccer, rugby, and hockey. Multiple organizations including the National Football League (NFL) have put forth guidelines for the initial evaluation of an athlete with suspected head trauma. Individuals with signs of loss of consciousness, confusion, ataxia, or amnesia are withheld from the remainder of the competition while patients with suspected severe injuries are triaged in the hospital.[15]

2.4.2 Computed Tomography

Skull fractures are best assessed on head CTs, both in cross-sectional two-dimensional images and in three-dimensional reconstructions (▶ Fig. 2.5). Almost all linear, nondisplaced skull fractures heal with nonoperative management, whereas surgical intervention is indicated for skull fractures depressed more than the thickness of the skull, fractures with significant mass effect or midline shift with or without underlying hematomas, open skull fractures, and skull base fractures with persistent cerebrospinal fluid (CSF) leaks lasting more than 24 hours.

In cases of mild TBI or concussion, the imaging resolution of CT is inadequate to demonstrate any abnormal intraparenchymal findings. Moderate TBIs may demonstrate small traumatic hematomas on head CT, such as traumatic subarachnoid hemorrhage, or even subdural or epidural hematomas (▶ Fig. 2.6). Traumatic subarachnoid hemorrhages have very low risk of clinical deterioration and are managed nonoperatively.[16] Epidural and subdural hematomas are rare in an athletic setting unless the injury was associated with significant velocity or height of fall.

2.4.3 Magnetic Resonance Imaging

MRI is superior to CT in evaluating soft tissue and intraparenchymal lesions specifically hematomas, contusions, or petechiae.

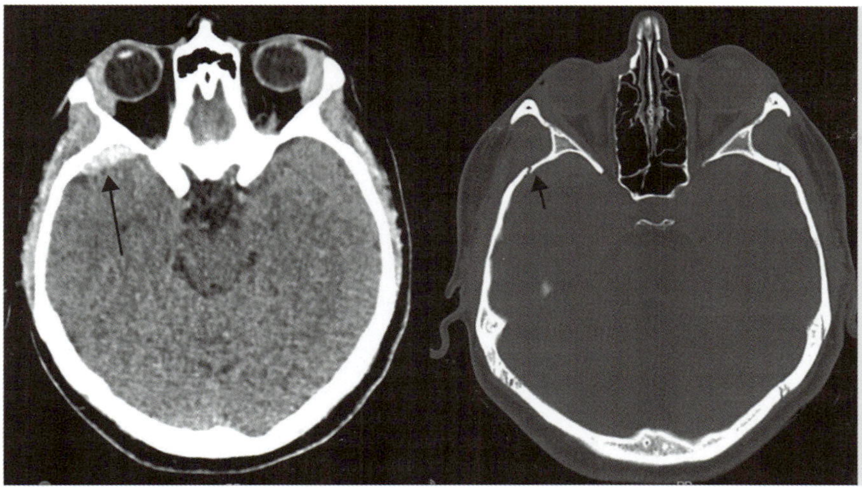

Fig. 2.5 Axial computed tomography (CT) images of an acute epidural hematoma of right temporal pole (left image, *long arrow*) with adjacent fracture extending into the squamosal suture of temporal bone (right image, *short arrow*).

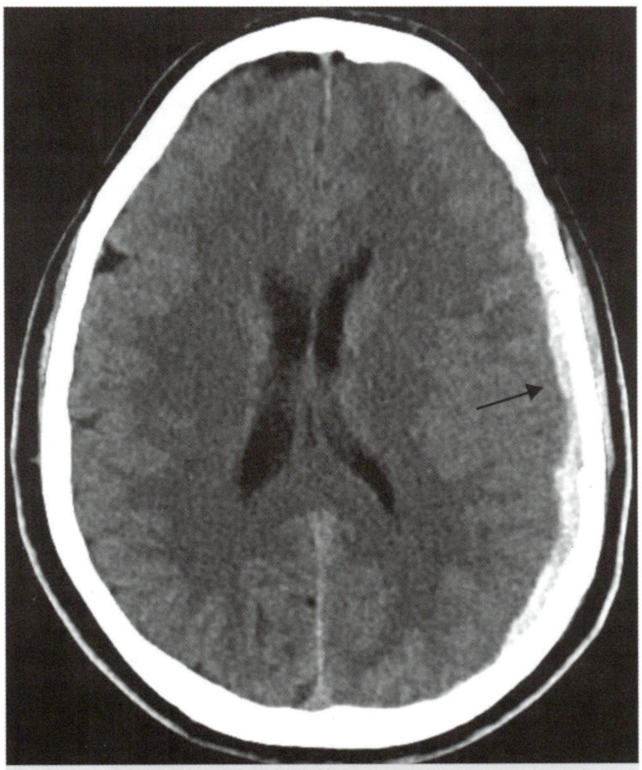

Fig. 2.6 Axial computed tomography (CT) image of a traumatic left frontoparietal convexity subdural hematoma (*arrow*).

MRI is most helpful in a patient with a low Glasgow coma score without a space-occupying lesion on CT to evaluate for alternative causes of impaired consciousness, namely, diffuse axonal injury, and is able to diagnose 10 to 20% of abnormalities missed on CT.[17] MRI is also useful in temporally characterizing intracranial hemorrhages as the oxygenated state of hemoglobin and its location (intracellular versus extracellular) affect the imaging findings of acute hemorrhage. Although the diagnostic specifics of chronic traumatic encephalopathy remain controversial, MRI may play a role in identifying individuals at risk for the condition.[18] The DETECT study found changes in thalamic volume and smaller amygdala, hippocampus, and cingulate gyrus volumes in former NFL football players compared to matched controls.[19]

In concussion and mild TBI patients, standard anatomical MRI often fails to demonstrate significant differences between these patients and normal controls. In post-concussion syndrome[20] and long-term follow-up of pediatric concussion patients,[21] standard anatomical MRI protocols did not detect any differences between concussed patients and age-matched controls. Recent interest in long-term sequelae of concussions and head trauma has led to research and development of improved imaging modalities such as diffusion tensor imaging (DTI) and resting state functional MRI (rsfMRI) that are better able to detect changes in brain anatomy and connectivity. In a study of 29 concussed and 48 healthy control university athletes, DTI and rsfMRI combined with cognitive evaluation resulted in overall accuracy of diagnosing concussion of 74% with a sensitivity of 64%.[22] Furthermore, DTI changes in the white matter persisted up to 6 months after injury in a separate study of 219 university athletes (82 concussed, 68 contact sport controls, and 69 noncontact sport controls). These persistent white matter changes were only seen in the concussed athletes at 6 months and not in either group of controls, and the extent of these changes was associated with clinical outcomes and delayed recovery time.[23]

2.4.4 Advanced Imaging

Advanced imaging modalities are currently being evaluated for potential utility in predicting the development of long-term neurologic sequelae in patients who suffer repetitive head trauma as discussed in the dedicated chapter 7 on chronic traumatic encephalopathy. Diffusion tensor MRI was studied in 14 cognitively impaired retired NFL football players.[18] It showed reductions of fractional anisotropy in the corpus callosum, and left temporal, bilateral frontal, and parietal regions compared to matched controls. Position emission tomography and MR spectroscopy may also have characteristic findings in patients suspected of having a long-term post-concussion syndrome; however, further work is needed to evaluate the predictive capacity of these techniques.[24,25]

2.5 Clinical Pearls

- Established guidelines and scoring systems can be used to determine which athletes require further imaging studies or clinical examinations.
- For assessing spinal injuries, radiographs and CT scans are best used for imaging bony elements, CTA is best for vascular elements, and MRI is best for ligamentous or spinal cord injuries.
- For assessing cranial trauma, CT scans are best used to evaluate skull fractures, and MRI is best for soft tissues and intraparenchymal injuries.
- With further research, advanced imaging modalities such as DTI and rsfMRI may become clinically significant tools for evaluating sports-related injuries.

2.6 Disclosure Statement

The authors have nothing to disclose.

References

[1] Prabhakar G, Mills G, Momtaz D, Ghali A, Chaput C. Survival rates in atlanto-occipital dissociation: a look at the past 20 years. Spine J. 2022; 22(9):1535–1539

[2] Wolf A, Levi L, Mirvis S, et al. Operative management of bilateral facet dislocation. J Neurosurg. 1991; 75(6):883–890

[3] Ball JR, Harris CB, Lee J, Vives MJ. Lumbar spine injuries in sports: review of the literature and current treatment recommendations. Sports Med Open. 2019; 5(1):26

[4] Choi JH, Ochoa JK, Lubinus A, Timon S, Lee YP, Bhatia NN. Management of lumbar spondylolysis in the adolescent athlete: a review of over 200 cases. Spine J. 2022; 22(10):1628–1633

[5] Basil GW, Burks SS, Green BA. Sports-related cervical spine injuries—background, triage, and prevention. J Craniofac Surg. 2021; 32(4):1643–1646

[6] Davidson RM, Burton JH, Snowise M, Owens WB. Football protective gear and cervical spine imaging. Ann Emerg Med. 2001; 38(1):26–30

[7] Copley PC, Tilliridou V, Kirby A, Jones J, Kandasamy J. Management of cervical spine trauma in children. Eur J Trauma Emerg Surg. 2019; 45(5): 777–789

[8] Beckmann NM, West OC, Nunez D, Jr, et al. Expert Panel on Neurological Imaging and Musculoskeletal Imaging. ACR Appropriateness Criteria® suspected spine trauma. J Am Coll Radiol. 2019; 16 5S:S264–S285

[9] Selden NR, Quint DJ, Patel N, d'Arcy HS, Papadopoulos SM. Emergency magnetic resonance imaging of cervical spinal cord injuries: clinical correlation and prognosis. Neurosurgery. 1999; 44(4):785–792, discussion 792–793

[10] Georgy BA, Hesselink JR. MR imaging of the spine: recent advances in pulse sequences and special techniques. AJR Am J Roentgenol. 1994; 162 (4):923–934

[11] Nidecker AE, Shen PY. Magnetic resonance imaging of the craniovertebral junction ligaments: normal anatomy and traumatic injury. J Neurol Surg B Skull Base. 2016; 77(5):388–395

[12] Stiell IG, Wells GA, Vandemheen K, et al. The Canadian CT Head Rule for patients with minor head injury. Lancet. 2001; 357(9266):1391–1396

[13] Mower WR, Hoffman JR, Herbert M, Wolfson AB, Pollack CV, Jr, Zucker MI, NEXUS II Investigators. Developing a decision instrument to guide computed tomographic imaging of blunt head injury patients. J Trauma. 2005; 59(4): 954–959

[14] Kuppermann N, Holmes JF, Dayan PS, et al. Pediatric Emergency Care Applied Research Network (PECARN). Identification of children at very low risk of clinically-important brain injuries after head trauma: a prospective cohort study. Lancet. 2009; 374(9696):1160–1170

[15] Jacobi J, Wasserman EB, Mack CD, et al. The National Football League Concussion Protocol: a review. HSS J. 2023; 19(3):269–276

[16] Griswold DP, Fernandez L, Rubiano AM. Traumatic subarachnoid hemorrhage: a scoping review. J Neurotrauma. 2022; 39(1–2):35–48

[17] Mittl RL, Grossman RI, Hiehle JF, et al. Prevalence of MR evidence of diffuse axonal injury in patients with mild head injury and normal head CT findings. AJNR Am J Neuroradiol. 1994; 15(8):1583–1589

[18] Hart J, Jr, Kraut MA, Womack KB, et al. Neuroimaging of cognitive dysfunction and depression in aging retired National Football League players: a cross-sectional study. JAMA Neurol. 2013; 70(3):326–335

[19] Schultz V, Stern RA, Tripodis Y, et al. Age at first exposure to repetitive head impacts is associated with smaller thalamic volumes in former professional American football players. J Neurotrauma. 2018; 35(2):278–285

[20] Panwar J, Hsu CC, Tator CH, Mikulis D. Magnetic resonance imaging criteria for post-concussion syndrome: a study of 127 post-concussion syndrome patients. J Neurotrauma. 2020; 37(10):1190–1196

[21] Virani S, Barton A, Goodyear BG, Yeates KO, Brooks BL. Susceptibility-weighted magnetic resonance imaging (MRI) of microbleeds in pediatric concussion. J Child Neurol. 2021; 36(10):867–874

[22] Ly MT, Scarneo-Miller SE, Lepley AS, et al. Combining MRI and cognitive evaluation to classify concussion in university athletes. Brain Imaging Behav. 2022; 16(5):2175–2187

[23] Wu YC, Harezlak J, Elsaid NMH, et al. Longitudinal white-matter abnormalities in sports-related concussion: a diffusion MRI study. Neurology. 2020; 95(7):e781–e792

[24] Alosco ML, Jarnagin J, Rowland B, Liao H, Stern RA, Lin A. Magnetic resonance spectroscopy as a biomarker for chronic traumatic encephalopathy. Semin Neurol. 2017; 37(5):503–509

[25] Mitsis EM, Riggio S, Kostakoglu L, et al. Tauopathy PET and amyloid PET in the diagnosis of chronic traumatic encephalopathies: studies of a retired NFL player and of a man with FTD and a severe head injury. Transl Psychiatry. 2014; 4(9):e441

3 Management of Sports-Related Head Injury in the Athlete

Margot Putukian

Summary

This chapter provides an overview of sports-related concussion (SRC), specifically reviewing the most recent consensus conference related to diagnosis and management issues. This serves as a guideline for the clinician and is based on current expert consensus and systematic reviews of the existing literature.

Keywords: concussion, sports-related concussion, head injury, traumatic brain injury, return to sport, management of concussion

Sports-related concussion (SRC) is a common injury in sport, and the body of knowledge regarding its assessment, diagnosis, and management has increased over the past two decades, with a majority in the last decade. SRC has been defined by the Concussion in Sport Group (CISG) and Consensus Statement[1] as "a traumatic brain injury caused by a direct blow to the head, neck or body resulting in an impulsive force being transmitted to the brain that occurs in sports and exercise-related activities. This initiates a neurotransmitter and metabolic cascade, with possible axonal injury, blood flow change and inflammation affecting the brain. Symptoms and signs may present immediately, or evolve over minutes or hours, and commonly resolve within days, but may be prolonged. No abnormality is seen on standard structural neuroimaging studies (computed tomography or magnetic resonance imaging T1- and T2-weighted images), but in the research setting, abnormalities may be present on functional, blood flow, or metabolic imaging studies. SRC results in a range of clinical symptoms and signs that may or may not involve loss of consciousness. The clinical symptoms and signs of concussion cannot be explained solely by (but may occur concomitantly with) drug, alcohol, or medication use, other injuries (such as cervical injuries, peripheral vestibular dysfunction) or other comorbidities (such as psychological factors or coexisting medical conditions)."[1] The American Congress of Rehabilitation Medicine has published diagnostic criteria for mild traumatic brain injury created by using a Delphi survey process of international interdisciplinary clinician-scientists which incorporate mechanisms of injury, symptoms, signs, and test findings.[2] These two definitions are in alignment with each other and can both be used for SRC, understanding that the diagnosis often requires clinical judgment.[3]

The leading proposed pathophysiological mechanisms of concussion is the shear strain of neural elements caused by rotational accelerations of the brain.[4] This causes a neurotransmitter and metabolic cascade, with changes in glucose, lactate, glutamate, and potassium; possible axonal injury; cerebral blood flow changes; and inflammation affecting the brain.

The incidence of SRC ranges from 1.6 to 3.8 million annually.[5,6,7] Concussions account for 4 to 10% of all American football injuries at the youth, high school, and collegiate levels.[8] It is estimated that 25 to 50% of concussions stem from sports and recreational activities. Men playing collision sports, such as American football, ice hockey, lacrosse, and rugby have the highest incidence of SRC. Among female athletes, the highest incidences occurred in those who played soccer, lacrosse, and field hockey.

In October 2022, the CISG, consisting of leading world experts in SRC, congregated in Amsterdam to discuss and refine the existing consensus statement with regards to concussion diagnosis and management in athletes.[1] According to the statement, there are 13 R's of SRC management: Recognize, Remove, Re-evaluate, Rest, Rehabilitation, Refer, Recover, Return-to-learn/return-to-sport, Reconsider, Residual effects, Reduce, Retire, and Refine.

3.1 Recognize and Remove

"Recognize" refers to identifying when a player may have sustained a concussion.[9] Players who have clear signs of SRC such as loss of consciousness or balance disturbance should be removed from play immediately. Clinical symptoms may not always involve loss of consciousness, and the onset of symptoms may be delayed for several minutes or even hours. Whenever an athlete is suspected of having sustained a concussion, he or she must be removed from play for assessment. Initial screening can be done on the sideline. There is no one test or marker currently available that can be used to diagnose concussion, though there are standardized assessment batteries/tools that, combined with clinical judgment, can assist the healthcare provider in making the diagnosis. SRC can include one or more of the following:

- Clinical symptoms: e.g., headache, memory dysfunction, and/or emotional lability
- Physical signs: e.g., loss of consciousness, ataxia, oculomotor–vestibular deficit
- Balance impairment
- Behavioral changes (e.g., irritability)
- Cognitive impairment (e.g., memory dysfunction, slowed reaction time)
- Sleep/wake disturbance

It is important to note that these symptoms and signs are nonspecific to concussion. A definitive sideline diagnosis may not be possible given many compounding factors; however, a preliminary clinical diagnosis can normally be made if these symptoms or signs occur after a mechanism of injury. In contrast to other sports-related injuries, a concussion must be excluded through a meticulous review of symptoms and a normal evaluation before participation return can be considered or initiated.

The CISG has updated the Concussion Recognition Tool-6 (CRT6) as well as several tools for the sideline assessment and follow-up office assessments https://www.concussioninsportgroup.com/scat-tool). The CRT6 is designed for athletes, coaches, and other stakeholders who are not healthcare providers. The Sport Concussion Assessment Tool-6 (SCAT6), ChildSCAT6, Sport Concussion Office Assessment Tool-6 (SCOAT6), and Child SCOAT6 are developed for use by healthcare providers. These tools are freely available https://www.concussioninsportgroup.com/scat-tool).

The SCAT6[10] is the most validated test battery that assesses possible SRC, and includes an on-field as well as an off-field component. The SCAT6 is aimed at athletes 13 years and older whereas the Child SCAT6[11] is a tool designed for children aged 8 to 12. The SCAT6 is most useful in the first 72 hours after injury to screen athletes, typically takes about 10 to 12 minutes to complete, and loses its ability to differentiate concussed versus nonconcussed individuals after 7 days from the initial injury.[10]

The on-field component of the SCAT6 includes identifying observable signs, the Glasgow Coma Scale (GCS), as well as other "red flags" for severe brain trauma, screening cervical spine, coordination and ocular/motor screens, as well as a test for memory assessment (the Maddocks questions) (see https://www.concussioninsportgroup.com/). The off-field component of the SCAT6 is ideally performed in a distraction-free environment such as the locker room or training room. This examination includes additional background information, a symptom checklist, and a brief neuropsychological battery (the Standardized Assessment of Concussion [SAC]) which includes orientation, concentration, and immediate and delayed memory, and an assessment of coordination and balance (i.e., mBESS, timed tandem gait).[12,13] To diagnose SRC, the symptoms should not be explained by drug, alcohol, or medication use, other injuries (such as cervical injuries, peripheral vestibular dysfunction, etc.), or other comorbidities (i.e., psychological factors or coexisting medical conditions).

Even if sideline screening is negative or early evaluation is normal, follow-up evaluations are advisable because SRC can have delayed onset of symptoms. Serial assessments are often required. The general consensus is conservative management in borderline or unclear cases, including keeping the athlete out of participation. It is often helpful to watch video review of the injury occurrence, if available, to help identify significant head-impact events.[14]

The player should not be left alone after sustaining an injury. An athlete diagnosed with SRC should not be allowed to return to play on the day of the injury, and should be assessed serially, and monitored and provided with instructions on symptoms or signs that might indicate complications (e.g., intracranial bleed) requiring emergency care. There is data that demonstrates that athletes who continue to play or are delayed in terms of seeing a healthcare provider are more likely to have a higher burden of symptoms as well as a delayed recovery and return to sport.[15] Historically, there has been concern for the possibility of second impact syndrome (SIS), where an athlete who continues to play with a concussion while the brain is vulnerable might sustain a second blow resulting in vascular congestion, cerebral edema, increased intracranial pressure, coma, or death. This has been reported in young athletes (< 20 years old) and though the existence of SIS is controversial, the importance of removing any player with possible SRC from play is unquestioned.

Based on clinical judgment, the clinician may opt to obtain further imaging or diagnostic studies to exclude a more severe brain injury including epidural hematoma, subdural hematoma, and parenchymal hemorrhage. Advanced neuroimaging is warranted in athletes with worrisome findings such as a focal neurologic deficit, basilar skull fracture, seizure, prolonged loss of consciousness, or a GCS (▶ Table 3.1) of less than 15. A GCS of 13 or higher correlates with mild brain injury, 9 to 12 with moderate injury, and a score of 8 or less represents a severe brain injury.

Table 3.1 Glasgow Coma Scale (GCS)

Eye opening	Verbal response	Motor response
None (1)	None (1)	None (1)
To pain (2)	Incomprehensible (2)	Extensor posturing (2)
To speech (3)	Inappropriate (3)	Abnormal flexion (3)
Spontaneous (4)	Confused (4)	Withdrawal (4)
	Oriented (5)	Localizes (5)
		Obeys commands (6)
	Total Points: 15	

3.2 Re-evaluate

A re-evaluation of the athlete should be performed in the emergency department or physician's office as soon as possible after the date of injury. One of the outcomes from the Consensus statement on concussion in sport conference was the development of the Sport SCOAT6[16] and Child SCOAT6[17] designed to assist healthcare providers in office-based assessment of the athletes with SRC who are 13 or older, or children age 8 to 12, respectively. The SCOAT6 (and Child SCOAT6) is a multimodal clinical management tool that aligns with the SCAT6[10] (and Child SCAT6,[11] respectively), and includes several components: symptoms, orthostatics, cervical spine examination, neurological examination, cognitive function, modified vestibular-oculomotor screening, screenings for anxiety, depression and sleep dysfunction, balance and tandem gait as well as dual task testing (tandem gait along with cognitive testing), and exercise testing. During the follow-up, a more thorough past medical history should be obtained specifically addressing if the patient has a history of any learning disabilities (e.g., ADHD), mood disorders, anxiety, headache disorders, or prior SRC. If the athlete has a history of SRC, information regarding quantity, specific injury characteristics, and return to play timing should be obtained. A detailed neurological examination should also be done including cognitive function, vestibular-ocular function, cranial nerve examination, sensorimotor examination, cerebellar examination, reflexes, and balance assessment to determine whether the patient's symptoms have changed since the time of injury. This may include asking parents, coaches, teammates, and roommates who know the patient best if they have noticed any changes.

Computerized cognitive evaluation tools such as the immediate post-concussion assessment and cognitive testing (IMPACT) are often used to assess athletes with SRC compared to their baseline. It should be used in conjunction with clinical assessment in determining when the athlete can return to play. Neuropsychological testing is not mandatory, but it can provide useful additional information for the clinician as well as serve as an educational tool to discuss the significance of the injury with the athlete. Formal neuropsychological testing should be performed by a trained and accredited neuropsychologist.

Advanced neuroimaging, fluid biomarkers, and genetic testing have been investigated over the past decade as possible methods for evaluating and tracking clinical recovery after SRC, but they require further validation to determine their clinical utility at this point in time.[18]

3.3 Rehabilitation

Historically, athletes who have sustained an SRC had been advised by their physicians to undergo complete rest. The most recent evidence shows that strict rest is not helpful, and after a very brief period (24–48 hours) of relative rest, patients should be encouraged to exercise and participate in low level cognitive loads as tolerated. Exercise and activities that include a change in direction and light strength training, as long as these do not significantly (more than 2 points on a 0–10 scale) increase symptoms for a prolonged (more than 30 minutes) period of time, can promote recovery from SRC.[1,15,19] Athletes recovering from SRC should not participate in activities that put them at risk for head contact until they are back to their pre-injury level of symptoms, cognitive function, balance, and neurological function. The return to sport (RTS) progression is a stepwise incremental increase in the intensity as well as the duration of exertion and sport-specific activities.[1,15] The first step considered in the treatment of SRC is submaximal exercise as it has been shown to be safe and in fact beneficial in the athlete's recovery.[19] This can be a brisk walk, stationary bicycling, or walking on the treadmill. Rehabilitation from SRC is best directly monitored by an athletic trainer, physical therapist, or other healthcare provider, in conjunction with a lead physician to oversee the RTS progression. The initial management of SRC is ideally a collaborative approach with targeted treatment as indicated.

3.4 Refer

Some patient athletes will have persisting symptoms after SRC[20,21] defined as symptoms that continue beyond the expected time frame of recovery (2–4 weeks).[15] Although this was previously defined as > 10 to 14 days in adults and > 4 weeks in children, the recent systematic review on recovery concluded that individuals should be treated individually, with all cohorts (age and sex) managed similarly.[15] Persisting symptoms are often nonspecific and may be related to preexisting, coexisting, or other confounding factors.[1,20,21] They do not necessarily indicate ongoing injury to the brain. A thorough clinical assessment should be performed to detect pathology that could be contributing to the persistent symptoms, including the components of the SCOAT6 or Child SCOAT6 which can help to target treatment. Currently, there is insufficient evidence to support the routine use of EEG, genetic testing, and advanced neuroimaging but research regarding their utility is ongoing.[18]

Current evidence-based treatment[19,20,21,22,23] for persisting post-concussive symptoms includes: a personalized approach utilizing a symptom-limited aerobic exercise program for those with autonomic instability or physical deconditioning, a physical therapy program addressing cervical spine or vestibular dysfunction, and cognitive therapy for those with persistent mood or behavioral symptoms.[1,19,22] Presently, there is limited evidence to support use of pharmacotherapy. If medication is deemed necessary, it is important to ensure that concussed athletes do not take anything that could mask symptoms of SRC, and the treating clinician should ensure to the best of their ability that such athletes are free from concussion-related symptoms before being cleared to return to contact play.

3.5 Recovery

Clinical recovery is defined as resolution of post-concussion related symptoms at rest and with physical and cognitive exertion as well as completion of the return to learn (RTL) (school/work) and RTS strategy.[15] In the recent systematic review on clinical recovery, RTL and RTS after SRC,[15] the pooled mean days until symptom free was 14.0 days (95% CI: 12.7, 15.4; n = 35 studies, I2 = 98.0%, Q statistic < 0.01) versus 19.8 days for days until RTS (95% CI: 18.8, 20.7; n = 57 studies, I2 = 99.3%, Q statistic < 0.01), with high heterogeneity between study subgroups. Importantly, though the majority of athletes have full RTL by 10 days, it can take twice that for RTS, and there is significant variability in the recovery trajectory, underscoring the importance of individualized management and RTL/RTS strategies.[15]

The strongest predictor of prolonged recovery after SRC is the initial burden and severity of symptoms.[15] Other factors to consider include:

- Burden of cognitive, balance, and oculomotor and vestibular abnormalities post injury
- Pre-existing history of depression and migraine history
- Continuing to participate after injury (versus immediate removal from play)
- Time taken to be seen by a healthcare provider

There were several other factors that were evaluated, and the findings were mixed as it related to previous history of SRCs, specific post-injury symptoms (e.g., dizziness, depressive symptoms, oculomotor symptoms), or specific post-injury signs (e.g., loss of consciousness and retrograde/post-traumatic amnesia). Having a low level of initial symptoms has been found to be a favorable prognostic indicator. A history of attention deficit hyperactivity disorder or learning disabilities or headache disorders may require more intervention regarding return to school.[15]

There is no established timeline for recovery. The management must be individualized for each athlete, and for each concussion, considering the current symptom burden, signs, and premorbid conditions. Care needs to be taken by the treating clinician to ensure the athlete is not allowed to return to contact play while there is ongoing brain dysfunction. Multiple studies suggest that physiological dysfunction may continue beyond clinical recovery. This supports the idea of a "buffer zone" of gradually increasing activity before full contact in sport. There are no modalities yet that have been found useful or reliable in predicting when it is safe for athletes to return to sport. Research is ongoing regarding such modalities measuring physiological changes after SRC such as functional MRI, diffusion tensor imaging, magnetic resonance spectroscopy, cerebral blood flow, electrophysiology, heart rate, measure of exercise performance, fluid biomarkers, and transcranial magnetic stimulation.[18]

3.6 Return to Sport (RTS) and Return to Learn (RTL)

The RTS recommendations (▶ Table 3.2) were modified,[1] yet they follow the concept of a gradual increase in the load and duration of activity occurring in a stepwise fashion concurrently with RTL. Step 1 is a brief period of relative rest (24–48 hours),

Table 3.2 Return-to-sport (RTS) strategy—each step typically takes a minimum of 24 hours

Step	Exercise strategy	Activity at each step	Goal
1	Symptom-limited activity	Daily activities that do not exacerbate symptoms (e.g., walking)	Gradual reintroduction of work/ school
2	Aerobic exercise **2A – Light** (up to approx. 55% maxHR) **then** **2B – Moderate** (up to approx. 70% maxHR)	Stationary cycling or walking at slow to medium pace; may start light resistance training that does not result in more than mild and brief exacerbation* of concussion symptoms	Increase heart rate
3	Individual sport-specific exercise Note: If sport-specific training involves any risk of inadvertent head impact, medical clearance should occur prior to step 3	Sport-specific training away from the team environment (e.g., running, change of direction and/or individual training drills away from the team environment); no activities at risk of head impact	Add movement, change of direction
Steps 4 to 6 should begin after the resolution of any symptoms, abnormalities in cognitive function, and any other clinical findings related to the current concussion, including with and after physical exertion.			
4	Noncontact training drills	Exercise to high intensity including more challenging training drills (e.g., passing drills, multiplayer training), can integrate into a team environment	Resume usual intensity of exercise, coordination, and increased thinking
5	Full-contact practice	Participate in normal training activities	Restore confidence and assess functional skills by coaching staff
6	Return to sport	Normal game play	

Abbreviations: HCP, healthcare professional; maxHR, predicted maximal heart rate according to age (i.e., 220 − age).
Note: * Mild and brief exacerbation of symptoms (i.e., an increase of no more than 2 points on a 0–10 point scale for less than an hour when compared with the baseline value reported prior to physical activity). Athletes may begin step 1 (i.e., symptom-limited activity) within 24 hours of injury, with progression through each subsequent step typically taking a minimum of 24 hours. If more than mild exacerbation of symptoms (i.e., more than 2 points on a 0–10 scale) occurs during steps 1 to 3, the athlete should stop and attempt to exercise the next day. Athletes experiencing concussion-related symptoms during steps 4 to 6 should return to step 3 to establish full resolution of symptoms with exertion before engaging in at-risk activities. Written determination of readiness to RTS should be provided by an HCP before unrestricted RTS as directed by local laws and/or sporting regulations.
Data from Patricios JS, Schneider KJ, Dvorak J, et al. Consensus statement on concussion in sport—the 6th international conference on concussion in sport - Amsterdam, October 2022. Br J Sports Med 2023;57:695–711.

followed by light activity (Step 2a), then moderate (Step 2b) aerobic activity, and sport-specific activity without risk for head contact (Step 3) all of which are considered treatment of acute concussion. Complete rest should be avoided, and athletes should be encouraged to participate in activities of daily life and in light cognitive challenges as tolerated. Importantly, the athlete can participate in steps 1 to 3 while symptomatic and can progress from one step to the next as long as the symptoms are not significant (increase by more than 2 on a scale of 0–10) or prolonged (longer than 1 hour). Once the athlete has returned to the baseline level of symptoms, cognitive function and clinical findings related to the current concussion, he or she should be evaluated by a healthcare provider and moved into the later steps (4–6) which re-introduce the athlete to contact and finally full sport activity. If at any point the athlete has significant concussion-related symptoms, he or she should drop back to the previous step and attempt to progress again after 24 hours. Each step typically takes at least 24 hours, and thus a minimum of 1 week to complete the full RTS strategy. This may vary depending on the individual's symptom burden, history, level of sport, and psychological readiness to return.[23,24] All athletes, whether elite or non-elite, should be managed using the same guidelines as stated above, and based on the most recent systematic review, can be applied to all other cohorts (both age and sex).[15]

For those under 18 years old, there is no evidence currently to suggest they should be managed differently from adults. The Child SCAT6 and Child SCOAT6 should be used for age-specific treatment. Otherwise, management guidelines are similar to those for adults (▶ Table 3.1). For SRC in children (aged 5–12 years) there is a paucity of data, though it is very common for symptoms to last for up to 4 weeks.

Schools are encouraged to have an RTL policy for SRC that includes education for teachers, staff, students, and parents on concussion prevention and management.[15] Academic dysfunction was reported in almost 40% of the studies included in the systematic review on RTL[15] and was greater in athletes who had a higher burden (number and severity of symptoms) at the time of their initial visit. These individuals also had a prolonged recovery (both in terms of RTL and RTS). In addition, there appears to be evidence that prolonged strict rest can delay RTL whereas early cognitive and physical activity improves RTL,[15] in alignment with the results for RTS.

Over 90% of student athletes will RTL by 10 days after injury, and not all athletes with SRC will need academic support.[15] Schools should offer academic support to recovering students if needed or requested and examples include (1) environmental adjustments (e.g., modified attendance, rest breaks or screen time limits), (2) physical adjustments (e.g., no activities with a risk for contact, collision, or falls, but allowing for safe,

Table 3.3 Return-to-learn (RTL) strategy

Step	Mental activity	Activity at each step	Goal
1	Daily activities that do not result in more than a mild exacerbation* of symptoms related to the current concussion	Typical activities during the day (e.g., reading) while minimizing screen time; start with 5–15 min at a time and increase gradually	Gradual return to typical activities
2	School activities	Homework, reading, or other cognitive activities outside of the classroom	Increase tolerance to cognitive work
3	Return-to-school part time	Gradual introduction of schoolwork; may need to start with a partial school day or with greater access to rest breaks during the day	Increase academic activities
4	Return-to-school full time	Gradually progress school activities until a full day can be tolerated without more than mild* symptom exacerbation	Return to full academic activities and catch up on missed work

Note: Following an initial period of relative rest (24–48 hours following injury at step 1), athletes can begin a gradual and incremental increase in their cognitive load. Progression through the strategy for students should be slowed when there is more than a mild and brief symptom exacerbation.
* Mild and brief exacerbation of symptoms is defined as an increase of no more than 2 points on a 0–10 point scale (with 0 representing no symptoms and 10 the worst symptoms imaginable) for less than an hour when compared with the baseline value reported prior to cognitive activity.
Data from Patricios JS, Schneider KJ, Dvorak J, et al. Consensus statement on concussion in sport—the 6th international conference on concussion in sport - Amsterdam, October 2022. Br J Sports Med 2023;57:695–711.

noncontact physical activity), (3) curriculum adjustments (e.g., extra time to complete assignments or reduced work, pre-printed notes), and (4) testing adjustments (e.g., exemption from, delaying, and/or permitting additional time for tests).[15] Student athletes may need regular medical follow-up to track their progress and collaboration between healthcare providers and stakeholders on education and school policies to facilitate academic support when needed.[1,15]

Child, adolescent, and university-level athletes should not return to sport until they have returned to school (▶ Table 3.3). However, early reintroduction of symptom-limited physical activity, as discussed above, is encouraged. Return to school is paramount to return to sport in school-aged individuals. These RTL and RTS strategies routinely overlap with each other as the athlete advances.

3.7 Reconsider—Potential Long-term Effects

There is significant media attention regarding the concern for possible long-term effects of SRC and whether there is an association with mental health problems, cognitive impairment, and neurological disorders (e.g., dementia) and neurodegenerative diseases (e.g., Parkinson's disease, Alzheimer's disease, amyotrophic lateral sclerosis [ALS]). These issues were reviewed in the most recent consensus statement[1] and the conclusions of the systematic review[25] were that related to mental health problems "1) former amateur athletes are not at increased risk for depression or suicidality during early adulthood or as older adults, 2) former professional soccer players are not at increased risk for psychiatric hospitalization during their adult life and 3) former professional football and soccer players are not at increased risk for death associated with having a psychiatric disorder or as a result of suicide." The systematic review[25] also found that "former male amateur athletes were not at increased risk for cognitive impairment, neurological disorders or neurodegenerative diseases compared with the general population." However, studies of former professional American football and professional soccer players reported a higher mortality rate from neurological diseases (ALS) and dementia compared to the general population.[1,25] The authors point out the significant limitations in methodology given the inability to control and/or adjust for many factors that can be associated with neurological outcomes, such as "genetic factors, educational attainment, socioeconomic status, smoking, hypertension and cardiovascular disease, diabetes, sleep apnea, white matter hyperintensities, social isolation, diet, PA or exercise."[25] They also state that in order to determine a causal association between exposure to contact sports and cognitive impairment or dementia later in life, well-designed case-control and cohort studies are essential.

There has also been increased interest regarding SRC or contact sports and the pathological entity of chronic traumatic encephalopathy (CTE). A cause-and-effect relationship between repetitive SRCs and CTE or contact sports and CTE has not yet been demonstrated. The consensus statement reviewed the literature regarding CTE and clarified the difference between CTE–neuropathological change (CTE-NC)[26] and a possible clinical condition, traumatic encephalopathy syndrome (TES), described in those with substantial exposure to repetitive head impacts through military service, or contact sports with clinical features of cognitive impairment, neurobehavioral dysregulation, and importantly, not explained by other neurologic, psychiatric, or medical conditions.[1,27] More research on CTE-NC and TES is needed to better characterize the prevalence, neuropathology, progression, differentiating neuropathological criteria between CTE-NC and Alzheimer's disease, and determine whether CTE-NC is progressive.[1]

3.8 Retire

The systematic review addressing when an athlete should consider retirement from contact or collision sport after SRC concluded that there are no absolute indicators specific to SRC that preclude participation.[1,28] There were no papers that specifically evaluated the question of "retirement" and instead the conclusions were based on situations where athletes had persisting symptoms, repeat concussions, abnormalities on physical examination or neurocognitive test, or findings on advanced imaging (some of which were identified incidentally and not necessarily related to SRC) where the decision to "retire" was considered.[28] The authors recommended "an individualized and collaborative approach to shared decision-making" as well as involving the athlete in the decision process, and stated that the clinicians involved in this decision should have expertise in managing SRC.[28] Making decisions on RTS and regarding participating in collision or contact sports require that the healthcare provider communicate with the athlete (and the parent/guardian) regarding what is known and unknown about the diagnosis and recovery trajectory, discuss the specific risks of return to the sport, and consider the athlete's personal preferences as well as risk tolerance.[23,28] It is also essential that athletes (and their parent/guardian) understand the positive benefits of exercise and sport, and they choose to avoid contact or collision sports, they should be are encouraged to remain physically active.

3.9 Risk Reduction

A detailed SRC history during the pre-participation examination is key in identifying athletes who are at high risk for SRC. Specific questions should include number of past SRCs, prior symptoms, length of recovery, and history of previous head, face, or cervical spine injuries. Sometimes prior SRCs could have been missed in the setting of concurrent head, face, or cervical spine injury. Questions investigating whether the impact is proportional to the severity of symptoms may alert clinicians to an athlete's increased vulnerability to injury. The pre-participation examination should also be used as an opportunity to educate the athlete on SRC prevention, the signs and symptoms of SRC, and the importance of early reporting and recognition of injury.

Concussion-prevention strategies can limit the number and severity of SRC in many sports. There is evidence for the following prevention strategies[29]: (1) mouthguards and helmet fit in child and adolescent ice hockey, (2) rules disallowing body checking in children and most adolescent ice hockey, (3) limiting contact practices and helmet fit in American football, (4) neuromuscular training warm up programs in rugby. Policies for stricter enforcement of red cards for high elbows in heading duels in professional soccer are associated with a nonsignificant reduction in SRC and a significant reduction in overall head injury.[29,30] Importantly, there does not appear to be statistically significant evidence supporting face shields, eyewear, headgear, or jugular vein compression collars in preventing SRC.

Nutrition and supplementation are being investigated as possible avenues for decreasing risk of neurocognitive deficits after SRC.[31] Thus far there has not been rigorous evidence from human studies, but in rodent models, the combination of omega-3 fatty acids and curcumin has shown promise for neuroprotective effects. The combination has been shown to be superior to either of them alone in animal models. More human studies still need to be done to support routine clinical use in athletes.

3.10 Refine—Para Sport and Pediatric Considerations

Participation in sport for people with disabilities has increased and is estimated to constitute 15 to 25% of the population around the globe. SRC is unique in the para athlete, with special considerations for wheelchair athletes or athletes with visual or hearing disabilities. The Concussion in Para Sport Group recently published its first statement on SRC assessment, prevention, and management that is a useful resource for providers caring for para athletes.[32] The consensus statement also addressed the pediatric athlete, and the unique considerations for both 5- to 12-year-olds and 13- to 18-year-olds.[1] In each systematic review, the pediatric considerations were also included, including authors with expertise in pediatric SRC population.[11,15,17,18,19,20,22,28,29]

SRC is a relatively common occurrence in athletes, and it is important for clinicians to be proficient in recognizing, diagnosing, and managing it. Despite the thousands of articles devoted to SRC, many of the systematic reviews found a very low number of high-quality studies, and a high number of articles with a high risk of bias. What we know about SRC continues to evolve, and more methodologically sound cohort and randomized control trials are needed. This chapter serves as a guideline for clinicians, summarizing the findings from the international consensus conference and companion systematic reviews.

3.11 Clinical Pearls

- An athlete suspected of having a concussion should be promptly removed from play and evaluated by a healthcare provider.
- Athletes with head injury should be immobilized and transported immediately to the nearest emergency facility if a concurrent cervical spine injury or serious intracranial injury (e.g., hemorrhage, skull fracture) is suspected.
- The SCAT and SCOAT are standardized tools that can be used to assist the healthcare provider in making the diagnosis of SRC and for targeted treatment.
- No athlete who has sustained a concussion should be allowed to return to play on the same day, even if the symptoms resolve and examination is normal.
- Each concussion is different, even in the same athlete. Individualized treatment, accounting for athlete-specific factors, the initial burden and severity of symptoms, and the recovery trajectory, is essential.
- Early exercise and sport-specific activities including change in direction (without risk for head contact) is an important component of treatment for SRC and can be introduced early in the RTS progression.
- RTL and RTS strategies can be useful in the management of SRC.

References

[1] Patricios JS, Schneider KJ, Dvorak J, et al. Consensus statement on concussion in sport: the 6th International Conference on Concussion in Sport - Amsterdam, October 2022. Br J Sports Med. 2023; 57(11):695–711

[2] Silverberg ND, Iverson GL, Cogan A, et al. ACRM Brain Injury Special Interest Group Mild TBI Task Force members, ACRM Mild TBI Diagnostic Criteria Expert Consensus Group. The American Congress of rehabilitation medicine

diagnostic criteria for mild traumatic brain injury. Arch Phys Med Rehabil. 2023; 104(8):1343–1355

[3] Davis GA, Patricios J, Schneider KJ, Iverson GL, Silverberg ND. Definition of sport-related concussion: the 6th International Conference on Concussion in Sport. Br J Sports Med. 2023; 57(11):617–618

[4] Giza CC, Hovda DA. The neurometabolic cascade of concussion. J Athl Train. 2001; 36(3):228–235

[5] Marar M, McIlvain NM, Fields SK, Comstock RD. Epidemiology of concussions among United States high school athletes in 20 sports. Am J Sports Med. 2012; 40(4):747–755

[6] Halstead ME, Walter KD, Moffatt K, Council on Sports Medicine and Fitness. Sport-related concussion in children and adolescents. Pediatrics. 2018; 142 (6):e20183074

[7] Nonfatal Traumatic Brain Injuries from Sports and Recreation Activities—United States. 2001–2005. Accessed October 29, 2023 at: https://www.cdc.gov/mmwr/preview/mmwrhtml/mm5629a2.htm

[8] Dompier TP, Kerr ZY, Marshall SW, et al. Incidence of concussion during practice and games in youth, high school, and collegiate American football players. JAMA Pediatr. 2015; 169(7):659–665

[9] Meehan WP, III, d'Hemecourt P, Collins CL, Comstock RD. Assessment and management of sport-related concussions in United States high schools. Am J Sports Med. 2011; 39(11):2304–2310

[10] Echemendia RJ, Brett BL, Broglio S, et al. Sport concussion assessment tool™ - 6 (SCAT6). Br J Sports Med. 2023; 57(11):622–631

[11] Davis GA, Echemendia RJ, Ahmed OH, et al. Child SCAT6. Br J Sports Med. 2023; 57(11):636–647

[12] Bell DR, Guskiewicz KM, Clark MA, Padua DA. Systematic review of the balance error scoring system. Sports Health. 2011; 3(3):287–295

[13] Hansen C, Cushman D, Anderson N, et al. A normative dataset of the balance error scoring system in children aged between 5 and 14. Clin J Sport Med. 2016; 26(6):497–501

[14] Davis GA, Makdissi M, Bloomfield P, et al. International consensus definitions of video signs of concussion in professional sports. Br J Sports Med. 2019; 53(20):1264–1267

[15] Putukian M, Purcell L, Schneider KJ, et al. Clinical recovery from concussion-return to school and sport: a systematic review and meta-analysis. Br J Sports Med. 2023; 57(12):798–809

[16] Patricios JS, Davis GA, Ahmed OH, et al. Introducing the Sport Concussion Office Assessment Tool 6 (SCOAT6). Br J Sports Med. 2023; 57(11):648–650

[17] Davis GA, Patricios JS, Purcell LK, et al. Introducing the Child Sport Concussion Office Assessment Tool 6 (Child SCOAT6). Br J Sports Med. 2023; 57(11):668–671

[18] Tabor JB, Brett BL, Nelson L, et al. Role of biomarkers and emerging technologies in defining and assessing neurobiological recovery after sport-related concussion: a systematic review. Br J Sports Med. 2023; 57 (12):789–797

[19] Leddy JJ, Burma JS, Toomey CM, et al. Rest and exercise early after sport-related concussion: a systematic review and meta-analysis. Br J Sports Med. 2023; 57(12):762–770

[20] Yeates KO, Räisänen AM, Premji Z, et al. What tests and measures accurately diagnose persisting post-concussive symptoms in children, adolescents and adults following sport-related concussion? A systematic review. Br J Sports Med. 2023; 57(12):780–788

[21] Broshek DK, Pardini JE, Herring SA. Persisting symptoms after concussion: time for a paradigm shift. PM R. 2022; 14(12):1509–1513

[22] Schneider KJ, Critchley ML, Anderson V, et al. Targeted interventions and their effect on recovery in children, adolescents and adults who have sustained a sport-related concussion: a systematic review. Br J Sports Med. 2023; 57(12):771–779

[23] Herring SA, Putukian M, Kibler WB, et al. Team Physician Consensus Statement: Return to Sport/Return to Play and the Team Physician: A Team Physician Consensus Statement-2023 Update. Med Sci Sports Exerc. 2024 May 1;56(5):767–775

[24] Herring S, Kibler WB, Putukian M, et al. Selected issues in sport-related concussion (SRC|mild traumatic brain injury) for the team physician: a consensus statement. Br J Sports Med. 2021; 55(22):1251–1261

[25] Iverson GL, Castellani RJ, Cassidy JD, et al. Examining later-in-life health risks associated with sport-related concussion and repetitive head impacts: a systematic reviewof case-control and cohort studies. Br J Sports Med. 2023; 57(12):810–821

[26] Bieniek KF, Cairns NJ, Crary JF, et al. TBI/CTE Research Group. The second NINDS/NIBIB consensus meeting to define neuropathological criteria for the diagnosis of chronic traumatic encephalopathy. J Neuropathol Exp Neurol. 2021; 80(3):210–219

[27] Katz DI, Bernick C, Dodick DW, et al. National Institute of Neurological Disorders and Stroke consensus diagnostic criteria for traumatic encephalopathy syndrome. Neurology. 2021; 96(18):848–863

[28] Makdissi M, Critchley ML, Cantu RC, et al. When should an athlete retire or discontinue participating in contact or collision sports following sport-related concussion? A systematic review. Br J Sports Med. 2023; 57(12):822–830

[29] Eliason PH, Galarneau J-M, Kolstad AT, et al. Prevention strategies and modifiable risk factors for sport-related concussions and head impacts: a systematic review and meta-analysis. Br J Sports Med. 2023; 57(12):749–761

[30] Beaudouin F, Aus der Fünten K, Tröß T, Reinsberger C, Meyer T. Head injuries in professional male football (soccer) over 13 years: 29% lower incidence rates after a rule change (red card). Br J Sports Med. 2019; 53 (15):948–952

[31] Oliver JM, Anzalone AJ, Turner SM. Protection before impact: the potential neuroprotective role of nutritional supplementation in sports-related head trauma. Sports Med. 2018; 48 Suppl 1:39–52

[32] Weiler R, Blauwet C, Clarke D, et al. Concussion in para sport: the first position statement of the Concussion in Para Sport (CIPS) Group. Br J Sports Med. 2021; 55(21):1187–1195

4 Post-concussion Syndrome Management

Benjamin L. Brett, Lindsay D. Nelson, and Michael A. McCrea

Summary

Development of persistent symptoms following sports-related concussion (SRC) or persistent post-concussion symptoms (PPCS) are often associated with a complex clinical presentation, which represents an intersection of preinjury (e.g., demographic and diagnostic), injury (e.g., mechanism of injury and presenting symptoms), and postinjury (e.g., method of initial injury management) factors that require a thorough diagnostic evaluation as part of a dynamic differential diagnosis process. Operationalizing a definition of the PPCS has been difficult due to the wide range and often nebulous presentation of symptoms post-injury (physical, emotional, and cognitive symptoms), as well as elevated base rates of concussion-like symptoms in noninjured athletes and high comorbidity of PPCS with other related conditions. Multidisciplinary management is considered the optimal approach to care following SRC, including for those experiencing prolonged symptoms. Variable evidence exists for the relationship between increased risk of developing PPCS and demographic and injury-related factors, with acute injury burden and preinjury history of a psychiatric diagnosis as the most consistent risk factors for prolonged recovery. A primary objective of post-injury management involves resumption of as many regular activities as possible without significant exacerbation of symptoms. Reintegration as soon as possible, even with accommodations, is likely to diminish the negative psychosocial effects of prolonged disruption of regular activities (sport, school, social pursuits). Extended, strict physical and cognitive rest beyond the acute phase of recovery is not recommended. Best practice, based on emerging research and multiple consensus guidelines, now indicates that reinitiating activity after 1 to 2 days of rest may facilitate the neurobiological recovery processes.

Keywords: post-concussion syndrome, PCS, Concussion, TBI, Rehabilitation, head injury, review

4.1 Post-concussion Syndrome

Although a large majority of athletes experience a rapid course of recovery following sports-related concussion (SRC), some continue to experience sequelae beyond 7–14; in an even more select percentage of injured athletes (2.5%), these symptoms persist beyond 90 days.[1] This persistence of sequelae associated with SRC beyond the typical course of recovery (i.e., acute and subacute periods) is commonly referred to as persistent post-concussion symptoms (PPCS). The exact mechanism that underlies prolonged recovery is not fully understood, although likely multifactorial. Currently, there are several hypotheses or models explaining the underlying mechanisms of persistent symptoms. These models include autonomic dysregulation, metabolic abnormalities not returned to preinjury homeostasis following the neurometabolic cascade of concussion (e.g., disruption in levels of glutamate, and myo-inositol, and N-acetylaspartate), disruption to the vestibulo-ocular system, cervical spine dysfunction, and possibly a persistent low-grade neuroinflammatory response. In all likelihood, PCS represents some combination of these various proposed etiologies, which may account for the high variability in clinical presentation across individuals.[2]

A number of demographic and preinjury (i.e., age, sex, preinjury headache/migraine, and psychiatric disorder) and injury-related factors (i.e., symptom burden) appear to confer increased risk of developing PCS (▶ Fig. 4.1).[3] However, there has been variability across studies in the degree to which these and other factors are associated with the incidence of PPCS. Of all factors, the most consistent and robust predictors of prolonged recovery following SRC include post-concussive symptom burden (i.e., severity and number of acute symptoms after injury). Among noninjury factors, there is increasing evidence for greater risk of PPCS among those with preinjury diagnoses of psychiatric disorders or higher preinjury levels of psychiatric symptoms, and the development of subacute headaches.[3]

Historically, the clinical persistence of symptoms following sport-related concussion was referred to as post-concussion syndrome (PCS). However, operationalization of a definition has been difficult due to the wide range and often nebulous presentation of symptoms associated with PCS, as well as elevated base rates of concussion-like symptoms in noninjured athletes and high comorbidity of PCS with other related conditions.[4] As such, the field has shifted focus toward treatment and management of individual symptoms that do not naturally resolve (i.e., persistent post concussion symptoms; PPCS) and away from the term PCS. It is vital for every clinician to take into account whether the

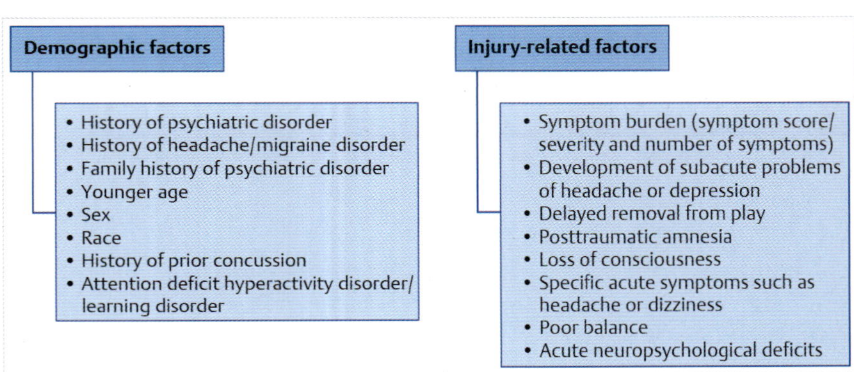

Fig. 4.1 Post-concussion syndrome and commonly investigated risk factors.

Table 4.1 Diagnostic criteria for post-concussion syndrome

DSM-IV	ICD-10
1. History of head trauma causing significant cerebral concussion	1. History of head trauma usually sufficiently severe to result in loss of consciousness
2. Three or more of the following symptoms occur shortly after trauma and last at least 3 months: • Becoming easily fatigued • Disordered sleep • Headache • Dizziness or vertigo • Irritability or aggression • Anxiety, depression, or affective lability • Changes in personality • Apathy or lack of spontaneity	2. Three or more of the following symptoms: • Headache, dizziness, malaise, fatigue, or noise intolerance • Irritability, emotional lability, depression, or anxiety • Subjective difficulty in concentration, mental tasks, or memory impairment • Insomnia • Reduced tolerance to alcohol • Preoccupation with the above symptoms or adoption of the sick role
3. Cognitive impairment in attention or memory based on objective testing 4. Symptoms started or significantly exacerbated after head trauma 5. Significant impairment in or interference with social or occupational functioning 6. Symptoms do not meet criteria for dementia due to head trauma and are not better explained by another disorder	3. Guidelines: • Careful evaluation with laboratory techniques (electroencephalography, brainstem evoked potentials, brain imaging, oculonystagmography) may yield objective evidence to substantiate the symptoms but results are often negative • The complaints are not necessarily associated with compensation motives • The etiology of these symptoms is not always clear, and both organic and psychological factors have been proposed to account for them. Some patients become hypochondriacal, embark on a search for diagnosis and cure, and may adopt a permanent sick role

Abbreviations: DSM-IV, Diagnostic and Statistical Manual of Mental Disorders-Fourth Edition; ICD-10, International Statistical Classification of Disease and Related Health Problems, 10th Revision.

presenting symptoms are a likely consequence of the target injury and whether other pre-existing or comorbid factors may be contributing to a patient's concerns. While terminology in the management of persistent symptoms has shifted away from PCS, diagnostic criteria still remain in use for the International Statistical Classification of Disease and Related Health Problems (ICD-10; ▶ Table 4.1). The most recent version of the Diagnostic and Statistical Manual of Mental Disorders-Fifth Edition (DSM-V) does not provide diagnostic criteria for PCS. The prior version DSM-Fourth Edition (DSM-IV)[5] are provided in ▶ Table 4.1 as well.[6]

Efforts have been made to establish distinct clinical profiles of acute concussion and prolonged recovery (i.e., clinical phenotypes), with the intention to improve treatment approaches based on precision medicine. However, given that symptom presentation following SRC can be variable, these phenotypes have yet to demonstrate reliability and validity across samples.[7] As such, persistent symptoms are generally categorized into broad domains, which include physical, emotional, and cognitive symptoms. Treatment of PPCS is generally based on individual symptoms within these domains. Growing evidence indicates that active rehabilitation, as opposed to extended rest following the initial injury, may be optimal for the prevention and treatment of PPCS.[8] In the following, we review the most commonly used methods of assessment and intervention for athletes with PPCS.

4.2 Management of PCS

Given the diverse clinical sequelae of concussion and multitude of factors that can influence recovery, multidisciplinary management is considered the optimal approach to care following SRC, including for those experiencing prolonged symptoms (▶ Fig. 4.2).[3,9] Professionals who frequently contribute to the management of athletes with PCS include athletic trainers (e.g., for monitoring of recovery and graded exertion/return-to-play programs), physicians (e.g., for neurologic and physical examinations, prescription of medications if relevant), neuropsychologists (e.g., for cognitive/neuropsychological and psychological health assessment), psychologists (e.g., for psychotherapy), and vestibular and other therapists. Irrespective of who manages a patient, taking a thorough history comprising questions about preinjury risk factors (e.g., psychiatric and headache history) as well as injury characteristics, activities, and ongoing symptoms is important for pinpointing factors that may be complicating recovery and, therefore, that may represent treatment target.

The management of athletes during the typical recovery phase and those experiencing prolonged symptoms has evolved from an emphasis on rest toward active treatment as part of recovery.[8] Greater weight being placed on active treatment is based upon a growing body of research that suggests rest has limited ability to effectively improve symptoms and may even be harmful beyond a certain point in recovery.[8] Although rest immediately following injury has potential benefits in the initial recovery from SRC by decreasing energy demands and restoring neurometabolic homeostasis, strict rest beyond 2 days has not been associated with additional benefits to recovery.

Strict rest beyond 5 days has been associated with exacerbation of psychological and behavioral symptoms among adolescents.[10] It is even hypothesized that over-prescribing rest may be a risk factor for persistent symptoms and development of PPCS especially psychological symptoms. As such, interest in the active treatment of SRC, such as prescribing regular, reduced-intensity physical activity, before becoming asymptomatic or fully recovered has grown. Although optimal management of SRC very

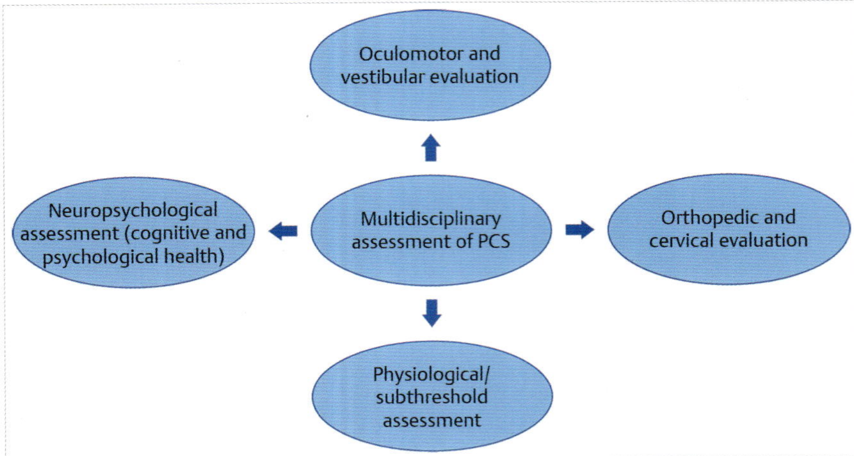

Fig. 4.2 Modalities and domains of assessment for post-concussion syndrome (PCS).

likely involves some combination of both (i.e., initial rest for restoration of neurometabolic and autonomic homeostasis and implementation of active treatment to facilitate the recovery process), it is still currently unclear as to exactly how much rest is required, when to initiate aspects of active recovery, and what is the optimal course of progressive challenge throughout active recovery. Given this uncertainty, most researchers and clinicians recommend encouraging rest for 1 to 2 days or until symptoms have stabilized, followed by a gradual increase in one's normal activities as tolerated.

With a number of active studies underway to advance the scientific support for differing clinical management practices, guidelines around how to prescribe rest versus activities after SRC are likely to continue to evolve. Individual factors may influence the optimal timing and dose of active rehabilitation, such as injury-related characteristics (e.g., severity), preexisting conditions, etc. An understanding of what exactly is therapeutic versus injurious is vital and initial attempts to identify therapeutic thresholds for athletes who can benefit from re-engaging in activity as part of the recovery process without detrimental exacerbation of symptoms are described in the following. Additionally, other empirically supported treatment methods for persistent symptoms are discussed.

4.3 Evaluation of PPCS

Although specific phenotypes or "subtypes" of PPCS are yet to be established, there are multiple means of evaluation that allow for identification and differentiation of primary and secondary symptoms.[11] For example, evaluating exercise tolerance (described in section 4.3.1) may help differentiate dizziness as a product of autonomic dysfunction and changes in cerebral blood flow (CBF).[2] Specifically, a lack of exacerbation of symptoms during exertional activity assessed through monitored subthreshold exercise suggests autonomic dysfunction does not underlie the persistent symptoms and other mechanisms driving symptoms should be considered (e.g., visual/oculomotor).[11] The following sections discuss current methods of evaluating and differentiating mechanisms of persistent symptoms, with the aim of informing treatment and intervention.

4.3.1 Subthreshold Exercise

Studies investigating the effectiveness of subthreshold aerobic exercise (i.e., exercise below the level of intensity that worsens symptoms) have suggested this method holds promise as a diagnostic tool. The implementation of subthreshold exercise is based upon the concept of exercise tolerance, which can be utilized as a means of identifying physiological/ autonomic dysfunction as the underlying mechanism of persistent symptoms.[12] Specifically, decoupling of the cardiovascular system and autonomic centers within the brain results in autonomic dysfunction, including discordance between the sympathetic and parasympathetic nervous system (e.g., decreased heart rate variability, HRV). Lower HRV results in exacerbated CBF in the natural direction, where lower than expected blood flow is observed at rest, and disproportionately higher CBF is observed during physical exertion. Exacerbation of symptoms or other indicators described below during subthreshold exercise suggests PPCS difficulties may be attributed, at least in part, to autonomic dysfunction.

The Buffalo Concussion Treadmill Test (BCTT) is a method that utilizes subthreshold exercise and involves a graded provocative exercise test assessing physiological recovery from concussion.[12] The BCTT assesses an athlete's ability to progress through increasingly demanding exercise leading to personal exhaustion or the maximum age-related HR. Athletes who reach either of these two targets, without significant symptom exacerbation, obvious physical distress, or a significant jump in cardiovascular activity from one stage to the next, are considered to have demonstrated physiological resolution of PCS symptoms. Additionally, by assessing exercise tolerance in those who are slow to recover from concussion, clinicians can differentiate physiological dysfunction from other characteristics of PPCS (e.g., vestibular dysfunction, emotional symptoms, etc.).

4.3.2 Neuropsychological Evaluation

Neuropsychological evaluation plays a vital role in the multidisciplinary evaluation of PPCS. Assessment in this realm can help identify deficits in cognition that persist during prolonged recovery from SRC.[13] Identifying specific domains of cognition that are affected following injury helps to inform practitioner-prescribed accommodations that may be necessary for returning to school. Given that one of the primary objectives of PCS management involves returning athletes to as many of their regular activities as possible without exacerbation of symptoms, detection of specific domains of cognitive dysfunction (e.g., reductions in learning and memory due to impaired processing speed) can inform appropriate academic accommodations (e.g., extra time for tests, assistance with note-taking, etc.), thereby allowing athletes to return to school without being negatively affected by their persisting cognitive symptoms.

Although not indicated for all cases acutely following SRC, comprehensive neuropsychological evaluation provides great benefit in most instances of PCS, especially for those with complex histories (e.g., pre-existing comorbidities, multiple concussions, etc.) or clinical presentations. Neuropsychological evaluation can help differentiate cognitive symptoms associated with PCS from other etiologies. For example, subjective reporting of trouble in concentrating may be associated with post-concussion headaches or psychiatric symptomology (e.g., anxiety), rather than a cognitive profile reflecting true deficits in attention. Additionally, comprehensive neuropsychological evaluation, which includes psychometrically validated measures of cognition and psychological symptomology/personality, can aid in differentiating symptoms among complex cases in which athletes have histories of conditions that often overlap with PCS (e.g., ADHD and inattention, learning disorders of language-based or mathematical abilities, premorbid depression, and postinjury emotional symptoms). Neuropsychological evaluation is at the intersection of neurology and psychiatry and is well-suited to facilitate treatment planning and referrals to appropriate specialties. For athletes never assessed prior to injury, clinical diagnostic interviews by a neuropsychologist or sports psychiatrist can also provide further clarification regarding preinjury diagnoses and emotional symptoms of PCS.

4.3.3 Oculomotor and Vestibular Assessment

Disruption in oculomotor and vestibular systems commonly presents clinically as various symptoms that can overlap across systems (e.g., dizziness, changes in balance, blurred vision). Physically, disruption to the oculomotor system results in several visual changes (i.e., difficulty with vergence eye movements and versional eye movements), while vestibular dysfunction can manifest as postural instability. Dysfunction within these two systems is common following SRC and there is some evidence to suggest that symptoms related to these systems are significant predictors of protracted recovery.[14] Identifying the underlying oculomotor or vestibular dysfunction is essential for informing individualized treatment and rehabilitation of related PPCS symptoms.

Evaluation of oculomotor or vestibular dysfunction is strongly dependent on the particular symptom or physical change being reported. For example, evaluation of athletes presenting with dizziness or balance problems may involve assessments such as the Dix-Hallpike test for benign paroxysmal positional vertigo or assessment of postural instability via the Balance Error Scoring System, Romberg's test, Functional Reach, etc. Signs and symptoms of oculomotor/visual changes can be assessed through various measures assessing saccade and smooth eye pursuits. A screening tool developed to evaluate different aspects of oculomotor and vestibular functioning following SRC has grown in popularity. The Vestibular/Ocular-Motor Screening (VOMS) tool measures symptom provocation across five domains (reevaluating symptoms after each domain), namely, smooth pursuit, horizontal and vertical saccades, convergence, horizontal and vertical vestibulo-ocular reflex (VOR), and visual motion sensitivity; however, several other measures are available.[15]

4.4 Treatment of PCS

4.4.1 Subthreshold Exercise

In addition to its use as a diagnostic tool, subthreshold exercise is also considered a rehabilitative tool for those experiencing prolonged symptoms. As part of the graduated return to play (GRTP) protocol put forth most recently by the Concussion in Sport Group,[9] initiation of low-level activity and aerobic exercise must occur following complete resolution of SRC-related symptoms. However, for those experiencing prolonged symptoms for an extended period of time, this is particularly problematic. As such, subthreshold exercise provides a means by which athletes can re-engage in physical activity in a safe manner that is much less likely to result in symptom exacerbation. By engaging in physical activity at safe and supervised levels, recovery is thought to be facilitated by resultant therapeutic processes, such as the release of brain-derived neurotrophic factor, as well as restoration of CBF and carbon dioxide sensitivity.

4.4.2 Oculomotor, Vestibular, and Cervical Rehabilitation

Interventions including oculomotor, vestibular, and cervical therapy are also paramount in the multidisciplinary approach for PPCS.[16] Providers with specialized training in concussion (e.g., physical therapist, optometrist/ophthalmologist) can implement these interventions in order to address some of the most common persistent symptoms of PPCS including visual and balance dysfunction, as well as headache. For example, vestibular and oculomotor assessment can identify specific mechanisms driving oculomotor dysfunction, such as problems with gaze stability, saccades, accommodative insufficiency, etc. Once a clinical profile has been identified, targeted treatments can address specific sources of dysfunction (e.g., alternating monocular and binocular tasks, visual pursuit/tracking tasks, gradual speeded saccade movements). This approach is similar for vestibular and orthopedic injury (often cervical) assessment and treatments as well. For example, changes in balance can be addressed with interventions such as gaze stability, coordination exercises, and visual motion sensitivity. Other interventions can address other related symptoms, such as cervical spine manual therapy for cervicogenic headache[17] or the Epley maneuver through physical therapy for persisting dizziness and vertigo, which are examples of other targeted treatments for persisting symptoms within this domain.

4.4.3 Pharmacological Management

Pharmacological management of symptoms during the acute and subacute periods of SRC recovery is rarely utilized. However, providers are more likely to prescribe medications in order to manage persisting symptoms that extend beyond typical recovery. A referral to a specialized provider may be necessary, depending on the particular symptoms that persist. A referral to a neurologist for evaluation and pharmacological consideration is appropriate in the context of persisting headache or migraine following SRC. Referrals to other providers may be appropriate based on the complexity of the presenting symptoms and patient history. For example, referral to a sports psychiatrist may be warranted if the persisting psychiatric symptoms are more severe or for an athlete who has a long-standing psychiatric history that was not managed pharmacologically prior to injury. Each provider must work with patients to determine risks and benefits of pharmacological management and practice on a case-by-case basis.

Recent findings indicate that the most commonly prescribed medications for the management of PPCS included amantadine (dopaminergic agent for attentional and other cognitive difficulties), amitriptyline (tricyclic antidepressant with off-label use for headache), and melatonin (for sleep).[18] The same study also found that female sex and higher acute symptom scores post-injury were more likely to result in pharmacological management of PPCS symptoms. As highlighted above, one of the primary aims in the multidisciplinary management of PPCS is to facilitate reengagement into regular day-to-day activities as much as possible. Although pharmacological management of PPCS symptoms may not necessarily completely "cure" the athlete, it can alleviate symptoms in a way that allows for at least partial resumption of normal activities, as well as initiation of other rehabilitative interventions (e.g., subthreshold exercise).

4.4.4 Psychological Interventions

As highlighted earlier, psychiatric difficulties (changes in mood or heightened anxiety) can occur following SRC and continue beyond the typical course of recovery. The underlying etiology of psychiatric symptoms commonly occurring in PPCS may vary by case and can be driven by biochemical mechanisms, adverse reactions to reduced participation in regular activities and decreased socialization, or exacerbation of preinjury psychiatric disorders and symptoms. Psychological interventions for persistent symptoms associated with PPCS can be classified into three primary categories, namely, cognitive behavioral therapy (CBT), education and reassurance, and mindfulness and relaxation.

CBT treatments can be modified in order to target the particular clinical presentation and emotional disruption experienced by the athlete. For example, treatments can focus on cognitive restructuring around athletes' expectations for recovery or irrational perceptions (e.g., catastrophizing) around the implications of their injury (e.g., loss of abilities, grave outcomes, limited chance of recovery). CBT can also aid in attenuating adverse reactions to physical symptoms and disruption of the negative feedback loop by which physical symptoms cause emotional distress, which elevates one's physiological stress response and exacerbates the symptoms. Similarly, variations of CBT, such as CBT for insomnia (CBTi), can target symptoms of insomnia and/or excessive daytime fatigue. Most randomized clinical trials (RCTs) show at least some benefit of CBT in the treatment of persistent symptoms.[19] Further, CBT holds promise as a preventative measure, as decreased prevalence of PPCS was recorded in an at-risk population when was CBT administered soon after injury.[20]

Education and reassurance have also been observed as having some efficacy in alleviating symptoms and aiding in athletes' recoveries. As an intervention, education and reassurance typically include providing information and counseling to the athlete on the typical type and course of symptoms assurance regarding the prognosis, common effective coping techniques, and means of reintegrating back into regular activities. Providing education resources shortly after injury has been shown to reduce the likelihood of developing PPCS as compared to those who did not receive similar resources.[21] Regarding mindfulness and relaxation strategies, there is currently limited evidence for their effectiveness in alleviating symptoms of PPCS due to a lack of RCTs.[19]

4.5 Clinical Pearls

- Development of persistent symptoms following SRC is often associated with complex clinical presentations comprising physical, emotional, and cognitive symptoms.
- Variable evidence exists for the relationship between increased risk of developing PPCS and demographic and injury-related factors, with injury burden (higher symptom score or more symptoms) and preinjury history of a psychiatric diagnosis as the most consistent risk factors for prolonged recovery.
- A primary objective of PPCS management involves resumption of as many regular activities as possible without significant exacerbation of symptoms. Reintegration as soon as possible, even with accommodations, is likely to diminish the negative psychosocial effects of prolonged disruption of regular activities (sport, school, social pursuits).
- Extended, strict physical and cognitive rest beyond the acute phase of recovery is not recommended. Best practice, based on emerging research and multiple consensus guidelines, now indicates that reinitiating activity after 1 to 2 days of rest may facilitate the neurobiological recovery processes.
- Concussion symptoms are nonspecific and can benefit from multidisciplinary evaluation and treatment.
- Development of persistent symptoms following SRC is often associated with complex clinical presentations which often represent an intersection of preinjury (e.g., demographic and diagnostic), injury (e.g., mechanism of injury and presenting symptoms), and postinjury (e.g., method of initial injury management) factors that require a thorough diagnostic evaluation as part of a dynamic differential diagnosis process.

4.6 Conflicts of Interest/Financial Disclosures

During the conduct of this work, B.L. Brett reports no conflicts of interest to disclose. M.A. McCrea reports grants from the Department of Defense, National Collegiate Athletic Association, and National Football League. L.D. Nelson reported grants from the Department of Defense, National Collegiate Athletic Association, National Football League, National Institute of Health, and Advancing a Healthier Wisconsin. He previously served as consultant to Neurotrauma Sciences, Inc. and is clinical consultant to the Green Bay Packers professional football club. He also reports honoria and travel support for professional speaking engagements.

References

[1] McCrea M, Guskiewicz K, Randolph C, et al. Incidence, clinical course, and predictors of prolonged recovery time following sport-related concussion in high school and college athletes. J Int Neuropsychol Soc. 2013; 19(1):22–33

[2] Pertab JL, Merkley TL, Cramond AJ, Cramond K, Paxton H, Wu T. Concussion and the autonomic nervous system: an introduction to the field and the results of a systematic review. NeuroRehabilitation. 2018; 42(4):397–427

[3] Iverson GL, Gardner AJ, Terry DP, et al. Predictors of clinical recovery from concussion: a systematic review. Br J Sports Med. 2017; 51(12):941–948

[4] Iverson GL, Silverberg ND, Mannix R, et al. Factors associated with concussion-like symptom reporting in high school athletes. JAMA Pediatr. 2015; 169(12):1132–1140

[5] Association AP. Diagnostic and Statistical Manual of Mental Disorders. 4th ed. Washington, DC: American Psychiatric Association; 1994

[6] ICD-10 T. The ICD-10 Classification of Mental and Behavioural Disorders—Clinical Descriptions and Diagnostic Guidelines. 1992. Accessed November 2, 2018 at: https://cdn.who.int/media/docs/default-source/classification/other-classifications/9241544228_eng.pdf?sfvrsn=933a13d3_1&download=true

[7] Nelson LD, Kramer MD, Patrick CJ, McCrea MA. Modeling the structure of acute sport-related concussion symptoms: a bifactor approach. J Int Neuropsychol Soc. 2018; 24(8):793–804

[8] Schneider KJ, Leddy JJ, Guskiewicz KM, et al. Rest and treatment/rehabilitation following sport-related concussion: a systematic review. Br J Sports Med. 2017; 51(12):930–934

[9] McCrory P, Meeuwisse W, Dvořák J, et al. Consensus statement on concussion in sport—the 5th international conference on concussion in sport held in Berlin, October 2016. Br J Sports Med. 2017; 51(11):838–847

[10] Thomas DG, Apps JN, Hoffmann RG, McCrea M, Hammeke T. Benefits of strict rest after acute concussion: a randomized controlled trial. Pediatrics. 2015; 135(2):213–223

[11] Ellis MJ, Leddy JJ, Willer B. Physiological, vestibulo-ocular and cervicogenic post-concussion disorders: an evidence-based classification system with directions for treatment. Brain Inj. 2015; 29(2):238–248

[12] Leddy JJ, Willer B. Use of graded exercise testing in concussion and return-to-activity management. Curr Sports Med Rep. 2013; 12(6):370–376

[13] Williams WH, Potter S, Ryland H. Mild traumatic brain injury and postconcussion syndrome: a neuropsychological perspective. J Neurol Neurosurg Psychiatry. 2010; 81(10):1116–1122

[14] Lau BC, Kontos AP, Collins MW, Mucha A, Lovell MR. Which on-field signs/symptoms predict protracted recovery from sport-related concussion among high school football players? Am J Sports Med. 2011; 39(11):2311–2318

[15] Kontos AP, Deitrick JM, Collins MW, Mucha A. Review of vestibular and oculomotor screening and concussion rehabilitation. J Athl Train. 2017; 52 (3):256–261

[16] Broglio SP, Collins MW, Williams RM, Mucha A, Kontos AP. Current and emerging rehabilitation for concussion: a review of the evidence. Clin Sports Med. 2015; 34(2):213–231

[17] Jull G, Trott P, Potter H, et al. A randomized controlled trial of exercise and manipulative therapy for cervicogenic headache. Spine. 2002; 27(17): 1835–1843, discussion 1843

[18] Pinto SM, Twichell MF, Henry LC. Predictors of pharmacological intervention in adolescents with protracted symptoms after sports-related concussion. PM R. 2017; 9(9):847–855

[19] Al Sayegh A, Sandford D, Carson AJ. Psychological approaches to treatment of postconcussion syndrome: a systematic review. J Neurol Neurosurg Psychiatry. 2010; 81(10):1128–1134

[20] Silverberg ND, Lange RT, Millis SR, et al. Post-concussion symptom reporting after multiple mild traumatic brain injuries. J Neurotrauma. 2013; 30(16): 1398–1404

[21] Ponsford J, Willmott C, Rothwell A, et al. Impact of early intervention on outcome after mild traumatic brain injury in children. Pediatrics. 2001; 108 (6):1297–1303

5 Congenital Cranial Anomalies and Implications for Athletics

Adam Ammar, Andrew M. Hersh, and Alan R. Cohen

Summary
Congenital cranial anomalies in children and adolescents can have implications for athletic participation. Given the benefits of sports participation for the physical, social, and emotional development of children, it is important to understand the specific considerations for various cranial anomalies. Some sports are entirely contraindicated due to the high risk of catastrophic injury in certain patients; however, many patients with cranial anomalies are still able to participate in sports to varying degrees. Patients should be counseled on their individual risks associated with sports participation, and in some instances, adjustments may be able to be made to reduce risk. This chapter will detail the considerations for patients with hydrocephalus, craniosynostosis, Chiari malformations, epilepsy, arachnoid cysts, vascular anomalies, and craniotomies.

Keywords: pediatrics, sports, hydrocephalus, craniosynostosis, arachnoid cyst, arteriovenous malformation, moyamoya, craniotomy, Chiari, epilepsy

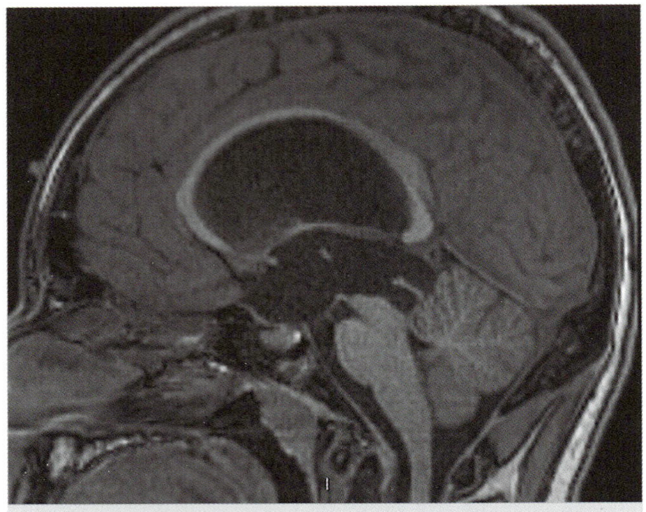

Fig. 5.1 Sagittal magnetic resonance imaging (MRI) of a child with hydrocephalus secondary to stenosis of the cerebral aqueduct of Sylvius.

5.1 Introduction

Pediatric and adolescent athletes are susceptible to acute and traumatic cranial injuries, which can be associated with significant limitations on their neurological function and participation in sports activities. The patterns of injury differ from those seen in adults owing to the unique features of the developing and growing cranial vault, such as a thinner calvarium in young children placing them at increased risk for traumatic brain injury (TBI). In addition, patients with congenital anomalies of the brain are at increased susceptibility to traumatic injuries and warrant additional considerations in evaluating them for participation in sports. Some sports are entirely contraindicated due to the high risk of catastrophic injury in certain patients; however, sports participation is overall beneficial to children's physical and emotional well-being, and their participation in sports should be encouraged when safe.

5.2 Hydrocephalus

Hydrocephalus is the abnormal increase in cerebrospinal fluid (CSF) of the ventricular system that can cause ventricular enlargement, accelerated head growth in infants, and clinical symptoms precipitating surgical intervention. It is a common but complex disease with heterogeneous etiologies that lead to physical or functional obstruction of the normal flow of CSF. The most common cause of acquired hydrocephalus in infants is hemorrhage, most often in premature births; other causes are myelomeningoceles, aqueductal stenosis, tumors, infection, and trauma (▶ Fig. 5.1). The clinical manifestations vary with age, but it often presents in infancy with enlarging head circumference, irritability, lethargy, and vomiting. Older children who can verbalize will often complain of headache before other symptoms.[1] Treatment is via CSF diversion, most commonly through ventricular shunt insertion or endoscopic third ventriculostomy.

There are several reasons why this population is thought to be at a higher risk for neurological sequelae during participation in sports. The main concern is shunt malfunction precipitating worsening of hydrocephalus. In addition, patients with long-standing hydrocephalus sometimes have a thinner cranium and can have a reduced physiological reserve of the central nervous system to respond to injury. CSF acts in part as a shock absorber for the brain, and in shunted patients the change in CSF flow dynamics could have a negative impact on this buffering effect. Nevertheless, reports of shunt-related complications in the literature for patients participating in sports or even SCUBA diving are exceedingly rare.[2,3] In fact, the medical literature suggests that there is no relationship between shunted hydrocephalus and risk of sports-related injuries, with reported sports-related shunt complications corresponding to a rate of less than 1%.[4] In addition, the risk of TBI was also found to be similar for children with and without shunted hydrocephalus.[5]

With this data in mind, there should be few or no restrictions on sports participation in patients with shunted hydrocephalus. If trauma occurs in the area of the shunt, evaluation can be performed to confirm functionality, but concern for complications should not preclude participation given the rarity of this occurrence. In a survey of 92 pediatric neurosurgeons, 90% did not restrict their patients' participation in noncontact sports, and one-third did not restrict participation in contact sports for children with CSF shunts.[6] In a survey of clinicians in the

United Kingdom, the following percentages advocated for participation in football, rugby, Taekwondo, and skiing to their patients: 96, 75, 77, and 97%, respectively.[7]

5.3 Craniosynostosis

Craniosynostosis is the premature fusion of one or more of the cranial sutures. The majority are spontaneous isolated defects, but 8% occur as a familial or syndromic form of synostosis.[8] They are classified according to the involved sutures, with sagittal synostosis accounting for the majority (approximately 60%) of cases, followed by coronal (25%) (▶ Fig. 5.2), metopic (15%), and then lambdoid (2%).[9] It is usually diagnosed early in infancy

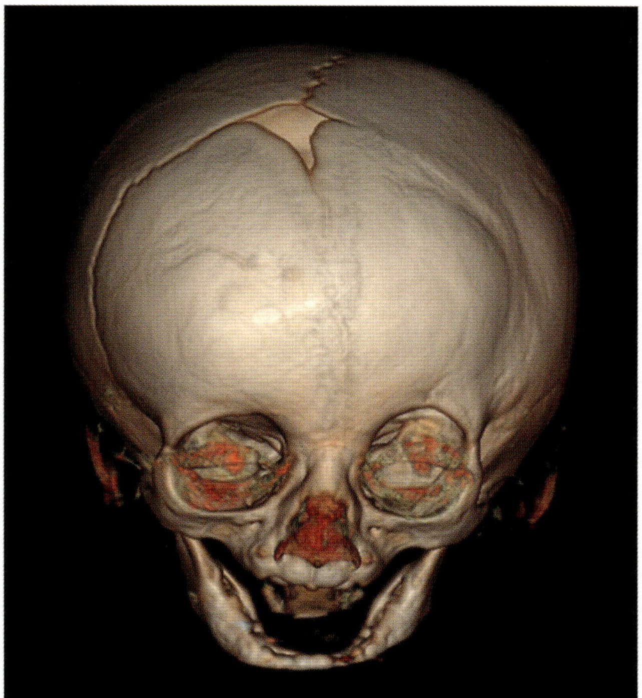

Fig. 5.2 Three-dimensional skull reconstruction demonstrating premature fusion of the coronal suture resulting in coronal craniosynostosis.

with parents noticing abnormal head shapes, and is treated with surgery, usually within the first year of life but some patients can have surgery as young children.

The main concern for sports participation is that the treatment of craniosynostosis sometimes results in a temporary cranial defect. Since most patients receive treatment in infancy, the cranial defect is often healed well before they participate in sports, limiting their risk. A study of 396 patients found the incidence of TBI in these patients was 0.[10] In a survey of children with craniosynostosis, a vast majority (88%) participated in sports, and although parental anxiety increased as the contact sustained during play increased, many children participated in heavy contact and combat sports with little evidence of harm.[11] In another nationwide survey of postsurgical craniosynostosis patients, sports participation was found to be exceedingly common, with contact sports being the most common sports category, and few head injuries reported (mostly concussions).[12] Given these findings, it is reasonable for children who have undergone craniosynostosis correction to participate in sports, including contact sports, once the cranial defect has filled.

5.4 Chiari Malformations

Chiari malformations encompass several distinct anatomical alterations of the posterior fossa. The most common malformation is the Chiari I, which features herniation of the cerebellar tonsils into the cervical spinal canal and is frequently accompanied by syringomyelia (▶ Fig. 5.3).[13,14] Chiari II malformations represent a more severe phenotype featuring herniation of the cerebellar vermis and brainstem through the foramen magnum, and are essentially always associated with myelomeningocele.[15] Chiari III and IV malformations are extremely rare and represent herniation of the posterior fossa along with an occipital encephalocele or severe cerebellar hypoplasia, respectively.[16,17]

Herniation of the tonsils ≥ 5 cm below the foramen magnum is typically considered diagnostic of a Chiari I malformation. Cerebellar herniation compresses neurological tissue and produces the classic symptoms of Chiari malformations, which are often nonspecific and include occipital headaches, neck pain, weakness, hyperreflexia, and ataxia. In some cases, syringomyelia results from obstruction of CSF causing myelopathy. Other symptoms arise from compression of cranial nerves coursing through the posterior fossa and include dysarthria and hearing loss.[18,19]

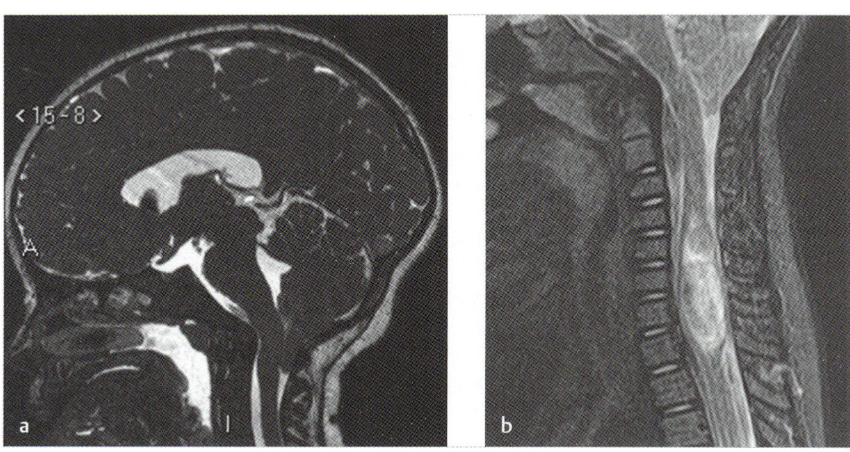

Fig. 5.3 **(a)** Sagittal magnetic resonance imaging (MRI) illustrating herniation of the cerebellar tonsils which is characteristic of a Chiari malformation. **(b)** Sagittal MRI in a patient with a Chiari malformation demonstrating a cervicothoracic syrinx.

However, although the radiographic findings of a Chiari I malformation are present in an estimated 1 to 3% of children, many patients will remain asymptomatic their entire lives.[20,21] Some athletes with a Chiari malformation are only identified after magnetic resonance imaging (MRI) is obtained following a concussion or other head injury.[22]

Uniform guidelines on sports participation in patients with an identified Chiari malformation are lacking. Several case reports describe injuries in athletes with Chiari I malformations, including sudden death following head or neck injury; however, the causality between the malformation and the severity of injury cannot be established from these limited reports, particularly given the high prevalence of Chiari malformations.[23] Concern has been raised that patients who incur a concussion may have worsening or recurrence of symptoms from their Chiari malformations.[22] Nonetheless, several studies involving hundreds of patients with Chiari I malformations have not identified an increased incidence of serious or permanent neurological deficits from sports participation.[24,25] Consequently, there seems to be little risk to full participation in sports in patients with Chiari I malformations, particularly asymptomatic patients without syringomyelia. Those who suffer a concussion but remain asymptomatic from the Chiari malformation can expect to return to sports following the proper conservative management of their injury.

Decision-making is more complicated for symptomatic patients and those with syringomyelia. Those who have undergone decompression with resolution of symptoms should be treated like asymptomatic patients; however, patients sometimes experience symptomatic recurrence after surgery and therefore warrant close follow-up and evaluation to determine safety during participation in sports. Decision-making should consider the symptoms experienced by the patient—certain "red-flag" symptoms, such as ataxia or myelopathy, should be considered contraindications for sports participation, in addition to the presence of a syrinx.[3,22] Shared decision-making with athletes on a case-by-case basis is critical with evaluation of radiographic findings, signs and symptoms, and nature of the sport.[24]

5.5 Epilepsy

Epilepsy, classically defined as two unprovoked seizures occurring > 24 hours apart, one unprovoked seizure with a high probability of recurrence, or diagnosis of an epilepsy syndrome, has a prevalence of approximately 1 to 2% worldwide.[26,27] The diagnosis of epilepsy reflects a predisposition toward recurrent unprovoked seizures, often genetic and/or syndromic in origin, indicating a structural epileptogenic lesion. Most epilepsy patients are treated medically; however, many patients suffer from drug-resistant epilepsy, and those with identifiable epileptogenic zones may be candidates for surgical resection.[28]

Severe head trauma can produce both focal and diffuse deficits in neurological tissue which may result in seizures, a phenomenon known as post-traumatic epilepsy.[29] Consequently, concern has been raised that head trauma or collisions during contact sports could exacerbate the severity of symptoms in patients with epilepsy, and historically patients with drug-resistant epilepsy were counseled to avoid even noncontact sports.[30] However, this concern does not hold true for most sports-related collisions or traumatic injuries, which are typically mild and do not affect epilepsy or induce seizures.[3,31] Indeed, physical activity and exercise have been associated with several positive effects on patients with epilepsy, including improved seizure control, mood, and overall health.[30] Studies of patients with epilepsy participating in contact sports have not identified an increased seizure frequency or risk of injury.[32] For several decades, official recommendations from the American Academy of Pediatrics have noted that epilepsy should not be a contraindication to participation in most sports. Recent guidelines from the International League Against Epilepsy encourage physical activity in most patients with epilepsy, excluding those who suffer from exercise-induced epilepsy.[33]

In addition to the concern for trauma worsening epilepsy, there is also consideration of injury from an unprovoked seizure during physical activity. Generalized tonic-clonic seizures impair consciousness and can cause injury from a sudden fall, while partial seizures can cause loss of control of body movements. Most patients with epilepsy can safely participate in most athletic activities, but patients should be counseled on risks from a seizure during an athletic event and advised to take measures to improve safety such as wearing helmets in collision sports.[30] Some exceptions that warrant closer consideration include activities involving heights, such as gymnastics, horseback riding, or rock climbing, where a seizure-induced fall can seriously injure the patient, and SCUBA diving or free climbing, where loss of consciousness can be fatal.[3,30] Guidelines from the International League Against Epilepsy which classify sports into three categories based on the degree of risk in patients with seizures are useful when counseling patients.[34]

5.6 Arachnoid Cysts

Arachnoid cysts are benign congenital cystic lesions of arachnoid membranes filled with CSF (► Fig. 5.4). They occur in approximately 1% of the general population, and are most often asymptomatic and diagnosed incidentally.[35] Although they are benign developmental anomalies, and asymptomatic patients are typically allowed to participate in sports, arachnoid cysts have been associated with multiple complications in the setting of trauma, including subdural and intracystic hemorrhage.[3] Several retrospective case series have reported on patients with arachnoid cysts presenting with symptoms following a traumatic event, most often due to the development of a subdural hygroma. Most of those reported post-traumatic hygromas, however, result from motor vehicle accidents, falls, or other trauma rather than sports injuries.[36] Rupture of an arachnoid cyst into the subdural space can sometimes lead to dangerous elevation of intracranial pressure. Larger size of the arachnoid cyst and head trauma have been identified as risk factors for symptomatic cyst rupture and hemorrhage. The higher rate of structural brain injury after trauma in patients with arachnoid cysts is postulated to be due to the presence of small bridging vessels between the dura and cyst membrane and the lower compliance of the arachnoid cyst compared to normal brain tissue, resulting in reduced cushioning following trauma.[35,37]

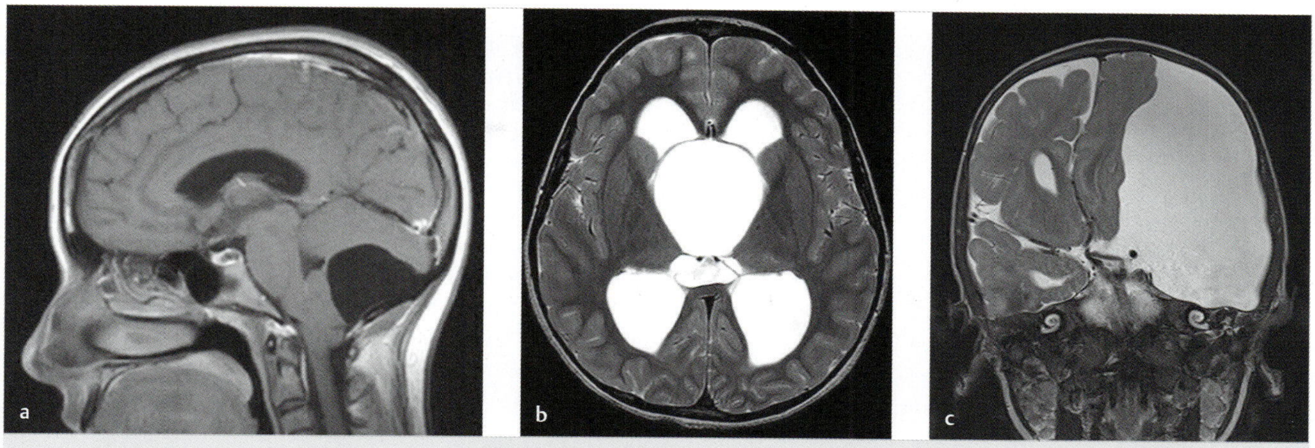

Fig. 5.4 (a) T1-weighted sagittal magnetic resonance imaging (MRI) illustrating a hypointense posterior fossa arachnoid cyst. (b) T2-weighted axial MRI illustrating a hyperintense suprasellar arachnoid cyst. (c) T2-weighted coronal MRI illustrating a hyperintense arachnoid cyst occupying the left hemisphere.

Individual opinions regarding sports participation vary widely, with some surgeons considering the presence of even an asymptomatic arachnoid cyst a contraindication to participation in sports, while others are more permissive. Sports organizations are also divided on the issue, with the Amateur Boxing Association of England preventing athletes with known arachnoid cysts from competing.[36] In a survey of 45 neurosurgeons on their management of an asymptomatic middle fossa arachnoid cyst, 22.1% of respondents advised against participation in contact sports.[38] Nonetheless, sports-related neurological injuries in patients with arachnoid cysts are rare, and although they may present an increased risk of injury, they are not an absolute contraindication to participation in contact sports. Patients and their family members, however, should be carefully counseled regarding the risk of a traumatically induced hemorrhage.

5.7 Intracranial Vascular Pathologies

5.7.1 Arteriovenous Malformations

Cerebral arteriovenous malformations (AVMs) are anomalous direct shunts between arteries and veins, creating a vascular parenchymal nidus. They are typically diagnosed during young adulthood with presentations including headache, seizure, and intracranial hemorrhage; however, with the increased frequency of neuroimaging, more incidental AVMs are being diagnosed.[39] The annual rupture rate for unruptured AVMs has been reported anywhere from 1 to 4%. Although ruptured lesions are usually treated, the management of unruptured AVMs remains controversial regarding whether or not to treat and what treatment modality should be adopted.[40]

Determination of return to play in these patients is difficult because there are limited published reports on resumption of contact activities after treatment of a hemorrhagic intracranial AVM, and none for unruptured and untreated AVMs. It is reasonable to wait for AVM obliteration before resumption of sports activities; this can be months in those treated with radiosurgery. Ultimately, any decision should include discussions between the athlete, family, athletic trainers, and physicians.[41]

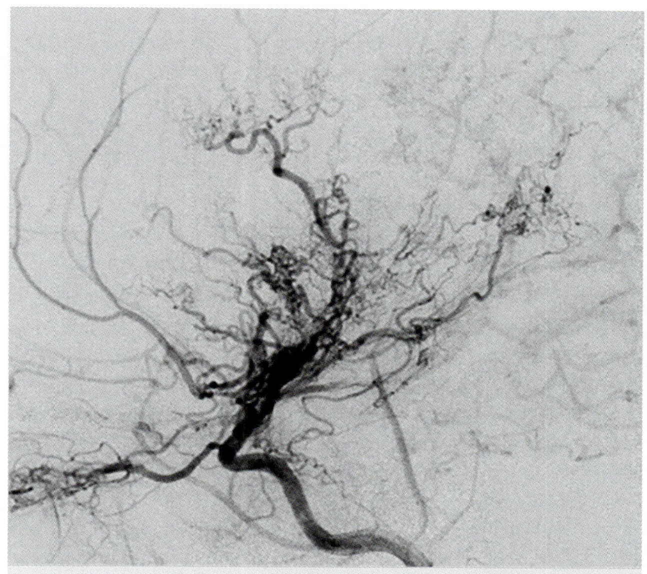

Fig. 5.5 Left common carotid cerebral angiogram in a child with moyamoya arteriopathy. The collateral vasculature appears as a "puff of smoke" on angiography, from which the disease derives its name.

5.7.2 Moyamoya Syndrome and Disease

Moyamoya syndrome is a cerebrovascular condition in which affected patients have progressive stenosis of the intracranial internal carotid arteries and their proximal branches, predisposing patients to strokes. The reduced blood flow leads to compensatory development of collateral vasculature by small vessels distally that look like a "puff of smoke" on angiography from which the syndrome's name is derived (▶ Fig. 5.5). It is called moyamoya disease when occurring in isolation and moyamoya syndrome when occurring secondary to another disease process such as radiotherapy to the head and neck or sickle cell disease. The most common presentations are ischemic stroke, hemorrhage, seizure, and headache.[42] Although there is no data on the safety of sports activities in children with moyamoya, hypovolemia from dehydration is a risk factor for ischemia, and so those who participate in sports activities should be vigilant to stay hydrated.

5.8 Prior Craniotomy

Craniotomies—the removal and replacement of the cranial bone—are performed for a variety of neurosurgical conditions. Fixation is often performed with titanium plates; however, in younger children, plating is also commonly performed using absorbable polymer plates and pins. Risks from sports participation and return to play in patients who have had a craniotomy vary tremendously based on the underlying pathology for which surgery was performed.

In regards to considerations for the bone flap, there are three main concerns for the safety of the skull to withstand impacts in the postoperative period: the strength of the bone flap to withstand direct pressure from blows to the head, the fragility of the brain tissue at the operative site either from the underlying insult or due to the surgical manipulation, and the alteration of the normal mechanics of the CSF to cushion the brain from impact. Healing of the bone flap with radiographic integration to the rest of the cranium usually occurs within 1 year of surgery. No studies exist comparing the effect of different fixation methods on this healing and time frame.[3] With these factors in mind, a conservative approach in regards to return to play after craniotomy has generally been taken in the past. One survey study of return to play practices among neurosurgeons in patients after craniotomy found that although the total number of patients allowed to return to play did not differ between pediatric and adult patients, there was a significant increase in return to play time for pediatric patients. Pediatric patients in the study were returned to play at a median of 6 months to 1 year compared with a median of 3 to 6 months for adults.[43] Before a patient can return to play after any craniotomy, radiographic partial or complete healing of the bone flap should be present along with documented neurologic and neuropsychological recovery. The decision should also depend on which sport the patient will participate in, with a more conservative approach for higher contact sports such as football and boxing. Any decision should be based on the input of a team, including a neurosurgeon, neuroradiologist, neuropsychologist, and/or sports medicine physician.[44]

5.9 Conclusions

Pediatric and adolescent athletes are susceptible to acute and traumatic cranial injuries, the patterns of which differ from those seen in adults. In addition, patients with congenital anomalies of the brain can be at increased risk of injury and warrant additional considerations in evaluating them for participation in sports. Some sports are entirely contraindicated due to the high risk of catastrophic injury in certain patients; however, sports participation is overall beneficial to children's physical, mental, and emotional well-being, and should be encouraged when safe. Decision-making on sports participation should consider the underlying disease pathology and its natural history, patient susceptibility to injury, and recovery after treatment. Discussions should include inputs from the patients, their family, and sports coach, as well as their team of providers including the surgeon, neurologist, radiologist, pediatrician, physical therapist, neuropsychologist, and/or sports medicine physician. Patients should be counseled on their individual risks associated with sports participation, and in some instances, adjustments may be able to be made to reduce risk.

5.10 Clinical Pearls

- Athletic activities should be encouraged in children when safe due to the positive impacts on development, health, and psychosocial well-being.
- Consideration of risks should include both how the disease increases risk of traumatic injury as well as how sports participation and athletic activity may worsen symptoms of a disease.
- Craniotomy and bone flap fixation should not be viewed as a contraindication to athletics. Return to play should be a gradual process with return to contact and collision sports occurring when bony fusion has occurred.

References

[1] Kestle JR. Pediatric hydrocephalus: current management. Neurol Clin. 2003; 21(4):883–895, vii

[2] Shastin D, Zaben M, Leach P. Can patients with a CSF shunt SCUBA dive? Acta Neurochir (Wien). 2016; 158(7):1269–1272

[3] Miele VJ, Bailes JE, Martin NA. Participation in contact or collision sports in athletes with epilepsy, genetic risk factors, structural brain lesions, or history of craniotomy. Neurosurg Focus. 2006; 21(4):E9

[4] Stanuszek A, Bębenek A, Milczarek O, Kwiatkowski S. Return to play in children with shunted hydrocephalus. J Neurosurg Pediatr. 2021; 29(1): 1–9

[5] Babl FE, Lyttle MD, Phillips N, et al. MBiostat. Mild traumatic brain injury in children with ventricular shunts: a PREDICT study. J Neurosurg Pediatr. 2020; 27(2):196–202

[6] Blount JP, Severson M, Atkins V, et al. Sports and pediatric cerebrospinal fluid shunts: who can play? Neurosurgery. 2004; 54(5):1190–1196, discussion 1196–1198

[7] Zaben M, Manivannan S, Petralia C, Bhatti I, Patel C, Leach P. Patient advice regarding participation in sport in children with disorders of cerebrospinal fluid (CSF) circulation: a national survey of British paediatric neurosurgeons. Childs Nerv Syst. 2020; 36(11):2783–2787

[8] Governale LS. Craniosynostosis. Pediatr Neurol. 2015; 53(5):394–401

[9] Kajdic N, Spazzapan P, Velnar T. Craniosynostosis—recognition, clinical characteristics, and treatment. Bosn J Basic Med Sci. 2018; 18(2):110–116

[10] Gilardino MS, Jandali S, Whitaker LA, Bartlett SP. Does the incidence of traumatic brain injury in children increase after craniofrontal surgery? J Craniofac Surg. 2011; 22(4):1284–1286

[11] Rotimi O, Jung GP, Ong J, Jeelani NUO, Dunaway DJ, James G. Sporting activity after craniosynostosis surgery in children: a source of parental anxiety. Childs Nerv Syst. 2021; 37(1):287–290

[12] Yengo-Kahn AM, Akinnusotu O, Wiseman AL, et al. Sport participation and related head injuries following craniosynostosis correction: a survey study. Neurosurg Focus. 2021; 50(4):E15

[13] Hersh DS, Groves ML, Boop FA. Management of Chiari malformations: opinions from different centers—a review. Childs Nerv Syst. 2019; 35(10): 1869–1873

[14] Zhao JL, Li MH, Wang CL, Meng W. A systematic review of Chiari I malformation: techniques and outcomes. World Neurosurg. 2016; 88:7–14

[15] Stevenson KL. Chiari type II malformation: past, present, and future. Neurosurg Focus. 2004; 16(2):E5

[16] Andica C, Soetikno RD. Chiari malformation type III: case report and review of the literature. Radiol Case Rep. 2015; 8(3):831

[17] Tubbs RS, Demerdash A, Vahedi P, Griessenauer CJ, Oakes WJ. Chiari IV malformation: correcting an over one century long historical error. Childs Nerv Syst. 2016; 32(7):1175–1179

[18] Hersh AM, Jallo G, Shimony N. Management of Chiari malformation. In: Shimony N, Jallo G, eds. Pediatric Neurosurgery Board Review. Springer, Cham; 2023:95–113

[19] Steinbok P. Clinical features of Chiari I malformations. Childs Nerv Syst. 2004; 20(5):329–331

[20] Aitken LA, Lindan CE, Sidney S, et al. Chiari type I malformation in a pediatric population. Pediatr Neurol. 2009; 40(6):449–454

[21] Leonard JR, Limbrick DD, Jr. Chiari I malformation: adult and pediatric considerations. Neurosurg Clin N Am. 2015; 26(4):xiii–xiv

[22] Turk ML, Schmidt K, McGrath ML. Diagnosis, management, and return to sport of a 16-year-old patient with a Chiari I malformation: a case report and literature review. J Athl Train. 2022; 57(2):177–183

[23] Spencer R, Leach P. Asymptomatic Chiari type I malformation: should patients be advised against participation in contact sports? Br J Neurosurg. 2017; 31(4):415–421

[24] Meehan WP, III, Jordaan M, Prabhu SP, Carew L, Mannix RC, Proctor MR. Risk of athletes with Chiari malformations suffering catastrophic injuries during sports participation is low. Clin J Sport Med. 2015; 25(2):133–137

[25] Strahle J, Geh N, Selzer BJ, et al. Sports participation with Chiari I malformation. J Neurosurg Pediatr. 2016; 17(4):403–409

[26] Falco-Walter J. Epilepsy—definition, classification, pathophysiology, and epidemiology. Semin Neurol. 2020; 40(6):617–623

[27] Fisher RS, Acevedo C, Arzimanoglou A, et al. ILAE official report: a practical clinical definition of epilepsy. Epilepsia. 2014; 55(4):475–482

[28] Thijs RD, Surges R, O'Brien TJ, Sander JW. Epilepsy in adults. Lancet. 2019; 393(10172):689–701

[29] Pitkänen A, Kyyriäinen J, Andrade P, Pasanen L, Ndode-Ekane XE. Epilepsy after traumatic brain injury. In: Pitkänen A, Buckmaster PS, Galanopoulou AS, Moshe SL, eds. Models of Seizures and Epilepsy. 2nd ed. Academic Press, Elsevier Inc.; 2017:661–681

[30] Sahoo SK, Fountain NB. Epilepsy in football players and other land-based contact or collision sport athletes: when can they participate, and is there an increased risk? Curr Sports Med Rep. 2004; 3(5):284–288

[31] Howard GM, Radloff M, Sevier TL. Epilepsy and sports participation. Curr Sports Med Rep. 2004; 3(1):15–19

[32] Alexander HB, Wright CJ, Taplinger DH, Fountain NB. Incidence of seizure exacerbation and injury related to football participation in people with epilepsy. Epilepsy Behav. 2020; 104 Pt A:106888

[33] van den Bogard F, Hamer HM, Sassen R, Reinsberger C. Sport and physical activity in epilepsy. Dtsch Arztebl Int. 2020; 117(1–2):1–6

[34] Capovilla G, Kaufman KR, Perucca E, Moshé SL, Arida RM. Epilepsy, seizures, physical exercise, and sports: a report from the ILAE Task Force on Sports and Epilepsy. Epilepsia. 2016; 57(1):6–12

[35] Zuckerman SL, Prather CT, Yengo-Kahn AM, Solomon GS, Sills AK, Bonfield CM. Sport-related structural brain injury associated with arachnoid cysts: a systematic review and quantitative analysis. Neurosurg Focus. 2016; 40(4):E9

[36] Strahle J, Selzer BJ, Geh N, et al. Sports participation with arachnoid cysts. J Neurosurg Pediatr. 2016; 17(4):410–417

[37] Wu X, Li G, Zhao J, Zhu X, Zhang Y, Hou K. Arachnoid cyst-associated chronic subdural hematoma: report of 14 cases and a systematic literature review. World Neurosurg. 2018; 109:e118–e130

[38] Tamburrini G, Dal Fabbro M, Di Rocco C. Sylvian fissure arachnoid cysts: a survey on their diagnostic workout and practical management. Childs Nerv Syst. 2008; 24(5):593–604

[39] Feghali J, Huang J. Updates in arteriovenous malformation management: the post-ARUBA era. Stroke Vasc Neurol. 2019; 5(1):34–39

[40] Mohr JP, Parides MK, Stapf C, et al. international ARUBA investigators. Medical management with or without interventional therapy for unruptured brain arteriovenous malformations (ARUBA): a multicentre, non-blinded, randomised trial. Lancet. 2014; 383(9917):614–621

[41] Smith MS, Friedman WA, Smith KB, Pass AN, Sr, Clugston JR. Intracranial arteriovenous malformation in a college football player and return-to-play considerations. Clin J Sport Med. 2014; 24(6):e62–e64

[42] Scott RM, Smith ER. Moyamoya disease and moyamoya syndrome. N Engl J Med. 2009; 360(12):1226–1237

[43] Saigal R, Batjer HH, Ellenbogen RG, Berger MS. Return to play for neurosurgical patients. World Neurosurg. 2014; 82(3–4):485–491

[44] Laker SR. Return-to-play decisions. Phys Med Rehabil Clin N Am. 2011; 22 (4):619–634, viii

6 Considerations for the Child with Sports-Related Head Injury

Gerard A. Gioia

Summary

This chapter addresses the key considerations for a child with sports-related head injury. Although the general model of evaluation and treatment is like that of adults, working with youth requires the clinician to frame the findings in a developmentally appropriate manner. Differences in language and cognitive capabilities including the youth's ability to describe their symptoms must be considered, using validated clinical tools for youth and likely recruiting parents as complementary informants. Symptom scales built specifically for youth have demonstrated the most effective ability to discriminate sports-related concussion (SRC) from uninjured. Systematic reviews conducted by the Concussion in Sport Group (CISG) and Centers for Disease Control and Prevention (CDC) have not found substantial support for the current cognitive and balance measures to distinguish injured from uninjured youth with the exception of early post-injury for adolescents. Recommendations were made for their improvement. The SCAT6 and SCOATT6 are new batteries emanating from the 6th international meeting of the CISG with recommendations for continued research validation. Treatment of concussion in youth follows a similar active rehabilitation model as with adults, with initiation of cognitive/school, physical, and social activity recommended in the first week although the unique contexts of treatment (family, school, peers) must be considered.

Keywords: concussion, child, adolescent, sports, head injury

6.1 Introduction

Evaluation and management of sports-related concussion (SRC) in children and adolescents (hereafter referred to as "youth") present a number of unique issues for the clinician.[1] The primary tasks of the concussion evaluation are to identify the mechanism and characteristics of the injury, define youth's post-concussion signs/symptoms and neurologic function relative to their preinjury status, delineate the impact of the symptoms on their everyday life, and formulate a treatment plan to guide active recovery. Concussion treatment and management should set the scene for the proper conditions to allow effective recovery and resolution of the presenting symptoms. The clinical process does not differ regardless of the age of the patient in that the fundamental domains to assess in youth parallel those of adults, i.e., post-concussion symptoms, neurocognition, balance, and ocular–motor functions.

However, a number of important differences must be taken into account for youth with concussion. The first unique difference is in the site and personnel involved in the evaluation. Unlike collegiate and professional athletes, most youth do not have the advantage of an onsite sports medicine professional to evaluate and diagnose the injury. Most youth sports are manned by nonmedical coaches and parents who have ideally been taught to "recognize and respond" to a suspected injury. In some cases, the parent may be the first person to identify a suspected concussion. Health care sites where the youth athlete might present must be prepared to conduct an appropriate examination with appropriate protocols in place.

The medical examination of the youth must be framed within the context of their developmental status, i.e., differences in physical, cognitive, behavioral, and emotional maturation. Like much of pediatric medicine, the concussion evaluation of the youth is not a simple "adult downsizing" but instead incorporates a developmental approach to understanding the presenting youth. For example, a concussive injury of a 7-year-old who collides with another player on a soccer field can be quite different from that of a 14-year-old skateboarder who strikes his or her head on concrete. Substantial differences exist at these two ages in their cognitive and linguistic capacities, emotional control, capability, and willingness to disclose the injury to adults, as well as academic, social, and familial demands. Younger age youth may have greater limitations identifying and articulating an internal symptom state (e.g., mental fogginess, irritability) relative to an adolescent.[2] This may result in reduced reliability of symptom reporting in younger reporters due to a concrete cognitive style, limited sense of time in which to reference the symptoms, lack of familiarity with symptom terminology, affirmative response style to please an inquiring adult, greater difficulties judging the severity of symptoms, and less developed social–emotional maturity.[3,4]

To address this issue, the use of developmentally appropriate language was incorporated in the Post-Concussion Symptom Inventory (PCSI)[5] for 5 to 12 years old such as, "Does your head hurt?" instead of "Do you have a headache?" and avoiding abstract terms such as "Do you feel mentally foggy?"—a symptom which appears on many symptom scales developed for adults—is important. Items with complex vocabulary that require perception of subtle internal states and that ask about sleep behaviors may also not be appropriate. Younger age youth may have greater difficulty linking events to time, such as "yesterday," "last week," or "before your injury." They are less adept at accurately reporting the precise timing of when an event occurred. Symptom assessment should focus on those more recently experienced by the child and not from a time point too distant from the evaluation date. For the above reasons, it is essential that parents serve as a complementary source of information regarding symptom presentation.[6]

With respect to response options for symptom reporting in youth, the commonly used seven-point graded scaling of symptoms is likely too complex for younger youth, necessitating response options with fewer choices. As such, the PCSI report scales for 5 to 12 years old use a three-point scale, asking whether the symptom is present "not at all," "a little," or "a lot" whereas the Health & Behavior Inventory (HBI)[7] uses a four-point response scaling. The PCSI symptom scales for 13- to 18-year-old youth and parents use a more traditional seven-point dimensional scale. The parent report form is framed from the observers' perspective (e.g., "Complains of headache" instead of "Headache") and includes four observable signs: appears dazed or stunned, becomes confused with directions or tasks, appears to move in a clumsy manner, and answers questions more slowly than usual.

In addition to the measures themselves, other factors should be taken into account in the concussion evaluation of youth. The postinjury demands of school or social situations may also vary significantly, requiring different recovery management strategies for the two age groups. These developmental dynamics and environmental demands are central to the evaluation and management of concussion in youth. The clinical diagnosis of concussion and its recovery must be understood within the context of the youth's injury history and preinjury developmental, medical, psychiatric, and family history where premorbid issues such as headaches, attentional issues, or anxiety must be factored into the current diagnostic consideration. Using clinical assessment tools with appropriate evidence substantially improves the clinician's ability to detect and quantify the presence versus absence of concussion effects. Parents of the youth are important partners in both the evaluation/diagnosis phase and the treatment phase. Use of parent- or school-reported[8] measures of concussion symptoms are often employed as central assessment tools, especially in elementary-age youth.

Over the past 15 years, relatively greater attention has been paid to the unique issues and needs of youth with concussion. Most recently, specific considerations for youth have been discussed in the Concussion in Sport Group 2022 Amsterdam meeting[9] and in the Centers for Disease Control and Prevention's (CDC) 2018 Pediatric Mild TBI Guidelines.[10] These systematic reviews provide the latest evidence-based recommendations for sports-related and general pediatric concussion care, respectively, including the available tools for evaluation and treatment. In keeping with standards for evidence-based medical practice,[11,12] three youth symptom measures have an evidence base to assist interpretation: Health and Behavior Inventory (HBI), Acute Concussion Evaluation (ACE), and the Post-Concussion Symptom Inventory (PCSI).

The Health and Behavior Inventory (HBI)[6] was developed as a 20-item concussion symptom scale for children 8 to 15 years of age seen in the emergency department. The measure is composed of three clinical scales—physical, cognitive, and sleep symptoms—with both self-report and parent report forms. It does not include emotional symptoms as these items do not discriminate concussions from the uninjured in the emergency department. The original version of the HBI includes a preinjury symptom rating and a postinjury rating to determine change from baseline. The HBI is incorporated within the Child SCAT tool described later. The HBI has published appropriate evidence of reliability and validity of its symptom scales with reliable change metrics to allow an empirical tracking of symptom change over time, a critical feature for the clinician. The HBI is included in the NINDS Pediatric TBI Common Data Elements.[13]

In 2003, the CDC identified a need to develop an evidence-based toolset for early and ongoing evaluation of symptoms in youth 5 to 18 years of age. This effort resulted in the development of the Acute Concussion Evaluation (ACE)[14] and the Post-Concussion Symptom Inventory[5,15] for the full youth age range. The ACE was developed to provide pediatric health care providers with a more systematic method to evaluate and diagnose concussion early post-injury as none existed at the time. The ACE tool was initially published in the CDC's 2007 "Heads Up: Brain Injury in Your Practice" www.cdc.gov/headsup) toolkit for health care providers from the emergency room to primary and specialty care. The intended respondent of the ACE was the parent and older child or adolescent. The ACE defines the injury characteristics including the mechanism of injury, presence of loss of consciousness, retrograde/anterograde amnesia, and early signs. It also assesses preinjury medical, developmental, and psychiatric history, which are important factors to take into consideration when rendering a diagnosis. The tool was developed to guide the health care provider with a systematic protocol for assessing these key elements of concussion and to guide the diagnosis. The ACE symptom scale consists of 21 symptoms to which patients respond "Yes/No" depending on whether they are experiencing the symptom "any more than usual." The question framed in this way considers the possibility of similar preinjury symptoms, an important feature to clarify given the nonspecific nature of many post-concussion symptoms. The symptom scale also inquires as to the possibility of "exertion effects" which are defined as the presence of increased symptoms with cognitive or physical demands, a condition frequently reported post-injury. The ACE was intended as a tool to be used together with a concussion-appropriate physical examination in the provider's office to establish the diagnosis. Psychometric evidence for the reliability of its scores and evidence of validity in its interpretation[14] have been established.

The PCSI was developed as a developmentally sensitive follow-up tool to assess the severity and progression of symptoms (not just their presence as in the ACE) over recovery. Three developmentally adapted versions of the PCSI and a companion parent report measure were developed taking the youth's vocabulary and understanding of symptoms into consideration: a 5-item measure for 5 to 7 years of age, 17-item version for 8 to 12 years of age, and 21-item measure for 13- to 18-year-old youth. As previously noted, a valid evaluation of post-concussion symptoms of a child or adolescent report requires developmentally sensitive measures suited to the appropriate cognitive level, reading skill and vocabulary, and capacity to perceive the symptoms accurately.[2] Whereas the HBI was developed for 8 to 15 years of age, the ACE and PCSI span the full age range from 5 to 18 years. Furthermore, it is the only youth measure to assess all four symptom domains commonly described in the concussion literature—physical, cognitive, emotional, and sleep/fatigue symptoms. To guide the individual's recovery, each of these domains should be fully assessed and tracked from early post-injury to recovery to document progress in the range and severity of symptoms, rate of recovery, and impact of symptoms on the child's everyday functioning. This symptom tracking also identifies the key targets for intervention. Because the symptoms of concussion are nonspecific and occur in other medical and developmental conditions, an explicit account of their preinjury presence and severity is deemed necessary to better understand the postinjury effects. Both the PCSI-2[15] and the HBI[7] take these preinjury symptoms directly into account.

6.2 SCAT6/SCOAT6

As part of the periodic systematic review of the literature conducted for the 2022 CISG meeting in Amsterdam,[16] the SCAT6 toolset was developed for health care professionals as a revision of the previous version (SCAT5) for the evaluation of suspected concussions in children, adolescents, and adults.[17] The Child SCAT6,[18] adapted for children 8 to 12 years of age, takes approximately 10 to 15 minutes to administer and is intended to be used ideally within 3 days and up to 7 days following injury. Unlike adolescent and adult athletes who have sports medicine personnel attending practices and games, the child athlete (less than 13 years of age) will likely be examined by a primary care provider or in the emergency department. The Child SCAT6 consists of: (1) brief background medical/developmental/psychiatric history, (2) symptom evaluation (parent, child), (3) cognitive screening including (a) immediate and delayed memory of a 10-item word list, (b) repeating digits backward, and (c) reciting days of the week in reverse order (timed), delayed recall of the word list, and (4) coordination and balance examination with the Balance Error Scoring System (BESS), timed tandem gait, complex tandem gait, and optional dual-task gait. Review of the Child SCAT6 finds the HBI symptom scale and elements of the balance examination to be most reliable although few validation studies have been conducted.[17] In fact, no evidence currently exists for the cognitive and balance tests in differentiating SRC in youth 5 to 12 years of age. Adolescents are administered the "adolescent/adult" version of the SCAT6 which includes: (1) documenting observable signs, (2) Glasgow Coma Scale, (3) cervical spine assessment, (3) finger to nose coordination examination, (4) Maddocks questions, (5) a similar cognitive battery as the Child SCAT6, and (6) the 22-item Post-Concussion Symptom Scale (PCSS).[19] The SCAT6 for 13- to 18-year-olds demonstrates relatively better evidence of reliability and validity in its use in the first 3 to 7 days post-injury,[17] although recommendations have been made to improve the cognitive and balance examinations. Further detail and the test protocol have been described by Echemendia et al.[17]

Given the limited demonstrated validity of the SCAT6 tools beyond 3 to 7 days, the CISG in Amsterdam developed a multimodal post-acute tool to be administered after 7 days post-injury to assess and track recovery, namely, the Sport Concussion Office Assessment Tool 6 (SCOAT6).[20] The Child SCOAT6 is designed for 8 to 12 years of age while the SCOAT6 applies to ages 13 and older. The child and adolescent/adult versions of the SCOAT6 were developed with the recognition that these tools require further evaluation to establish their valid clinical utility across the recovery continuum. The multiple dimensions include the following domains: (1) symptom scales (HBI with 11 additional items from the Melbourne Pediatric Symptom Scale[21]); (2) the PACE-Self-Efficacy Scale to assess patient's confidence in the recovery process; (3) a cognitive battery including a memory of a 10-item word list, digits backward, days in reverse order (errors, time to completion), and processing speed with the Symbol Digit Modalities test; (4) orthostatic tests including blood pressure, heart rate, and associated symptom assessment with positional changes; (5) cervical spine examination; (6) neurological examination; (7) balance assessments including the modified BESS, tandem gait/complex tandem gait (backward, forward—eyes open, eyes closed), dual task tandem gait (serial 3's/7's, months or days backward); (8) visio-vestibular examination (smooth pursuits, fast saccades [horizontal/vertical], gaze stability [vestibular–ocular reflex] [vertical/horizontal], near point convergence, left/right monocular accommodation); and (9) a set of mental health measures including anxiety, depression, sleep disturbance, and fear avoidance after TBI. Recovery guidance is provided including a graduated return to school strategy and a return to sport strategy. Not all of these measures are administered to each patient at each visit but are available when clinically indicated.

6.3 Treatment and Management of Concussion in Youth

A critical component of concussion management is the provision of targeted treatments to assist recovery. Treatment and management of concussion has evolved substantially over the past 10 years from a passive "rest" model to an active rehabilitation model that is now the basis of a positive recovery.[22,23] Since 2012, the international CISG consensus statements[24] have explicitly called for an active model of concussion rehabilitation. Early on, Leddy et al[25] and Gagnon et al[26] reported positive findings with postinjury physical activity in patients with persisting symptoms for more than 4 weeks post-injury. These findings resulted in a paradigm shift suggesting that subsymptom threshold levels of physical activity may promote concussion recovery. A consensus meeting in Pittsburgh[22] focused on targeted treatment outlined key points in support of an active rehabilitation model for concussion. Within the pediatric realm, the CDC treatment guidelines for pediatric mild traumatic brain injury[10] further reinforced the active, individualized, symptom-limited gradual reintroduction of activity during recovery. The active rehabilitation model of concussion applies directly to youth of all ages although parents and teachers play an important role in assisting them with these recovery-enhancing activities.

To set the scene for recovery, the clinician should guide the youth with concussion to focus on essential lifestyle factors. Appropriate sleep hygiene is an essential foundation for a proper recovery program. Youth should be encouraged to get adequate sleep at night, aiming for 9 hours per night with no late nights or overnights. Bedtime on weekdays and weekends should be within 1 to 2 hours. All electronics should be turned off 1 hour before bedtime. Daytime naps should be brief (45 minutes at most) if they feel very tired or fatigued, but parents should ensure they do not interfere with falling asleep at night. Next, recovering youth should eat three meals per day to provide the necessary fuel for recovery. Hydration is also critical and should be approximately equal to one's body weight in ounces, not exceeding 100 ounces per day. Daily exercise is not found to be detrimental and is strongly recommended[23] toward the end of the first week, starting slow and building up as symptoms are tolerated. Finally, managing one's stress during recovery is also critically important to preserve energy and positive focus.

The development of an individualized, targeted, post-injury management strategy for the youth rests upon a thorough assessment of their symptom-related status in the context of their history, using the tools recommended above. The management plan is uniquely individualized to the youth's presentation. In planning an individualized management strategy, one must take the developmental level of the youth athlete into account as younger versus older youth experience different levels and types of social, cognitive/school, and physical demands. The involvement of the parent and the school personnel becomes essential.

In guiding recovery, the clinician should assess the patient's symptom tolerance for various cognitive, social, and physical activities, and assist the patient in managing the activity type and intensity to minimize significant symptom exacerbation.[1] One must take care not to reinforce underactivity in the recovering athlete despite the presence of symptoms as inactivity can result in adverse consequences such as depressed mood and anxiety as well as social isolation.[27] The treatment strategy is, therefore, to encourage the youth athlete to engage in balanced cognitive, social, and physical activities to the extent they do not significantly worsen the symptoms.

6.4 Return to School

School represents a significant factor to manage in the recovering youth athlete. Returning a student to school within the first 2 to 3 days post-injury was found to be associated with a lower overall symptom burden and was beneficial for recovery.[28] The first paper to empirically examine school-related problems[29] describes the range of academic problems experienced by students following a concussion, including aspects of impaired cognition (attention/concentration, working memory, new learning and memory, speed of information processing, executive functioning) and social–emotional functioning (increased irritability, moodiness, emotional overreaction), necessitating an explicit assessment of how they may impact academic learning and performance.[8]

Planning for the youth's return to school is a significant aspect of concussion management, requiring the attention of the clinician.[30] There is a growing evidence base upon which to guide the return to school process. A systematic review of available evidence, following the 2016 Berlin conference,[31] summarized six recommendations to facilitate an appropriate return to school, namely: (1) employing a school concussion management policy to guide the support process, (2) using a medical letter to the school to facilitate academic supports, (3) ongoing medical re-evaluation with regular communication of student's status with the school and family, (4) the possibility of temporary absence from school after concussion, (5) screening for symptoms that may affect return to school (e.g., vestibular problems) and require symptom-specific academic accommodations, and (6) high-quality research to further guide the return process.

In planning for the return of a symptomatic student to school, one should assess the status of the symptom and identify activities that increase the symptoms (i.e., exertional effects). Guidance should be provided to the student and school regarding the amount of time and degree of intensity the student is able to tolerably engage in their class schedule before symptoms worsen. Strategies can be recommended to reduce these exertional effects such as taking a 10- to 15-minute rest break periodically and allowing the student to re-engage in the school program to a moderate degree while employing symptom management strategies. To support recovery in the student-athlete's return to school, specific accommodations can be tailored to the student's management plan, such as the use of the Symptom Targeted Academic Management Plan (STAMP[29]).

6.5 Returning the Youth Athlete to Sport

The return to play (RTP) process in youth athletes will differ significantly depending on the level of play and the availability of appropriate medical personnel to assess and monitor the athlete's RTP response. While collegiate and professional sports teams and some high schools have sports medicine professionals including athletic trainers and team physicians to guide the RTP process systematically, athletes in youth sports and a certain percentage of high schools do not have these resources. In many cases, the clinician must rely on coaches and parents to oversee the RTP progression. Every state in the US plus the District of Columbia has an active "Return to Play" law that requires written medical clearance by a health care provider trained in the evaluation and management of concussion. These laws apply to all public high school sports, and some states have extended this law to youth sports programs. The recent 2022 CISG meeting reviewed the return to sport literature[32] and found that for adolescents and adults, the time to recovery (14.0 days) and RTP (19.8 days) has lengthened since the last meeting, possibly due to greater surveillance and active management. It is good practice to provide a standard written document stating that the youth athlete has met all criteria for recovery and can return to "risk" activities such as sports, physical education class, and recess. The use of a structured gradual RTP protocol is recommended to guide the parent/coach through the systematic steps, providing written documentation of successful completion at each stage of the process (► Fig. 6.1).

Physical Activity & Gradual Return to Play (RTP) Progression General

Athlete name: ______________________ Completed by: ______________________

Following a concussion, a medically supervised 5 STEP Gradual Return to Play progression must be successfully completed (symptom-free) before final medical clearance to return to competition.

Instructions: The physical activity program following concussion takes place in two parts. Steps 1 and 2 start when the person is still symptomatic with the focus on helping with recovery. Step 3 begins when the athlete has been fully asymptomatic with Step 2 activities. Beginning with Step 3, assess the athlete for any symptoms occurring during the physical activity and over the next 24 hours. In the **RTP Status Box,**circle response (Symptom/No Symptom), record the date, and initials. If no symptoms are reported over the 24 hours, go to the next step. If any symptoms return at any time during steps 3-5, return to the previous step and proceed. If symptoms worsen, seek medical attention. Steps 3-5 must be completed with no symptoms, and FINAL WRITTEN MEDICAL CLEARANCE must be obtained, before return to full competition.

Player can start Step 1 after 48 hours post-injury Date Step 1 started______________

RTP Status

Step 1: Light general conditioning exercises:

- NO CONTACT
- Begin with a sport specific warm-up.
- Do a (15-20 minutes) workout which can include: stationary bicycle, fast-paced walking or light jog, rowing or freestyle swimming.

Step 1 Date:__________
Symptoms No Symptoms
(Circle one)
Initials:

Step 2: General conditioning and sport-specific skill work; Individually:

- NO CONTACT
- Continue with the sport-specific warm-up.
- Slowly increase intensity and duration of workout (20-30 minutes).
- Begin skill work within the workout.
- Begin sport-specific skill work within the workout, but no spins, dives, or jumps.

Step 2 Date:__________
Symptoms No Symptoms
(Circle one)
Initials:

Player must be asymptomatic to begin Step 3. Indicate date player became asymptomatic______________

Step 3: General conditioning, skill work; individually and with a team-mate:

- NO CONTACT
- Continue with general conditioning (up to 60 minutes). Increase intensity and duration. Begin interval training.
- Continue with individual skill work.
- May begin skill work with a partner.
- May start beginner level spins, dives, and jumps.

Step 3 Date:__________
Symptoms No Symptoms
(Circle one)
Initials:

Step 4: General conditioning, skill work and team drills:

- **NO CONTACT:** Do not play live scrimmages.
- Resume regular conditioning and duration of practice.
- Increase interval training and skill work as required.
- Gradually increase skill level of spins, dives, and jumps.
- Review team plays with no contact.

Step 4 Date:__________
Symptoms No Symptoms
(Circle one)
Initials:

Step 5: Full team practice with body contact:

- Join team in a full practice with controlled body contact.
- If a full practice is completed with no symptoms, get Final Medical Clearance form signed. Give to the coach. You are ready to return to competition.

Step 5 Date:__________
Symptoms No Symptoms
(Circle one)
Initials:

Final Medical Clearance Instructions: For final medical clearance, send this completed form to your medical provider at the successful completion of the 5-step program.

Provider: ________ Email: ______________________

Phone: ______________________ Fax: ______________________

Fig. 6.1 Sample medical clearance document for supervised five-step gradual return to play after head injury.

References

[1] Gioia GA. Multimodal evaluation and management of children with concussion: using our heads and available evidence. Brain Inj. 2015; 29(2): 195–206

[2] Fritz GK, Yeung A, Wamboldt MZ, et al. Conceptual and methodologic issues in quantifying perceptual accuracy in childhood asthma. J Pediatr Psychol. 1996; 21(2):153–173

[3] De Los Reyes A, Kazdin AE. Informant discrepancies in the assessment of childhood psychopathology: a critical review, theoretical framework, and recommendations for further study. Psychol Bull. 2005; 131(4):483–509

[4] Varni JW, Limbers CA, Burwinkle TM. How young can children reliably and validly self-report their health-related quality of life?: an analysis of 8,591 children across age subgroups with the PedsQL 4.0 Generic Core Scales. Health Qual Life Outcomes. 2007; 5:1

[5] Sady MD, Vaughan CG, Gioia GA. Psychometric characteristics of the postconcussion symptom inventory in children and adolescents. Arch Clin Neuropsychol. 2014; 29(4):348–363

[6] Varni JW, Limbers CA, Burwinkle TM. Parent proxy-report of their children's health-related quality of life: an analysis of 13,878 parents' reliability and validity across age subgroups using the PedsQL 4.0 Generic Core Scales. Health Qual Life Outcomes. 2007; 5:2

[7] Ayr LK, Yeates KO, Taylor HG, Browne M. Dimensions of postconcussive symptoms in children with mild traumatic brain injuries. J Int Neuropsychol Soc. 2009; 15(1):19–30

[8] Gioia GA, Babikian T, Barney BJ, et al. Identifying school challenges following concussion: psychometric evidence for the Concussion Learning Assessment & School Survey, 3rd Ed. (CLASS-3). J Pediatr Neuropsychol. 2020; 6:203–217

[9] Davis GA, Schneider KJ, Anderson V, et al. Pediatric sport-related concussion: recommendations from the Amsterdam Consensus Statement 2023. Pediatrics 2023.

[10] Lumba-Brown A, Yeates KO, Sarmiento K, et al. Centers for Disease Control and Prevention guideline on the diagnosis and management of mild traumatic brain injury among children. JAMA Pediatr. 2018; 172(11): e182853

[11] Chelune GJ. Evidence-based research and practice in clinical neuropsychology. Clin Neuropsychol. 2010; 24(3):454–467

[12] Iverson GL. Evidence-based neuropsychological assessment in sport-related concussion. In: Webbe F, ed. The Handbook of Sport Neuropsychology. New York: Springer Publishing Company; 2012:131–153

[13] McCauley SR, Wilde EA, Anderson VA, et al. Pediatric TBI Outcomes Workgroup. Recommendations for the use of common outcome measures in pediatric traumatic brain injury research. J Neurotrauma. 2012; 29(4): 678–705

[14] Gioia GA, Collins MW, Isquith PK. Improving identification and diagnosis of mild traumatic brain injury with evidence: psychometric support for the acute concussion evaluation. J Head Trauma Rehabil. 2008; 23(4):230–242

[15] Gioia GA, Vaughan CG, Sady MD. PostConcussion Symptom Inventory-2: Technical Manual. Lutz, FL: Psychological Assessment Resources, Inc.; 2019

[16] Patricios JS, Schneider KJ, Dvorak J, et al. Consensus statement on concussion in sport: the 6th International Conference on Concussion in Sport-Amsterdam, October 2022. Br J Sports Med. 2023; 57(11):695–711

[17] Echemendia RJ, Burma JS, Bruce JM, et al. Acute evaluation of sport-related concussion and implications for the Sport Concussion Assessment Tool (SCAT6) for adults, adolescents and children: a systematic review. Br J Sports Med. 2023; 57(11):722–735

[18] Davis GA, Echemendia RJ, Ahmed OH, et al. Child SCAT6. Br J Sports Med. 2023; 57(11):636–647

[19] Lovell MR, Iverson GL, Collins MW, et al. Measurement of symptoms following sports-related concussion: reliability and normative data for the post-concussion scale. Appl Neuropsychol. 2006; 13(3):166–174

[20] Patricios JS, Schneider GM, van Ierssel J, et al. Beyond acute concussion assessment to office management: a systematic review informing the development of a Sport Concussion Office Assessment Tool (SCOAT6) for adults and children. Br J Sports Med. 2023; 57(11):737–748

[21] Davis GA, Rausa VC, Babl FE, et al. Improving subacute management of post concussion symptoms: a pilot study of the Melbourne Paediatric Concussion Scale parent report. Concussion. 2020; 7(1):CNC97

[22] Collins MW, Kontos AP, Okonkwo DO, et al. Statements of agreement from the Targeted Evaluation and Active Management (TEAM) Approaches to Treating Concussion Meeting held in Pittsburgh, October 15-16, 2015. Neurosurgery. 2016; 79(6):912–929

[23] Leddy JJ, Burma JS, Toomey CM, et al. Rest and exercise early after sport-related concussion: a systematic review and meta-analysis. Br J Sports Med. 2023; 57(12):762–770

[24] McCrory P, Meeuwisse WH, Aubry M, et al. Consensus statement on concussion in sport: the 4th International Conference on Concussion in Sport held in Zurich, November 2012. Br J Sports Med. 2013; 47(5):250–258

[25] Leddy JJ, Kozlowski K, Donnelly JP, Pendergast DR, Epstein LH, Willer B. A preliminary study of subsymptom threshold exercise training for refractory post-concussion syndrome. Clin J Sport Med. 2010; 20(1):21–27

[26] Gagnon I, Galli C, Friedman D, Grilli L, Iverson GL. Active rehabilitation for children who are slow to recover following sport-related concussion. Brain Inj. 2009; 23(12):956–964

[27] Silverberg ND, Iverson GL. Is rest after concussion "the best medicine?": recommendations for activity resumption following concussion in athletes, civilians, and military service members. J Head Trauma Rehabil. 2013; 28(4): 250–259

[28] Vaughan CG, Ledoux AA, Sady MD, et al. PERC 5P Concussion Team. Association between early return to school following acute concussion and symptom burden at 2 weeks postinjury. JAMA Netw Open. 2023; 6(1): e2251839

[29] Ransom DM, Vaughan CG, Pratson L, Sady MD, McGill CA, Gioia GA. Academic effects of concussion in children and adolescents. Pediatrics. 2015; 135(6):1043–1050

[30] Gioia GA. Return to school: When and how should return to school be organized after a concussion? In: Gagnon I, Ptito A, eds. Sports Concussions: A Complete Guide to Recovery and Management. New York: CRC Press; 2018:241–261

[31] Purcell LK, Davis GA, Gioia GA. What factors must be considered in "return to school" following concussion and what strategies or accommodations should be followed? A systematic review. Br J Sports Med. 2019; 53(4):250

[32] Putukian M, Purcell L, Schneider KJ, et al. Clinical recovery from concussion-return to school and sport: a systematic review and meta-analysis. Br J Sports Med. 2023; 57(12):798–809

7 Concussion: Long-term Sequelae

Ryan G. Eaton, Joshua L. Wang, and Russell R. Lonser

Summary
Concussion is a common neurologic condition resulting from traumatic impact to the head and neck area. Athletes participating in contact sports and military personnel are commonly affected. Exposure to repetitive head injury has been linked to long-term cognitive and behavioral changes which Bowman and Blau termed "chronic traumatic encephalopathy (CTE)" in 1940. Although the link between this long-term neurologic sequela and evidence of neuropathologic damage was initially purposed a century ago by Dr. Harrison Martland, public interest in CTE significantly increased recently as a result of two case studies published by Dr. Bennet Omalu. He studied the brains of two National Football League (NFL) players who had exhibited cognitive and mood symptoms while alive and found evidence of "diffuse amyloid plaques as well as sparse neurofibrillary tangles (NFTs) and tau-positive neuritic threads." Currently, CTE can only be diagnosed post-mortem through the pathognomonic features defined as "p-tau aggregates in neurons, astrocytes, and cell processes around small vessels in an irregular pattern at the depths of the cortical sulci." The clinical syndrome is heterogenous and may include mood or behavioral changes, gradual cognitive deterioration, and/or a Parkinson-like syndrome. Current research is focused on establishing a consensus on clinical criteria using advanced imaging to help risk-stratify individuals. Treatment of suspected CTE is supportive with multimodal rehabilitation and treatment of cognitive and mood symptoms.

Keywords: concussion, long-term sequelae, chronic traumatic encephalopathy, traumatic brain injury, tauopathy, neurodegenerative disease

7.1 Introduction

Concussion is a common cause of mild traumatic brain injury (mTBI) in athletes. Although concussion-related signs/symptoms often resolve within 7 to 10 days in adults, children and adolescents may require therapy for persistent (weeks to months) symptomatology.[1,2] Recently, groups have associated sports-related concussion with chronic traumatic encephalopathy (CTE). What is now known as CTE was first described by a pathologist, Harrison Martland, MD in 1928 in brains of boxers at autopsy.[3] The premortem clinical syndrome found in the boxers was characterized by evidence of memory loss, disorientation, cognitive dysfunction, and behavioral decline in an individual with a history of repetitive head trauma. However, the diagnosis of CTE can only be made on postmortem examination of the brain.[4] In this chapter, we describe the historic, clinical, histologic, and management features of the long-term sequalae of concussions as well as current controversies in the field.

7.2 History

The clinical effects of repetitive head trauma were initially described by Martland (in 1928) in a series of boxers who demonstrated a pattern of cognitive and behavioral signs/symptoms following repetitive head injury.[3] He termed this "punch drunk syndrome," which has also been referred to as "dementia pugilistica." Punch drunk syndrome is defined by a gradual progression from "uncertainty in equilibrium" to, in severe cases, "propulsive gait with facial characteristics of Parkinsonian syndrome" after repetitive head injury.[5] Later in 1940, Bowman and Blau introduced the term "chronic traumatic encephalopathy" based on histologic observations of a 28-year-old boxer who experienced persistent confusion, memory impairment, and emotional lability without improvement over 18 months.[6] The long-term neurologic sequelae of repetitive head injury was further described by Critchley (in 1957) in a series of 69 boxers. He found that these boxers experienced persistent mental confusion and amnesia with impaired motor ability that appeared to "advance steadily" with evidence of reversal.[7]

The neuropathologic process that formed the presumed basis for the clinical syndrome of CTE was first described by Corsellis in 1973. His description of the "Aftermath of Boxing" highlighted neuropathologic changes such as ventricular dilation, neurofibrillary tangles, and cavum septum pellucidum.[8] Although reports of persistent post-traumatic neurologic sequalae continued over the next 40 years, it was not until 2005 when Omalu and colleagues described the autopsy findings of retired National Football League (NFL) player, Mike Webster, that the term Chronic Traumatic Encephalopathy became popularized.[9,10] Before death, this football player exhibited signs/symptoms, including mood disorder, cognitive impairment, and parkinsonism. At autopsy, his brain demonstrated "diffuse amyloid plaques as well as sparse neurofibrillary tangles (NFTs) and tau-positive neuritic threads" that were thought to be associated with his repetitive head trauma.[9] Omalu and colleagues published a second case of a retired professional football player who was diagnosed with severe major depressive disorder and autopsy demonstrated tau-positive neurofibrillary tangles present in varying degrees in all regions of the brain.[11] These early cases expanded interest and understanding into the potential long-term impact of repetitive head injury in athletes.

7.3 Epidemiology

Sports-related concussions affect approximately 300,000 young American adults annually.[12] High-risk sports include boxing, American football, wrestling, ice hockey, martial arts, rugby, and soccer.[12] Similarly, military personnel frequently experience work-related concussions. A study of the incidence and prevalence of long-term neurologic problems and pathologic findings in 202 deceased former football players found that 56% of collegiate and 86% of professional football players had severe pathology, while only 21% of high school players had evidence of CTE (all mild pathology).[13] A similar pathologic review of 266 pathologic samples of former NFL players estimated that the odds of CTE double every 2.6 years of football played.[14] The clinical significance of these pathologic findings, however, remains unclear as a study by Braak and colleagues of 2,332 brains from individuals older than 24 years found that all had some degree of abnormally phosphorylated tau.[15]

7.4 Pathologic Features

7.4.1 Gross Findings

The most commonly observed gross pathologic finding in CTE is generalized cerebral atrophy, typically involving the frontal and temporal lobes.[16,17] Shrinkage of the mammillary bodies and atrophy of the thalamus and hypothalamus often occur, resulting in enlargement of the lateral and third ventricles.[16,17] The septum pellucidum has been frequently described as taking on a cavum appearance or containing a fenestration.[16,17] Deep brain structures, including the substantia nigra and locus coeruleus, lose pigmentation and can have a pale appearance.[16,17] However, scarring of the cerebellum that was initially described by Corsellis in 1973 does not appear to be a reliable finding in recent autopsy series of patients with repetitive head injury.[16,17]

7.4.2 Histologic Features

Histologically, CTE has been classically described as a tauopathy with evidence of hyperphosphorylated tau (p-tau) found throughout the brain.[9,11,17,18,19,20,21] Tau is a microtubule-associated protein that assists in normal trafficking of cellular contents.[22] Tau becomes hyperphosphorylated in pathologic conditions causing it to dissociate from the microtubule and aggregate into NFTs. NFTs form the presumed pathologic basis for multiple degenerative neurologic conditions, including Alzheimer's disease, corticobasal degeneration, Pick's disease, frontotemporal lobe degeneration, and progressive supranuclear palsy.[23] Although tau hyperphosphorylation appears to play a role in the pathogenesis of CTE, its significance is controversial as abnormally phosphorylated tau is commonly found in the aging brain in patients with no history of trauma.[15,24]

Researchers have focused on using the specific location of key pathologic features including hyperphosphorylated tau, NFTs, neuritic threads, and amyloid plaques to characterize CTE. McKee and colleagues described four potential stages of the distribution of the hyperphosphorylated tau pathology.[4] In stage I, there is focal tau deposition as neurofibrillary tangles form around small blood vessels in the depth of the sulci in the frontal cortex.[25] In stage II, the neurofibrillary tangles spread to the superficial cortex with staining reflecting larger concentrations of affected regions. Stage III reflects widespread p-tau deposition now densely affecting the medial temporal structures. In stage IV, nearly the entire superficial and deep cerebral cortex is affected with resultant neuronal loss, gliosis, and tau deposition in astrocytes. The visual cortex is spared.[18] Omalu and colleagues also proposed a four-class system based on the anatomic distribution of NFTs, amyloid plaques, and neuritic threads that did not have a clear progression from one stage to the other.[26] Davis and colleagues challenged the findings of McKee and colleagues suggesting that the stage I and II findings were consistent with normal aging while the stage III and IV findings likely represented a form of frontotemporal lobar dementia.[26,27]

To establish consistent pathologic criteria for CTE, the NIH convened a consensus conference of CTE pathologic experts in 2015. This consensus group noted that the most specific feature for CTE was the regional distribution of tau aggregates with the pathognomonic finding being abnormal perivascular accumulation of tau in the cortical sulci (▶ Table 7.1).[4,28] The pathognomonic finding of CTE was defined as "abnormal perivascular accumulation of tau in neurons, astrocytes and cell process in an irregular pattern at the depths of the cortical sulci". This classification emphasized the importance of the regional distribution of the tau aggregates.[4]

The neuropathologic findings in CTE share several important histologic characteristics with other disease states. A subset of patients with CTE can present with predominantly parkinsonian symptoms. Adams and colleagues compared postmortem samples from contact sports athletes to individuals from the community and found that longer time of playing contact sports was associated with a stronger neocortical distribution of alpha-synuclein deposits, the pathologic finding in Parkinson's disease.[29] Amyloid-beta peptide deposits may also be seen in later stages of CTE but in a lower density than what is seen in Alzheimer's disease.[18] Microglia activation and astrocytosis commonly occur and their role may be mechanistically similar to other neurodegenerative states.[30] Lastly, TDP-43 immunoreactive inclusions found in neurons and glial cells caused by disrupted nucleocytoplasmic transport are a potential mechanistic driver of neurodegenerative disease such as amyotrophic lateral sclerosis, Parkinson's disease, Alzheimer's disease, and CTE.[16,31]

7.5 Clinical Syndrome

Presumptive CTE is suggested by a constellation of symptoms including impaired cognition, memory, and executive function with disturbances in mood and behavior.[18,32,33] Patients may experience nonspecific symptoms such as headache, irritability, and/or difficulty concentrating.[34] In severe cases, mood symptoms may manifest as depression, suicidality, apathy, and poor impulse control. These clinical findings can progress to dementia with severe loss of attention.[18,32] Nevertheless, overall understanding of the clinical presentation is limited, as many of these clinical features can be found in persons in the normal population (including those without a history of head injury). Attempts to characterize the antemortem clinical features of CTE are limited by the retrospective nature of data collection, including interviews with family members that are limited by recall bias. Furthermore, families of individuals with behavior changes are more likely to donate the individual's brain for specimen analysis than family members of asymptomatic individuals. Finally, it is not clear the extent to which these findings differ from individuals with other neurodegenerative conditions who were not exposed to concussions. Prospective longitudinal studies are needed to define the clinical features associated with CTE finding at autopsy.

7.6 Diagnostic Modalities

7.6.1 Imaging

Although the official diagnosis of CTE can only be made at autopsy, neuroimaging modalities may help in diagnosing or

Table 7.1 Pathologic classifications of CTE

Feature	Omalu et al[26]	McKee et al[18]	NIH Consensus Statement[4]
Pathologic features	"Multifocal/diffuse tauopathy (may be accompanied by low-grade multifocal white matter rarefaction, microglial activation, parenchymal histiocytes)" "Topographically distributed NFTs/Neuritic tangles (NTs) (+/– diffuse amyloid plaques)" "Absence of classic/neuritic amyloid plaques" "Absence of pathognomonic histomorphology of other tauopathies"	"Perivascular foci of p-tau immunoreactive NFTs and Astrocytic tangles (ATs) in the neocortex" "Irregular distribution of p-tau immunoreactive NFTs and Ats at the depths of cerebral sulci" "NFTs in the cerebral cortex located preferentially in the superficial layers (often most pronounced in temporal cortex)" "Supportive, non-diagnostic features: Clusters of subpial Ats in the cerebral cortex, most pronounced at the sulcal depths"	"Abnormal p-tau immunoreactive pretangles and NFTs preferentially affecting superficial layers (layers II–III)" "Pretangles, NFTs or extracellular tangles primarily in CA2 and CA4 of the hippocampus, NFTs in subcortical nuclei" "p-tau immunoreactive thorned astrocytes at the glial limitans in the subpial and periventricular regions" "p-tau immunoreactive large grain-like and dot-like structures and TDP-43 immunoreactive neuronal cytoplasmic inclusions and dot-like structures in the hippocampus, anteromedial temporal cortex and amygdala"
Pathognomonic finding	"Sparse, moderate, or frequent band-shaped, flame-shaped, small globose, large globose NFTs accompanied by sparse moderate, or frequent NTs"	Not discussed	"p-tau aggregates in neurons, astrocytes, and cell processes around small vessels in an irregular pattern at the depths of the cortical sulci"
Classification system	Phenotype 1: sparse to frequent NFTs and NTs in cerebral cortex and brainstem, no NFTs and NTs in cerebellum, no diffuse amyloid plaques Phenotype 2: similar to phenotype 1 except diffuse amyloid plaques present Phenotype 3: NFTs and NTs predominantly in brainstem; no diffuse amyloid plaques Phenotype 4: none to sparse NFTs and NTs in the cerebral cortex, subcortical structures, and brainstem; no NFTs and NTs in the cerebellum; no diffuse amyloid plaques	Stage I: perivascular p-tau at depths of sulci primarily in frontal cortex Stage II: NFTs in superficial cortical layers (adjacent to focal epicenters) Stage III: dense p-tau in medial temporal lobe structures and widespread regions of cortex; mild cerebral atrophy macroscopically Stage IV: p-tau densely deposited throughout neuroaxis with further cerebral atrophy	Not discussed
Progression	Nonprogressive	Progression over years	Not discussed

Abbreviations: CTE, chronic traumatic encephalopathy; NFTs, neurofibrillary tangles; NTs, neuropil threads.

stratifying the risk of developing CTE in high-risk persons in the future.[35] A magnetic resonance (MR) imaging study of 86 NFL football players revealed decreased thalamic volume in participants who had played football longer and had an earlier first exposure to head injury.[36] NFL players had smaller amygdala, hippocampus, and cingulate gyrus volumes than that of controls.[36] Moreover, MR spectroscopy has shown a decrease in N-acetyl aspartate in mixed martial art athletes and increase in choline, myo-inositol, and glutathione in former soccer players.[37,38,39] Hart and colleagues performed a diffusion tensor MR imaging based analysis on 14 cognitively impaired retired NFL players and 14 matched controls and found significant differences in white matter abnormalities with reductions of fractional anisotropy in frontal and parietal regions bilaterally, as well as in the left temporal lobe and corpus callosum.[40] Finally, positron emission tomography can utilize ligand binding to detect the accumulation of abnormal biomarkers associated with CTE.[41] [18F] flortaucipir binds directly to the tau constituent of the NFT while [11C]DPA-713 binds to the translocator protein (TSPO), a transmembrane protein associated with brain injury.[42,43] These are being investigated as potential imaging biomarkers for CTE.

7.6.2 Molecular Biomarkers

Significant research interest has centered on the investigation of potential molecular biomarkers in concussion and traumatic brain injury.[44,45,46,47] Molecular biomarkers can be sampled from salivary secretions, blood, and cerebrospinal fluid (CSF). Cheng and colleagues sampled salivary secretions of patients who experienced head trauma and healthy controls. They examined the extracellular vesicle contents in these samples for expression of several genes known to be involved in amyloid processing, tau hyperphosphorylation, and microglial activation. They found increased expression of CDC2, CSNK1A1, and cathepsin D (CTSD) in the injured patients compared to healthy controls.[48] A study of serum biomarkers found both higher concentrations of plasma t-tau and plasma exosomal tau in former NFL players compared to the general population.[37,49] Spinal fluid biomarkers have shown less promise. A study comparing the CSF extracellular vesicle protein profile of former NFL players to healthy controls found no difference between the two groups. Investigation of other potential CSF biomarkers such as triggering receptor expressed on myeloid cells 1 and p-tau181 is underway.[50,51,52] Despite extensive preclinical analysis, biomarkers have failed to establish a practical role clinically to date.

7.7 Treatment

There are no approved medications or therapies for those who suffer from the long-term sequalae of concussions. Prophylactic utilization of protective head attire is the first-line prevention strategy. It is recommended that individuals suspected of experiencing a concussion cognitively and physically rest until the acute symptoms resolve followed by a gradual re-introduction into exertion prior to medical clearance.[53] Patients suspected of having severe concussions or suspected long-term neurologic sequala are managed primarily with supportive measures including cognitive rehabilitation, motor and vestibular therapies, and treatment of comorbid mood disorders.[54]

Preclinical studies are underway targeting molecular pathways in patients with presumed CTE.[55] Salsalate has been shown to inhibit tau acetylation while methylene blue minimized neuronal degeneration in TBI rodents.[56,57] Glycogen synthase 3 beta, which promotes tau phosphorylation, has also been targeted successfully in preclinical models using dimethyl fumarate, intravenous simvastatin, valproate, and lithium.[58,59,60,61] Immunotherapeutics have also been successful in preclinical work. An adeno-associated virus vector coding for anti-pTau antibody was able to reduce central nervous system (CNS) p-tau levels in TBI rodents while the antibody 6C5 was shown to prevent neuronal tau uptake.[62,63] Other work has investigated targeting the metabolic changes and complex inflammatory cascade that underly the pathogenesis of CTE.[64,65,66]

7.8 Conclusion

Concussions occur frequently in both athletes and military personnel. The long-term neurologic sequelae of repetitive head injury are not clearly understood. In the future, imaging and molecular biomarkers may play a supplementary role in the clinical assessment and prognosis of patients with suspected CTE. Treatment is primarily supportive although continued research is underway in identifying potential therapeutic targets.

7.9 Clinical Pearls

- Concussion is a common neurologic condition resulting from traumatic impact to the head and neck area.
- Athletes participating in contact sports and military personnel are most affected.
- Repetitive head injury has been linked to long-term neurologic sequalae characterized by cognitive and behavioral changes broadly regarded as chronic traumatic encephalopathy (CTE).
- CTE can only be diagnosed post-mortem with the pathognomonic feature being "p-tau aggregates in neurons, astrocytes, and cell processes around small vessels in an irregular pattern at the depths of the cortical sulci."
- Current research is focused on establishing a consensus clinical criteria and using advanced imaging to help risk-stratify individuals with a history of exposure to repeated head injuries.
- Treatment of suspected CTE is supportive.

7.10 Disclosure Statement

The authors have nothing to disclose.

References

[1] Makdissi M, Darby D, Maruff P, Ugoni A, Brukner P, McCrory PR. Natural history of concussion in sport: markers of severity and implications for management. Am J Sports Med. 2010; 38(3):464–471

[2] Babcock L, Byczkowski T, Wade SL, Ho M, Mookerjee S, Bazarian JJ. Predicting postconcussion syndrome after mild traumatic brain injury in children and adolescents who present to the emergency department. JAMA Pediatr. 2013; 167(2):156–161

[3] Martland HS. Punch drunk. JAMA. 1928; 91(15):1103–1107

[4] McKee AC, Cairns NJ, Dickson DW, et al. TBI/CTE group. The first NINDS/NIBIB consensus meeting to define neuropathological criteria for the diagnosis of chronic traumatic encephalopathy. Acta Neuropathol. 2016; 131(1):75–86

[5] Cantu RC, Bernick C. History of chronic traumatic encephalopathy. Semin Neurol. 2020; 40(4):353–358

[6] Bowman K, Blau A. Psychotic states following head and brain injury in adults and children. In: Brock S, ed. Injuries of the Skull, Brain and Spinal Cord: Neuro-psychiatric, Surgical and Medico-legal Aspects. Williams & Wilkins Co; 1940:309–360

[7] Critchley M. Medical aspects of boxing, particularly from a neurological standpoint. BMJ. 1957; 1(5015):357–362

[8] Corsellis JA, Bruton CJ, Freeman-Browne D. The aftermath of boxing. Psychol Med. 1973; 3(3):270–303

[9] Omalu BI, DeKosky ST, Minster RL, Kamboh MI, Hamilton RL, Wecht CH. Chronic traumatic encephalopathy in a National Football League player. Neurosurgery. 2005; 57(1):128–134, discussion 128–134

[10] Kasper BS, Taylor DC, Janz D, et al. Neuropathology of epilepsy and psychosis: the contributions of J.A.N. Corsellis. Brain. 2010; 133(Pt 12):3795–3805

[11] Omalu BI, DeKosky ST, Hamilton RL, et al. Chronic traumatic encephalopathy in a national football league player: part II. Neurosurgery. 2006; 59(5): 1086–1092, discussion 1092–1093

[12] Noble JM, Hesdorffer DC. Sport-related concussions: a review of epidemiology, challenges in diagnosis, and potential risk factors. Neuropsychol Rev. 2013; 23(4):273–284

[13] Mez J, Daneshvar DH, Kiernan PT, et al. Clinicopathological evaluation of chronic traumatic encephalopathy in players of American football. JAMA. 2017; 318(4):360–370

[14] Mez J, Daneshvar DH, Abdolmohammadi B, et al. Duration of American football play and chronic traumatic encephalopathy. Ann Neurol. 2020; 87 (1):116–131

[15] Braak H, Thal DR, Ghebremedhin E, Del Tredici K. Stages of the pathologic process in Alzheimer disease: age categories from 1 to 100 years. J Neuropathol Exp Neurol. 2011; 70(11):960–969

[16] McKee AC, Gavett BE, Stern RA, et al. TDP-43 proteinopathy and motor neuron disease in chronic traumatic encephalopathy. J Neuropathol Exp Neurol. 2010; 69(9):918–929

[17] McKee AC, Cantu RC, Nowinski CJ, et al. Chronic traumatic encephalopathy in athletes: progressive tauopathy after repetitive head injury. J Neuropathol Exp Neurol. 2009; 68(7):709–735

[18] McKee AC, Stern RA, Nowinski CJ, et al. The spectrum of disease in chronic traumatic encephalopathy. Brain. 2013; 136(Pt 1):43–64

[19] Geddes JF, Vowles GH, Nicoll JA, Révész T. Neuronal cytoskeletal changes are an early consequence of repetitive head injury. Acta Neuropathol. 1999; 98 (2):171–178

[20] Omalu BI, Bailes J, Hammers JL, Fitzsimmons RP. Chronic traumatic encephalopathy, suicides and parasuicides in professional American athletes: the role of the forensic pathologist. Am J Forensic Med Pathol. 2010; 31(2):130–132

[21] Saing T, Dick M, Nelson PT, Kim RC, Cribbs DH, Head E. Frontal cortex neuropathology in dementia pugilistica. J Neurotrauma. 2012; 29(6): 1054–1070

[22] Brunden KR, Trojanowski JQ, Lee VM. Advances in tau-focused drug discovery for Alzheimer's disease and related tauopathies. Nat Rev Drug Discov. 2009; 8(10):783–793

[23] Katsumoto A, Takeuchi H, Tanaka F. Tau pathology in chronic traumatic encephalopathy and Alzheimer's disease: similarities and differences. Front Neurol. 2019; 10:980

[24] Crary JF, Trojanowski JQ, Schneider JA, et al. Primary age-related tauopathy (PART): a common pathology associated with human aging. Acta Neuropathol. 2014; 128(6):755–766

[25] Falcon B, Zivanov J, Zhang W, et al. Novel tau filament fold in chronic traumatic encephalopathy encloses hydrophobic molecules. Nature. 2019; 568(7752):420–423

[26] Omalu B, Bailes J, Hamilton RL, et al. Emerging histomorphologic phenotypes of chronic traumatic encephalopathy in American athletes. Neurosurgery. 2011; 69(1):173–183, discussion 183

[27] Davis GA, Castellani RJ, McCrory P. Neurodegeneration and sport. Neurosurgery. 2015; 76(6):643–655, discussion 655–656

[28] Ban VS, Madden CJ, Bailes JE, Hunt Batjer H, Lonser RR. The science and questions surrounding chronic traumatic encephalopathy. Neurosurg Focus. 2016; 40(4):E15

[29] Adams JW, Alvarez VE, Mez J, et al. Lewy body pathology and chronic traumatic encephalopathy associated. rom contact sports. J Neuropathol Exp Neurol. 2018; 77(9):757–768

[30] Hickman S, Izzy S, Sen P, Morsett L, El Khoury J. Microglia in neurodegeneration. Nat Neurosci. 2018; 21(10):1359–1369

[31] Anderson EN, Morera AA, Kour S, et al. Traumatic injury compromises nucleocytoplasmic transport and leads to TDP-43 pathology. eLife. 2021; 10: e67587

[32] Stern RA, Daneshvar DH, Baugh CM, et al. Clinical presentation of chronic traumatic encephalopathy. Neurology. 2013; 81(13):1122–1129

[33] Baugh CM, Stamm JM, Riley DO, et al. Chronic traumatic encephalopathy: neurodegeneration following repetitive concussive and subconcussive brain trauma. Brain Imaging Behav. 2012; 6(2):244–254

[34] Daneshvar DH, Riley DO, Nowinski CJ, McKee AC, Stern RA, Cantu RC. Long-term consequences: effects on normal development profile after concussion. Phys Med Rehabil Clin N Am. 2011; 22(4):683–700, ix

[35] Lin A, Charney M, Shenton ME, Koerte IK. Chronic traumatic encephalopathy: neuroimaging biomarkers. Handb Clin Neurol. 2018; 158:309–322

[36] Schultz V, Stern RA, Tripodis Y, et al. Age at first exposure to repetitive head impacts is associated with smaller thalamic volumes in former professional American football players. J Neurotrauma. 2018; 35(2):278–285

[37] Alosco ML, Jarnagin J, Rowland B, Liao H, Stern RA, Lin A. Magnetic resonance spectroscopy as a biomarker for chronic traumatic encephalopathy. Semin Neurol. 2017; 37(5):503–509

[38] Mayer AR, Ling JM, Dodd AB, Gasparovic C, Klimaj SD, Meier TB. A longitudinal assessment of structural and chemical alterations in mixed martial arts fighters. J Neurotrauma. 2015; 32(22):1759–1767

[39] Koerte IK, Lin AP, Muehlmann M, et al. Altered neurochemistry in former professional soccer players without a history of concussion. J Neurotrauma. 2015; 32(17):1287–1293

[40] Hart J, Jr, Kraut MA, Womack KB, et al. Neuroimaging of cognitive dysfunction and depression in aging retired National Football League players: a cross-sectional study. JAMA Neurol. 2013; 70(3):326–335

[41] Villemagne VL, Doré V, Burnham SC, Masters CL, Rowe CC. Imaging tau and amyloid-β proteinopathies in Alzheimer disease and other conditions. Nat Rev Neurol. 2018; 14(4):225–236

[42] Mitsis EM, Riggio S, Kostakoglu L, et al. Tauopathy PET and amyloid PET in the diagnosis of chronic traumatic encephalopathies: studies of a retired NFL player and of a man with FTD and a severe head injury. Transl Psychiatry. 2014; 4(9):e441

[43] Coughlin JM, Wang Y, Munro CA, et al. Neuroinflammation and brain atrophy in former NFL players: an in vivo multimodal imaging pilot study. Neurobiol Dis. 2015; 74:58–65

[44] Papa L, Akinyi L, Liu MC, et al. Ubiquitin C-terminal hydrolase is a novel biomarker in humans for severe traumatic brain injury. Crit Care Med. 2010; 38(1):138–144

[45] Wang KK, Yang Z, Zhu T, et al. An update on diagnostic and prognostic biomarkers for traumatic brain injury. Expert Rev Mol Diagn. 2018; 18(2): 165–180

[46] Saatman KE, Duhaime AC, Bullock R, Maas AI, Valadka A, Manley GT, Workshop Scientific Team and Advisory Panel Members. Classification of traumatic brain injury for targeted therapies. J Neurotrauma. 2008; 25(7): 719–738

[47] Dambinova SA, Bettermann K, Glynn T, et al. Diagnostic potential of the NMDA receptor peptide assay for acute ischemic stroke. PloS One. 2012; 7 (7):e42362

[48] Cheng Y, Pereira M, Raukar N, et al. Potential biomarkers to detect traumatic brain injury by the profiling of salivary extracellular vesicles. J Cell Physiol. 2019; 234(8):14377–14388

[49] Stern RA, Tripodis Y, Baugh CM, et al. Preliminary study of plasma exosomal tau as a potential biomarker for chronic traumatic encephalopathy. J Alzheimers Dis. 2016; 51(4):1099–1109

[50] Muraoka S, Jedrychowski MP, Tatebe H, et al. Proteomic profiling of extracellular vesicles isolated. rom cerebrospinal fluid of former National Football League players at risk for chronic traumatic encephalopathy. Front Neurosci. 2019; 13:1059

[51] Donat CK, Scott G, Gentleman SM, Sastre M. Microglial activation in traumatic brain injury. Front Aging Neurosci. 2017; 9:208

[52] Bergauer A, van Osch R, van Elferen S, Gyllvik S, Venkatesh H, Schreiber R. The diagnostic potential of fluid and imaging biomarkers in chronic traumatic encephalopathy (CTE). Biomed Pharmacother. 2022; 146: 112602

[53] McCrory P, Meeuwisse WH, Aubry M, et al. Consensus statement on concussion in sport: the 4th International Conference on Concussion in Sport held in Zurich, November 2012. Br J Sports Med. 2013; 47(5):250–258

[54] Kontos AP, Deitrick JM, Collins MW, Mucha A. Review of vestibular and oculomotor screening and concussion rehabilitation. J Athl Train. 2017; 52 (3):256–261

[55] Pierre K, Dyson K, Dagra A, Williams E, Porche K, Lucke-Wold B. Chronic traumatic encephalopathy: update on current clinical diagnosis and management. Biomedicines. 2021; 9(4):415

[56] Fenn AM, Skendelas JP, Moussa DN, et al. Methylene blue attenuates traumatic brain injury-associated neuroinflammation and acute depressive-like behavior in mice. J Neurotrauma. 2015; 32(2):127–138

[57] Lagraoui M, Sukumar G, Latoche JR, Maynard SK, Dalgard CL, Schaefer BC. Salsalate treatment following traumatic brain injury reduces inflammation and promotes a neuroprotective and neurogenic transcriptional response with concomitant functional recovery. Brain Behav Immun. 2017; 61:96–109

[58] Rojo AI, Sagarra MR, Cuadrado A. GSK-3beta down-regulates the transcription factor Nrf2 after oxidant damage: relevance to exposure of neuronal cells to oxidative stress. J Neurochem. 2008; 105(1):192–202

[59] Cuadrado A, Kügler S, Lastres-Becker I. Pharmacological targeting of GSK-3 and NRF2 provides neuroprotection in a preclinical model of tauopathy. Redox Biol. 2018; 14:522–534

[60] Mountney A, Boutté AM, Gilsdorf J, Lu XC, Tortella FC, Shear DA. Intravenous administration of simvastatin improves cognitive outcome following severe traumatic brain injury in rats. J Neurotrauma. 2016; 33(16):1492–1500

[61] Yu F, Wang Z, Tanaka M, et al. Posttrauma cotreatment with lithium and valproate: reduction of lesion volume, attenuation of blood-brain barrier disruption, and improvement in motor coordination in mice with traumatic brain injury. J Neurosurg. 2013; 119(3):766–773

[62] Sacramento CB, Sondhi D, Rosenberg JB, et al. Anti-Phospho-Tau gene therapy for chronic traumatic encephalopathy. Hum Gene Ther. 2020; 31 (1–2):57–69

[63] Nobuhara CK, DeVos SL, Commins C, et al. Tau antibody targeting pathological species blocks neuronal uptake and interneuron propagation of tau in vitro. Am J Pathol. 2017; 187(6):1399–1412

[64] Logsdon AF, Lucke-Wold BP, Nguyen L, et al. Salubrinal reduces oxidative stress, neuroinflammation and impulsive-like behavior in a rodent model of traumatic brain injury. Brain Res. 2016; 1643:140–151

[65] Wang Y, Liu Y, Nham A, et al. Calpain-2 as a therapeutic target in repeated concussion-induced neuropathy and behavioral impairment. Sci Adv. 2020; 6(27):eaba5547

[66] Zhang J, Teng Z, Song Y, Hu M, Chen C. Inhibition of monoacylglycerol lipase prevents chronic traumatic encephalopathy-like neuropathology in a mouse model of repetitive mild closed head injury. J Cereb Blood Flow Metab. 2015; 35(3):443–453

Part II

Spine

II

8 Sports-Related Spine Injuries

Andrew M. Hersh, Michael D. White, and Nicholas Theodore

Summary

Sports are the fourth most common cause of spine injuries, whose effects can range from a short-term suspension of play to permanent neurological deficits preventing safe return to play. The cervical spine is the most common location of sports-related spine injuries, especially in the pediatric population. A brief overview of spine biomechanics is presented in this chapter to aid in understanding the nature of spine injuries across different sports. Spine injuries in contact sports are readily understood to result from collisions and violent impacts, but even sports without contact, such as gymnastics and diving, can have a high risk of injury to the spine. Moreover, repetitive microtrauma to the spine occurs from the extreme forces placed on the spine from vigorous athletic participation, increasing the prevalence of neck and back pain and predisposing to injury. The chapter also reviews several classification systems intended to assist with communication about the injury and operative decision-making.

Keywords: spine injury, spinal cord injury, trauma, athlete, sports, contact sports, biomechanics

8.1 Introduction

Sports are the fourth most common cause of spine injuries following motor vehicle crashes, violence, and falls, with nearly 15% of spine injuries occurring in the context of athletic activities.[1,2] In addition to injuries to the bony spine and ligaments, traumatic spinal cord injury (SCI) is a feared outcome in acute sports-related injury, with 10% of SCIs attributable to sports.[3] Furthermore, the prevalence of low back and neck pain is higher in the athletic population than the general population, with approximately 10 to 15% of athletes suffering from low back pain and a lifetime prevalence of 48% for neck pain.[4,5] Spine injuries and SCI are a significant source of morbidity, can entail prolonged recovery times, and may incapacitate athletes from returning to play. Catastrophic injuries can cause significant and permanent impairment in functional status or even be fatal, with athletes facing a higher mortality rate when hospitalized for spine injuries compared to other sports-related injuries.[2,6]

Most spinal trauma injures the cervical spine, which can be neurologically devastating for athletes, followed by the lumbar and thoracic spine.[1] Unfortunately, the incidence of traumatic spine injuries has increased over time in both the pediatric and adult populations.[6,7] Particularly in the pediatric population, athletic injuries are the cause of nearly 25% of all pediatric cervical spine injuries presenting to the emergency department.[8] Indeed, pediatric spine injuries have been reported more frequently in the cervical spine compared to adults, reflecting differences in spine anatomy, including laxity of the ligamentous structures and multiple vertebral ossification centers in children, and mechanism of injury.[9] SCI attributable to athletic activity is more commonly seen in the second decade of life compared to other causes of SCI that typically occur in older individuals.[3]

A review of the National Trauma Data Bank identified 1,723 cases of pediatric sports-related traumatic spine injuries from 2011 to 2014, with a median age of 15 years. Most injuries (81%) occurred in males, with cycling and contact sports as the most common etiologies. These injuries were associated with longer hospitalizations and the need for ICU-level care compared to other sports injuries.[10] Other sex differences in spine injuries have been noted. A review of the National Electronic Injury Surveillance System from 2009 to 2018 identified snowboarding and weightlifting as the most common causes of traumatic lumbar injuries in males, whereas horseback riding and skiing were the most common causes in females. The overall incidence was also higher in males.[11]

8.2 Association of Sports with Spine Injuries

Full-contact sports are associated with a high risk of severe spine injuries. Although football accounts for many sports-related spine injuries seen in the United States, this finding is at least partly attributable to the sheer number of athletes playing football, and thus at risk of injury. Some estimates place the number of football players suffering from cervical spine injuries to be as high as 10 to 15%, although most of these result in full recovery. Still, players with cervical injuries often have persistent radiographic changes evident on follow-up imaging.[12] Data from the National Center for Catastrophic Sports Injury Research across 1989 to 2002 shows an incidence of six quadriplegic events annually for football players at the high school and college level.[13] An updated analysis of professional American football players from 2000 to 2010 found that injuries to the spine or axial skeleton accounted for 7% of all injuries, with cervical spine injuries representing 45% of these injuries.[14] Unfortunately, rates of spine injuries in the National Football League remain high, with an incidence of 2.47 spine/core injuries per 1,000 exposures in 2021, increasing from 1.63 per 1,000 exposures during 2018–2020.[15] Ice hockey and wrestling are other significant sources of spine injuries from contact sports.[16]

Sports without contact or with only limited contact between players can also result in catastrophic spinal injuries, including diving, baseball, cheerleading, skiing, and snowboarding.[1,3,16] For example, diving headfirst into a shallow pool or lake can cause a devastating neurological injury from the axial compression force to the cervical spine. The injury is frequently a complete SCI, with total loss of motor function below the level of the injury.[17] Devastating cervical spine injuries have also been reported from high-energy beach breaking waves in shallow water.[18]

In contrast to full-contact sports and diving, most spine injuries incurred by baseball players affect the lumbar spine, rather than the cervical spine, and pitchers have the highest rates of injuries.[19] These injuries primarily result from degenerative conditions brought on by vigorous baseball playing, as well as collision impacts between players.[20] A review of a Major League Baseball database identified 172 spine injuries from 2011 to 2016, of which 73% were localized to the lumbar spine. The authors estimated that 1.3% of spine injuries are season-ending for the player, a low rate but one which nevertheless highlights the ever-present potential for devastating damage.[19]

Separately, a study from the Canadian Hospitals Injury Reporting and Prevention Program database identified 125 cases of neck and spine injuries over a 20-year period among cheerleaders, including sprains, fractures, and dislocations. These injuries were primarily related to falls from heights or tosses.[21] Gymnasts have a high incidence of low back pain, with some studies estimating spinal derangements in up to 75% of pediatric gymnasts owing to the extreme forces placed on the spine from gymnastic activities.[22]

A detailed description of the types and treatments of spine injuries and SCI will be presented for different sports in later chapters. Here we will briefly review the biomechanical properties of the spine contributing to injury and provide an overview of the types of spine injuries that can occur in athletes.

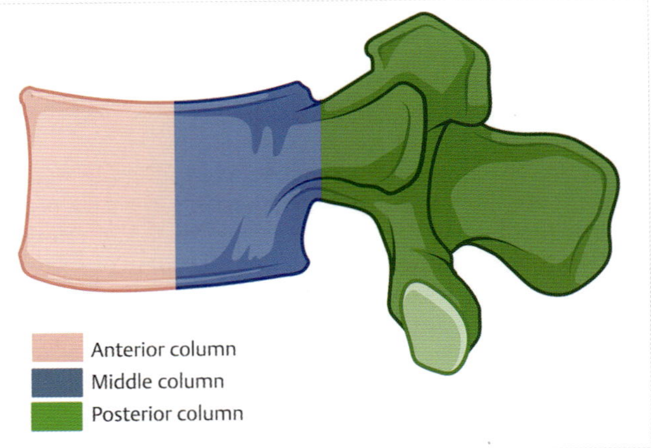

Fig. 8.1 Representation of the three-column model of the spine, illustrating the anterior, middle, and posterior columns. Instability occurs with damage to two columns. (Created with BioRender.com.)

8.3 Spine Anatomy and Properties

An understanding of the unique biomechanical properties of the bony spine is critical to grasping the distinct injury patterns produced across different sports and age groups. The study of spine biomechanics centers around the concepts of spinal stability and instability, which can be difficult to define clinically but are understood to represent the capacity of spinal units to work together to protect neurological tissue and limit displacement under physiological loads.[23] A spinal unit consists of two adjacent vertebral bodies, an intervertebral disk, cartilaginous endpoints, and bridging ligamentous tissues. Each spinal unit presents biomechanical characteristics similar to those of the entire spine.[24]

The craniocervical and thoracolumbar junctions are important transition zones that are prone to injury. The craniocervical junction, consisting of the occiput–C1 and C1–C2 joints, stabilizes the skull base to the spine. Several unique ligamentous structures provide stability in this region, including the alar ligament, cruciate ligament, tectorial membrane, and the anterior and posterior atlanto-occipital ligaments. Disruption of these ligaments, as may occur from extreme hyperextension or hyperflexion, as well as congenital defects and inflammatory conditions, can produce craniocervical instability. A severe consequence of this instability is atlanto-occipital dislocation, which can produce severe neurological impairment including cranial nerve deficits and quadriplegia.[25,26] The thoracolumbar junction spans T10–L2 and is a highly mobile area of the spine, thus accounting for a substantial proportion of spine injuries and fractures.[27]

The spine, as originally proposed by Denis, can be conceptualized as divided into three distinct columns—anterior, middle, and posterior (▶ Fig. 8.1). The anterior column includes the anterior longitudinal ligament and the anterior two-thirds of the vertebral body and intervertebral disk, the middle column includes the posterior one-third of the vertebral body and intervertebral disk, along with the posterior longitudinal ligament, while the posterior column includes all structures posterior to the middle column including the posterior ligamentous complex (PLC), the pedicles, facets, and spinous processes. The central thesis of the three-column model is that disruption of two or more columns is needed for instability.[28] Injuries that disrupt the PLC alone, for example, are not inherently unstable. This model emphasizes the importance of the middle column, which includes the neutral axis of the spine, as a source of stability.[29]

Athletic activities often require movements beyond the "normal" range of physiological motion. Instability of the athletic spine can result from acute traumatic injuries and chronic degenerative changes incurred from overuse and improper mechanics. Acute traumatic injuries more commonly occur in full-contact sports, while chronic injuries are most common and are frequently seen in low-contact sports, although all athletic activities can result in chronic spine changes.[30] Repetitive movement patterns of the spine during an athletic event or training session, such as axial rotations and lateral bending during baseball, golf, or tennis, can cause microtrauma to the functional spine units, particularly when inadequate recovery time is provided.[31] For example, baseball pitching involves repeated pelvic rotation, trunk rotation, and angular velocities, with transmission of forces to the lower limbs through external rotation of the legs. Improper pitching mechanics and overuse can cause costovertebral joint dysfunction and thoracic spine pain.[31] Extreme lumbar flexion, extension, and lateral bending during tennis can contribute to low back pain, while asymmetric loading of the spine during golf can stem from lateral bending during swinging.[32] Symptoms from overuse injuries can accumulate gradually and may initially be unnoticed.[30] Endurance training, core strength, and dynamic stabilization exercises can improve coordination among muscle groups and mitigate against injury.[31,32]

Chronic overuse injuries in older athletes are exacerbated by normal age-related degenerative changes and reduction in bone mass. Adults with sports-related spine injuries are less likely to exhibit a full recovery compared to younger pediatric patients.[6] Osteoporosis increases the risk for compression fractures and kyphotic deformities, although athletic activities that involve loading forces to the spine and weight-bearing activities may protect against age-related bone loss. In contrast, low-impact sports, such as cycling, may increase the risk of osteoporosis.[32]

8.4 Sports-Related Spine Injuries

Many types of spine injuries can occur due to sports including strains, stress fractures, compression fractures, dislocations, and disk herniations, among others. Strains are common and can result from low-grade forces to the spine, causing paravertebral muscle pain, and can usually be treated with conservative management and nonsteroidal anti-inflammatory drugs.[33] A study of sports-related traumatic spinal injuries in the adult population found that water sports and contact sports were associated with the highest rates of SCI (over 40% each). Importantly, 39% of patients also presented with traumatic brain injury, which was associated with adverse discharge, demonstrating the complexity of many of these injuries which are not limited solely to the spine.[6]

8.4.1 Cervical Spine Injuries

Unstable fractures and dislocations in the cervical spine generally occur in the sub-axial spine and can cause permanent neurological deficits.[33] Falls and whiplash injuries can produce cervical hyperextension.[34] Neck flexion produces straightening of the cervical spine and diminishes the capacity of the vertebral column to resist axial forces, so that an axial force applied to the head during neck flexion can produce a flexion or compression fracture.[33,34] Burst fractures can result from severe compression causing failure of the anterior and middle spinal columns.[35] Instability of the bony spine from these axial forces can cause protrusion of bone fragments into the spinal canal and injure the cord, risking quadriplegia.[33] The C5 and C6 vertebral levels are the most common site of flexion fractures in adolescents, and often result from helmet-first football tackles ("spearing") and violent collisions.[34]

Transient deficits can also occur following cervical trauma, defined as cervical cord neurapraxia, including paresthesias, numbness, weakness, and paralysis. Symptoms typically last less than 15 minutes but can persist for several days.[36] Cervical cord neurapraxia is estimated to occur in 1.3 to 6 per 10,000 athletes and can result from a variety of positions, including hyperextension, hyperflexion, or axial load mechanisms, with cervical stenosis as a predisposing factor.[33,36]

8.4.2 Thoracic and Lumbar Spine Injuries

Below the cervical spine, the thoracolumbar junction is most vulnerable to injury due to its high mobility and flexibility. Compression fractures are a common cause of injury, and can result from hyperflexion, hyperextension, axial loading, and violent collisions. Traumatic injuries can also cause avulsion fractures of the posterior elements. A rare avulsion fracture known as a clay-shoveler's fracture can occur from rotational movements and most frequently affects the spinous processes of C7 or T1, although it can occur at other lower cervical or upper thoracic levels.[37]

Spondylolysis, or a defect of the pars interarticularis, is one of the most common etiologies of low back pain in athletes, particularly in the pediatric athletic population, where it presents up to 9 × more frequently than the adult population. In contrast, diskogenic causes are more commonly responsible for low back pain in adult athletes.[22] Nearly all cases of pediatric spondylolysis occur at the L5 vertebra, followed by L4, and can be unilateral or bilateral. Repetitive flexion and extension movements have been associated with the development of spondylolysis. Bilateral pars defects and mechanical stress on the posterior elements can predispose to spondylolisthesis, or displacement of the vertebral body.[34]

8.4.3 Back Pain

Beyond traumatic etiologies, repetitive microtrauma from vigorous training regimens and high-intensity forces on the spine render athletes susceptible to sprains, degenerative disk disease, spondylolysis, and spondylolisthesis, all of which contribute to back pain. Such pain can incapacitate athletes from competitive events and places professional players at risk for early career retirement.[38] Although most people will eventually develop back pain during their lifetime, athletes usually experience such pain at a younger age. Estimates of incidence of back pain in athletes vary widely, ranging from approximately 10 to 30%, although this number varies widely across sports, genders, and athletic intensity. For example, around 30 to 50% of football players are believed to experience back pain, while the rate in gymnasts reaches as high as 50 to 86%.[39,40] Skiing and rowing are associated with the highest incidences of low back pain, owing to the rotation and flexion forces placed on the spine for long periods of time.[41] Sports requiring hyperextension movements, such as gymnastics and diving, are associated with higher rates of spondylolysis in athletes than their peers, and competitive runners are at risk for sacral stress fractures.[42] Sports that require extreme rotation of the lumbar spine and place high compressive loads on the spine, such as baseball and golf, also contribute to lumbar strain, facet joint pain, and disk degeneration. Indeed, low back pain is believed to affect 3 to 15% of baseball players.[38]

Most cases of low back pain will improve over time and can be managed with conservative therapy, including physical therapy, exercise, and pain medication. Around 80% of athletes with spondylolysis will improve with nonoperative treatment.[42] Direct repair of the pars is a surgical option for persistent cases and is described in later chapters. Athletes with herniated disks contributing to low back pain can benefit from diskectomies.[42] Unfortunately, some athletes will suffer from chronic back pain not alleviated by conservative or surgical intervention.

8.4.4 Spinal Cord Injuries

The most catastrophic spinal injuries cause damage to the spinal cord, which can cause permanent paralysis of the upper and/or lower extremities. Sports-related injuries are one of the most common causes of SCI, responsible for approximately 7 to 9% of all SCIs in the United States.[2,16] Naturally, the greatest risk for SCI is presented by contact sports, including hockey, football, and wrestling, but SCI can arise from other mechanisms. Head strikes during diving cause a sudden halt in velocity and transmit significant forces to the cervical spine, which can cause bony fractures or dislocations that compress and injure the spinal cord. These injuries typically affect young, healthy males and can cause severe quadriparesis.[43] Similarly, horseback riding and skiing are not contact sports but can cause severe SCI from violent falls at fast speeds. Indeed, a systematic review by the Spinal Cord Injury Research Evidence Team identified diving as being responsible for the greatest percentage of sports-related SCIs in the United States, with nearly twice as many SCIs attributable to diving compared to football. Diving was also identified as the principal cause in Canada, Japan, China, and Denmark.[44]

8.5 Injury Classification and Scoring Systems

Prompt evaluation and treatment of traumatic spinal injuries are critical to improve an athlete's chances of recovery. The athlete should be evaluated for life-threatening injuries and a limited on-field examination performed to identify neurological deficits and severity of injury, followed by transport to a hospital. Radiographs are critical in the diagnosis of unstable injuries, with CT scans helping to illustrate bony injuries and determine fracture morphology, while MRIs are useful in the workup of ligamentous injury and SCI. Several classification and scoring systems incorporate data from the neurological examination and imaging and are useful in the operative decision-making process.

The most detailed classification systems are those proposed by the AOSpine Knowledge Forum Trauma, with unique classifications for injuries to the upper cervical spine (C0–C2), subaxial cervical spine, thoracolumbar spine, and sacral spine. Additionally, the upper cervical spine is separated into three distinct anatomical regions: (1) the occipital condyle and craniocervical junction, (2) the C1 ring and C1–C2 joint, and (3) C2 and the C2–C3 joint. For each spinal region, injuries are subdivided into three categories: Type A injuries are isolated bony injuries, such as compression injuries, affecting individual vertebral levels; Type B injuries refer to ligamentous and tension band injuries; and Type C injuries are translation injuries owing to failure of all elements. Classification of sacral fractures differs, with Type A injuries referring to lower sacrococcygeal injuries, Type B injuries referring to posterior pelvic injuries, and Type C injuries referring to spino-pelvic injuries. Subaxial cervical spine injuries have an additional morphological classification—Type F—referring to facet injuries, which can either be nondisplaced fractures (F1), fractures with potential for instability (F2), floating lateral mass (F3), or pathologic subluxation of dislocated facet (F4).[45]

For each injury morphology, injuries can be further classified based on the neurological status at the time of initial examination and clinical modifiers. Neurological status includes intact (N0), transient with complete recovery at the time of examination (N1), nerve root injury or radiculopathy (N2), incomplete SCI or incomplete cauda equina injury (N3), and complete SCI (N4). Clinical modifiers vary across the spinal regions and reflect patient-specific characteristics that influence treatment, such as patient comorbidities, bone disease, and vascular injury.[45]

The AOSpine classifications are detailed and can produce an impressive array of injury combinations, helping to communicate precisely about the nature of the injury, but several scoring systems have been proposed to simplify surgical decision-making, including the Thoracolumbar Injury Classification and Severity Score (TLICS) and the Subaxial Injury Classification (SLIC) and Severity Scale. TLICS grades thoracolumbar injuries according to three components—(1) injury morphology, (2) integrity of the posterior ligamentous complex (PLC), and (3) neurological status (▶ Table 8.1).[46] Morphology includes compression fracture, burst fracture, translational/rotational injury, and distraction injury. Compression (or wedge) fractures involve only the anterior column of Denis' three-column model and, barring involvement of the PLC, are therefore stable injuries, while burst fractures also involve the middle column and should therefore be worked up as unstable injuries. Translation/rotation injuries can result from high-energy traumas causing vertebral fractures with unilateral or bilateral facet dislocation leading to spinal column subluxation, visible on imaging as horizontal displacement of the spinal column or a shift in the midline sagittal plane. They are severe, unstable injuries that almost always cause SCI. Distraction injuries include flexion-distraction injuries (also known as Chance fractures) which are horizontal fractures that disrupt the middle and posterior columns, often occurring concomitantly with anterior column injuries and separating parts of the spinal column. They are unstable injuries with circumferential disruption of the spinal cord and often result from motor-vehicle accidents with rapid deceleration, leading to the common term "seatbelt fractures" to describe flexion-distraction injuries.[47,48] The other two components of TLICS are the PLC integrity and the patient's neurological status. The PLC is graded as intact, suspected or indeterminate disruption, or definitely disrupted, while the neurological status is graded as intact, nerve root injury, complete SCI, incomplete SCI, or cauda equina injury.[47] Note that a complete SCI receives fewer points than an incomplete SCI, as surgical intervention is considered less effective for complete injuries due to the lower likelihood of restoring neurological function.

Table 8.1 The TLICS grading system[47]

Injury category	Component	Points
Morphology	Compression	1
	Burst	2
	Translation/Rotation	3
	Distraction	4
Integrity of the PLC	Intact	0
	Suspected/Indeterminate	2
	Injured	3
Neurological status	Intact	0
	Nerve root injury	2
	Complete SCI	2
	Incomplete cord	3
	Cauda equina	3
		0–3: nonoperative 4: indeterminate 5+: operative

Abbreviations: PLC, posterior ligamentous complex; SCI, spinal cord injury; TLICS, Thoracolumbar Injury Classification and Severity Score.

The SLIC scoring system is similar to TLICS but adapted for the subaxial cervical spine. Once again, the system comprises the three principal components of injury, morphology, disko-ligamentous complex, and neurological status. Distraction injuries in the subaxial spine here include facet perch and hyperextension injuries, while rotational/translational injuries include facet dislocation and unstable teardrop injuries. The disko-ligamentous complex and neurological status are also graded as in TLICS, except cauda equina injuries are naturally excluded from the neurological status classification. Summing the points for both TLICS and SLIC produces a useful heuristic for decision-making, with scores of 3 points or less considered nonoperative, scores of 5 points or more considered operative, and scores of 4 points considered indeterminate.[49] Although these systems provide a clear and concise way to classify thoracolumbar spine injuries, the indeterminate cases where patients receive a score of 4 points are often the most challenging, and surgeons need to consider other clinical tools and imaging to guide decision-making.

Finally, the American Spinal Injury Association (ASIA) Impairment Scale is the most commonly used classification system for SCI. Complete injuries are categorized as Grade A, while patients without neurological injury are considered Grade E (▶ Table 8.2). The remaining Grades B, C, and D are for incomplete injuries. Grade C and D injuries refer to cases where motor function is preserved below the level of injury, with Grade D injuries referring to cases where half of the muscle groups below the injury level have a strength grade of at least 3/5, and Grade C injuries referring to cases where most of the muscles below the injury level have a grade less than 3/5. Lastly, loss of motor function with preservation of sensory function below the injury level are categorized as Grade B.[50] Patients with Grade A injuries have a poor prognosis and traditionally are not considered operative candidates, with surgical intervention typically targeted at Grade B to D injuries, although some studies suggest there may be some residual nerve function even in apparently complete injuries that can show improvement over time.[51,52] Repeat assessment of the ASIA score at each visit helps in monitoring injury progression and recovery. However, a limitation of the scoring system is that two patients can have vastly different functional limitations even though they have the same grade, depending on the anatomical region of the spine (e.g., high cervical Grade C injuries cause more debilitating deficits compared to lumbar Grade C injuries).

Table 8.2 ASIA impairment scale grading system[50]

Grade	Injury	Definition
A	Complete	No motor or sensory function below level of injury
B	Incomplete	Motor function not preserved but sensory function is preserved below level of injury
C	Incomplete	Motor function preserved with at least 50% of muscles below level of injury lower than grade 3/5
D	Incomplete	Motor function preserved with at least 50% of muscles below level of injury grade 3/5 or greater
E	Normal	Normal motor and sensory function, neurologically intact

Abbreviation: ASIA, American Spinal Injury Association.

8.6 Conclusion

Sports, whether recreational or professional, contact or no-contact, can cause traumatic spine injuries incapacitating athletes and requiring urgent intervention. The most feared outcome of a spinal injury is SCI, which can cause permanent neurological deficits. Moreover, the extreme forces placed on the spine from participation in sports increase the risk of spondylosis and predispose the athlete to spine injury. Many athletes suffer from neck and back pain at a younger age compared to their nonathletic peers, and workup requires careful assessment to determine if they would benefit from surgical intervention. Athletes with traumatic spinal injuries often require surgery for stabilization and clinical improvement, but unfortunately return-to-play is not always safe. The evaluation, workup, and surgical and nonsurgical treatments of athletic spinal injuries, along with return-to-play guidelines, will be discussed in detail in the following chapters.

8.7 Clinical Pearls

- Sports represent the fourth most common cause (approximately 15%) of spine injuries in the United States.
- Although contact sports are responsible for a large number of sports-related spine injuries, other athletic activities are not without risk, with a high proportion of SCI occurring in the context of diving.
- Athletes have a high prevalence of neck and back pain and experience these conditions at a younger age than their nonathletic peers, owing to the unique biomechanical forces placed on their spines in the context of sports.
- Spondylolysis is one of the most common causes of low back pain in pediatric athletes.
- The AOSpine classifications, TLICS, and SLIC grading systems are all valuable tools in the workup and decision-making of spinal injuries.

References

[1] Menzer H, Gill GK, Paterson A. Thoracic spine sports-related injuries. Curr Sports Med Rep. 2015; 14(1):34–40

[2] Puvanesarajah V, Qureshi R, Cancienne JM, Hassanzadeh H. Traumatic sports-related cervical spine injuries. Clin Spine Surg. 2017; 30(2):50–56

[3] Basil GW, Burks SS, Green BA. Sports-related cervical spine injuries—background, triage, and prevention. J Craniofac Surg. 2021; 32(4):1643–1646

[4] Ball JR, Harris CB, Lee J, Vives MJ. Lumbar spine injuries in sports: review of the literature and current treatment recommendations. Sports Med Open. 2019; 5(1):26

[5] Noormohammadpour P, Farahbakhsh F, Farahbakhsh F, Rostami M, Kordi R. Prevalence of neck pain among athletes: a systematic review. Asian Spine J. 2018; 12(6):1146–1153

[6] Hauser BM, Gupta S, Hoffman SE, et al. Adult sports-related traumatic spinal injuries: do different activities predispose to certain injuries? J Neurosurg Spine. 2021; 1:1–7

[7] Verhofste BP, Hedequist DJ, Birch CM, et al. Operative treatment of cervical spine injuries sustained in youth sports. J Pediatr Orthop. 2021; 41(10):617–624

[8] Alas H, Pierce KE, Brown A, et al. Sports-related cervical spine fracture and spinal cord injury: a review of nationwide pediatric trends. Spine. 2021; 46 (1):22–28

[9] Leonard JR, Jaffe DM, Kuppermann N, Olsen CS, Leonard JC, Pediatric Emergency Care Applied Research Network (PECARN) Cervical Spine Study Group. Cervical spine injury patterns in children. Pediatrics. 2014; 133(5): e1179–e1188

[10] Gupta S, Hauser BM, Zaki MM, et al. Morbidity after traumatic spinal injury in pediatric and adolescent sports-related trauma. J Neurosurg Spine. 2019; 32(5):1–7

[11] Cheng R, Kahan JB, Li D, Schneble CA, Gardner EC. Sex- and sports-specific epidemiology of traumatic lumbar spine injuries sustained during sporting activities: male snowboarders and female horseback riders at greatest risk. Arthrosc Sports Med Rehabil. 2021; 3(2):e515–e520

[12] Thomas BE, McCullen GM, Yuan HA. Cervical spine injuries in football players. J Am Acad Orthop Surg. 1999; 7(5):338–347

[13] Boden BP, Tacchetti RL, Cantu RC, Knowles SB, Mueller FO. Catastrophic cervical spine injuries in high school and college football players. Am J Sports Med. 2006; 34(8):1223–1232

[14] Mall NA, Buchowski J, Zebala L, Brophy RH, Wright RW, Matava MJ. Spine and axial skeleton injuries in the National Football League. Am J Sports Med. 2012; 40(8):1755–1761

[15] Platt B, Abed V, Khalily C, et al. Injury rates remained elevated in the second national football league season after the onset of the COVID-19 pandemic. Arthrosc Sports Med Rehabil. 2023; 5(2):e325–e329

[16] Boden BP, Prior C. Catastrophic spine injuries in sports. Curr Sports Med Rep. 2005; 4(1):45–49

[17] Yun JH, Yi YG, Lee J, Bang MS. Rehabilitation outcome in people with spinal cord injuries resulting from diving in South Korea. Spinal Cord Ser Cases. 2022; 8(1):40

[18] Griepp DW, De la Garza Ramos R, Lee J, et al. Beach breaking waves and related cervical spine injuries: a level one trauma center experience and systematic review. World Neurosurg. 2022; 160:e471–e480

[19] Makhni MC, Curriero FC, Yeung CM, et al. Epidemiology of spine-related neurologic injuries in professional baseball players. Spine. 2022; 47(6): E265–E271

[20] Morimoto M, Okada R, Sugiura K, et al. Low back pain and lumbar degeneration in Japanese professional baseball players. Orthop J Sports Med. 2022; 10(10):23259671221125513

[21] Hardy I, McFaull S, Saint-Vil D. Neck and spine injuries in Canadian cheerleaders: an increasing trend. J Pediatr Surg. 2015; 50(5):790–792

[22] Micheli LJ, Wood R. Back pain in young athletes. Significant differences from adults in causes and patterns. Arch Pediatr Adolesc Med. 1995; 149 (1):15–18

[23] Izzo R, Guarnieri G, Guglielmi G, Muto M. Biomechanics of the spine. Part I: spinal stability. Eur J Radiol. 2013; 82(1):118–126

[24] Somovilla-Gómez F, Lostado-Lorza R, Corral-Bobadilla M, Escribano-García R. Improvement in determining the risk of damage to the human lumbar functional spinal unit considering age, height, weight and sex using a combination of FEM and RSM. Biomech Model Mechanobiol. 2020; 19(1):351–387

[25] Theodore N, Aarabi B, Dhall SS, et al. The diagnosis and management of traumatic atlanto-occipital dislocation injuries. Neurosurgery. 2013; 72 Suppl 2:114–126

[26] Finn MA, Bishop FS, Dailey AT. Surgical treatment of occipitocervical instability. Neurosurgery. 2008; 63(5):961–968, discussion 968–969

[27] Beisse R. Endoscopic surgery on the thoracolumbar junction of the spine. Eur Spine J. 2006; 15(6):687–704

[28] Denis F. The three column spine and its significance in the classification of acute thoracolumbar spinal injuries. Spine. 1983; 8(8):817–831

[29] Benzel EC. Biomechanics of Spine Stabilization. 2nd ed. In: Benzel EC, ed. Georg Thieme Verlag; 2001

[30] de Jonge MC, Kramer J. Spine and sport. Semin Musculoskelet Radiol. 2014; 18(3):246–264

[31] Donatelli R, Dimond D, Holland M. Sport-specific biomechanics of spinal injuries in the athlete (throwing athletes, rotational sports, and contact-collision sports). Clin Sports Med. 2012; 31(3):381–396

[32] Borg-Stein J, Elson L, Brand E. The aging spine in sports. Clin Sports Med. 2012; 31(3):473–486

[33] Boden BP, Jarvis CG. Spinal injuries in sports. Neurol Clin. 2008; 26(1): 63–78, viii

[34] Maxfield BA. Sports-related injury of the pediatric spine. Radiol Clin North Am. 2010; 48(6):1237–1248

[35] Rajasekaran S. Thoracolumbar burst fractures without neurological deficit: the role for conservative treatment. Eur Spine J. 2010; 19(Suppl 1):S40–S47

[36] Clark AJ, Auguste KI, Sun PP. Cervical spinal stenosis and sports-related cervical cord neurapraxia. Neurosurg Focus. 2011; 31(5):E7

[37] Hoong WTJ, Kaliya-Perumal AK. Multiple clay shoveler's fractures of the thoracic spine. Diagnostics (Basel). 2022; 12(9):2190

[38] Wasser JG, Zaremski JL, Herman DC, Vincent HK. Assessment and rehabilitation of chronic low back pain in baseball: part II. Res Sports Med. 2017; 25(2):231–243

[39] Lawrence JP, Greene HS, Grauer JN. Back pain in athletes. J Am Acad Orthop Surg. 2006; 14(13):726–735

[40] De Luigi AJ. Low back pain in the adolescent athlete. Phys Med Rehabil Clin N Am. 2014; 25(4):763–788

[41] Farahbakhsh F, Rostami M, Noormohammadpour P, et al. Prevalence of low back pain among athletes: a systematic review. J Back Musculoskeletal Rehabil. 2018; 31(5):901–916

[42] Bono CM. Low-back pain in athletes. J Bone Joint Surg Am. 2004; 86(2): 382–396

[43] Yılmaz M, Ikizoglu E, Arslan M, Ozgiray E, Calıskan KE, Erbayraktar RS. An overview of spinal injuries due to dive or fall into shallow water: our long-term, double-center experience from the Aegean Coast. Emerg Med Int. 2021; 2021:9937730

[44] Chan CWL, Eng JJ, Tator CH, Krassioukov A, Spinal Cord Injury Research Evidence Team. Epidemiology of sport-related spinal cord injuries: a systematic review. J Spinal Cord Med. 2016; 39(3):255–264

[45] Divi SN, Schroeder GD, Oner FC, et al. AOSpine-spine trauma classification system: the value of modifiers: a narrative review with commentary on evolving descriptive principles. Global Spine J. 2019; 9(1) Suppl:77S–88S

[46] Doerr SA, Weber-Levine C, Hersh AM, et al. Automated prediction of the Thoracolumbar Injury Classification and Severity Score from CT using a novel deep learning algorithm. Neurosurg Focus. 2022; 52(4):E5

[47] Vaccaro AR, Lehman RA, Jr, Hurlbert RJ, et al. A new classification of thoracolumbar injuries: the importance of injury morphology, the integrity of the posterior ligamentous complex, and neurologic status. Spine. 2005; 30(20): 2325–2333

[48] Whitney E, Alastra AJ. Vertebral Fracture. StatPearls. Published online April 3, 2023. Accessed November 21, 2023 at: https://www.ncbi.nlm.nih.gov/books/NBK547673/

[49] Vaccaro AR, Hulbert RJ, Patel AA, et al. Spine Trauma Study Group. The subaxial cervical spine injury classification system: a novel approach to recognize the importance of morphology, neurology, and integrity of the disco-ligamentous complex. Spine. 2007; 32(21):2365–2374

[50] Roberts TT, Leonard GR, Cepela DJ. Classifications in brief: American Spinal Injury Association (ASIA) Impairment Scale. Clin Orthop Relat Res. 2017; 475 (5):1499–1504

[51] Angeli CA, Boakye M, Morton RA, et al. Recovery of over-ground walking after chronic motor complete spinal cord injury. N Engl J Med. 2018; 379 (13):1244–1250

[52] Choe AS, Belegu V, Yoshida S, et al. Extensive neurological recovery from a complete spinal cord injury: a case report and hypothesis on the role of cortical plasticity. Front Hum Neurosci. 2013; 7(JUN):290

9 Biomechanics of the Head and Spine in Sports

Declan A. Patton and Kristy B. Arbogast

Summary

Over 80 years ago, the mechanism of the head injury was investigated using physical models and it was determined that linear and angular kinematics were responsible for focal and diffuse shear strains, respectively. Since then, the biomechanics of the head when loaded has been investigated by conducting cadaveric experiments, scaling animal models to humans, reconstructing impacts using anthropomorphic test devices (ATD), and using in vivo devices to monitor head loading of volunteers in the laboratory and on-field during sporting contests. The likelihood of head injury depends on the loading conditions, such as whether the impact was directly to the head or indirectly to the body, the duration of the impact pulse, and the direction of the resultant loading. The hierarchy of hazard controls (e.g., from elimination to protective equipment) can be applied to impact biomechanics in a sporting setting to reduce the risk of head injury. Traditional helmets were designed to prevent focal injuries, such as skull fractures, but novel helmet technologies aimed at reducing rotational loads have been developed more recently. Although significant disabling injuries to the cervical spine are rare, minor injuries to the cervical and lumbar spine in sport are common and derive from strain on the muscles and activation of the pain receptors in the facet joints, often from overuse or poor mechanics.

Keywords: prevention, helmets, acceleration, thresholds

9.1 Introduction

Research in fundamental biomechanics increases our understanding of the mechanisms of brain and spine injury in sports and allows for the development of effective mitigation strategies. This chapter will focus primarily on the biomechanics of injury to the head and brain, as these injuries are much more common in athletes than those to the spine and represent increasing concern for both short- and long-term consequences.

9.2 Fundamental Brain Biomechanics

Sports participation involves motion and acceleration of the head during activities such as running, jumping, and stopping that can inertially load the brain[1,2] and provide potential for direct head impact, especially in contact and collision sports,[3,4,5] increasing the likelihood of head injuries including those to the brain and skull. ▶ Fig. 9.1 is a flow diagram redrawn from Ommaya et al,[6] which relates the mechanical loading of the head to biomechanical responses of the brain. Static mechanical loads are present only during head crush and are rarely seen in sports. In contrast, dynamic mechanical loads to the head are common in sports and cause head motions that surpass a kinematic tolerance limit and cause tissue loads that surpass some tissue-level functional tolerance limit, resulting in clinical manifestation of injury. Head motions resulting from dynamic mechanical loads are some a combination of translation (i.e., linear) and rotational (i.e., angular) loading conditions.

9.2.1 Translational Kinematics

The biomechanical response of the head to impacts has been investigated using human volunteers and physical, animal, cadaver, and mathematical models. Over 80 years ago, Holbourn[7] investigated the biomechanical response of the brain using physical

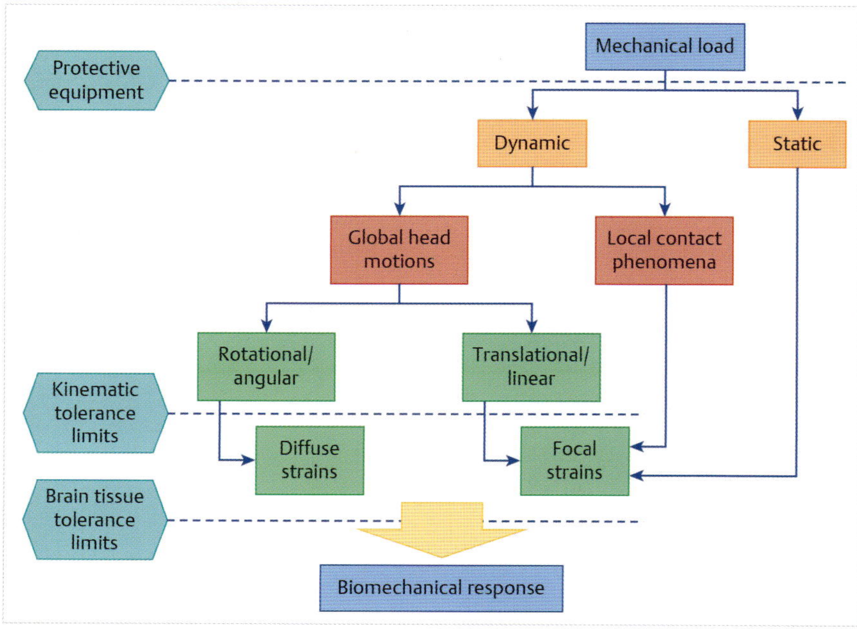

Fig. 9.1 Flow diagram of mechanical load to biomechanical response. (Redrawn from Ommaya et al.[6])

models of gelatin "brains" in wax "skulls" and hypothesized that linear acceleration was only responsible for local contusions and skull fracture. Lissner et al[8] performed drop tests of cadaver heads and concluded that the linear acceleration tolerance for skull fracture is reduced if the time duration is increased, which led to the development of the Wayne State Tolerance Curve (WSTC). The WSTC is the basis for the Gadd Severity Index (GSI),[9] which is used by the National Operating Committee on Standards for Athletic Equipment (NOCSAE) for testing the performance of American football helmets,[10] and the Head Injury Criterion (HIC),[11] which is used widely in the automotive industry, among others, to evaluate head protection.

9.2.2 Rotational Kinematics

Holbourn[7] also hypothesized that rotational kinematics were the main cause of shear strains in the brain and indicative of the probability of injury in that region. In a primate model, Pudenz and Shelden[12] replaced a section of the skull with a window through which the motion of the brain was recorded using a high-speed camera. Impacts to the head were observed to cause rotations of the brain within the cranial cavity. However, when the head of the animal was limited to linear acceleration, brain motion was reduced. In a subsequent primate model, Ommaya et al[13] found that brain injury was more easily produced in tests in which the head was free to rotate compared with tests in which cervical collars were worn to prevent flexion of the neck and subsequent rotation of the head. It was concluded that the use of a cervical collar reduced the angular acceleration of the head and, therefore, reduced shear strains in the brain. Similar to linear acceleration, there is an interplay between angular acceleration magnitude and duration; Ommaya and Hirsch[14] demonstrated that the angular acceleration tolerance for brain injury is reduced if the time duration is increased. Gennarelli et al[15] directly tested the rotational hypothesis for the mechanism of brain injury and reported that animals subjected to purely rotational head motions experienced traumatic unconsciousness, but no animal subjected to purely translational head motions were rendered unconscious. Therefore, it was concluded that widely distributed shear strains produced by rotational head motions were the primary mechanism of diffuse brain injury.

9.3 Direct versus Indirect Loads

Dynamic mechanical loads can be direct or indirect head acceleration events (HAEs). Both can generate rotational and translational head motion. Indirect HAEs induce inertial head motions after an impact remote from the head (e.g., body check in hockey), whereas direct HAEs induce head motions via direct contact with the head (e.g., punch to the jaw in boxing) and, therefore, involve contact phenomena.[16] In general, indirect HAEs have lower peak head kinematics compared with direct events; evidence rooted in fundamental primate models of brain injury[16] and examples from high school female lacrosse and collegiate ice hockey players illustrates this point.[12,13] The further an indirect impact is from the head, the less energy is transmitted to the head, as more energy is attenuated by the body. An example of this is a rugby tackle, for which a lower point of initial contact on the body (e.g., waist) results in lower peak head kinematics compared with a tackle with a higher point of contact (e.g., chest).[17] This translates to injury-causing scenarios, as well. In professional ice hockey and American football, over 95% and over 99% of concussions, respectively, involve direct head contact.[14,15] Concussions due to indirect contact are rare.

9.4 Techniques to Determine Injury Thresholds

9.4.1 Physical Reconstructions

Early animal models of brain injury used brain size, mass, or inertia to scale kinematic injury tolerance values to humans[14,18,19]; however, such traditional techniques lack validation[20] and did not incorporate the viscoelastic properties and morphological features of the brain.[21] In recent decades, sporting impacts have been reconstructed to investigate the head kinematics associated with concussion and nonconcussion cases and gain insight into thresholds. Newman et al[22,23,24] reconstructed 31 head impact cases in professional American football using anthropomorphic test devices (ATDs) after previously using video analysis to determine the configuration of the impacts and the representative velocities involved. A value of 78 g was associated with a 50% likelihood of concussion. Sanchez et al[25] reanalyzed the reconstructions of Newman et al,[22,23,24] highlighting errors in the rotational kinematic calculations, and determined the median concussion case had a peak resultant angular velocity and acceleration of 41.5 rad/s and 6.5 rad/s^2, respectively. McIntosh et al[26] reconstructed 40 head impact cases in Australian football using video analysis and rigid body modeling. Tolerance values of 65 g, 22 rad/s, and 4.0 krad/s^2 were associated with a 50% likelihood of concussion for peak linear acceleration, angular velocity, and angular acceleration, respectively.

9.4.2 Head Impact Sensors

Recent advances in technology have enabled the development of head impact sensors, which facilitate the study of the head impact biomechanics of athletes in vivo and calculation of injury risk curves.[27] Using instrumented American football helmets to monitor the head impacts of collegiate athletes, Rowson and Duma[28] and Rowson et al[29] reported tolerance values of 193 g, 28.3 rad/s, and 6.4 krad/s^2 were associated with a 50% likelihood of concussion for peak linear acceleration, angular velocity, and angular acceleration, respectively. Tolerance values associated with a 50% likelihood of concussion have also been calculated based on data from instrumented helmets in youth American football: 164 g and 6.9 krad/s^2 for peak linear and angular acceleration, respectively.[30] However, such tolerance limits are likely overestimated considering previous cadaver tests in which 165 g resulted in probable damage to brain tissue[31] and 200 g was associated with a 10% risk of skull fracture.[32] Further, average kinematic values associated with concussion in American football have been measured to be approximately 60 g to 100 g and 2,600 to 6,400 rad/s^2 for playing levels ranging from youth to professional.[28,29,30,33]

There is considerable debate as to whether an actual threshold of concussive injury can be determined.[34] Mihalik et al[35] evaluated this possibility using data from instrumented helmets in college football, comparing the sensor data to actual player diagnosis of concussion. It was determined that any choice of threshold value would result in many unnecessary negative evaluations if sensor data were the sole diagnostic criteria. A large-scale study using instrumented helmet sensor data from multiple collegiate football teams has suggested that head impact thresholds for concussions need to be considered at the individual level.[36,37] Others have postulated that the density of impacts before the injurious impact influences the likelihood for injury.[38,39] These data point to challenges in identifying a single biomechanical value that is associated with a particular injury risk.

Contributing to this uncertainty is a series of laboratory validation studies using ATD headforms wearing instrumented helmets that identified the errors associated with measurements from instrumented helmet sensors, attributed to relative motion between the helmet and the head.[40,41,42] Instrumented skin patch and headband sensors have also been used to monitor head impacts in sports[43,44]; however, laboratory studies involving ATDs[42,45,46] and human volunteers[47] have demonstrated that these sensors also overestimate peak kinematics. Instrumented mouthguards have been found to have superior accuracy compared with other instrumented impact sensors due to improved sensor–skull coupling.[47,48] Sufficient data from instrumented mouthguards have not been collected to date to generate injury thresholds.

Another consideration for data generated from head impact sensors is the issue of false-positive events, i.e., when an event is recorded by the sensor but is not associated with an HAE.[44] Although it has limitations, time-stamped video serves as an independent data source that can be used to verify HAEs recorded by sensors and provide valuable contextual information.[16] However, in a review of studies from 2000 to 2019 that reported head impact sensor data, including some in which injury thresholds were calculated, only 20% used video to verify all HAEs.[27] More recently, advanced postprocessing techniques, such as machine learning algorithms, have been developed to verify HAEs.[49] In 2022, the Consensus Head Acceleration Measurement Practices (CHAMP) group was founded to develop and recommend best practices for collecting, analyzing, and reporting head acceleration measurement data in sport[50] such that future data collection using head impact sensors will use rigorous and robust methods.

9.4.3 Computational Models

Finite element (FE) analysis is another powerful tool for investigating the biomechanical response during impact and identifying important thresholds for tissue-level damage. FE analysis is the method of dividing geometry into a convenient number of elements and imposing the basic physical laws and kinematics, in addition to certain assumptions and boundary conditions, directly to each element. FE head models must use appropriate material properties and be validated to achieve accurate results.[51] One such model is the Kungliga Tekniska Högskolan (KTH) FE head model, which has been extensively compared to experimental cadaveric data for intracranial pressure, intracerebral acceleration, relative brain–skull motion, skull fracture, and brain tissue strain.[52,53] Kleiven[54] used the KTH model to simulate head impacts in American football and found that strains in the gray matter and corpus callosum were significantly correlated with concussion. Patton et al[55,56] used the KTH model to simulate head impacts in Australian football and found that impacts to the temporal region of the head caused coronal rotations, which render injurious stresses and strains in the brain, specifically in the thalamus, corpus callosum, and white matter regions. More recent studies have used head impact kinematic data recorded using instrumented mouthguards during sports participation to drive FE head models.[57] One of the main limitations of FE analysis is that it is computationally intensive; therefore, current efforts use machine learning to rapidly estimate brain tissue strain.[58,59] Another limitation is that many models represent the anatomy of the 50th percentile male, which is why some studies have explored the development of subject-specific models[60,61] A recent review of contemporary brain FE models provides a discussion of their individual strengths and limitations.[51]

FE models provide helpful visual representation of the relative contribution of translational and rotational loading to injury in the brain. **Video 9.1** shows maximum principal strain in the brain from a pulse with a peak linear acceleration of 35 g with both low and high rotational kinematics.[62] Given similar linear acceleration, the loading condition with high rotational acceleration results in much higher strains in the brain.

9.5 Role of Impact Direction

There is strong evidence that the threshold of injury varies by direction of head motion. Using a primate head injury model, Gennarelli et al[63] found that the injury severity increased as the loading plane varied from sagittal to coronal. Subsequent porcine studies have also found similar direction-dependent differences in injury outcomes.[64] Such findings are supported by video analysis studies of concussions in Australian[65] and American[66] football, which reported the side of the head as the most common impact site for concussions, suggesting that tolerance may be lower for impacts that lead to coronal head movement. This concept is well illustrated using an FE model of the brain. **Video 9.2** depicts the maximum principal strain in the brain from rotational impacts with peak kinematics of 40 rad/s and 4 krad/s^2 applied in different planes.[62] The highest strains are observed from rotational loading in the transverse plane, followed by the coronal and sagittal planes.

9.6 Biomechanics of Injury Prevention

Armed with the knowledge of the fundamental biomechanics of head protection, one can apply the National Institute for Occupational Safety and Health (NIOSH) hierarchy of hazard controls to head impacts in contact and collision sports (▶ Table 9.1). The most effective hazard control method, elimination, may not be the ideal choice due to the health and social benefits of physical activity and sports participation[67]; however, substituting a combat, collision, or contact sport with a low- or noncontact sport may be a more beneficial option (e.g., flag football instead of tackle football[68]). Engineering controls on the environment are intended to isolate players from potential hazards, such as padding rugby goal posts.[69] Ground hardness is another potential environmental hazard for brain injury, which has been investigated by various studies.[70] Administrative controls via modification of

Table 9.1 The hierarchy of hazard controls applied to head injury biomechanics

Effectiveness	Level	Intervention
Higher	Elimination	Stop playing contact sport
	Substitution	Play a sport with a lower risk of head injury
	Engineering controls	Ensure playing fields are suitable and safe
	Administrative controls	Implement rules of the sport to ensure player safety
Lower	Personal protective equipment	Wear effective head protection

Abbreviation: NIOSH, National Institute for Occupational Safety and Health.

the laws and rules of the game are one of the most common methods of injury prevention in sport. Examples exist across multiple sports where changes to how often teams practice, how current rules are enforced, and governance on how opposing players can interact with one another have resulted in concussion reduction.[71,72,73,74] Technique and training are other examples of administrative controls; training programs aiming to increasing neck strength appear to demonstrate benefits in reduced peak head kinematics.[75]

The last level of the hierarchy of hazard control is protective equipment. The main goal of protective equipment is to reduce the mechanical load on the body. The obvious example of protective equipment for the head is a helmet. A typical sports helmet comprises an outer shell to distribute the load and resist penetration, an inner liner to attenuate the energy of the impact, a comfort liner to provide a comfortable fit on the head, and a retention system to maintain the helmet on the head (▶ Fig. 9.2).

Helmets have different designs, materials, and features depending on the requirements of the sport.[76] Traditionally, they were designed to prevent focal injuries, such as skull fractures, which are associated with linear acceleration.[77] As such, many helmets initially used inexpensive foams, such as expanded polystyrene or polypropylene, for the energy-attenuating inner liner.[78] More recently, novel helmet technologies have been developed with rotation-damping systems, created through innovative materials or structures, that have demonstrated effectiveness in reducing rotational kinematics during oblique laboratory impacts.[79,80,81,82,83]

The impact performance standards for most helmets typically involve a drop test onto a flat anvil with a linear acceleration–based pass/fail threshold.[84] Some helmet standards have added rotational performance criteria to test requirements, such as the NOCSAE standard for American football helmets.[10] Helmet rating programs aimed at consumers, such as the Virginia Tech Summation of Tests for the Analysis of Risk (STAR), also incorporate rotational performance criteria.[28] **Video 9.3** illustrates the test setup for the Virginia Tech test program. STAR ratings exist for helmets from a wide range of sports, including football, hockey, and equestrian, among others. There is a need for other helmet standards to complement current linear drop test requirements with rotational performance criteria.[77,85] Helmet evaluation test conditions must mimic those observed on the field for the sport in question so that better-performing helmets in the laboratory correlate to lower injury risk on-field.[86]

More recently, there have been innovations around helmet add-ons that provide additional protection, often directed

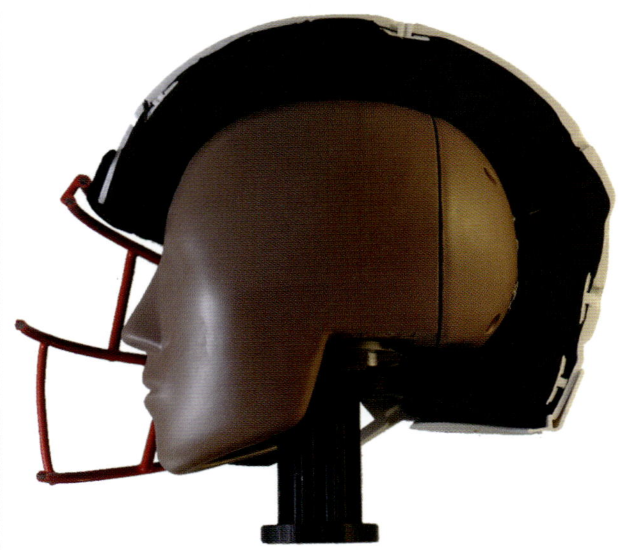

Fig. 9.2 Sagittal view of a Riddell SpeedFlex Precision football helmet showing relative dimensions of a helmet compared with the 50th percentile adult head. (Reproduced with permission by Biocore LC.)

toward the practice setting. While benefits have been demonstrated in the laboratory by reducing metrics of linear and angular kinematics,[87,88,89,90] on-field studies have reported mixed results.[88,89,91] It is important to note that even within a given product, there are multiple versions, and not all published on-field evaluations, nor discussions in the lay press, are clear which version is being evaluated.[91]

Soft-shelled helmets, which are commonly referred to as headgear, are allowed in other sports, such as soccer, rugby union, rugby league, and Australian football.[92] Older laboratory studies concluded that headgear was ineffective at reducing the linear acceleration of the head associated with concussion,[93,94] which was attributed to a lack of, or inadequate, impact performance standards.[92] Similar to helmet add-ons in American football, prototype rugby headgear demonstrated that small design changes resulted in significant improvements in impact energy attenuation.[95] More recently, advances in material technology have resulted in modern headgear designs performing well in laboratory studies.[96] However, headgear has not been found to reduce the risk of concussion in field studies of soccer,[97] rugby union,[98,99] and Australian football.[100,101]

9.7 Prevention of Long-term Consequences of Repetitive Head Impacts

As more is understood about how to prevent brain injury in sport, concern about the potential for negative effects from repetitive head impact exposure (RHIE), in the absence of diagnosed injury, has intensified, and strategies to prevent the consequences of RHIE are being sought. A critical barrier to progress in our understanding of RHIE from a prevention standpoint is the subjective symptom-based nature of concussion diagnosis. To date, there is no universally deployed diagnostic biomarker for concussive neurodysfunction and, therefore, no simple means by which to measure when a player's impact exposure is too much. As a result, biomechanical interventions to minimize the effect of RHIE have simply been focused on reducing the frequency and density of impacts, assuming that less is better. For example, contact practices have been limited in American football,[72,102] and the introduction of heading in soccer practices and games has been delayed into later adolescence.[103] Future advancements in this area depend on the development of objective biomarkers that can be used to help regularly monitor (e.g., after a game or practice or weekly through a season) the effects of sport participation on neurofunction. Armed with these new tools, prevention strategies can be developed and evaluated to reduce the short- and long-term effects of head impact, in the absence of diagnosed injury, in sport.

9.8 Biomechanics of Spinal Injury in Sport

Consideration of spinal injury in sport focuses on injury primarily to the cervical and lumbar spine. From a cervical spine perspective, minor injuries such as stingers and cervical strains are the most frequent and result in limited time missed.[104,105] Stingers occur from either traction to the brachial plexus or direct nerve root compression,[106] while cervical strains are due to single or repetitive movements that strain the muscles in the cervical spine and activate the mechanically sensitive pain receptors in facet joints.[107] No clear prevention strategies exist to address these mechanisms.

While significant disabling injuries to the cervical spine are rare, they are often initiated by head contact resulting in sharp deceleration of the head and continued inertia of the torso, leading to buckling, axial compression, and flexion of the cervical spine.[108,109] This mechanism is typically seen in spearing injuries in football or rugby (e.g., leading with the head in a tackle) or direct head contact in other sports, such as diving, equestrian, gymnastics, and wrestling. Such loading results in both ligamentous and bony injuries to the posterior elements of the spine as well as compressive and often wedged failure of the vertebral bodies. These loading conditions increase the likelihood of spinal instability and injury to the spinal cord itself. Extension cervical spine injuries in sport are less common than flexion injuries, result in less spinal instability, and are often caused by a direct impact to the forehead or mandible or a high-severity impact to the posterior torso. The primary prevention strategy for both axial compression/flexion or extension injuries of the cervical spine is to minimize the head impact that creates these loading conditions on the spine.[110] In sports, this takes the form of rules of the game designed to eliminate leading with the head, training in heads-up tackling and blocking techniques, environmental constraints that limit diving in shallow water, and the introduction of spotters in gymnastics.

The incidence of disabling cervical spine injuries is much less than the incidence of crown impacts to the head in sports. This is due to the ability of the cervical spine to bend "out of the way" of the moving torso, without injury, once the head has been decelerated.[110] Any aspect of the environment that further constrains the head limits this natural protective motion of the spine. From a prevention perspective, consider the material characteristics of the impact surface and the helmet. Increased padding allows the head to pocket and changes the vector and duration over which the loads to the cervical spine are applied, thus increasing risk to the spine.[110] Surfaces and helmets must balance the benefit of increased compliance to mitigate head injury with unintended negative consequences to the cervical spine.

Lumbar spine injury in sport encompasses primarily low back pain, minor fractures of the spinal processes, and disk herniation—all rising from the repetitive motions of flexion, extension, and torsion required for some sports (e.g., golf, baseball, figure skating).[111] Low back pain is particularly prevalent, with some sport-specific studies reporting that nearly all athletes experience it at some point during athletic career.[112,113] From a biomechanical perspective, the two primary causes are overuse and poor mechanics. Prevention strategies often center around increasing core muscle strength to better support the repetitive movement demand of the sport and improving technique to leverage the strengthened core muscles.

9.9 Clinical Pearls

- Understanding fundamental biomechanics of brain and spinal injury in sport gives insight into the mechanisms of injury and spurs the development of prevention strategies.
- Both linear and rotational accelerations contribute to brain injury; however, rotational head motion more directly leads to diffuse brain injuries such as concussion.
- The likelihood of injury depends on the direction of head acceleration, with coronal and axial loading being more injurious than movement in the sagittal plane.
- An absolute biomechanical threshold of brain injury may not exist. Evidence suggests that loading conditions that cause brain injury may be individualized and dependent on an athlete's impact density, previous injury history, and other personalized characteristics such as genetics.
- Strategies to minimize brain injury in sport should consider all levels in the hierarchy of hazard control. These include elimination (e.g., removal from sport), substitution (e.g., flag football for contact football), engineering controls (e.g., high-quality playing surfaces), administrative controls (e.g., improved and enforced rules of the game), and personalized protective equipment (e.g., helmets).
- Contemporary head protection, including helmets, soft headgear, and helmet add-ons, that uses innovative materials or structure shows promise in mitigating the head loading that leads to concussion. Further research must link

demonstrated benefits in the laboratory to injury reductions on-field.

- Minor injuries to the cervical and lumbar spine in sport are common and derive from strain on the muscles and activation of the pain receptors in the facet joints, often from overuse or poor mechanics.
- Disabling sports injuries of the cervical spine are rare. Prevention strategies focus on environmental and administrative controls that limit scenarios of direct head impact where the cervical spine is required to withstand the forces and moments caused by the continued momentum of the moving torso.

References

[1] Funk JR, Cormier JM, Bain CE, Guzman H, Bonugli E, Manoogian SJ. Head and neck loading in everyday and vigorous activities. Ann Biomed Eng. 2011; 39(2):766–776

[2] Miller LE, Urban JE, Whelan VM, Baxter WW, Tatter SB, Stitzel JD. An envelope of linear and rotational head motion during everyday activities. Biomech Model Mechanobiol. 2020; 19(3):1003–1014

[3] Reynolds BB, Patrie J, Henry EJ, et al. Comparative analysis of head impact in contact and collision sports. J Neurotrauma. 2017; 34(1):38–49

[4] Nguyen JVK, Brennan JH, Mitra B, Willmott C. Frequency and magnitude of game-related head impacts in male contact sports athletes: a systematic review and meta-analysis. Sports Med. 2019; 49(10):1575–1583

[5] Huber CM, Patton DA, McDonald CC, et al. Sport- and gender-based differences in head impact exposure and mechanism in high school sports. Orthop J Sports Med. 2021; 9(3):2325967120984423

[6] Ommaya AK, Thibault L, Bandak F. Mechanisms of impact head injury. Int J Impact Eng. 1994; 15(4):535–560

[7] Holbourn AHS. Mechanics of head injuries. Lancet. 1943; 242(6267): 438–441

[8] Lissner HR, Lebow M, Evans FG. Experimental studies on the relation between acceleration and intracranial pressure changes in man. Surg Gynecol Obstet. 1960; 111(3):329–338

[9] Gadd CW. Use of a weighted-impulse criterion for estimating injury hazard. Paper presented at: 10th Stapp Car Crash Conference. Otero County, NM: SAE; 1966:164–174

[10] National Operating Committee on Standards for Athletic Equipment. Standard Performance Specification for Newly Manufactured Football Helmets. NOCSAE (ND)002-17m19. Overland Park, KS: NOCSAE; 2019

[11] NHTSA. Occupant Crash Protection - Head Injury Criterion. FMVSS 208. Washington, DC: Office of Regulatory Analysis, Plans and Policy; 1972

[12] Pudenz RH, Shelden CH. The lucite calvarium; a method for direct observation of the brain; cranial trauma and brain movement. J Neurosurg. 1946; 3(6):487–505

[13] Ommaya AK, Rockoff SD, Baldwin M. Experimental concussion; a first report. J Neurosurg. 1964; 21(4):249–265

[14] Ommaya AK, Hirsch AE. Tolerances for cerebral concussion from head impact and whiplash in primates. J Biomech. 1971; 4(1):13–21

[15] Gennarelli TA, Thibault LE, Ommaya AK. Comparison of translational and rotational head motions in experimental cerebral concussion. Paper presented at: 15th Stapp Car Crash Conference. Coronado, CA: SAE; 1971:797–803

[16] Kuo C, Patton D, Rooks T, et al. On-field deployment and validation for wearable devices. Ann Biomed Eng. 2022; 50(11):1372–1388

[17] Tierney GJ, Simms CK. Can tackle height influence head injury assessment risk in elite rugby union? J Sci Med Sport. 2018; 21(12):1210–1214

[18] Ommaya AK, et al. Scaling of experimental data on cerebral concussion in sub-human primates to concussion threshold for man. Paper presented at: 11th Stapp Car Crash Conference. Anaheim, CA: SAE; 1967:73–80

[19] Margulies SS, Thibault LE. A proposed tolerance criterion for diffuse axonal injury in man. J Biomech. 1992; 25(8):917–923

[20] Panzer MB, Wood GW, Bass CR. Scaling in neurotrauma: how do we apply animal experiments to people? Exp Neurol. 2014; 261:120–126

[21] Wu T, Antona-Makoshi J, Alshareef A, Giudice JS, Panzer MB. Investigation of cross-species scaling methods for traumatic brain injury using finite element analysis. J Neurotrauma. 2020; 37(2):410–422

[22] Newman JA, Beusenberg MC, Fournier E, et al. A new biomechanical assessment of mild traumatic brain injury: part 1 - methodology. Paper presented at: International Research Council on the Biomechanics of Impact Conference. Sitges, Spain: IRCOBI; 1999:17–36

[23] Newman JA, Barr C, Beusenberg MC, et al. A new biomechanical assessment of mild traumatic brain injury: part 2 - results and conclusions. Paper presented at: International Research Council on the Biomechanics of Impact Conference. Montpellier, France: IRCOBI; 2000:223–233

[24] Newman JA, Beusenberg MC, Shewchenko N, Withnall C, Fournier E. Verification of biomechanical methods employed in a comprehensive study of mild traumatic brain injury and the effectiveness of American football helmets. J Biomech. 2005; 38(7):1469–1481

[25] Sanchez EJ, Gabler LF, Good AB, Funk JR, Crandall JR, Panzer MB. A reanalysis of football impact reconstructions for head kinematics and finite element modeling. Clin Biomech (Bristol, Avon). 2019; 64:82–89

[26] McIntosh AS, Patton DA, Fréchède B, Pierré PA, Ferry E, Barthels T. The biomechanics of concussion in unhelmeted football players in Australia: a case-control study. BMJ Open. 2014; 4(5):e005078

[27] Patton DA, Huber CM, Jain D, et al. Head impact sensor studies in sports: a systematic review of exposure confirmation methods. Ann Biomed Eng. 2020; 48(11):2497–2507

[28] Rowson S, Duma SM. Development of the STAR evaluation system for football helmets: integrating player head impact exposure and risk of concussion. Ann Biomed Eng. 2011; 39(8):2130–2140

[29] Rowson S, Duma SM, Beckwith JG, et al. Rotational head kinematics in football impacts: an injury risk function for concussion. Ann Biomed Eng. 2012; 40(1):1–13

[30] Campolettano ET, Gellner RA, Smith EP, et al. Development of a concussion risk function for a youth population using head linear and rotational acceleration. Ann Biomed Eng. 2020; 48(1):92–103

[31] Daniel RP, Patrick LM. Instrument panel impact study. Paper presented at: 9th Stapp Car Crash Conference. Minneapolis, MN: SAE; 1965:165–179

[32] Mertz HFJ Jr, Prasad P, Nusholtz GS. Head injury risk assessment for forehead impacts. Paper presented at: International Congress & Exposition. Detroit, MI: SAE; 1996:1–21

[33] Pellman EJ, Viano DC, Tucker AM, Casson IR, Waeckerle JF. Concussion in professional football: reconstruction of game impacts and injuries. Neurosurgery. 2003; 53(4):799–812, discussion 812–814

[34] Guskiewicz KM, Mihalik JP. Biomechanics of sport concussion: quest for the elusive injury threshold. Exerc Sport Sci Rev. 2011; 39(1):4–11

[35] Mihalik JP, Lynall RC, Wasserman EB, Guskiewicz KM, Marshall SW. Evaluating the "threshold theory": can head impact indicators help? Med Sci Sports Exerc. 2017; 49(2):247–253

[36] Rowson S, Duma SM, Stemper BD, et al. Correlation of concussion symptom profile with head impact biomechanics: a case for individual-specific injury tolerance. J Neurotrauma. 2018; 35(4):681–690

[37] Rowson S, Campolettano ET, Duma SM, et al. Accounting for variance in concussion tolerance between individuals: comparing head accelerations between concussed and physically matched control subjects. Ann Biomed Eng. 2019; 47(10):2048–2056

[38] Beckwith JG, Greenwald RM, Chu JJ, et al. Head impact exposure sustained by football players on days of diagnosed concussion. Med Sci Sports Exerc. 2013; 45(4):737–746

[39] Broglio SP, Lapointe A, O'Connor KL, McCrea M. Head impact density: a model to explain the elusive concussion threshold. J Neurotrauma. 2017; 34 (19):2675–2683

[40] Jadischke R, Viano DC, Dau N, King AI, McCarthy J. On the accuracy of the Head Impact Telemetry (HIT) system used in football helmets. J Biomech. 2013; 46(13):2310–2315

[41] Allison MA, Kang YS, Maltese MR, Bolte JH, IV, Arbogast KB. Measurement of Hybrid III head impact kinematics using an accelerometer and gyroscope system in ice hockey helmets. Ann Biomed Eng. 2015; 43(8): 1896–1906

[42] Siegmund GP, Guskiewicz KM, Marshall SW, DeMarco AL, Bonin SJ. Laboratory validation of two wearable sensor systems for measuring head impact severity in football players. Ann Biomed Eng. 2016; 44(4):1257–1274

[43] McIntosh AS, Willmott C, Patton DA, et al. An assessment of the utility and functionality of wearable head impact sensors in Australian Football. J Sci Med Sport. 2019; 22(7):784–789

[44] Patton DA, Huber CM, McDonald CC, Margulies SS, Master CL, Arbogast KB. Video confirmation of head impact sensor data from high school soccer players. Am J Sports Med. 2020; 48(5):1246–1253

[45] Tyson AM, Duma SM, Rowson S. Laboratory evaluation of low-cost wearable sensors for measuring head impacts in sports. J Appl Biomech. 2018; 34(4): 320–326

[46] Patton DA, Huber CM, Douglas EC, Seacrist T, Arbogast KB. Laboratory assessment of a head impact sensor for youth soccer ball heading impacts using an anthropomorphic test device. Proc Inst Mech Eng P J Sport Eng Technol. 2024; 238(1): 36–43

[47] Wu LC, Nangia V, Bui K, et al. In vivo evaluation of wearable head impact sensors. Ann Biomed Eng. 2016; 44(4):1234–1245

[48] Kieffer EE, Begonia MT, Tyson AM, Rowson S. A two-phased approach to quantifying head impact sensor accuracy: in-laboratory and on-field assessments. Ann Biomed Eng. 2020; 48(11):2613–2625

[49] Wu LC, Kuo C, Loza J, et al. Detection of American football head impacts using biomechanical features and support vector machine classification. Sci Rep. 2017; 8(1):855

[50] Arbogast KB, Caccese JB, Buckley TA, et al. Consensus Head Acceleration Measurement Practices (CHAMP): origins, methods, transparency and disclosure. Ann Biomed Eng. 2022; 50(11):1317–1345

[51] Ji S, Ghajari M, Mao H, et al. Use of brain biomechanical models for monitoring impact exposure in contact sports. Ann Biomed Eng. 2022; 50 (11):1389–1408

[52] Kleiven S. Evaluation of head injury criteria using a finite element model validated against experiments on localized brain motion, intracerebral acceleration, and intracranial pressure. Int J Crashworthiness. 2006; 11 (1):65–79

[53] Zhou Z, Li X, Kleiven S, Shah CS, Hardy WN. A reanalysis of experimental brain strain data: implication for finite element head model validation. Stapp Car Crash J. 2018; 62(07):293–318

[54] Kleiven S. Predictors for traumatic brain injuries evaluated through accident reconstructions. Stapp Car Crash J. 2007; 51:81–114

[55] Patton DA, McIntosh AS, Kleiven S. The biomechanical determinants of concussion: finite element simulations to investigate brain tissue deformations during sporting impacts to the unprotected head. J Appl Biomech. 2013; 29(6):721–730

[56] Patton DA, McIntosh AS, Kleiven S. The biomechanical determinants of concussion: finite element simulations to investigate tissue-level predictors of injury during sporting impacts to the unprotected head. J Appl Biomech. 2015; 31(4):264–268

[57] Cecchi NJ, Domel AG, Liu Y, et al. Identifying factors associated with head impact kinematics and brain strain in high school American football via instrumented mouthguards. Ann Biomed Eng. 2021; 49(10): 2814–2826

[58] Zhan X, Liu Y, Raymond S, et al. Rapid estimation of entire brain strain using deep learning models. IEEE Trans Biomed Eng. 2021; 68(11):3424–3434

[59] Ghazi K, Wu S, Zhao W, Ji S. Instantaneous whole-brain strain estimation in dynamic head impact. J Neurotrauma. 2021; 38(8):1023–1035

[60] Alshareef A, Wu T, Giudice JS, Panzer MB. Toward subject-specific evaluation: methods of evaluating finite element brain models using experimental high-rate rotational brain motion. Biomech Model Mechanobiol. 2021; 20(6): 2301–2317

[61] Ho J, Von Holst H, Kleiven S. Automatic generation and validation of patient-specific finite element head models suitable for crashworthiness analysis. Int J Crashworthiness. 2009; 14(6):555–563

[62] Mao H, Zhang L, Jiang B, et al. Development of a finite element human head model partially validated with thirty five experimental cases. J Biomech Eng. 2013; 135(11):111002

[63] Gennarelli TA, Thibault LE, Adams JH, Graham DI, Thompson CJ, Marcincin RP. Diffuse axonal injury and traumatic coma in the primate. Ann Neurol. 1982; 12(6):564–574

[64] Eucker SA, Smith C, Ralston J, Friess SH, Margulies SS. Physiological and histopathological responses following closed rotational head injury depend on direction of head motion. Exp Neurol. 2011; 227(1):79–88

[65] McIntosh AS, McCrory P, Comerford J. The dynamics of concussive head impacts in rugby and Australian rules football. Med Sci Sports Exerc. 2000; 32(12):1980–1984

[66] Lessley DJ, Kent RW, Funk JR, et al. Video analysis of reported concussion events in the National Football League during the 2015–2016 and 2016–2017 seasons. Am J Sports Med. 2018; 46(14):3502–3510

[67] Fentem PH. ABC of sports medicine. Benefits of exercise in health and disease. BMJ. 1994; 308(6939):1291–1295

[68] Lynall RC, Lempke LB, Johnson RS, Anderson MN, Schmidt JD. A comparison of youth flag and tackle football head impact biomechanics. J Neurotrauma. 2019; 36(11):1752–1757

[69] Mills NJ. Foam protection in sport. In: Jenkins M, ed. Materials in Sports Equipment. Boca Raton, FL: CRC Press; 2003:9–46

[70] Kent R, Forman J, Bailey AM, et al. The biomechanics of concussive helmet-to-ground impacts in the National Football league. J Biomech. 2020; 99: 109551

[71] Baker HP, Volchenko E, Athiviraham A. Does the MLB's collision at home plate rule change prevent concussion injuries in catchers? Phys Sportsmed. 2020; 48(3):354–357

[72] Stemper BD, Shah AS, Harezlak J, et al. And the CARE Consortium Investigators. Repetitive head impact exposure in college football following an NCAA rule change to eliminate two-a-day preseason practices: a study from the NCAA-DoD CARE consortium. Ann Biomed Eng. 2019; 47(10): 2073–2085

[73] Raftery M, Tucker R, Falvey ÉC. Getting tough on concussion: how welfare-driven law change may improve player safety-a Rugby Union experience. Br J Sports Med. 2020; 55(10):527–529

[74] Williamson RA, Kolstad AT, Krolikowski M, et al. Incidence of head contacts, penalties, and player contact behaviors in youth ice hockey: evaluating the "zero tolerance for head contact" policy change. Orthop J Sports Med. 2021; 9(3):2325967121992375

[75] Wahlquist VE, Glutting JJ, Kaminski TW. Examining the influence of the Get aHEAD Safely in Soccer™ program on head impact kinematics and neck strength in female youth soccer players. Res Sports Med. 2024; 32 (1):17–27

[76] McIntosh AS, Andersen TE, Bahr R, et al. Sports helmets now and in the future. Br J Sports Med. 2011; 45(16):1258–1265

[77] Kleiven S. Why most traumatic brain injuries are not caused by linear acceleration but skull fractures are. Front Bioeng Biotechnol. 2013; 1:15

[78] Newman JA. Biomechanics of human trauma: head protection. In: Nahum AM, Melvin JW, eds. Accidental Injury: Biomechanics and Prevention. New York, NY: Springer; 1993:292–310

[79] Hansen K, Dau N, Feist F, et al. Angular impact mitigation system for bicycle helmets to reduce head acceleration and risk of traumatic brain injury. Accid Anal Prev. 2013; 59:109–117

[80] Bottlang M, Rouhier A, Tsai S, Gregoire J, Madey SM. Impact performance comparison of advanced bicycle helmets with dedicated rotation-damping systems. Ann Biomed Eng. 2020; 48(1):68–78

[81] DiGiacomo G, Tsai S, Bottlang M. Impact performance comparison of advanced snow sport helmets with dedicated rotation-damping systems. Ann Biomed Eng. 2021; 49(10):2805–2813

[82] Chung VWJ, Dias L, Booth G, Cripton PA. Incorporating neck biomechanics in helmet testing: evaluation of commercially available WaveCel helmets. Clin Biomech (Bristol, Avon). 2022; 94:105628

[83] Patton DA, Mohammadi R, Halldin PH, et al. Radial and oblique impact testing of alpine helmets onto snow surfaces. Appl Sci (Basel). 2023; 13 (6):3455

[84] Whyte T, Stuart C, Mallory A, et al. A review of impact testing methods for headgear in sports: considerations for improved prevention of head injury through research and standards. J Biomech Eng. 2019; 141(7):070803

[85] Halldin P, Kleiven S. The development of next generation test standards for helmets. Paper presented at: 1st International Conference on Helmet Performance and Design. London, England; 2013:1–8

[86] Diekfuss JA, Yuan W, Dudley JA, et al. Evaluation of the effectiveness of newer helmet designs with emergent shell and padding technologies versus older helmet models for preserving white matter following a season of high school football. Ann Biomed Eng. 2021; 49(10):2863–2874

[87] Breedlove KM, Breedlove E, Nauman E, Bowman TG, Lininger MR. The ability of an aftermarket helmet add-on device to reduce impact-force accelerations during drop tests. J Athl Train. 2017; 52(9):802–808

[88] Cecchi NJ, Callan AA, Watson LP, et al. Padded helmet shell covers in American football: a comprehensive laboratory evaluation with preliminary on-field findings. Ann Biomed Eng. 2023; e-pub ahead of print. DOI: 10.1007/s10439-023-03169-2

[89] O'Connell K, Brown C, Tripp PM. American Football soft-shell helmet covers reduce head impact severity: a critically appraised topic. Int J Athl Ther Train. 2023; 28:228–233

[90] Bailey AM, Funk JR, Crandall JR, Myers BS, Arbogast KB. Laboratory evaluation of shell add-on products for american football helmets for professional linemen. Ann Biomed Eng. 2021; 49(10):2747–2759

[91] National Football League. Guardian Cap results: "exceeded our expectations". Accessed July 10, 2023 at: https://www.nfl.com/playerhealthandsafety/equipment-and-innovation/engineering-technology/guardian-cap-results-exceeded-our-expectations. Published September 2022

[92] Patton DA, McIntosh AS. Considerations for the performance requirements and technical specifications of soft-shell padded headgear. Proc Inst Mech Eng P J Sport Eng Technol. 2016; 230(1):29–42

[93] McIntosh AS, McCrory P. Impact energy attenuation performance of football headgear. Br J Sports Med. 2000; 34(5):337–341

[94] Hrysomallis C. Impact energy attentuation of protective football headgear against a yielding surface. J Sci Med Sport. 2004; 7(2):156–164

[95] McIntosh A, McCrory P, Finch CF. Performance enhanced headgear: a scientific approach to the development of protective headgear. Br J Sports Med. 2004; 38(1):46–49

[96] Stitt D, Kabaliuk N, Alexander K, Draper N. Potential of soft-shell rugby headgear to mitigate linear and rotational peak accelerations. Ann Biomed Eng. 2022; 50(11):1546–1564

[97] McGuine T, Post E, Pfaller AY, et al. Does soccer headgear reduce the incidence of sport-related concussion? A cluster, randomised controlled trial of adolescent athletes. Br J Sports Med. 2020; 54(7):408–413

[98] McIntosh AS, McCrory P, Finch CF, Best JP, Chalmers DJ, Wolfe R. Does padded headgear prevent head injury in rugby union football? Med Sci Sports Exerc. 2009; 41(2):306–313

[99] Stokes KA, Cross M, Williams S, et al. Padded headgear does not reduce the incidence of match concussions in professional men's rugby union: a case-control study of 417 cases. Int J Sports Med. 2021; 42(10):930–935

[100] Willmott C, Reyes J, K Nguyen JV, et al. A pilot case crossover study of the use of padded headgear in junior Australian football. Concussion. 2023; 7(4):CNC99

[101] Makovec Knight J, Mitra B, McIntosh A, et al. The association of padded headgear with concussion and injury risk in junior Australian football: a prospective cohort study. J Sci Med Sport. 2022; 25(4):312–320

[102] Broglio SP, Williams RM, O'Connor KL, Goldstick J. Football players' head-impact exposure after limiting of full-contact practices. J Athl Train. 2016; 51(7):511–518

[103] Chrisman SPD, Ebel BE, Stein E, Lowry SJ, Rivara FP. Head impact exposure in youth soccer and variation by age and sex. Clin J Sport Med. 2019; 29 (1):3–10

[104] Chung AS, Makovicka JL, Hassebrock JD, et al. Epidemiology of cervical injuries in NCAA football players. Spine. 2019; 44(12):848–854

[105] Deckey DG, Makovicka JL, Chung AS, et al. Neck and cervical spine injuries in National College Athletic Association athletes: a 5-year epidemiologic study. Spine. 2020; 45(1):55–64

[106] Kepler CK, Vaccaro AR. Injuries and abnormalities of the cervical spine and return to play criteria. Clin Sports Med. 2012; 31(3):499–508

[107] Cavanaugh JM, Lu Y, Chen C, Kallakuri S. Pain generation in lumbar and cervical facet joints. J Bone Joint Surg Am. 2006; 88 Suppl 2:63–67

[108] McElhaney JH, Myers BS. Biomechanical aspects of cervical trauma. In: Nahum AM, Melvin JW, eds. Accidental Injury: Biomechanics and Prevention. New York, NY: Springer; 1993:311–361

[109] Myers BS, Winkelstein BA. Epidemiology, classification, mechanism, and tolerance of human cervical spine injuries. Crit Rev Biomed Eng. 1995; 23 (5–6):307–409

[110] Winkelstein BA, Myers BS. The biomechanics of cervical spine injury and implications for injury prevention. Med Sci Sports Exerc. 1997; 29(7) Suppl: S246–S255

[111] Ball JR, Harris CB, Lee J, Vives MJ. Lumbar spine injuries in sports: review of the literature and current treatment recommendations. Sports Med Open. 2019; 5(1):26

[112] Wilson F, Ardern CL, Hartvigsen J, et al. Prevalence and risk factors for back pain in sports: a systematic review with meta-analysis. Br J Sports Med. 2020; 55(11):601–607

[113] Trompeter K, Fett D, Platen P. Prevalence of back pain in sports: a systematic review of the literature. Sports Med. 2017; 47(6):1183–1207

10 Nonsurgical Treatment of Spinal Injuries

Mitchell J. Christiansen, Michael D. White, Jeff Ehresman, Joseph D. DiDomenico, and Randall W. Porter

Summary

Athletes at both elite and amateur levels are subjected to unique forces to the spinal column that can lead to injuries uncommon in the general population. Injuries can range in severity from mild cervical or lumbar strain and sprain injuries, disk herniations, bulges, and ligamentous injuries to debilitating three-column injuries that result in spinal cord injury. Nonoperative management is often the preferred modality for treating less serious injuries. However, deciding whether to operate requires consideration of neurologic integrity, spinal stability, spinal alignment, and how the injury responds to conservative measures. Imaging and complete physical examinations with close follow-up are imperative in this patient population to allow for safe short return-to-play intervals. Despite improvements in managing the wide array of sports-related spine injuries, clear return-to-play guidelines remain poorly defined in this population.

Keywords: cervical, fracture, herniation, lumbar, nonsurgical, return-to-play, sports, thoracic

10.1 Introduction

Spine injuries are a significant problem faced by both elite athletes and physically active members of the general population.[1,2] A meta-analysis of six studies found that the lifetime prevalence of back pain in athletes across any anatomic region of the spine is between 47 and 90%.[2] These injuries can range from mild cervical strain to neuropraxia or complete spinal cord injury (SCI). The focus of this chapter is to describe the management of nonsurgical spine injuries, which may include strains or sprains to the supporting muscles, ligaments, and tendons; disk bulges; foraminal compromise; annular tears; and disk herniations.

It is well known that physical activity can increase the risk of back pain.[3,4] However, there is also evidence that strenuous exercise can prevent back pain.[5,6] Studies have hypothesized a U-shaped dose–response curve, indicating that, although a sedentary lifestyle can have deleterious effects on spine health, there are also potential risks associated with highly strenuous activity.[3,4,7] Athletes, especially those involved in contact sports, can be subjected to high levels of physical strain and high-speed force imparted on the cervical, thoracic, and lumbar spine, which places them at increased risk of injury to the spine and surrounding structures.

Spine injuries among athletes can differ from those in the general population in that there are often specific forces exerted on an athlete's spine related to the particular sport played. Generally, back and neck pain among athletes leads to increased treatment costs, lost playing time, decreased quality of life, and decreased performance.[8] Contact sports, in particular, can lead to axial load injuries of the cervical spine. Lumbar and thoracic soft-tissue injuries can result from axial load, a direct blow to the anatomy of the spine, hyperflexion, hyperextension, or rotational forces.

10.2 General Considerations and Initial Assessment

If an injury to the spine is suspected in an athlete, initial evaluation should begin with an on-field or sideline evaluation. On-field assessments should begin with identification of any neurological deficits through a detailed examination of the player's motor function, sensation, and reflexes. Although rare, more serious injuries, such as SCI, should be ruled out prior to further workup. If the player is exhibiting radicular symptoms or soft-tissue injury, the athlete can be escorted to the sidelines for further evaluation by the medical staff and athletic trainer. The context in which the injury occurred should be determined, and it can be helpful to review video of the incident when available. The patient's symptoms and location of any pain should also be clearly identified to help localize the region of injury.

Further evaluation on the sideline can focus on assessing the location and severity of pain, aggravating and alleviating factors, active and passive range of motion, and gait. Of note, players with suspected cervical spine injuries should also be assessed for concussion using the Sport Concussion Assessment Tool, because these injuries can often occur simultaneously. Imaging with anteroposterior and lateral radiographs can assess for bony fractures or malalignment. However, computed tomography is generally recommended because it provides higher resolution to evaluate for traumatic pathology. Players who are experiencing neurological deficits or symptoms should undergo magnetic resonance imaging (MRI), which permits better assessment for disk herniation and bulging, integrity of ligamentous structures, and neural compression. In the following sections, management of nonsurgical injuries involving the cervical, thoracic, and lumbar spine will be discussed in further detail.

10.3 Cervical Spine

10.3.1 Epidemiology

Cervical spine injuries without SCI are common in contact sports and can range in severity from minor muscle sprains and strains to ligamentous strain, disk herniations, annular tears, symptomatic radiculopathy, and stingers and burners. These injuries are more common among athletes who participate in contact sports, but noncontact cervical spine injuries can also occur. American football, wrestling, and gymnastics have the highest incidence of cervical spine injuries in the United States.[9,10] In Canada, ice hockey is the sport that is associated with the highest number of cervical spine injuries, whereas in Europe, rugby has the highest incidence of such injuries.[11,12] A study of 11 National Football League (NFL) seasons found that 987 of 2,208 (44.7%) spine injuries occurred in the cervical spine, more than in any other area of the spine.[13]

10.3.2 Strain and Sprain

The most common cervical injuries are to the soft tissue and muscles of the neck. These injuries often present with neck pain, restricted range of motion, and unilateral muscle spasm. The mechanism of these injuries often involves whiplash, with rapid flexion-extension or lateral flexion-extension causing trauma to the soft tissue of the neck. These injuries are managed with conservative measures, including rest, physical therapy, muscle relaxants, and nonsteroidal anti-inflammatory drugs (NSAIDs).[14]

10.3.3 Ligamentous Injuries

The stability of the cervical spine relies heavily on ligamentous structures. Disruption of these structures often results in neurological compromise. Some of the more severe ligamentous injuries of the upper cervical spine include atlanto-occipital dislocations, atlantoaxial dislocations, transverse ligament disruptions, C2–C3 disk space disruption, and locked facet joints. These injuries are rare in the low-energy setting of most sports. The craniocervical junction is stabilized primarily by the ligamentous structures in the region, so injury involvement of these structures generally necessitates surgical intervention to prevent catastrophic neurological injury.[15]

10.3.4 Disk Bulge and Herniation

Cervical disk herniations, disk bulges, annular tears, and spondylosis are common throughout many sports but are particularly common in football, baseball, and soccer players.[16,17,18] These findings can have a significant impact on players' ability to participate in their sport. Schroeder et al[19] found that college football players entering the NFL draft with a history of cervical disk herniation were less likely to be drafted and played less total time professionally. Prior studies have found that the rate of cervical disk herniations is significantly higher in contact athletes than in the general population.[20] Additionally, the patterns of this pathology differ; cervical disk herniations in contact sports like football are most commonly seen at C3–C4 and C5–C6, whereas in the general population, the most common level is C6–C7.[21,22] Presenting symptoms will often include cervical neck pain, radicular pain, upper extremity numbness, myelopathy, weakness, or transient quadriplegia. Diagnosis is established with MRI, the imaging modality of choice for cervical disk herniation.[23]

Nonoperative management is recommended for the initial treatment of cervical disk herniation in athletes without neurological deficits or myelopathy. Conservative measures should include a trial of NSAIDs, physical therapy, suspension of participation and contact, and epidural steroid injections. Despite conflicting evidence, much of the literature recommends operative management after 6 months of conservative management if symptoms persist or if imaging reveals evidence of spinal cord or symptomatic root compression.[24] However, soft disk herniations will almost always resolve with conservative measures, although resolution can take up to 6 months. Studies in football players, rugby players, and Major League Baseball pitchers have found that superior outcomes are associated with operative management in cervical herniation refractory to conservative management.[12,25,26]

Case Example: Cervical Disk Herniation

A professional running back in his early 30 s was evaluated for injury during a game after experiencing hyperflexion of his neck while being tackled by another player. Upon sideline assessment, he was full strength with no neurological deficits, but he did report significant left trapezius pain and spasms. Further workup with MRI of his cervical spine demonstrated a C4–C5 cervical disk herniation eccentric to the left and causing foraminal stenosis (► Fig. 10.1). The player opted to be managed conservatively with rest, NSAIDs, and a cervical collar. The player was reevaluated 3 months after the injury, with complete resolution of his symptoms. Repeat MRI 3 months after the injury showed almost complete resolution of the disk. The successful recovery of this player with conservative management highlights the importance of trialing nonsurgical approaches for athletes with acute cervical disk herniations and the potential resolution of symptoms on radiographic findings with time.

10.3.5 Definition of Cervical Stenosis

Cervical stenosis has been defined in a variety of ways over the years in the literature, reflecting the evolving understanding of the condition and its clinical manifestations. One of the earliest definitions involved sagittal measurement of the spinal canal diameter.[27] A recent study found that a minimal disk-level diameter cutoff of 0.8 cm had the greatest positive predictive value (84%) for SCI following minor trauma.[28] Another historically prominent definition is the Torg ratio, calculated by dividing the sagittal diameter of the spinal canal by the sagittal diameter of the vertebral body.[29] A ratio of less than 0.8 is defined as significant spinal stenosis and associated with higher risk for neurological injury.[30] A third definition is based on the space available for the cord (SAC) ratio, which measures the sagittal diameter of the spinal cord divided by the sagittal diameter of the spinal canal. The SAC ratio theoretically provides a more accurate definition of cervical spinal stenosis. Some literature suggests that the sagittal diameters of vertebral disks are larger in athletic populations than in the general population, thus yielding lower Torg ratios.[31] The SAC ratio is not affected by this possibly confounding variable. In a study of 1,211 subjects, anteroposterior cervical spinal cord diameters were found to be independent of spinal canal diameter, and SAC ratios of 62% or greater were found to increase the risk of spinal cord compression.[32] This study implies that using only spinal cord diameter may not accurately assess the risk of cord compression. When choosing a particular method, the choice should be based on the specific clinical context and the aspects of cervical stenosis that need to be assessed.

10.3.6 Neuropraxia, Stingers, and Burners

Cervical cord neuropraxia is most common among football players.[30] This injury involves sensory symptoms such as burning, radiating pain, and tingling involving the extremities in a

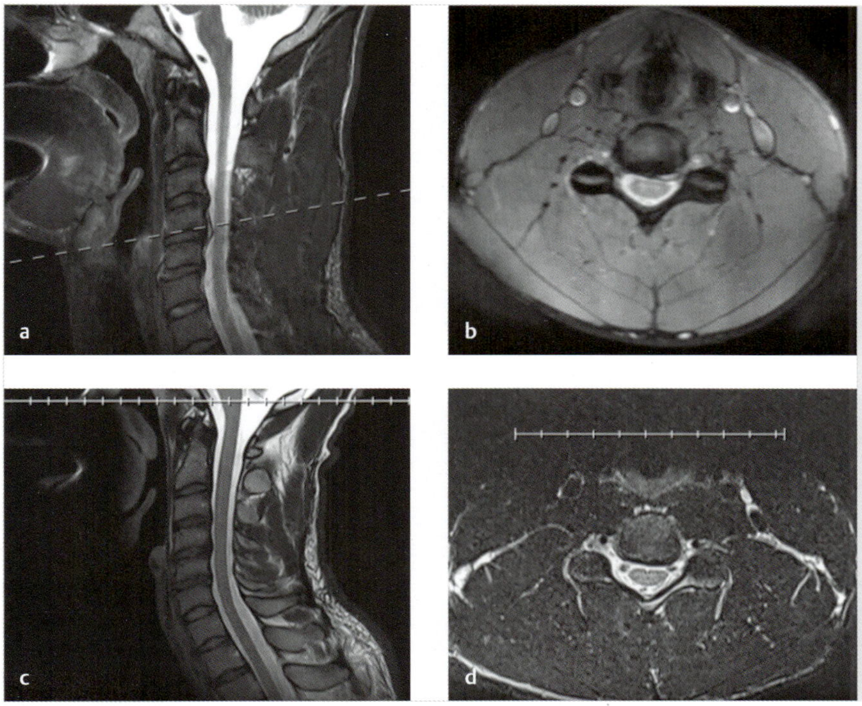

Fig. 10.1 Magnetic resonance imaging (MRI) of a football player in his early 30s with a C4–C5 cervical disk herniation after hyperflexing his neck following a tackle. Sagittal **(a)** and axial **(b)** T2-weighted MRI sequences show a C4–C5 cervical disk herniation that is eccentric to the left and causing foraminal stenosis at the time of injury. Sagittal **(c)** and axial **(d)** T2-weighted MRI sequences obtained at 3 months after the injury show almost complete resolution. (Used with permissions from Barrow Neurological Institute, Phoenix, Arizona.)

variety of distributions, including in the upper, lower, or ipsilateral extremities or all four extremities. Motor symptoms follow a similar anatomic distribution and can range in severity from paresthesia to weakness to paralysis. Importantly, neuropraxia usually resolves in less than 15 minutes and rarely lasts longer than 48 hours.[33] These injuries usually result from hyperextension or lateral compression of the cervical spine in which the canal diameter is narrowed. Preexisting cervical stenosis can put athletes at risk for neuropraxic injuries. Cervical traumatic neuropraxia is often managed conservatively if the symptoms resolve, but if the patient has persistent symptoms and a canal diameter of less than 8 mm, surgical intervention may be necessary.

Stingers and burners are common injuries that specifically refer to clinically mild cervical neuropraxia with more transient symptoms. In a study of 201 college football players, 65% reported having a stinger or burner in their 4-year career.[34] A stinger is often unilateral and is thought to be due to trauma to the brachial plexus, often caused by a tackle. Symptoms include sudden, sharp, stinging pain that radiates down the arm and then resolves in a matter of seconds to minutes. A burner injury exhibits a characteristic burning, radiates pain bilaterally, and can indicate underlying cervical stenosis. Stinger and burner injuries respond well to conservative management.

Case Example: Cervical Traumatic Neuropraxia

A professional football player in his mid-20s experienced loss of consciousness and transient quadriplegia after attempting a tackle on a kickoff. MRI following the injury did not show any T2 cord signal or other signs of traumatic injury, and the patient's cervical canal diameter at C5–C6 was measured at 10.4 mm at the time of initial injury. Repeat MRI 3 months later showed a canal diameter of 7.1 mm at the same C5–C6 level (▶ Fig. 10.2). This underscores the importance of exercising caution in treating players with small cervical canal diameter and their heightened susceptibility to neuropraxia. This player was cleared to return to play following resolution of symptoms and unremarkable imaging findings.

10.3.7 Fractures without SCI

Fractures of the upper cervical spine, such as hangman's or Jefferson fractures, are rare in sports. Injuries sustained while mountain biking have been reported as the most common cause of an upper cervical spine fracture in sports. In a Canadian study, 14 of 79 cervical spine injuries in mountain bikers were upper cervical fractures.[35] Odontoid fractures appear to be the most common upper cervical fracture.[35] In patients younger than 30 years, use of a hard cervical collar or halo vest is appropriate. For type I and III odontoid fractures without displacement or ligamentous injury, the use of a hard cervical collar or halo vest can promote healing of the fracture and high rates of fusion. The same conservative management can be used to treat type II fractures but is associated with a high rate of nonunion because such fractures occur at the watershed zone at the base of the dens. If there is no displacement or ligamentous disruption, other isolated C1 or C2 fractures, including bilateral hangman's fractures, can be treated conservatively with a hard cervical collar or halo vest for 6 to 12 weeks and may not require surgical intervention.[36]

One controversial pathology is that of incidentally found os odontoideum, a congenital abnormality of C2 with an isolated ossicle superior to and independent of a hypoplastic dens. Although the natural history of patients with os odontoideum in contact sports is not well-described, it is generally accepted

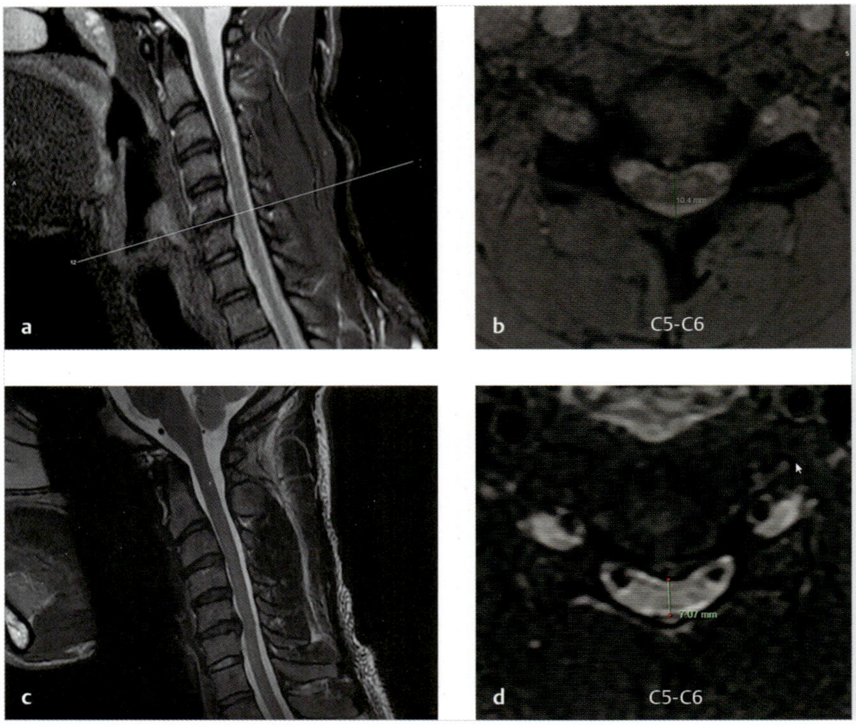

Fig. 10.2 Magnetic resonance imaging (MRI) of a football player in his mid-20s who experienced loss of consciousness and transient quadriplegia after attempting a tackle on a kickoff. Sagittal **(a)** and axial **(b)** MRI obtained at the time of the injury shows the spinal canal to be 10.4 mm in diameter. Sagittal **(c)** and axial **(d)** MRI obtained at 6 months after the injury showing a smaller canal diameter of 7 mm at C5–C6. (Used with permissions from Barrow Neurological Institute, Phoenix, Arizona.)

that these patients should refrain from playing contact sports given the high rate of instability at C1–C2 and higher risk for SCI.[37,38] Although definitive return-to-play guidelines have been difficult to establish, there is a general consensus that players who demonstrate radiographic healing of the fracture with normal alignment, unremarkable neurological examination findings, and pain-free full range of motion are able to safely resume training, followed by return to play.[36] Many surgeons will also recommend obtaining an MRI to ensure that there is no T2 cord signal before clearing the player to return to activities.[20,39] The presence of persistent T2 cord signal is considered a contraindication for returning to play even for asymptomatic patients.[20]

Compression and burst fractures of the cervical, thoracic, and lumbar spine can occur among athletes when a neutrally aligned spine is subjected to an axial load.[40] These injuries are often seen in mountain bikers and rugby players.[35,41] Most compression and burst fractures can be managed conservatively with a hard cervical orthosis. Surgical fixation is indicated for patients with three-column injuries, instability, severe canal compromise, or neurological deficits. These treatment decisions can be guided by the subaxial cervical spine injury classification score.[42] This score incorporates three categories for the surgeon to assess: the morphology of the fracture, the integrity of the diskoligamentous complex, and the patient's neurologic status and deficits. The scores from each category are added together, with a score of 3 or less suggesting nonoperative management, a score of 4 being indeterminate, and a score of 5 or more indicating the need for surgical treatment. Additionally, fractures involving more than 1 cm in height, causing a significant kyphotic deformity, or having greater than 40% lateral mass involvement should be managed operatively.[42] Return to play can be initiated for players with no neurological deficits, no cervical pain, full range of motion, and radiographic evidence of fusion and healing without T2 cord signal.

Unilateral and bilateral facet fractures can present with symptomatic cervical pain without neurological symptoms. Unilateral and nondisplaced facet fractures can be managed conservatively with a rigid cervical collar in many cases. Cervical spine MRI can be obtained to assess for disruption of the joint capsule. In addition, dynamic flexion-extension radiographs can show translation of the vertebral bodies suggesting instability. Unilateral facet fractures without disruption of the facet joint capsule and without instability on dynamic radiographs can be managed with a rigid cervical collar. Some players may experience persistent neck pain after 6 to 12 weeks despite wearing a collar. Persistent neck pain after a trial of rigid cervical collar constitutes failure of conservative management, and the patient should consider surgery. Players with no neurological symptoms, full range of motion, no neck pain, and healing of the fracture on radiographic follow-up can be cleared to return to play. Once again, MRI can be obtained before a return to team activities to ensure the absence of T2 cord signal. Fractures involving the bilateral facets will often present with some level of instability and are not generally amenable to nonoperative management. Similarly, injuries that include capsular disruption or dislocation are best treated surgically.

10.3.8 Return-to-Play Recommendations

Athletes with strains and sprains must have resolution of symptoms and normal range of motion before return to play. For individuals with stinger injuries, return to play can be immediate if symptoms last less than 5 minutes. Bilateral symptoms, such as in burners, or persistent neurological symptoms warrant removal from play and further imaging to assess the extent of injury. Generally, athletes with cervical neuropraxia of all clinical varieties should be allowed to return to play in the absence of neurological symptoms if they have full strength and range of motion and if cervical stenosis is absent on imaging.[43] Cervical canals should normally be 10 to 14 mm in diameter. Athletes whose cervical spinal canals measure less than 8 mm are at high risk for injury and should be considered on a case-by-case basis for return to play.

Players with cervical disk herniation often return to play after treatment, whether treatment is conservative or operative. The primary indication for operative management after conservative management is persistent symptomatic disk herniation despite conservative measures for at least 3 months, signal changes, or evidence of cord compression on MRI. Return to play is permitted for players with improved symptoms and imaging findings showing a lack of cord compression.

For individuals with sports-related fractures in the upper cervical spine, such as odontoid and C1/C2 fractures, return to play after conservative treatment emphasizes radiographic healing, unremarkable neurological examination findings, absence of T2 cord signal, and return of full range of motion. Similarly, for compression and burst fractures of the cervical spine that are managed conservatively, return to play is permitted with radiographic evidence of fusion and absent T2 signal along with no neurological deficits, full range of motion, and no pain. The same principles for return to play apply to players with unilateral and bilateral facet fractures.

10.4 Thoracic Injuries

10.4.1 Epidemiology

Sports-related injuries of the thoracic spine are less common than those of the cervical and lumbar spine. However, one study has shown that injuries to the thoracic spine may involve the greatest loss of playing time.[16] Anatomically, the thoracic spine has a "fourth" column consisting of the rib cage, costosternal, and costovertebral junctions, providing stability to T1–T8.[44] As a result, 75% of spinal fractures occur below the T8 level.[44]

10.4.2 Strain and Sprain

Strain and sprain generally result from overuse or overstretching of certain muscles. Muscle tenderness, localized pain, and limited range of motion are common in these injuries. Many of the superficial muscles, including latissimus dorsi, rhomboids, and trapezius, have significant interaction with thoracic spinous processes; consequently, sports that involve significant use of these muscles are associated with musculoligamentous injury. In sports that involve a violent rotational motion, it is common to experience a sprain injury on the side contralateral to the dominant throwing arm.[45] Sprain injuries are treated conservatively with rest, ice and heat, and NSAIDs.

10.4.3 Ligamentous Injuries

Ligamentous injuries can represent more serious injuries and can be diagnosed by the evidence of instability on plain films or short tau inversion recovery changes on MRI. The notable anatomy in this region includes the supraspinous ligament, interspinous ligament, facet joint capsules, and ligamentum flavum. These ligaments compose the posterior ligament complex that limits flexion of the spine. Most injuries to the posterior ligament complex involve high-energy trauma with seat belts. These injuries are rarely seen in sports. MRI remains the gold standard in diagnosis and assessment of the posterior ligamentous complex stability.[46]

10.4.4 Disk Bulge and Herniation

Thoracic disk herniation is relatively uncommon and unlikely to be symptomatic. Notably, the thoracic disk is more likely to have calcification or complete ossification.[47] Most thoracic herniations respond well to conservative management, with the exceptions of giant herniated disks and giant calcified herniated disks, which often cause progressively worsening myelopathy.

10.4.5 Neuropraxia

Neuropraxia involving the thoracic spine is not widely reported or extensively studied in the literature. The thoracic spine is relatively stable and, compared with other regions, is less prone to those injuries that cause nerve compression or neuropraxia.

10.4.6 Fractures without SCI

Although fractures in the thoracic region caused by high-energy trauma are relatively common in the general population, such fractures are rare in sports. The posterior elements can be injured with flexion injuries or direct blows. One such injury is the clay shoveler's fracture, which is an avulsion fracture of the spinous process of the lower cervical or upper thoracic vertebrae. It has been reported in a variety of sports, including golf, baseball, wrestling, running, and volleyball, to name a few. It can be caused by either a direct blow or repetitive overload causing a stress fracture.[48,49,50,51] Among rowers, it is common to have strains and stress fractures at T4–T7 due to rhomboid, latissimus dorsi, and erector spinae contraction.[45] These fractures have a high rate of union and are managed nonoperatively with rest, analgesics, and physical therapy.[48]

Compression fractures of the thoracic spine have also been reported in sports, such as in a report of T12 compression fracture in a teenage basketball player by McHugh-Pierzina et al.[52] These fractures are usually treated conservatively with a thoracolumbar spinal orthosis for 6 to 12 weeks and activity restriction.[53] Long-term considerations for these types of fractures include monitoring over time for the development kyphotic deformity, which is evaluated on standing scoliosis radiographs.

10.4.7 Return-to-Play Recommendations

The stability of the thoracic spine makes it less prone to injury. For strains and sprains, if symptoms are relatively mild, the player may be returned to play during the game. The thoracic spine fractures that happen in athletes, such as avulsions of spinous process and compression fractures, are often managed conservatively with excellent results. Adequate healing should be demonstrated on follow-up radiographs before the athlete returns to play.

10.5 Lumbar Injuries

10.5.1 Epidemiology

Injuries of the lumbar spine are common among athletes, and low back pain is estimated to affect 10 to 15% of athletes.[54] Low back pain is a common complaint in the general population, with a lifetime prevalence estimated at 75 to 84%, with the 1-year point prevalence for adults being 28.4%.[55,56] Compared to the thoracic spine, the lumbar spine is significantly more mobile, constituting a risk of fracture in a low-energy and repetitive-stress setting. The lower lumbar spine is also subjected to the greatest static axial forces, which predisposes it to disk degeneration. Athletes who perform squats or similar exercises and repetitive actions, such as rowing, are predisposed to disk herniations or annular tears.

10.5.2 Strain and Sprain

Sudden twisting or bending motions can injure the muscles and soft tissues of the lumbar spine. These injuries result in lower back pain and stiffness. These injuries are treated conservatively with rest, ice and heat, and NSAIDs. The player may return to play when they are asymptomatic for 2 weeks if imaging demonstrates absence of a disk herniation. Patients with disk degeneration and disk bulges may return to play when they report 2 weeks of no symptoms while participating in practice.

10.5.3 Ligamentous Injuries

Among athletes, the most commonly injured ligaments in the lumbar region are the sacroiliac joints, interspinous ligaments, and supraspinous ligaments. Sprains and tears of interspinous and supraspinous ligaments and tendons commonly occur in athletes and cause acute-onset back pain with localized tenderness and thickening.[57] Treatment of these sprains is conservative, involving rest until asymptomatic for at least 1 week. Sacroiliac joint dysfunction is another common problem for athletes in sports with repetitive and asymmetric loading of the joint, such as football, basketball, powerlifting, gymnastics, and golf.[58] Treatment is conservative, with activity modification.

10.5.4 Disk Bulge and Herniation

Lumbar disk herniation is highly prevalent among athletes and is a significant source of low back pain. Disk herniations account for 28% of lumbar spine injuries in football, usually in the L4–L5 or L5–S1 disk.[16] Among football players, lumbar spine injuries are most common among offensive and defensive linemen.[59] A study of 342 professional athletes found no significant difference in outcomes for nonsurgical and surgical treatments of lumbar disk herniation.[60] The same study found that Major League Baseball players who underwent microdiskectomy had significantly shorter careers.[60] A study from Japan that included 308 athletes found that 59.7% of college baseball players showed signs of disk degeneration, and 89.5% had low back pain at some point in their life.[61] A 17-year study of players in the National Basketball Association, which included 12,594 injuries among 6,145 players, found that 10.2% of all injuries (1,279 of 12,594 injuries) were lumbar spine injuries.[62] Lumbar disk degeneration comprised 0.9% of total injuries (110 of 12,594 injuries) but accounted for 2,151 (3.6%) of total games missed (2,151 of 59,179 games).[62]

Lumbar disk herniations can present with low back pain, radicular pain, and occasionally weakness. Some provocative tests, such as the straight leg raise (Lesgue test), can be used to test for lumbosacral nerve root irritation. Although this test may have positive results in the setting of a herniated lumbar disk, it is not specific and can have positive results in patients with many other lumbar pathologies. Initial treatments for herniated lumbar disks are conservative and include activity modification, anti-inflammatory medications, core strengthening, physical therapy, and epidural steroid injections.[60,63,64] Surgery is generally reserved for players for whom initial conservative management fails.

Careful consideration should be given to cases in which young athletes who participate in baseball, basketball, and gymnastics present with signs of spondylosis. Generally, spondylosis is managed conservatively in the absence of neurological signs or radiculopathy. The approach to management of lumbar disk herniation should be tailored to the individual athlete. Current guidelines support conservative management for 1 week to 6 months, followed by consultation with a spine surgeon if symptoms persist.

10.5.5 Spondylolysis and Spondylolisthesis

Several studies have shown increased radiographic degenerative changes in younger athletes who participate in baseball, basketball, swimming, and gymnastics.[61,62,65,66] Furthermore, the prevalence of spondylolysis is high in the athlete population, with an estimated 47% of young athletes who present with low back pain receiving a diagnosis of spondylolysis.[67] Lumbar isthmic spondylolysis is especially common among gymnasts due to repetitive hyperextension of the lumbar spine, resulting in chronic joint stress. The incidence of this injury is notably higher among gymnasts than among the general population (11% vs. 2.3%).[68] Definitive diagnosis of spondylolysis begins with anterior–posterior and lateral radiographs, followed by computed tomography to better view the pars interarticularis.[69] Conservative management with a hard brace has been shown to yield favorable results in 94% of patients with early spondylolysis, with the effectiveness of the treatment dependent on computed tomography and MRI signal intensities.[70] Bilateral pars defects, which progress to spondylolysis in approximately 85% of cases, can be initially managed through a combination of stabilization and physical therapy.[71,72] This treatment protocol typically involves use of a stabilization brace for 8 to 12 weeks in conjunction with a graduated exercise program featuring isometric core and hamstring exercises. If conservative measures fail, injection of the pars defect can be considered. If the latter does not provide relief, or if instability of greater than 4 mm is observed, consideration should be given to direct pars repair or lumbar fusion.

Lumbar isthmic spondylolisthesis refers to the displacement of lumbar vertebrae anteriorly with respect to the lower vertebrae and represents a more severe pathology on the continuum of spondylolysis injuries. For low-grade spondylolisthesis, treatment is nonoperative. Reports of unilateral acute pars defects in pediatric patients have demonstrated osseous healing with bracing for 3 to 6 months.[72,73] However, it is generally advised to discontinue bracing once symptoms have resolved, regardless of whether radiographic evidence of healing is found.[74]

10.5.6 Definition of Spinal Stenosis

Lumbar spinal stenosis, a condition characterized by narrowing of the spinal canal, can pose unique challenges to athletes, subjecting the vertebrae, ligaments, and disks to unique forces. Spinal stenosis is differentiated into three main types: central stenosis, lateral recess stenosis, and midzone stenosis. Central stenosis involves narrowing of the vertebral foramen due to bulging disks, osteophytes, and thickened yellow ligament. Lateral recess stenosis involves compression of the nerve roots in the foramen. Midzone stenosis refers to compression within the foraminal zone located anterior to the pars interarticularis. This type of stenosis is more commonly a result of spondylolysis.

10.5.7 Fractures without Instability

Severe unstable fractures and injuries to all three columns are rare in sports. More commonly seen are minor fractures involving the pars interarticularis, articular process, transverse process, vertebral end plate, or spinous process that can result from repetitive activity or low-energy impacts. Almost all of these fractures are treated conservatively with rest, ice, NSAIDs, muscle relaxants, and bracing.[64] Isolated unilateral facet fractures in the lumbar spine are treated in the same manner and rarely require surgical intervention.[75] When there is concern for a more severe thoracolumbar fracture that is potentially unstable, the thoracolumbar injury classification and severity score can help guide further treatment. This score is calculated by assessing the fracture morphology, the integrity of the posterior ligamentous complex, and the patient's neurological status (▶ Fig. 10.3). Points for each category are assigned, and the total number of points determines whether the fracture is stable and can be managed conservatively, indeterminate, or unstable and requires surgery. The thoracolumbar injury classification and severity score is detailed in Chapter 8.

10.5.8 Return-to-Play Recommendations

A systematic review found that, among athletes with lumbar disk herniation, operative and nonoperative groups have comparable return-to-play outcomes.[64] Two studies showed that the number of players who returned to play and the number of games played were lower for National Basketball Association players who received surgical treatment for lumbar disk herniation.[76,77] The return-to-play criteria for lumbar disk herniation involve symptom resolution, restoration of full range of motion, and the ability to perform sport-specific movement without pain regardless of operative or nonoperative management.

Return-to-play guidelines are varied after nonsurgical treatment of spondylolysis, but returning to competitive play after 2 to 12 weeks of treatment and symptom resolution has been effective.[72,73,78] In a study of 73 patients with spondylolysis managed conservatively with a Boston Overlap Brace, 80% returned to play in 4 to 6 weeks.[79] Miller et al reported excellent long-term outcomes and high return-to-play rates (91%) in patients with spondylolysis and spondylolisthesis managed

TLICS: Three Independent predictors				
1	**Morphology** Immediate stability	- Compression - Burst - Translation/rotation - Distraction	1 2 3 4	- Radiographs - CT
2	**Integrity of PLC** Long-term stability	- Intact - Suspected - Injured	0 2 3	- MRI
3	**Neurological status**	- Intact - Nerve root - Complete cord - Incomplete cord - Cauda equina	0 2 2 3 3	- Physical examination
	Predicts	**- Need for surgery**	0–3 4 >4	- Nonsurgical - Surgeon's choice - Surgical

Fig. 10.3 Thoracolumbar Injury Classification and Severity Score (TLICS). CT, computed tomography; MRI, magnetic resonance imaging; PLC, posterior ligamentous complex. (Reproduced with permission from Radiology Assistant www.radiologyassistant.nl]).

nonoperatively if the initial slip was less than 30%.[80] All of the patients in this cohort improved with conservative management and returned to their respective sports; at longest follow-up, only 22% of athletes limited their recreational activities.[80] An important return-to-play consideration in spondylolysis is to confirm bony union with radiographs.[81]

Fractures of the lumbar spine are often conservatively managed with bracing, and patients should expect to return to play when their preinjury activity level is possible without pain and there is radiographic evidence of bone healing.

10.6 Conclusion

Activity in various sports introduces unique mechanisms of force that can lead to spinal injuries in a young population. The decision regarding operative versus nonoperative management is often guided by the principles of neurologic integrity, stability, and alignment. Regardless of the treatment, imaging and close clinical follow-up are important, especially when the patient's return to play is being considered. Generally, the decision to allow an athlete to return to play is made when the player is neurologically intact, free of symptoms, and has a full range of motion without pain.

10.7 Clinical Pearls

- Sprains, strains, burners, and stingers are spine injuries that can often be managed conservatively with rest, physical therapy, and NSAIDs.
- Nonoperative management is recommended for the initial treatment of disk herniations in patients without myelopathy, with operative management generally recommended if symptoms persist after 6 months.
- Neuropraxia is common among football players and includes burning, radiating pain, and tingling, often stemming from hyperextension. Although they may initially raise concern for cord injury, symptoms usually resolve quickly.
- Return-to-play recommendations vary based on the athletic sport and type of injury, but generally require resolution of symptoms and normal range of motion before return can be considered. Athletes with fractures should show evidence of healing on radiographic imaging before returning to play.

10.8 Disclosures

The authors have no personal, financial, or institutional interest in any of the drugs, materials, or devices described in this manuscript.

Acknowledgments

We thank the staff of Neuroscience Publications at Barrow Neurological Institute for assistance with manuscript preparation.

References

[1] Fett D, Trompeter K, Platen P. P-27 Epidemiology of back pain in sports: a cross-sectional study. Br J Sports Med. 2016; 50 Suppl 1:A46.1–A46

[2] Trompeter K, Fett D, Platen P. Prevalence of back pain in sports: a systematic review of the literature. Sports Med. 2017; 47(6):1183–1207

[3] Vuori IM. Dose-response of physical activity and low back pain, osteoarthritis, and osteoporosis. Med Sci Sports Exerc. 2001; 33(6) Suppl: S551–S586, discussion 609–610

[4] Heneweer H, Staes F, Aufdemkampe G, van Rijn M, Vanhees L. Physical activity and low back pain: a systematic review of recent literature. Eur Spine J. 2011; 20(6):826–845

[5] Rainville J, Hartigan C, Martinez E, Limke J, Jouve C, Finno M. Exercise as a treatment for chronic low back pain. Spine J. 2004; 4(1):106–115

[6] Shiri R, Coggon D, Falah-Hassani K. Exercise for the prevention of low back pain: systematic review and meta-analysis of controlled trials. Am J Epidemiol. 2018; 187(5):1093–1101

[7] Newcomer K, Sinaki M. Low back pain and its relationship to back strength and physical activity in children. Acta Paediatr. 1996; 85(12):1433–1439

[8] Mortazavi J, Zebardast J, Mirzashahi B. Low back pain in athletes. Asian J Sports Med. 2015; 6(2):e24718

[9] Bailes JE, Hadley MN, Quigley MR, Sonntag VK, Cerullo LJ. Management of athletic injuries of the cervical spine and spinal cord. Neurosurgery. 1991; 29(4):491–497

[10] Deckey DG, Makovicka JL, Chung AS, et al. Neck and cervical spine injuries in National College Athletic Association athletes: a 5-year epidemiologic study. Spine. 2020; 45(1):55–64

[11] Tator CH, Provvidenza C, Cassidy JD. Spinal injuries in Canadian ice hockey: an update to 2005. Clin J Sport Med. 2009; 19(6):451–456

[12] Andrews J, Jones A, Davies PR, Howes J, Ahuja S. Is return to professional rugby union likely after anterior cervical spinal surgery? J Bone Joint Surg Br. 2008; 90(5):619–621

[13] Mall NA, Buchowski J, Zebala L, Brophy RH, Wright RW, Matava MJ. Spine and axial skeleton injuries in the National Football League. Am J Sports Med. 2012; 40(8):1755–1761

[14] Boden BP, Jarvis CG. Spinal injuries in sports. Neurol Clin. 2008; 26(1):63–78, viii

[15] Joaquim AF, Ghizoni E, Tedeschi H, et al. Upper cervical injuries—a rational approach to guide surgical management. J Spinal Cord Med. 2014; 37(2):139–151

[16] Gray BL, Buchowski JM, Bumpass DB, Lehman RA, Jr, Mall NA, Matava MJ. Disc herniations in the National Football League. Spine. 2013; 38(22):1934–1938

[17] Makhni MC, Curriero FC, Yeung CM, et al. Epidemiology of spine-related neurologic injuries in professional baseball players. Spine. 2022; 47(6): E265–E271

[18] Abdalkader M, Guermazi A, Engebretsen L, et al. MRI-detected spinal disc degenerative changes in athletes participating in the Rio de Janeiro 2016 Summer Olympics games. BMC Musculoskelet Disord. 2020; 21(1):45

[19] Schroeder GD, Lynch TS, Gibbs DB, et al. The impact of a cervical spine diagnosis on the careers of National Football League athletes. Spine. 2014; 39 (12):947–952

[20] Fryhofer GW, Smith HE. Return to play for cervical and lumbar spine conditions. Clin Sports Med. 2021; 40(3):555–569

[21] Mai HT, Burgmeier RJ, Mitchell SM, et al. Does the level of cervical disc herniation surgery affect performance-based outcomes in National Football League athletes? Spine. 2016; 41(23):1785–1789

[22] Radhakrishnan K, Litchy WJ, O'Fallon WM, Kurland LT. Epidemiology of cervical radiculopathy. A population-based study from Rochester, Minnesota, 1976 through 1990. Brain. 1994; 117(Pt 2):325–335

[23] Tempel ZJ, Bost JW, Norwig JA, Maroon JC. Significance of T2 hyperintensity on magnetic resonance imaging after cervical cord injury and return to play in professional athletes. Neurosurgery. 2015; 77(1):23–30, discussion 30–31

[24] Meredith DS, Jones KJ, Barnes R, Rodeo SA, Cammisa FP, Warren RF. Operative and nonoperative treatment of cervical disc herniation in National Football League athletes. Am J Sports Med. 2013; 41(9):2054–2058

[25] Hsu WK. Outcomes following nonoperative and operative treatment for cervical disc herniations in National Football League athletes. Spine. 2011; 36(10):800–805

[26] Roberts DW, Roc GJ, Hsu WK. Outcomes of cervical and lumbar disk herniations in Major League Baseball pitchers. Orthopedics. 2011; 34(8): 602–609

[27] Wilkinson HA, LeMay ML, Ferris EJ. Roentgenographic correlations in cervical spondylosis. Am J Roentgenol Radium Ther Nucl Med. 1969; 105(2):370–374

[28] Aebli N, Rüegg TB, Wicki AG, Petrou N, Krebs J. Predicting the risk and severity of acute spinal cord injury after a minor trauma to the cervical spine. Spine J. 2013; 13(6):597–604

[29] Pavlov H, Torg JS, Robie B, Jahre C. Cervical spinal stenosis: determination with vertebral body ratio method. Radiology. 1987; 164(3):771–775

[30] Torg JS, Corcoran TA, Thibault LE, et al. Cervical cord neurapraxia: classification, pathomechanics, morbidity, and management guidelines. J Neurosurg. 1997; 87(6):843–850
[31] Torg JS, Naranja RJ, Jr, Pavlov H, Galinat BJ, Warren R, Stine RA. The relationship of developmental narrowing of the cervical spinal canal to reversible and irreversible injury of the cervical spinal cord in football players. J Bone Joint Surg Am. 1996; 78(9):1308–1314
[32] Nakashima H, Yukawa Y, Suda K, Yamagata M, Ueta T, Kato F. Relatively large cervical spinal cord for spinal canal is a risk factor for development of cervical spinal cord compression: a cross-sectional study of 1211 subjects. Spine. 2016; 41(6):E342–E348
[33] Torg JS, Pavlov H, Genuario SE, et al. Neurapraxia of the cervical spinal cord with transient quadriplegia. J Bone Joint Surg Am. 1986; 68(9): 1354–1370
[34] Levitz CL, Reilly PJ, Torg JS. The pathomechanics of chronic, recurrent cervical nerve root neurapraxia. The chronic burner syndrome. Am J Sports Med. 1997; 25(1):73–76
[35] Dodwell ER, Kwon BK, Hughes B, et al. Spinal column and spinal cord injuries in mountain bikers: a 13-year review. Am J Sports Med. 2010; 38 (8):1647–1652
[36] Cantu RC, Li YM, Abdulhamid M, Chin LS. Return to play after cervical spine injury in sports. Curr Sports Med Rep. 2013; 12(1):14–17
[37] Arvin B, Fournier-Gosselin MP, Fehlings MG. Os odontoideum: etiology and surgical management. Neurosurgery. 2010; 66(3) Suppl:22–31
[38] Wu X, Wood KB, Gao Y, et al. Surgical strategies for the treatment of os odontoideum with atlantoaxial dislocation. J Neurosurg Spine. 2018; 28(2): 131–139
[39] Schroeder GD, Canseco JA, Patel PD, et al. Updated return-to-play recommendations for collision athletes after cervical spine injury: a modified Delphi consensus study with the Cervical Spine Research Society. Neurosurgery. 2020; 87(4):647–654
[40] Allen BL, Jr, Ferguson RL, Lehmann TR, O'Brien RP. A mechanistic classification of closed, indirect fractures and dislocations of the lower cervical spine. Spine. 1982; 7(1):1–27
[41] Banerjee R, Palumbo MA, Fadale PD. Catastrophic cervical spine injuries in the collision sport athlete, part 1: epidemiology, functional anatomy, and diagnosis. Am J Sports Med. 2004; 32(4):1077–1087
[42] Vaccaro AR, Hulbert RJ, Patel AA, et al. Spine Trauma Study Group. The subaxial cervical spine injury classification system: a novel approach to recognize the importance of morphology, neurology, and integrity of the disco-ligamentous complex. Spine. 2007; 32(21):2365–2374
[43] Weinberg J, Rokito S, Silber JS. Etiology, treatment, and prevention of athletic "stingers". Clin Sports Med. 2003; 22(3):493–500, viii
[44] Stillerman CB, Chen TC, Couldwell WT, Zhang W, Weiss MH. Experience in the surgical management of 82 symptomatic herniated thoracic discs and review of the literature. J Neurosurg. 1998; 88(4):623–633
[45] Watkins RG. The Spine in Sports. Mosby; 1996:657
[46] Haba H, Taneichi H, Kotani Y, et al. Diagnostic accuracy of magnetic resonance imaging for detecting posterior ligamentous complex injury associated with thoracic and lumbar fractures. J Neurosurg. 2003; 99(1) Suppl:20–26
[47] Quint U, Bordon G, Preissl I, Sanner C, Rosenthal D. Thoracoscopic treatment for single level symptomatic thoracic disc herniation: a prospective followed cohort study in a group of 167 consecutive cases. Eur Spine J. 2012; 21(4): 637–645
[48] Hetsroni I, Mann G, Dolev E, Morgenstern D, Nyska M. Clay shoveler's fracture in a volleyball player. Phys Sportsmed. 2005; 33(7):38–42
[49] Sorell R, Wieschhaus K, Simons SM. A nontraumatic clay shoveler's fracture in a runner. Curr Sports Med Rep. 2021; 20(1):7–9
[50] Kang DH, Lee SH. Multiple spinous process fractures of the thoracic vertebrae (clay-shoveler's fracture) in a beginning golfer: a case report. Spine. 2009; 34(15):E534–E537
[51] Yamaguchi KT, Jr, Myung KS, Alonso MA, Skaggs DL. Clay-shoveler's fracture equivalent in children. Spine. 2012; 37(26):E1672–E1675
[52] McHugh-Pierzina VL, Zillmer DA, Giangarra CE. Thoracic compression fracture in a basketball player. J Athl Train. 1995; 30(2):163–164
[53] Horton WC, Kraiwattanapong C, Akamaru T, et al. The role of the sternum, costosternal articulations, intervertebral disc, and facets in thoracic sagittal plane biomechanics: a comparison of three different sequences of surgical release. Spine. 2005; 30(18):2014–2023
[54] De Luigi AJ. Low back pain in the adolescent athlete. Phys Med Rehabil Clin N Am. 2014; 25(4):763–788
[55] Cassidy JD, Carroll LJ, Côté P. The Saskatchewan health and back pain survey. The prevalence of low back pain and related disability in Saskatchewan adults. Spine. 1998; 23(17):1860–1866, discussion 1867
[56] Heliövaara M, Sievers K, Impivaara O, et al. Descriptive epidemiology and public health aspects of low back pain. Ann Med. 1989; 21(5):327–333
[57] Valat JP, Rozenberg S. Local corticosteroid injections for low back pain and sciatica. Joint Bone Spine. 2008; 75(4):403–407
[58] Peebles R, Jonas CE. Sacroiliac joint dysfunction in the athlete: diagnosis and management. Curr Sports Med Rep. 2017; 16(5):336–342
[59] Gatt CJ, Jr, Hosea TM, Palumbo RC, Zawadsky JP. Impact loading of the lumbar spine during football blocking. Am J Sports Med. 1997; 25(3): 317–321
[60] Hsu WK, McCarthy KJ, Savage JW, et al. The professional athlete spine initiative: outcomes after lumbar disc herniation in 342 elite professional athletes. Spine J. 2011; 11(3):180–186
[61] Hangai M, Kaneoka K, Hinotsu S, et al. Lumbar intervertebral disk degeneration in athletes. Am J Sports Med. 2009; 37(1):149–155
[62] Drakos MC, Domb B, Starkey C, Callahan L, Allen AA. Injury in the national basketball association: a 17-year overview. Sports Health. 2010; 2(4): 284–290
[63] Weinstein JN, Lurie JD, Tosteson TD, et al. Surgical vs nonoperative treatment for lumbar disk herniation: the Spine Patient Outcomes Research Trial (SPORT) observational cohort. JAMA. 2006; 296(20):2451–2459
[64] Ball JR, Harris CB, Lee J, Vives MJ. Lumbar spine injuries in sports: review of the literature and current treatment recommendations. Sports Med Open. 2019; 5(1):26
[65] Goldstein JD, Berger PE, Windler GE, Jackson DW. Spine injuries in gymnasts and swimmers. An epidemiologic investigation. Am J Sports Med. 1991; 19 (5):463–468
[66] Katz DA, Scerpella TA. Anterior and middle column thoracolumbar spine injuries in young female gymnasts. Report of seven cases and review of the literature. Am J Sports Med. 2003; 31(4):611–616
[67] Micheli LJ, Wood R. Back pain in young athletes. Significant differences from adults in causes and patterns. Arch Pediatr Adolesc Med. 1995; 149(1):15–18
[68] Jackson DW, Wiltse LL, Cirincoine RJ. Spondylolysis in the female gymnast. Clin Orthop Relat Res. 1976(117):68–73
[69] Campbell RS, Grainger AJ, Hide IG, Papastefanou S, Greenough CG. Juvenile spondylolysis: a comparative analysis of CT, SPECT and MRI. Skeletal Radiol. 2005; 34(2):63–73
[70] Sairyo K, Sakai T, Yasui N, Dezawa A. Conservative treatment for pediatric lumbar spondylolysis to achieve bone healing using a hard brace: what type and how long? Clinical article. J Neurosurg Spine. 2012; 16(6):610–614
[71] Kalichman L, Hunter DJ. Diagnosis and conservative management of degenerative lumbar spondylolisthesis. Eur Spine J. 2008; 17(3):327–335
[72] Radcliff KE, Kalantar SB, Reitman CA. Surgical management of spondylolysis and spondylolisthesis in athletes: indications and return to play. Curr Sports Med Rep. 2009; 8(1):35–40
[73] Morita T, Ikata T, Katoh S, Miyake R. Lumbar spondylolysis in children and adolescents. J Bone Joint Surg Br. 1995; 77(4):620–625
[74] Standaert CJ, Herring SA. Expert opinion and controversies in musculoskeletal and sports medicine: core stabilization as a treatment for low back pain. Arch Phys Med Rehabil. 2007; 88(12):1734–1736
[75] Wood KB, Li W, Lebl DR, Ploumis A. Management of thoracolumbar spine fractures. Spine J. 2014; 14(1):145–164
[76] Anakwenze OA, Namdari S, Auerbach JD, et al. Athletic performance outcomes following lumbar discectomy in professional basketball players. Spine. 2010; 35(7):825–828
[77] Minhas SV, Kester BS, Larkin KE, Hsu WK. The effect of an orthopaedic surgical procedure in the National Basketball Association. Am J Sports Med. 2016; 44(4):1056–1061
[78] El Rassi G, Takemitsu M, Woratanarat P, Shah SA. Lumbar spondylolysis in pediatric and adolescent soccer players. Am J Sports Med. 2005; 33(11): 1688–1693
[79] d'Hemecourt PA, Zurakowski D, Kriemler S, Micheli LJ. Spondylolysis: returning the athlete to sports participation with brace treatment. Orthopedics. 2002; 25(6):653–657
[80] Miller SF, Congeni J, Swanson K. Long-term functional and anatomical follow-up of early detected spondylolysis in young athletes. Am J Sports Med. 2004; 32(4):928–933
[81] Li Y, Hresko MT. Lumbar spine surgery in athletes: outcomes and return-to-play criteria. Clin Sports Med. 2012; 31(3):487–498

11 Emergent Management of the Athlete with Spinal Cord Injury

Kelly Jiang, Andrew M. Hersh, and Nicholas Theodore

Summary

Successful emergent management of spinal cord injury (SCI) relies on comprehensive pregame preparation by the medical team. In the field, providers should prioritize spinal immobilization with a cervical collar and backboard, and only removing athletic equipment when necessary for medical intervention. Transport to a capable facility as quickly as possible is critical for improving long-term outcomes. Once at the hospital, athletes with SCI should receive a thorough neurological examination. SCI can be treated by mean arterial pressure (MAP) augmentation and decompressive surgery. Treatment recommendations for patients with acute SCI remain controversial, and further studies are necessary to improve the safety and long-term functioning of athletes who suffer traumatic SCI.

Keywords: spinal cord injury, emergency medical services, sports injuries

11.1 Introduction

On September 9, 2007, Buffalo Bills tight end Kevin Everett suffered a career-ending spinal cord injury (SCI). After making a tackle, Everett fell face down on the field, paralyzed below the neck. Within 13 minutes, Everett was immobilized, loaded into an ambulance, and in transit to a hospital. Everett suffered a cervical fracture dislocation, but due to the swift, coordinated care of the National Football League medical team, he received timely decompression surgery. After 3 months of his injury, Everett began walking unassisted and regained most of his neurologic function.

Although Everett's story garnered significant attention for SCIs in sports, concern for the spinal protection of athletes began in 1976 when the National Football League banned head-first tackling after it was found to cause cervical spine injuries resulting in quadriplegia. Several years later, the National Hockey League followed suit, banning checking from behind, which previously caused players to collide head-first with the boards or ice. Even after significant changes in safety rules and advancements in protective equipment, 12,000 athletes suffer an SCI each year, making sports the fourth leading cause of SCI.[1,2] Everett's story is a testament to the importance of medical preparedness. Appropriate emergent management of athletes with SCI may determine whether an athlete survives or ever walks again.

11.2 Pregame Planning

Successful field management of the athlete with SCI begins with appropriate pregame planning. Prior to the event, the medical team should confirm the availability of an immobilization backboard, tools for sporting equipment removal, and a cervical collar, in addition to standard emergency medical supplies.[3] Consistent review and rehearsal of spinal precaution protocols are vital for coordinating an effective response. Medical teams covering athletic events should have regular practice of log-rolling patients, cutting off and unscrewing face masks, removing helmets and shoulder pads, and securing patients to immobilization devices. In addition, transport protocol should be in place and rehearsed to ensure that the player with an acute SCI is safely transported to a Level-1 trauma center with 24-hour neurosurgical coverage and the ability to perform advanced imaging (computed tomography [CT] and magnetic resonance imaging [MRI]) expeditiously as well as getting a patient to the operating theater as quickly as possible if needed.

11.3 Initiating Spinal Precautions

After traumatic contact in sports, spine injury should be considered in the presence of any altered mental status, bilateral neurologic findings, significant midline spine pain, or spinal column deformity.[3] Because athletes may be eager to return to the game by downplaying their injury, it is important to have the medical team perform a thorough neurological examination before clearing the player.

Catastrophic injuries may be readily apparent, but evaluating more minor spinal injuries can be challenging in the field. Stingers are transient neuropraxias caused by trauma to the cervical nerve roots or brachial plexus that can appear similar to true SCI. Stingers cause symptoms lasting minutes to hours, and they always affect the upper extremities unilaterally.[4] They are usually caused by a stretching force on the shoulder with the head flexed in the opposite direction. Although there are no standardized return-to-play guidelines following a stinger, the physician can consider clearing an athlete if the patient has no pain, intact neurovascular function, full cervical spine and shoulder range of motion, and a negative Spurling test.[5] Spinal precautions should be performed if an athlete shows signs or symptoms deviating from the typical presentation of a stinger, has significant neck pain, or if symptoms persist.[2]

11.4 On-Field Management

Up to 25% of SCIs occur during the initial manipulation of a patient following a traumatic event.[6] Minimization of spinal movement immediately after injury is, therefore, critical to long-term outcomes. Athletes with suspected SCI should be treated by qualified providers using the Advanced Trauma Life Support guidelines addressing airway, breathing, circulation, then disability. Pre-hospital management of SCI should prioritize rapid transport to a capable facility, and transport should not be delayed for additional treatment like intubation and artificial ventilation when possible.[7]

Upon reaching the athlete, providers should immediately provide manual stabilization of the head and neck.[3] The athlete should be placed into a neutral supine position for appropriate assessment and immobilization.[8] If athletes are found in a position in which they must be moved, they should be log rolled to supine position.[9] If the athlete experiences pain, airway compromise, neurologic symptoms, or resistance during realignment attempts, the cervical spine should be manually stabilized in the position found.[9] Face masks should be removed in athletes wearing protective equipment, but the helmet and shoulder pads should remain in place unless directly inhibiting medical care.[3] Helmets and shoulder pads worn together provide neutral alignment in the supine position and can serve as immobilization when secured to a board.[10] When necessary, helmet and shoulder pads should be removed simultaneously to maintain neutral spine alignment. A cervical collar should be placed, if possible, when equipment is removed, and manual stabilization with the collar in place should be maintained. Once the cervical spine has been stabilized, the athlete should be secured to a full-body immobilization board, transferred to an ambulance, and transported to the closest capable facility.[3]

11.5 In-Hospital Management

Once the athlete has reached an emergency department, airway, breathing, and circulation continue to take priority over the spinal injury. Cervical cord injuries render patients especially susceptible to respiratory depression, temperature dysregulation, and neurogenic shock, which may require intubation and fluid resuscitation.[11] These immediate life-threatening concerns should be addressed first. Once the athlete has been stabilized, a thorough neurologic examination, including mental status, cranial nerve function, and American Spinal Injury Association Impairment Scale score, should be performed as early as possible to determine the level and severity of the injury.

Further diagnosis requires prompt radiographic imaging. Helmets and shoulder pads should be removed in the emergency department by trained providers only prior to imaging, as protective equipment can hinder radiographic visualization of the cervical spine.[3] CT scans are the preferred imaging modality because they have improved sensitivity for detecting spine fractures and the ability to assess soft tissues compared to plain radiographs.[12] They are also preferred in the acute setting over MRI due to their increased availability and speed at most institutions and compatibility with athletic and medical equipment. When MRIs can be obtained, they provide superior quality imaging of the spinal cord, ligaments, disks, and soft tissues, which is helpful supplementation to the CT.[13]

Treatment of acute SCI involves mean arterial pressure (MAP) augmentation to improve spinal cord perfusion and surgery for decompression of the spinal cord and stabilization of the spine. However, there are currently no guidelines standardizing the timing or method.[14,15] Patients with acute SCI are susceptible to disruption of the sympathetic response, resulting in bradycardia and hypotension. To prevent hypoperfusion of the spinal cord, maintaining MAP at a target greater than 85 to 90 mmHg through vasopressors is recommended.[16] In general, the decision to perform a decompression intervention is based on the instability of the fracture, degree of ongoing compression of nervous tissue, or the presence of neurological deficits. Decompression can be performed surgically or through closed reduction. If decompression is indicated, timing is critical and the procedure should occur within 24 hours of the injury to improve long-term neurological outcomes.[17] Surgery can be considered for spinal fractures of any location and involves the decompression of neural elements, reduction of dislocations, and stabilization of the spine.[18] Closed reduction is indicated only in cervical fractures with misalignment of the spine such as in the case of bilateral locked facets. In closed reduction, traction is applied longitudinally across the spine by Gardner-Wells tongs or halo devices. Weight is increased incrementally with intermittent radiographic and neurologic examinations to monitor the patient until adequate traction is achieved. Closed reduction can be performed quickly and may prevent the need for urgent surgery but is only possible in awake and examinable patients.[19]

11.6 Additional Treatment Options

Hypothermia and high-dose methylprednisolone have been suggested to improve outcomes for acute spinal injury. Hypothermia is hypothesized to reduce damage in the spinal cord by decreasing oxygen demand and slowing down the inflammatory cascade after injury.[20] However, it is unclear what cooling regimen is most beneficial and whether rewarming can cause further damage.[21] Hypothermia is currently considered an experimental treatment and is not recommended in field or acute hospital management of acute SCI at this time.[3] High-dose methylprednisolone has also been explored as an early treatment strategy for SCI. Some evidence has shown neurological improvement compared to placebo, but others have found an increased risk of respiratory complications, infections, and death.[22,23,24] Like hypothermia, methylprednisolone use is controversial and is not adequately supported as standard protocol.[25]

11.7 Conclusion

SCI is one of the most catastrophic injuries that athletes can sustain while participating in their sport. Although uncommon, they can be deadly or result in permanent paralysis. Medical provider competency should be maintained through regular rehearsal of spinal protection protocol as the emergency response to an athlete with suspected SCI is critical to long-term neurological outcome. Treatment recommendations for patients with acute SCI remain controversial and are not well standardized, and further studies are necessary to improve the safety and long-term functioning of athletes who suffer traumatic SCI.

11.8 Clinical Pearls

- SCI is an uncommon but potentially deadly or catastrophic injury that athletes can sustain during their sport.
- Successful emergent management of SCI relies on comprehensive pregame preparation by the medical team.
- In the field, providers should prioritize spinal immobilization with a cervical collar and backboard, and only removing athletic equipment when necessary for medical intervention. Transport to a capable facility as quickly as possible is critical for improving long-term outcomes.
- Once at the hospital, athletes with SCI should receive a thorough neurological examination. SCI can be treated by MAP augmentation and decompressive surgery or closed reduction.

11.9 Disclosures

Kelly Jiang: None.
Andrew M. Hersh: None.
Nicholas Theodore: Royalties from Globus Medical. Stock Ownership in Globus Medical. Consultant for Globus Medical. On Scientific Advisory Board/Other Office for Globus Medical.

References

[1] Sekhon LHS, Fehlings MG. Epidemiology, demographics, and pathophysiology of acute spinal cord injury. Spine. 2001; 26(24) Suppl:S2–S12

[2] Assenmacher B, Schroeder GD, Patel AA. On-field management of spine and spinal cord injuries. Oper Tech Sports Med. 2013; 21(3):152–158

[3] Swartz EE, Boden BP, Courson RW, et al. National athletic trainers' association position statement: acute management of the cervical spine-injured athlete. J Athl Train. 2009; 44(3):306–331

[4] Weinberg J, Rokito S, Silber JS. Etiology, treatment, and prevention of athletic "stingers". Clin Sports Med. 2003; 22(3):493–500, viii

[5] Bowles DR, Canseco JA, Alexander TD, Schroeder GD, Hecht AC, Vaccaro AR. The prevalence and management of stingers in college and professional collision athletes. Curr Rev Musculoskelet Med. 2020; 13(6):651–662

[6] Theodore N, Hadley MN, Aarabi B, et al. Prehospital cervical spinal immobilization after trauma. Neurosurgery. 2013; 72 Suppl 2:22–34

[7] Gardner BP, Watt JW, Krishnan KR. The artificial ventilation of acute spinal cord damaged patients: a retrospective study of forty-four patients. Paraplegia. 1986; 24(4):208–220

[8] Ahn H, Singh J, Nathens A, et al. Pre-hospital care management of a potential spinal cord injured patient: a systematic review of the literature and evidence-based guidelines. J Neurotrauma. 2011; 28(8):1341–1361

[9] De Lorenzo RA. A review of spinal immobilization techniques. J Emerg Med. 1996; 14(5):603–613

[10] Laprade RF, Schnetzler KA, Broxterman RJ, Wentorf F, Gilbert TJ. Cervical spine alignment in the immobilized ice hockey player. A computed tomographic analysis of the effects of helmet removal. Am J Sports Med. 2000; 28(6):800–803

[11] Karlsson AK. Overview: Autonomic dysfunction in spinal cord injury: clinical presentation of symptoms and signs. In: Weaver LC, Polosa C, eds. Progress in Brain Research. Vol. 152. Autonomic Dysfunction After Spinal Cord Injury. Elsevier; 2006:1–8

[12] Antevil JL, Sise MJ, Sack DI, Kidder B, Hopper A, Brown CVR. Spiral computed tomography for the initial evaluation of spine trauma: a new standard of care? J Trauma. 2006; 61(2):382–387

[13] Demaerel P. Magnetic resonance imaging of spinal cord trauma: a pictorial essay. Neuroradiology. 2006; 48(4):223–232

[14] Fehlings MG, Perrin RG. The role and timing of early decompression for cervical spinal cord injury: update with a review of recent clinical evidence. Injury. 2005; 36 Suppl 2:B13–B26

[15] Karsy M, Hawryluk G. Modern medical management of spinal cord injury. Curr Neurol Neurosci Rep. 2019; 19(9):65

[16] Hadley MN, Walters BC. Introduction to the guidelines for the management of acute cervical spine and spinal cord injuries. Neurosurgery. 2013; 72 Suppl 2:5–16

[17] Early versus Delayed Decompression for Traumatic Cervical Spinal Cord Injury: Results of the Surgical Timing in Acute Spinal Cord Injury Study (STASCIS) | PLOS ONE. Accessed October 29, 2023 at: https://journals.plos.org/plosone/article?id=10.1371/journal.pone.0032037

[18] Bagnall AM, Jones L, Duffy S, Riemsma RP. Spinal fixation surgery for acute traumatic spinal cord injury. Cochrane Database Syst Rev. 2008(1):CD004725

[19] Grant GA, Mirza SK, Chapman JR, et al. Risk of early closed reduction in cervical spine subluxation injuries. J Neurosurg. 1999; 90(1) Suppl:13–18

[20] Guest JD, Dietrich WD. Spinal cord ischemia and trauma. In: Tisherman SA, Sterz F, eds. Therapeutic Hypothermia: Molecular and Cellular Biology of Critical Care Medicine. Springer US; 2005:101–118

[21] Hansebout RR, Hansebout CR. Local cooling for traumatic spinal cord injury: outcomes in 20 patients and review of the literature. J Neurosurg Spine. 2014; 20(5):550–561

[22] Bracken MB, Shepard MJ, Collins WF, et al. A randomized, controlled trial of methylprednisolone or naloxone in the treatment of acute spinal-cord injury. Results of the Second National Acute Spinal Cord Injury Study. N Engl J Med. 1990; 322(20):1405–1411

[23] Hurlbert RJ. The role of steroids in acute spinal cord injury: an evidence-based analysis. Spine. 2001; 26(24) Suppl:S39–S46

[24] Bracken MB. Steroids for acute spinal cord injury. Cochrane Database Syst Rev. 2012; 1(1):CD001046

[25] Hurlbert RJ, Hadley MN, Walters BC, et al. Pharmacological therapy for acute spinal cord injury. Neurosurgery. 2013; 72 Suppl 2:93–105

12 Physical Examination of the Athletic Spine

Stephanie Van, Faisel M. Zaman, and Mark I. Ellen

Summary

A consistent approach when performing a physical examination is essential when providing coverage to athletes. In combination with a thorough knowledge of the athlete's needs, a systematically performed physical examination leads to a timely assessment of an injury and reduced errors of diagnosis and judgment.

Keywords: sideline spine examination, sideline coverage, athlete spinal examination, athletic spinal assessment

12.1 Introduction

Injuries to the back can significantly impact an athlete's ability to participate maximally in the sport. Spinal cord injuries (SCIs) resulting from sports now represent nearly 9% of all causes of SCI.[1] Spinal injuries in an athlete can result in significant morbidity and mortality. Prompt and proper assessment, triage, and management of this type of injury can help an athlete preserve the maximum function possible. This chapter will detail each phase of a comprehensive yet concise spine evaluation and review basic differences between the office-based setting and the sideline examination for sports medicine and general medicine physicians who practice in both environments.[2]

12.2 The Spine Examination

Standardization of the spine examination requires consistency and versatility so that evolving, rare, or catastrophic pathologies are not missed. On the field, the location and severity of an acute injury must be deduced quickly to determine if an athlete can return to play or else be safely transported off the field for a more detailed assessment. Once on the sideline, it is best to evaluate the asymptomatic region first for a baseline normal examination, and then evaluate the abnormal or painful region.

Whenever possible, the spine should always be seen on physical examination free from layers of clothing. In an office setting, a patient should be gowned. On the sideline, athletic wear should be removed as appropriate.

The importance of knowing athletes well, including past medical history, cannot be overemphasized. Special considerations may exist and can influence risk of injury during participation in sports. For example, patients with Down's syndrome have a tendency for atlantoaxial instability that may be evident on flexion and extension X-rays, but clinically asymptomatic. In these cases, consultation with a spine surgeon may be warranted before clearance for sports participation can be safely guaranteed. Counseling of athletes and their families about the risks and appropriate precautions should be individualized and is crucial to their decision-making. The family of a patient with Down's syndrome may decide that the risk of playing volleyball, despite the low but potential risk of catastrophic SCI, does not outweigh the risk of limiting recreation. Discussions about short- and long-term goals can help patients and families with decisions regarding sports participation.

The sideline assessment focuses on where an athlete is experiencing acute symptoms. Although the covering physician may not have witnessed the injury, a timely but thorough evaluation, assessment, and plan should be influenced by the clinical concern and an athlete's need for acute management, and not by pressure from the injured athlete, team, or coach to return to play.[3] It is important to assess immediately whether or not the athlete will need basic life support or expedited medical transport to a trauma center. Emergent management of an athlete with spinal injury is described in detail later in this book. Neurological compromise that indicates SCI can be detected on physical examination alone. Triage to the most appropriate level of care may happen without the need for on-site imaging. Optimal conditions for sideline evaluation include designated medical tents which minimize crowd noise, improve communication among the patient and the care team, and allow for privacy when a full head-to-toe spine examination is warranted. The sideline physician should also have all of the necessary tools at hand to perform a comprehensive neurological assessment, including a reflex hammer and alcohol swabs for a detailed sensory exam (these can assess sensation of light touch, pinprick, and cold/wet).[4]

12.3 Phases of the Physical Examination of the Spine and Corresponding Pathologies

12.3.1 Cervical Spine

Inspection

Resting neck position, shoulder height, muscle atrophy, surgical scars, and skin and tissue quality can be assessed with visual inspection. If there is concern for a cervical spine injury, a careful shoulder evaluation should also be performed.

Range of Motion

Forward flexion, backwards extension, left- and right-side bending, and axial rotation of the neck should be assessed for limitations with active and passive movement. In the athletic patient with a neck injury, pain or limitations in neck range of motion are commonly caused by neck muscle strain, stinger injuries, herniated or torn intervertebral disks, facet joint injury, vertebral subluxation, or fracture. Many athletes may notice a delay in onset of neck stiffness, with gradually increasing axial pain after several hours or even days post-performance.

Palpation

Although palpation provides nonspecific data, it is an important part of the physical examination. Taut bands and tenderness along muscle fibers can signify trigger points, myofascial pain, and cervical strain. Tenderness over the occipital nerves can signify the patient may have occipital neuralgia. Exquisite tenderness over bony prominences such as the midline spinous processes may signify bony injury such as a vertebral compression fracture or cervical spinous process fracture (Clay Shoveler's fracture).

Neurological Assessment and Provocative Maneuvers

Traditional dermatomal mapping corresponds to sensory nerve root innervation but does not necessarily correlate with dynatomal patterns, or the distribution of referred symptoms from an irritated nerve root.[5] When there is focal weakness or paresthesia, a thorough motor and sensory examination can help identify and localize a nerve root, plexus, or cord injury. Focal weakness, reflex changes or altered sensation in the upper extremities suggest acute neurological compromise. Hyperreflexia, reflex asymmetry, or Hoffman's sign (flexion of the thumb after flick of the ipsilateral third digit nail) may indicate an upper motor neuron injury.

Spurling's test assesses for radicular symptoms that can arise from cervical nerve root impingement but should not be performed in cases when a cervical fracture is suspected. With the neck extended and head rotated to the affected side, the physician applies an axial load down onto the cervical spine, which, if positive, may produce pain or paresthesias along the arm, forearm, and fingers (▶ Fig. 12.1). This provocative maneuver is not only highly sensitive, but 93% specific for cervical radiculopathy and can help confirm this diagnosis.[6] A provocative maneuver reproducing shoulder or upper extremity symptoms above the elbow is also significant, and should be noted, since a delayed positive test can occur in many cases.

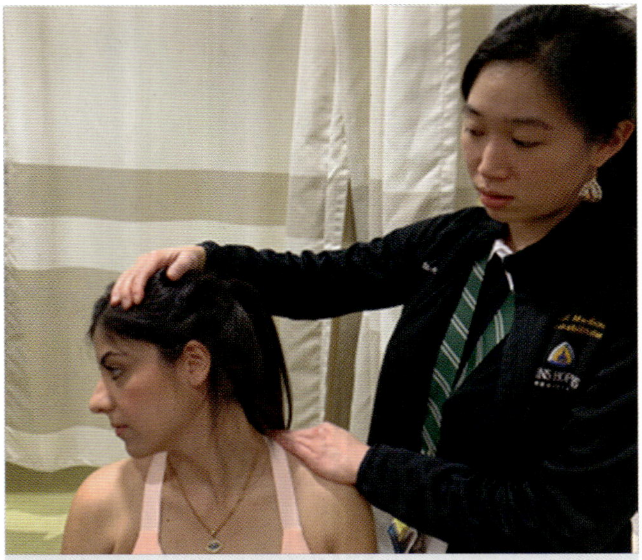

Fig. 12.1 Spurling's test where the patient is asked to rotate his or her neck all the way to one side and slightly extend backwards, while the examiner applies downward pressure at the top of the head. This test is positive for cervical radiculopathy when the maneuver provokes pain radiating down the upper extremity.

Plain radiographs or higher level imaging are warranted in athletes with persistent spine pain, neurological signs and symptoms, radicular pain, or clinical suspicion for more alarming etiology.[7]

Any athlete who has neck pain, is unconscious, or is motionless must be treated as having an SCI until proven otherwise. Movement of an athlete suspected of having suffered an SCI should be performed only to maintain basic life support and safety in a neutral, supine position with a backboard.[8] Emergent management of this type of injury is detailed in later chapters. Again, a thorough neurological assessment can help identify and localize a nerve root or cord injury. Serial assessments should be performed as signs and symptoms of neurological injury may have delayed onset.

Cervical spine injuries due to sports participation are rare but can be catastrophic. They are seen predominantly in diving, football, gymnastics, and ice hockey, but can occur in any sport.[9] Anterior neck flexion with high velocity axial loading can result in cervical compression fractures, commonly seen at C5. Bone fragments from these fractures can project directly into the spinal canal and cause SCI. Acute hyperextension of the neck can result in a central cord syndrome, most commonly seen at the C4–C5 levels.[10] Repetitive axial loading on a straightened cervical spine (as seen often in football) can result in neck pain, cervical canal stenosis, and loss of lordosis, a syndrome known as Spear Tackler's spine. This is why spear tackling, or the deliberate use of the top of the helmet as the initial point of contact, has been banned from high school and collegiate-level sports since 1976, a policy that has significantly reduced rates of cervical neurological injury.[11]

Acute neck and shoulder pain in a contact sport athlete is commonly caused by a "stinger injury" involving a peripheral nerve injury of either a cervical nerve root or brachial plexus. These types of peripheral nerve injuries warrant a thorough assessment of the shoulder. Bilateral "stinger" type symptoms, or history of multiple previous "stinger injuries" affecting the neck or causing lower extremity weakness, raise concern for a cervical SCI. Typically, most of these injuries cause only transient symptoms, and if symptoms resolve and full strength returns, athletes may be permitted to return to play. Only a small percentage of "stinger injuries" (approximately 5–10%) are serious enough to result in prolonged neurological deficits.[8]

Acute concussion or traumatic brain injury (TBI) may occur concomitantly with cervical spine injuries and should always be considered during sideline evaluation. These injuries are covered in detail in the "Brain" portion of this text.

12.3.2 Thoracic Spine

Inspection

Scoliosis can be identified by assessing the symmetry of the thorax, shoulders, and hips in standing and with Adam's forward bending test. Thoracic hyperkyphosis may be a sign of Scheuermann's disease, a likely genetic condition that commonly occurs during growth spurts and can cause back pain and limited range of motion in a young athlete. In severe cases of scoliosis or hyperkyphosis, respiratory insufficiency and diminished aerobic capacity can limit participation in sports and other physical activity.[12]

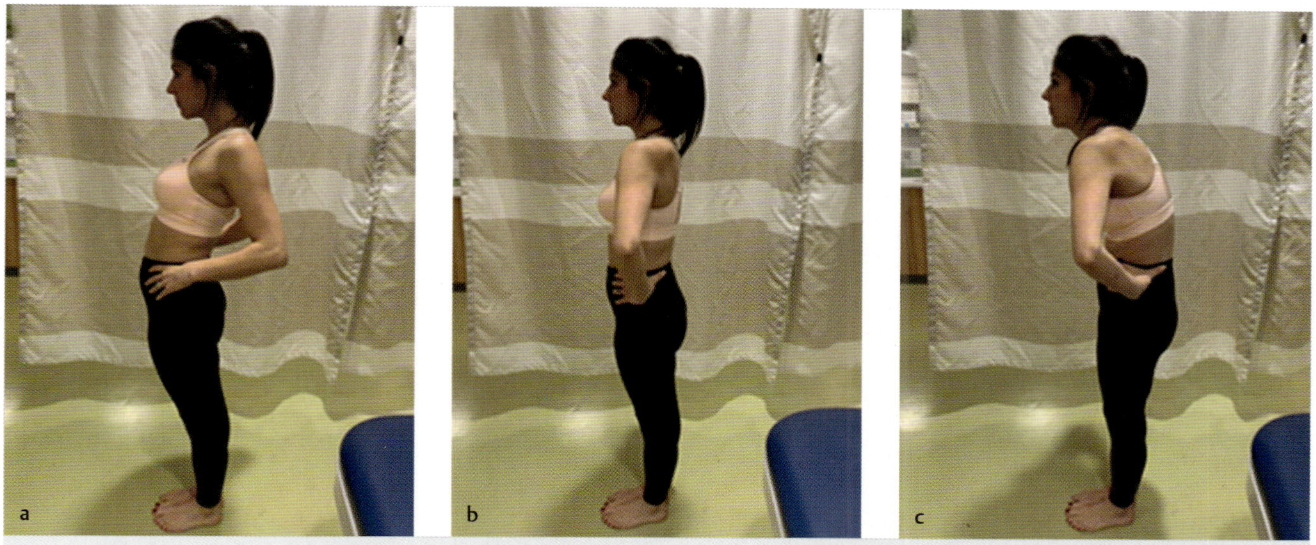

Fig. 12.2 (a–c) Thoracic spine range of motion in backwards extension, neutral spine, and forward flexion.

Range of Motion

Forward flexion, backwards extension, left- and right-side bending, and axial rotation of the thoracic spine should be assessed (▸ Fig. 12.2). Pain with extension may indicate a pars interarticularis fracture (spondylolysis), though this is more commonly seen in the lumbar spine. Facet loading may provoke painful facet arthropathy (usually seen in older patients), but there is little evidence to support the sensitivity and specificity of this test.[13]

Palpation

Taut bands and tenderness along muscle fibers can signify trigger points, myofascial pain, and thoracic strain. These are commonly related to cervical pathology given that the thoracic spine is involved in maintaining neck posture and mobility, as shown in studies examining whiplash-associated disorders.[14] Exquisite tenderness over bony prominences such as the spinous processes may signify bony injury such as a pars interarticularis fracture or vertebral compression fracture.[7]

Neurological Assessment and Provocative Maneuvers

In most situations, new focal weakness, reflex changes, altered sensation in the lower extremities, or bowel or bladder incontinence is indicative of spine pathology. In exceedingly rare cases, these findings could suggest acute spinal cord compromise in the thoracic spine.

Thoracolumbar strain injuries can be commonly seen in sports such as snowboarding and motocross. One study found over 20% of presentations to the emergency department (ED) after motocross injury could be attributed to thoracolumbar strain.[15,16] Acute thoracic compression fractures in athletes during sports participation have been described only in case reports.[7] Overall, thoracic pathology due to sports injury is quite rare given the reduced rotational range of motion and protection of the rib cage at these levels compared to the cervical or lumbar regions.[7,16]

12.3.3 Lumbar Spine

Inspection

A truncal lean or lumbar shift with ambulation or seated posture can indicate intervertebral disk pathology. Increased axial loads to the lumbar spine can be seen in weight lifters, wrestlers, and football linemen. Lumbar hyperlordosis is a predisposing factor for developing spondylolysis and, if observed, should trigger workup including standing full-length radiographs of the spine to rule out associated thoracic hyperkyphosis, including Scheuermann's disease.[17]

Range of Motion

Forward flexion, backwards extension, left- and right-side bending, and axial rotation of the lumbar spine should be assessed (▸ Fig. 12.3). Pain with extension may indicate a pars interarticularis fracture (spondylolysis). These are most commonly seen at L5 and L4, likely due to the higher degree of mobility and range of motion at these levels. Herniated disks impinging upon exiting nerve roots or the spinal cord itself will elicit pain with these simple range of motion maneuvers. Traumatic injuries to the disks themselves can also cause pain.

Palpation

Similar to higher levels within the spine, taut bands and tenderness along muscle fibers can signify trigger points, myofascial pain, and lumbar strain. Exquisite tenderness over bony prominences such as the midline spinous processes may signify bony injury such as a pars interarticularis fracture, vertebral compression fracture, and chance fracture (usually due to traumatic crush injuries resulting in hyperflexion of the spine).

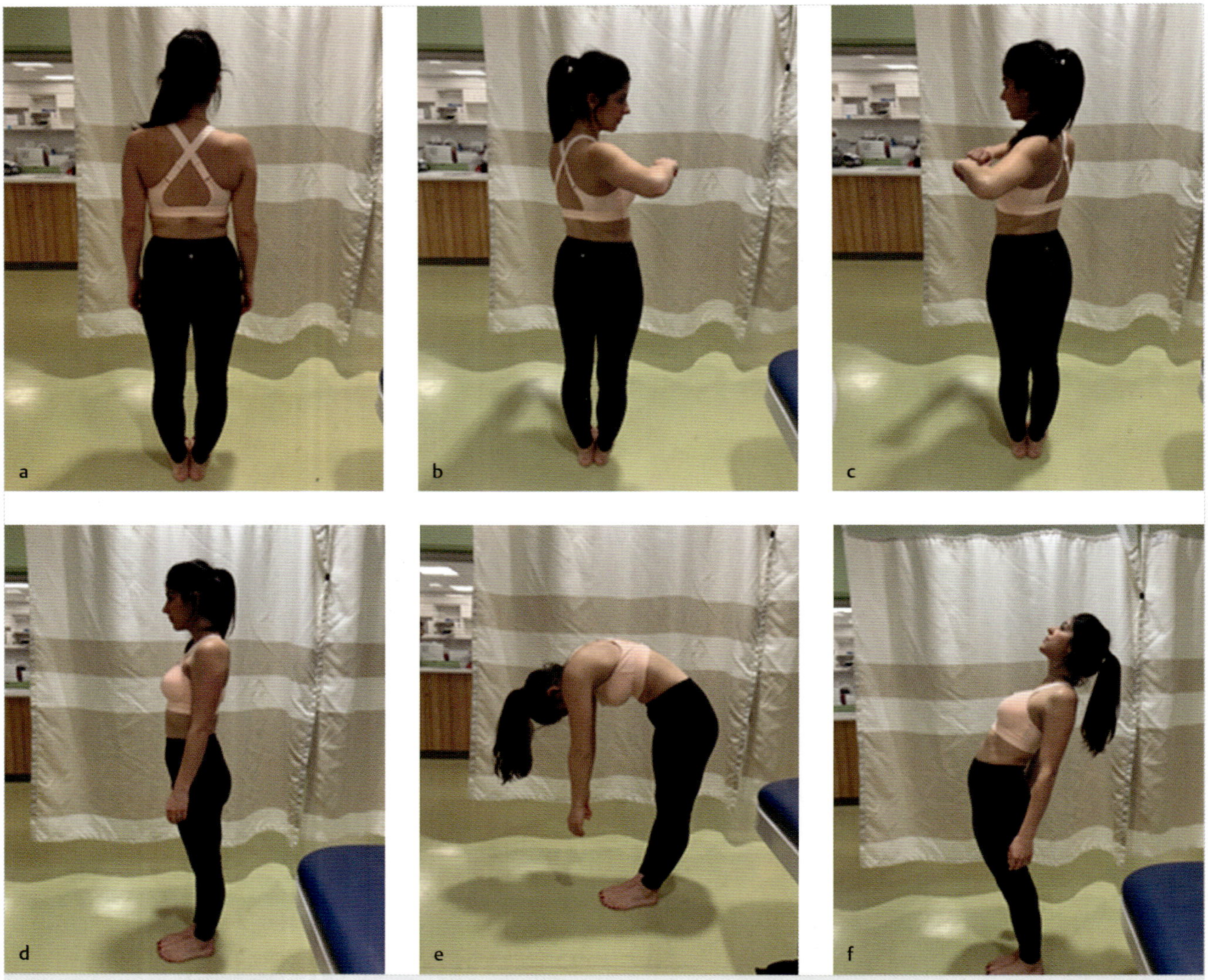

Fig. 12.3 (a–c) Lumbar spine range of motion in neutral, right and left rotation. **(d–f)** Lumbar spine in neutral, forward flexion, and backwards extension.

Neurological Assessment and Provocative Maneuvers

Specific to the lumbar spine are the straight leg raise (► Fig. 12.4) and slump tests (► Fig. 12.5), which induce stretch upon the nerve roots exiting at the level of the lumbar disks. The slump test involves the patient seated and slumped over while the examiner passively raises each leg and assesses for reproduction of radicular distribution of pain. This test is more sensitive but just as specific as the straight leg test for lumbar radiculopathy due to disk herniation.[18] The straight leg raise test is performed while the patient is supine and the examiner passively raises each leg while the opposite extremity lies flat. Radicular pain provoked between 30 and 70 degrees of flexion in either test suggests nerve root impingement, and higher level imaging may be warranted.

The sports in which athletes are at greatest risk for low back and lumbar spine injuries include gymnastics, weightlifting, and football, though they are also common in wrestling and skiing. Herniated disks are seen most commonly in elite gymnasts and football linemen.[7] Athletes with immature skeletons who participate in any sport with aggressive axial rotation of the spine, such as gymnastics, swimming, discus, javelin, baseball, and golf, are most susceptible to unilateral or bilateral pars interarticularis fractures (spondylolysis or spondylolisthesis). These injuries, particularly spondylolisthesis, can result in anterior displacement of vertebrae and subsequent spinal instability. Concern for these injuries warrants initial workup involving plain films in flexion and extension, and possibly higher level imaging.[7] If there is concern for radicular injury on the sideline, generally either a straight leg or slump test is sufficient for the assessment of radicular symptoms.

12.3.4 Shoulder, Hip, and Sacroiliac Joints

An athlete primarily complaining of shoulder pain should still be assessed for cervical spine injury, as cervical radicular pain could contribute to these symptoms. The base of the lumbar spine is closely associated with the sacroiliac joints and hips

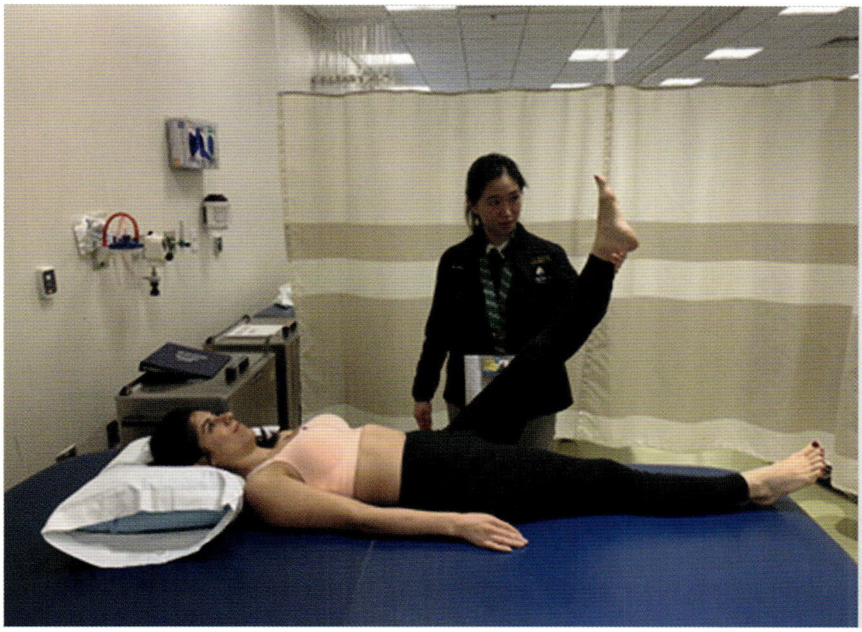

Fig. 12.4 The straight leg raise test is performed while the patient is supine and the examiner passively raises each leg while the opposite extremity lies flat. If radicular pain is provoked between 30 and 70 degrees of flexion in either test, this suggests nerve root impingement, and higher level imaging may be warranted.

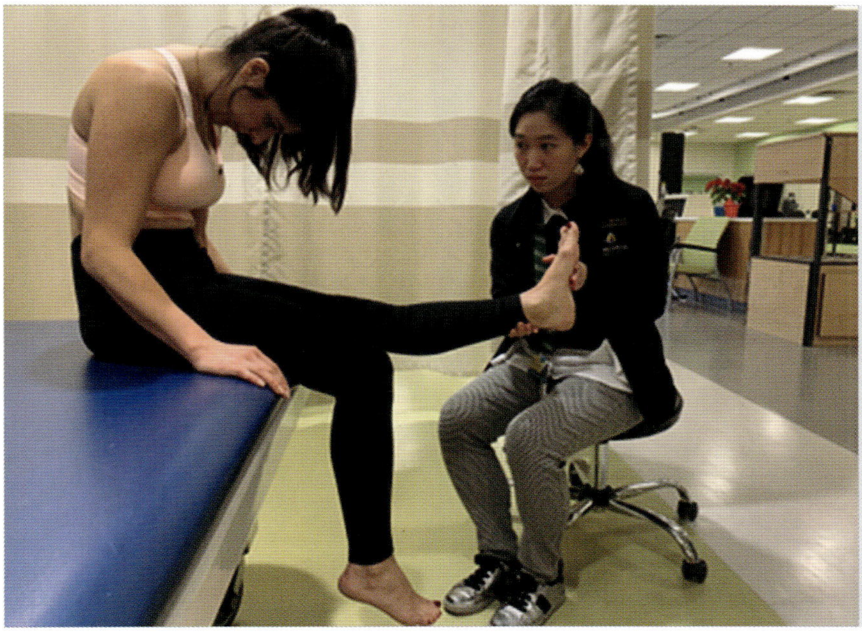

Fig. 12.5 The slump test is performed with the patient seated and slumped over while the examiner passively raises each leg and assesses for reproduction of radicular distribution of pain.

where concomitant pathology could contribute to the presentation of an athlete with suspected low back or spinal injury. Pain or dysfunction at the inguinal, gluteal, or sacral sulcus regions warrants subsequent examination and testing to evaluate for nonspinal injury.

12.4 Clinical Pearls

- Thorough and efficient evaluation of the athletic spine can help quickly diagnose acute injury and rule out rare but potentially catastrophic injury.
- A thorough evaluation of the athletic spine requires a private, enclosed setting, appropriate exposure of the spine, a reflex hammer, and alcohol swabs or other method to adequately assess light touch, pinprick, and temperature sensation.
- Essential elements of a thorough evaluation of the athletic spine are a detailed history, visual inspection, palpation, active and passive range of motion, neurological assessment, and provocative maneuvers specific to the area of injury and differential diagnoses.
- Signs and symptoms of neurological compromise and potential spinal cord injury include new focal weakness,

numbness, reflex changes (hyperreflexia or asymmetry), or bladder or bowel incontinence. Any of these should trigger removal from play and emergent workup and triage in an otherwise healthy athlete.

- Frequent serial assessments should be performed to monitor for evolution or progression of symptoms, and there should be a high threshold to provide clearance for athletes to return to play.
- Be aware of peripheral pathology that can be associated with or appear as spine or cord injury such as shoulder, brachial plexus, sacroiliac joint, or hip injuries.

References

[1] Cantu RC, Li YM, Abdulhamid M, Chin LS. Return to play after cervical spine injury in sports. Curr Sports Med Rep. 2013; 12(1):14–17

[2] Anderson S, Schnebel B. Sideline neurological evaluation: a detailed approach to the sideline, in-game neurological assessment of contact sport athletes. Curr Pain Headache Rep. 2016; 20(7):46

[3] Putukian M. Clinical evaluation of the concussed athlete: a view from the sideline. J Athl Train. 2017; 52(3):236–244

[4] Kirshblum SC, Waring W, Biering-Sorensen F, et al. Reference for the 2011 revision of the International Standards for Neurological Classification of Spinal Cord Injury. J Spinal Cord Med. 2011; 34(6):547–554

[5] Slipman CW, Plastaras CT, Palmitier RA, Huston CW, Sterenfeld EB. Symptom provocation of fluoroscopically guided cervical nerve root stimulation. Are dynatomal maps identical to dermatomal maps? Spine. 1998; 23(20):2235–2242

[6] Tong HC, Haig AJ, Yamakawa K. The Spurling test and cervical radiculopathy. Spine. 2002; 27(2):156–159

[7] Huang P, Anissipour A, McGee W, Lemak L. Return-to-play recommendations after cervical, thoracic, and lumbar spine injuries: a comprehensive review. Sports Health. 2016; 8(1):19–25

[8] Rihn JA, Anderson DT, Lamb K, et al. Cervical spine injuries in American football. Sports Med. 2009; 39(9):697–708

[9] Betz RR, Mulcahey MJ, D'Andrea LP, Clements DH. Acute evaluation and management of pediatric spinal cord injury. J Spinal Cord Med. 2004; 27 Suppl 1:S11–S15

[10] Cuccurullo SJ. Physical Medicine and Rehabilitation Board Review. 3rd ed. Demos Medical Publishing; 2014

[11] Torg JS, Sennett B, Pavlov H, Leventhal MR, Glasgow SG. Spear tackler's spine. An entity precluding participation in tackle football and collision activities that expose the cervical spine to axial energy inputs. Am J Sports Med. 1993; 21(5):640–649

[12] Lorente A, Barrios C, Lorente R, Tamariz R, Burgos J. Severe hyperkyphosis reduces the aerobic capacity and maximal exercise tolerance in patients with Scheuermann disease. Spine J. 2019; 19(2):330–338

[13] Revel ME, Listrat VM, Chevalier XJ, et al. Facet joint block for low back pain: identifying predictors of a good response. Arch Phys Med Rehabil. 1992; 73 (9):824–828

[14] Heneghan NR, Smith R, Tyros I, Falla D, Rushton A. Thoracic dysfunction in whiplash associated disorders: a systematic review. PLoS One. 2018; 13(3): e0194235

[15] Silva LOJE, Fernanda Bellolio M, Smith EM, Daniels DJ, Lohse CM, Campbell RL. Motocross-associated head and spine injuries in adult patients evaluated in an emergency department. Am J Emerg Med. 2017; 35(10):1485–1489

[16] Hubbard ME, Jewell RP, Dumont TM, Rughani AI. Spinal injury patterns among skiers and snowboarders. Neurosurg Focus. 2011; 31(5):E8

[17] Omidi-Kashani F, Ebrahimzadeh MH, Salari S. Lumbar spondylolysis and spondylolytic spondylolisthesis: who should be have surgery? An algorithmic approach. Asian Spine J. 2014; 8(6):856–863

[18] Majlesi J, Togay H, Unalan H, Toprak S. The sensitivity and specificity of the Slump and the Straight Leg Raising tests in patients with lumbar disc herniation. J Clin Rheumatol. 2008; 14(2):87–91

13 Rehabilitation of Athletic Spinal Injuries

Alexis M. Coslick and Mark I. Ellen

Summary

Athletic spinal injuries range from acute injury to overuse injury and can vary in time missed from sport. Depending on the athlete's diagnosis and goals, an individualized treatment plan can be developed. This program is continually re-evaluated with regard to regression or progression. The principles of rehabilitation for the spine follow the same general progression for other body parts. Initially there is a period of relative rest while undergoing pain control modalities. The rehabilitation progression consists of assessing the athlete for impaired biomechanics and asymmetries, working on core stabilization and spinal mobilization, stretching, followed by strengthening. Strengthening can further advance to include increased weight or intensity, adding balance and proprioception, and progressing to sport-specific exercises. Full clearance for return to play occurs after the athlete completes the rehabilitation program and achieves full range of motion and strength, and after completion of the sport-specific progression.

Keywords: athlete spine rehabilitation, sports rehabilitation, athlete spine injuries, spine rehabilitation, spine exercises, spine therapy

13.1 Introduction

Spinal injuries can be categorized by mechanism and timeline, such as acute versus overuse injuries.[1] Overuse injuries usually occur secondary to a training error[2] or fatigue due to repetitive stressors and/or excessive loads placed upon the body.[3,4]

Athletes undergo complex physical stressors with increased biomechanical forces at unique joint angles for specific athletic motions.[5] This causes the athlete to be susceptible to specific spinal injuries associated with the sport. Athletes experience increased compressive, rotational, and shear forces, along with tensile stress about the spinal column[5] as compared to their sedentary counterparts. Strength and flexibility impairments can alter an athlete's biomechanics, which may result in pain.[6] This can create a cycle leading to inhibition and disuse, resulting in further muscle atrophy,[7] weakness,[1] and neuromuscular impairments.[1,7]

The rehabilitation team must pay careful attention to the demands of the athlete's sport and then develop a sport-specific rehabilitation and maintenance program. Athletes may also challenge clinicians by not fully disclosing the severity of their symptoms for fear of lost playing time or compensation.[4] In addition, the coach may place pressure on the athlete to return to play as quickly as possible. This urgency may vary depending on the time of season versus the offseason. Therefore, one must be thorough in the evaluation and take into account not just the actual injury, but all of the factors which may influence an athlete's decision-making.

It is important to make as accurate a diagnosis as possible in order to develop a well-defined and individualized treatment plan[5,8,9,10] based on the particular injury and athletic endeavor.[2] Relative rest of the involved area may be necessary; however, total immobilization should only be utilized sparingly,[5,10] if ever. In some cases, it may be possible to rehabilitate the athletes while they continue to participate in their sport.[11,12] For mechanical low back pain, potential activity modifications may be trialed[13] as the natural course is typically self-limiting.[11] More significant pain or injury to the spine such as spondylolysis[13] will require time away from the athlete's sport.[11] Most etiologies of back[4] and neck pain[14] can be managed well nonoperatively with a comprehensive functional rehabilitation program[4,15] that corrects biomechanics[1,2,3,7,16] and strength imbalances, improves flexibility, and incorporates a spine stabilization program.[1,3,7,16]

13.2 General Rehabilitation Overview

The development of the rehabilitation program begins with evaluation of the athlete's current abilities and limitations.[11,12,16] The goals of rehabilitation are to combat deconditioning, prevent further impairment, and return the athlete to the sport safely and as soon as reasonably possible[4,5,10,11,12] while minimizing the risk of future injury.[11] Regardless of the injury, the spine rehabilitation program for athletes should follow the same general progression to return to play while making adjustments for each individual.[11] Clinicians should utilize the athlete's pain level, activity tolerance, and improvements in strength and flexibility to guide their progression or regression of the rehabilitation program.

13.3 Acute Phase

Rehabilitation of athletically induced spinal injuries uses the same principles that exist for other injuries such as peripheral joints. Initially, treatment should focus on decreasing pain[7] and inflammation[5,10,17] while protecting the injured segment.[5,17] The athlete should utilize cryotherapy[3,14] as a mainstay due to its anti-inflammatory properties. Anti-inflammatory medications are helpful as adjunct therapy during the acute phase[5,14,15] to decrease inflammation and pain often associated with injuries. This reduction in pain can allow the athlete to better participate in rehabilitation, prevent immobility, and minimize deconditioning and disuse.

13.4 Therapeutic Modalities

Therapeutic modalities should also be integrated during the acute phase and continued throughout rehabilitation to alleviate pain and inflammation. Manual therapy, in the hands of an experienced certified practitioner, has been shown to be beneficial in the short term to reduce pain[14,17] as well as promote healing.[17] Manual therapy strategies include soft tissue massage,[1,3] soft tissue mobilization, myofascial release, and traction.[3] Athletic trainers and physical therapists may incorporate neural glides, taping,[3] ultrasound, or transcutaneous electrical stimulation (TENS).[1,3]

13.5 Biomechanics

Assessment of an athlete's biomechanics helps to identify underlying factors that contribute to injury.[1,2,3,7,16] The spine supports muscular forces transmitted between the upper and lower extremities,[4] allowing the body to function as a cohesive unit. Therefore, poor neck and back biomechanics can negatively affect force production by the extremities[2] and lead to impairments elsewhere in the body. Improper technique places undue demand upon the spine and overcomes the spine and surrounding musculature's ability to withstand external forces.[2] Retraining of the musculature with proper techniques for each particular sport and skill is essential.[16]

13.6 Core Stabilization

Since the 1980s, stabilization of the core has been a basic tenet of spinal rehabilitation.[2,12] The core consists of the spine, hips, pelvis, proximal lower extremities, and abdomen,[9] as well as the musculature that surrounds these structures. It functions to maintain stability of the body during functional movements.[8] Strengthening core musculature optimizes dynamic multiplanar spine stabilization and force transfer to the extremities during sports activities.[2,8] Rehabilitation of the core consists of progressive activation, strengthening, and coordination of the trunk musculature[6,9,18] to address balance,[8,9] flexibility,[6,9,18] endurance,[9] motor relearning,[8] and proprioception deficits.[18]

It is recommended that all spinal rehabilitation programs commence with the athlete placed in a pain-free non-weight-bearing (prone or supine) neutral spine position,[5,10,16] which decreases the stress placed on the spine[19] (▶ Fig. 13.1). This posture should be maintained throughout all upper and lower body exercises to improve spinal alignment and protect the injured segment.[5] Neutral spine is a position that can be maintained with slight exertion by the body's structures[19] and optimizes balance and power.[7] Implementing proprioceptive training into the rehabilitation program improves joint position sense, which may help with posture and maintaining the spine in a neutral position. The neutral spine position is found by gently flexing and extending the spine to achieve a position of comfort. It is necessary for the athlete to initially avoid axial loading of the injured segments and spine movements that provoke pain. These maneuvers will be reintroduced later in a controlled manner[17] as the athlete progresses through the rehabilitation program.

13.7 Spine Mobility

Early mobilization should be implemented to restore range of motion of the spine[3] and to improve flexibility of the extremities. This will decrease the stress applied through the lumbar spine.[5] There are various exercises to increase cervical and lumbar spinal mobility. Cervical extension mobilization utilizes the athlete's fingers or a strap to act as a fulcrum about the posterior neck at different spinal levels[20] (▶ Fig. 13.2). Targeting the superior cervical flexors and extensors is accomplished with nodding against gravity.[20] The cat/cow exercise consists of the patient in the quadruped position with the palms and knees in contact with the floor. Gentle mobilization is achieved as the athlete slowly arches and rounds the spine. Dead bug exercise are performed with the athlete in supine position (▶ Fig. 13.3). One shoulder is flexed to 180 degrees while the opposite hip and knee are flexed to 90 degrees. Both the limbs are lowered, and the remaining two limbs follow the same pattern, alternating to create a marching movement. Stretching should also target the soft tissues adjacent to the injured spinal segment including the hips,[4,7,17] pelvis,[4] extremities,[7] and abdomen. The abdominal musculature is elongated in the upward dog pose where the athlete is prone and pushes up onto the elbows or palms with the elbows in full extension (▶ Fig. 13.4). The spinal musculature is stretched in child's pose where the athlete is in a kneeling position with the hips externally rotated and the trunk is flexed in order to place the chest and shoulders on the floor with the shoulders flexed to 180 degrees (▶ Fig. 13.5), or by performing supine unilateral and bilateral hip and knee flexion into the chest. Athletes should let pain guide their level of activity and should avoid any positions that exacerbate their symptoms.

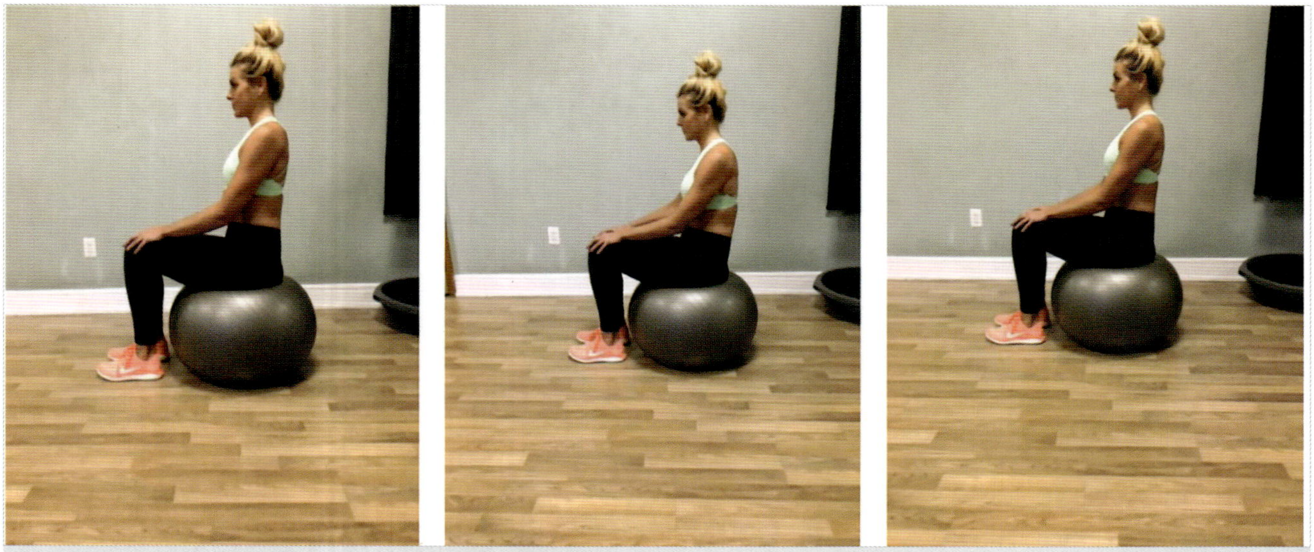

Fig. 13.1 Finding neutral (neutral, flexion, extension) spine position.

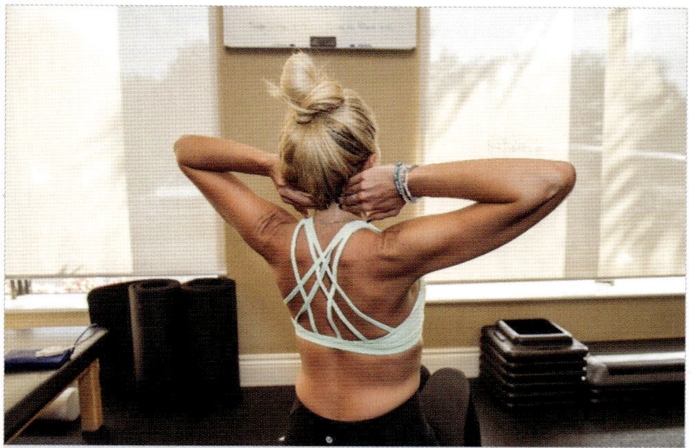

Fig. 13.2 Cervical extensor musculature stretching using the fingers as a fulcrum.

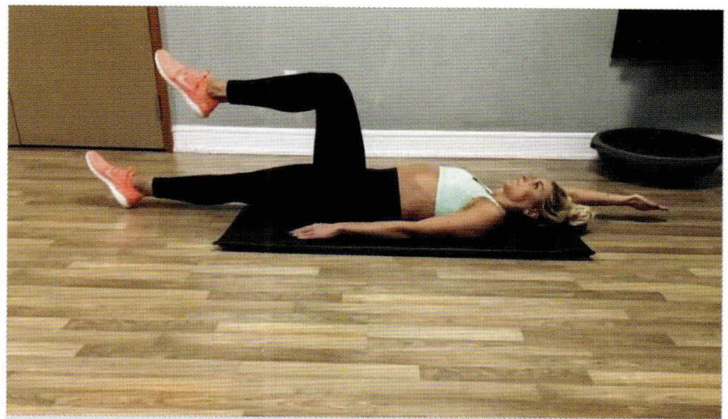

Fig. 13.3 Dead bug exercise.

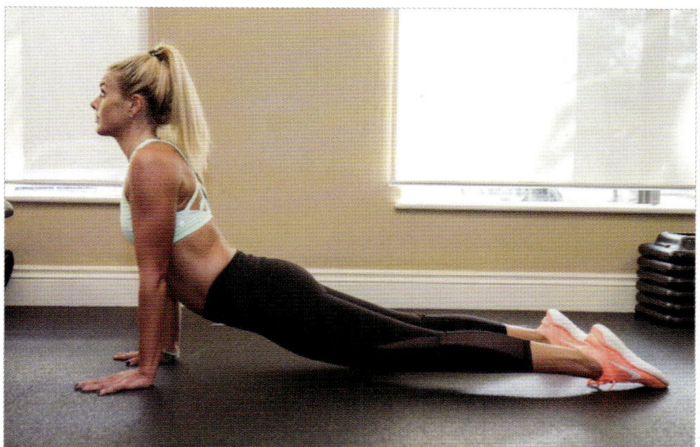

Fig. 13.4 Stretching of the abdominal musculature in upward facing dog pose.

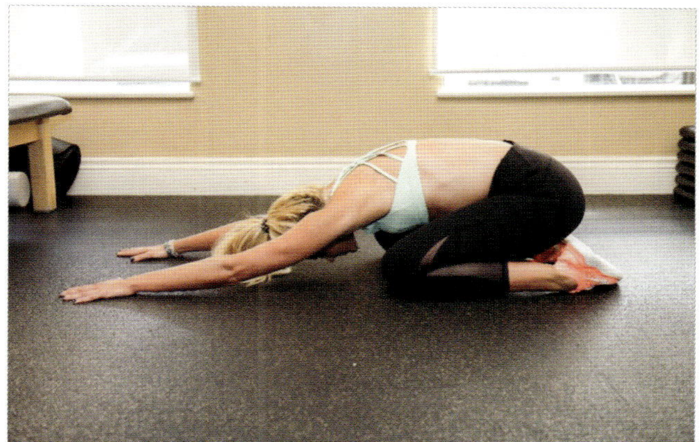

Fig. 13.5 Stretching the back musculature in child's pose.

13.8 Muscle Activation and Motor Control

Coordination of motor activity allows the body to perform as a unit.[2,10] However, patients with back pain are more likely to exhibit impaired muscle activation.[6,18] The athlete should activate isolated muscles, paying particular attention to the activation of the gluteal muscles.[6] The individual[17] and sequential activation of core and extremity musculature maximizes force production and transmission to the extremities,[5,9] while decreasing the stress applied to the distal joints.[9] Learning new patterns of motor control will alter the athlete's biomechanics and result in dynamic stabilization of the spine.[2] This neuromuscular control should be maintained as the athlete progresses through spine stabilization and more functional exercises. This may diminish the risk of future back pain.[5]

The athletes should be assessed for any strength imbalances within their core musculature while performing both single-plane and triplanar (transverse, coronal, and sagittal) activities.[3] These muscle groups include the paraspinal muscles,[7] transverse abdominis,[2,3,7] quadratus lumborum, multifidi,[2,7,9] latissimus dorsi, and scapular stabilizers.[2,7] In addition to the back and abdominal musculature, the quadriceps, hamstrings, and gluteal muscles[5] are paramount in the force transfer between the trunk and extremities.[7]

13.9 Adaptive Progression

Rehabilitation exercises may be modified and adapted as the athlete progresses from the acute phase prior to returning to sport. Isometric spine stabilization exercises can be implemented early on in the rehabilitation program,[3,5,10] especially if pain-free range of motion is limited.[21] Isometric exercises involve maintaining a constant muscle length, which prevents the injured segment from being loaded at weak points throughout different joint angles. The transverse abdominis and multifidus should be targeted early[2,3] with partial sit-ups and "Supermans." Supermans are performed in a prone position, lifting an upper extremity and the opposite lower extremity off the ground as the athlete isometrically contracts the posterior spinal muscles. The athlete then slowly lowers the extremities to the ground and elevates the opposite two extremities. As the athlete's strength increases, the Superman can progress to a dynamic lift of all four extremities at the same time (▶ Fig. 13.6). Partial sit-ups require the athlete

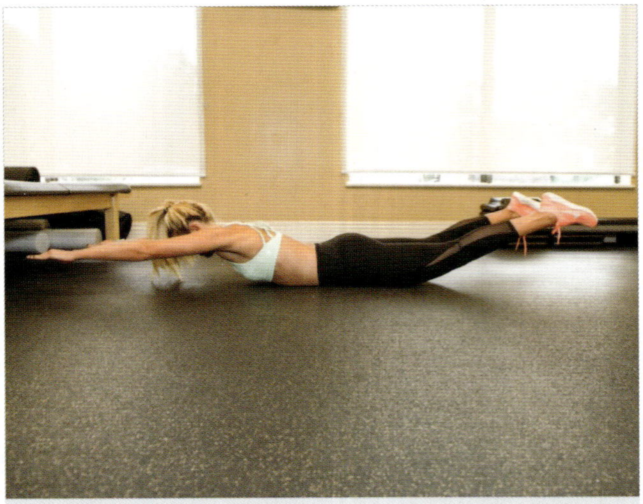

Fig. 13.6 Superman with all four extremities elevated emphasizing back musculature and neuromuscular coordination.

to lead with the chest elevating both the shoulders and back and then holding this position (▶ Fig. 13.7). Other exercises that can be added include planks, quadrupeds, and cervical nodding. Planks are performed in a prone or side-lying position initially on the elbows and feet and advancing to contacting the ground with the palms and feet. Quadrupeds are performed with the athlete on all fours while elevating the extremities similarly to Supermans. Cervical flexors are activated when nodding the head against resistance.[3] The aforementioned exercises can initially be performed as isometric exercises and then advanced to more fluid movements. Next, progression to performing these exercises on a stability ball can continue to challenge strength and neuromuscular control[22] (▶ Fig. 13.8).

Both upper and lower extremity exercises should accompany truncal exercises. For the upper extremities, athletes can perform unweighted shoulder shrugs, shoulder rolls, and arm rolls with their shoulders abducted to 90 degrees and the elbows fully extended. From this same position, the athlete can then adduct his or her upper extremities to midline.[22] Lower extremity exercises can begin with wall slides to strengthen the thigh musculature. The athlete's back rests against the wall and flexes the hips and knees to 90 degrees into a sitting position.[22] In bridging, athletes are supine with two feet on the floor and lift their pelvis off the floor. Progression includes elevating one lower extremity with the hip and knee extended as the athlete leaves the other foot on the ground to act as the bridge when the athlete lifts the pelvis.

As the athlete continues to recover, the exercises advance to further challenge the athlete. The volume of exercise increases as the athlete performs a greater number of repetitions or sets of each exercise. The concluding phase of these exercises involves increased intensity with the addition of ankle weights and light hand weights.[22]

As the athlete's strength increases, balance work should be added to the rehabilitation program to further challenge the athlete.[10] Core stability exercises can incorporate balance and proprioceptive training by altering the surface on which the athlete is working with the addition of a Bosu ball or stability ball. Yoga[23,24] and Pilates[23] are added later during rehabilitation. Yoga relies on a series of positions and exercises that integrate

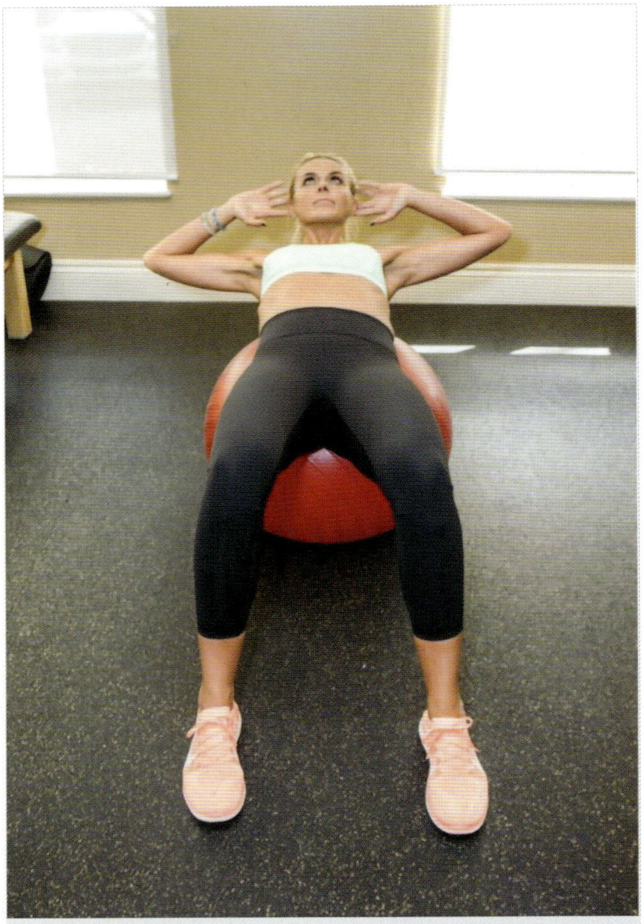

Fig. 13.7 Partial sit-up on a stability ball, strengthening abdominal musculature.

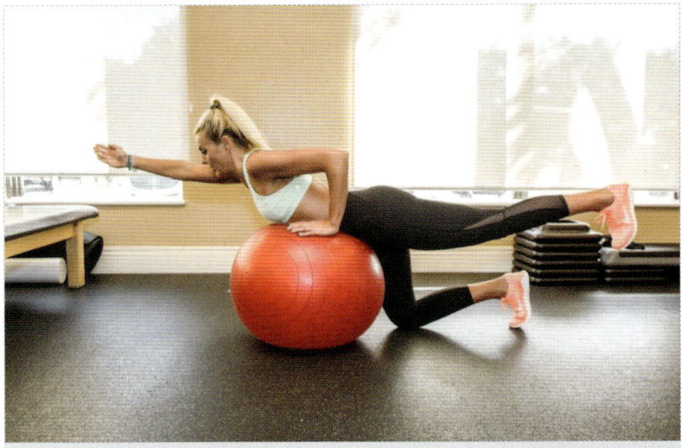

Fig. 13.8 Quadruped on a stability ball.

strength with balance while loading the joints at various angles to improve range of motion.[24]

As the athlete progresses through each phase of the rehabilitation program, frequent assessments by the training staff and physician are conducted to gauge the athlete's response to treatment and the athlete's readiness for proceeding to the next phase.[11,12] The successful completion of each phase is dictated by the alleviation of the athlete's pain and improvement in strength and flexibility.

The athlete advances to closed kinetic chain[3] and triplanar[8,17] activities to simulate functional movements. It is necessary to increase the demands placed on the athlete's body in a controlled environment to prepare the athlete for future stresses.[17] This phase of rehabilitation introduces therapeutic exercises that mimic athletic performance[2,17] and sport-specific activities.[1,2,3,7,16]

13.10 Aerobic Excercise

Aerobic exercise should be added throughout the rehabilitation program as tolerated to prevent deconditioning.[1,3] Aerobic conditioning strengthens musculoskeletal structures[10,11] and improves cardiovascular fitness.[10] There are multiple modalities for cardiovascular conditioning including aquatic therapy, antigravity treadmill, stationary bicycle, and elliptical trainer. It is important to select a cardiovascular activity that is individualized for the athlete to offload the stress placed upon the spine.[5]

13.11 Aquatic Rehabilitation

Aquatic-based rehabilitation, termed aquatic therapy or hydrotherapy, can also be utilized to promote recovery from injury,[5,11,25,26] increase strength,[11,26] and improve range of motion.[26] Although there is limited literature to support a specific aquatic therapy rehabilitation program, this is a valuable option for athletes who are unable to tolerate full weight-bearing. Water-based exercise enables sport-specific actions while minimizing impact.[25,26] This may also diminish the athlete's anxiety about reinjury during recovery and rehabilitation.[25] Aquatic exercises can be used to specifically target core musculature and improve neuromuscular control while offloading the body. Aquatic therapy allows the athlete to gradually increase the loading experienced by the body as the athlete transitions from deeper to shallower water and finally to land.[26] As land-based therapy is introduced, aquatic-based therapy can continue to be incorporated on alternating days if needed, with the progression to more frequent land-based training.[26]

In order to return to competition, athletes must be able to perform all of the sport-specific skills[1,3,7,17] at their preinjury intensity and skill level.[7] This requires successful completion of the entire rehabilitation program, which is defined by full pain-free range of motion, normal strength,[1,3,4,7,14] and the ability to appropriately stabilize the core musculature with all tasks.[1,3,4,7] This is accomplished first in a controlled practice setting and advances to competition, signifying readiness for return to play. Once the athlete has made enough progress to return to play, a maintenance program should be added to the athlete's daily routine to diminish the risk of future injuries.[2]

13.12 Rehabilitation Progression

- Find neutral spine position:
  - Seated: gentle rounding and arching of the spine until the athlete finds the position of comfort with the least stress applied to the spine.
    - This can also be performed on a stability ball.
  - The exercises below should be performed while maintaining a neutral spine.
- Range of motion and gentle mobilization:
  - Cervical spine:
    - Gentle flexion, extension, side-bending, rotation.
    - Using the fingers as a fulcrum on the posterior spine will stretch the cervical flexors.
  - Lumbar spine:
    - Mobilization:
      - Cat/cow mobilization.
      - Seated arching and rounding of the spine on a stability ball.
      - Deadbugs.
    - Stretching:
      - Child's pose.
      - Supine hugging of one knee or bilateral knees to the chest.
      - Upward dog on elbows or palms with elbows extended.
- Core strengthening:
  - Isometrics:
    - Cervical nodding against the athlete's hands or clinician's hands.
    - Planks: progress from elbows to palms in prone and lateral positions.
    - Quadruped: initially either single upper extremity or lower extremity and progress to opposite upper and lower extremity simultaneously.
    - Superman: initially either single upper extremity or lower extremity and progress to opposite upper and lower extremity simultaneously and then elevating all four extremities.
    - Partial sit-ups: on the floor or stability ball.
  - Strengthening with mobility and coordination:
    - Partial sit-ups.
    - Superman: similar to isometric strengthening, but now as a flow movement coordinating all four extremities.
    - Quadruped: similar to isometric strengthening, but now as a flow movement coordinating all four extremities.
- Extremity strengthening:
  - Upper extremity:
    - Shoulder shrugs.
    - Shoulder rolls.
    - Arm rolls.
    - Arm adduction.
      - Progression includes increasing the number of sets and repetitions and adding handheld weights.
  - Lower extremity:
    - Fire hydrants.
    - Donkey kicks.
    - Wall sits.
    - Bridging.
      - Initially two feet are placed on the floor with the hips and pelvis lifted in the air.

        - The athlete progresses to elevate one extremity and performs single extremity bridging.
    - The progression includes increasing the number of sets or repetitions and the addition of ankle weights or using a weighted vest or holding a medicine ball for wall sits.
- Balance and proprioception:
    - Superman: progress to a stability ball.
    - Yoga and Pilates: different postures and positions will incorporate stretching, mobility, coordination, and strengthening.
- Aerobic exercise:
    - Elliptical.
    - Stationary bicycle.
    - Aquatic jogging.
    - Swimming laps.
    - Anti-gravity treadmill:
        - The intensity and distance can be gradually increased.
        - This can be implemented earlier in the rehabilitation progression as tolerated by the athlete to prevent deconditioning.
- Aquatic exercise:
    - Range of motion of the shoulders and hips.
    - Utilizing the resistance of the water to strengthen shoulder and hips.
        - Performing the same shoulder mobility exercises as on land listed above.
        - Hip flexion, extension, abduction, adduction.
- Return to play:
    - Reintroducing sport-specific exercises such as jumping, sprinting, pivoting, sports-specific footwork.
    - Maximum intensity sport-specific drills without contact including reintroducing a ball or other sports equipment.
    - Full contact in practice in a somewhat controlled environment.
    - Return to full competition.

13.13 Clinical Pearls

- The rehabilitation program relies on an accurate diagnosis and considers the athlete's preinjury physical abilities, the skills required for the position, and the timing during the season or off-season.
- The goals of rehabilitation are to decrease pain, prevent deconditioning, return the athlete to a level that exceeds his or her prior physical abilities as quickly as possible while correcting suboptimal biomechanics, and preventing future injury.
- Rehabilitation is initially aimed at pain control and anti-inflammation. Therapeutic modalities such as neural glides, transcutaneous electrical stimulation, ultrasound, and iontophoresis can be incorporated.
- Emphasis is placed on core stabilization, which encompasses strengthening, motor coordination, flexibility, balance, and proprioceptive neuromuscular facilitation.
- The athlete begins the rehabilitation in neutral spine position and maintains this posture throughout the program, including returning to sport.
- Spine rehabilitation includes restoring range of motion, progressive strengthening, and advancing to multiplanar functional and sport-specific activities.
- Aerobic activity is added to prevent cardiovascular deconditioning. The exact modality is individualized to reduce the stress placed on the athlete's spine.
- Aquatic therapy can be used for aerobic conditioning or to improve range of motion, strength, and core stabilization while offloading the injured segment.
- In order to return to play, the athlete must achieve pain-free full range of motion, full strength, and the ability to perform the sport-specific skills at the highest intensity required for the sport.

References

[1] d'Hemecourt PA, Gerbino PG, II, Micheli LJ. Back injuries in the young athlete. Clin Sports Med. 2000; 19(4):663–679

[2] Standaert CJ, Herring SA, Pratt TW. Rehabilitation of the athlete with low back pain. Curr Sports Med Rep. 2004; 3(1):35–40

[3] Sampsell E. Rehabilitation of the spine following sports injury. Clin Sports Med. 2010; 29(1):127–156

[4] Trainor TJ, Trainor MA. Etiology of low back pain in athletes. Curr Sports Med Rep. 2004; 3(1):41–46

[5] Watkins RG, Dillin WH. Lumbar spine injury in the athlete. Clin Sports Med. 1990; 9(2):419–448

[6] Kruse D, Lemmen B. Spine injuries in the sport of gymnastics. Curr Sports Med Rep. 2009; 8(1):20–28

[7] Krabak B, Kennedy DJ. Functional rehabilitation of lumbar spine injuries in the athlete. Sports Med Arthrosc Rev. 2008; 16(1):47–54

[8] Akuthota V, Nadler SF. Core strengthening. Arch Phys Med Rehabil. 2004; 85 (3) Suppl 1:S:86–92

[9] Kibler WB, Press J, Sciascia A. The role of core stability in athletic function. Sports Med. 2006; 36(3):189–198

[10] Watkins RG. Lumbar disc injury in the athlete. Clin Sports Med. 2002; 21(1): 147–165, viii

[11] White AA, Voy RO, Ryan EJ, Beeten R. A program for the evaluation and management of the high performance athlete with acute low back pain. J Athl Train. 1990; 25(3):228–229, 230, 231, 232

[12] Hopkins TJ, White AA, III. Rehabilitation of athletes following spine injury. Clin Sports Med. 1993; 12(3):603–619

[13] De Luigi AJ. Low back pain in the adolescent athlete. Phys Med Rehabil Clin N Am. 2014; 25(4):763–788

[14] Krabak BJ, Kanarek SL. Cervical spine pain in the competitive athlete. Phys Med Rehabil Clin N Am. 2011; 22(3):459–471, viii

[15] Mautner KR, Huggins MJ. The young adult spine in sports. Clin Sports Med. 2012; 31(3):453–472

[16] Watkins RG, III. Great rehabilitation and great physical bodies allow professional athletes undergoing lumbar discectomy to return to sport at a high rate. Spine J. 2011; 11(3):187–189

[17] Vangelder LH, Hoogenboom BJ, Vaughn DW. A phased rehabilitation protocol for athletes with lumbar intervertebral disc herniation. Int J Sports Phys Ther. 2013; 8(4):482–516

[18] Renkawitz T, Boluki D, Grifka J. The association of low back pain, neuromuscular imbalance, and trunk extension strength in athletes. Spine J. 2006; 6(6):673–683

[19] Panjabi MM. The stabilizing system of the spine. Part II. Neutral zone and instability hypothesis. J Spinal Disord. 1992; 5(4):390–396, discussion 397

[20] Durall CJ. Therapeutic exercise for athletes with nonspecific neck pain: a current concepts review. Sports Health. 2012; 4(4):293–301

[21] Vegso JJ, Torg E, Torg JS. Rehabilitation of cervical spine, brachial plexus, and peripheral nerve injuries. Clin Sports Med. 1987; 6(1):135–158

[22] Watkins III RG, Watkins IV RG. Watkins spine email document. 07/25/2018

[23] Sorosky S, Stilp S, Akuthota V. Yoga and Pilates in the management of low back pain. Curr Rev Musculoskelet Med. 2008; 1(1):39–47

[24] Polsgrove MJ, Eggleston BM, Lockyer RJ. Impact of 10-weeks of yoga practice on flexibility and balance of college athletes. Int J Yoga. 2016; 9(1):27–34

[25] Wicker A. Sport-specific aquatic rehabilitation. Curr Sports Med Rep. 2011; 10(2):62–63

[26] Thein JM, Brody LT. Aquatic-based rehabilitation and training for the elite athlete. J Orthop Sports Phys Ther. 1998; 27(1):32–41

14 Spinal Manipulation

Michael A. Miller

Summary
The intent of this chapter is to offer insight into how chiropractic relates to treating many musculoskeletal injuries with emphasis on spinal misalignments, referred to as subluxations, and the relationship to the nervous system. I have attempted to incorporate some of my observations as it relates to treatment of professional athletes from my experience over the past 38 years with the New England Patriots. The team approach to injury control has been the most effective with evaluation and treatment protocols. The entire medical team including physicians, trainers, physical therapists, nutritionists, massage therapists, and allied health professionals understand their role as specialists designed to foster optimum performance from the athlete. We also understand our limitations and realize we are all team members dependent upon each other's expertise. The players' confidence in our skills allow them to perform at their maximum potential and creates an environment of trust that we will maintain their health, and if injuries occur, we will design an appropriate rehabilitation and strengthening program customized to allow them to return to play. Chiropractic has proven its efficacy in treating these sports-related injuries and has gained national recognition among all 32 teams in the National Football League.

Keywords: sports chiropractic, spinal manipulation, subluxation and effects of spinal misalignment, concussion, chronic traumatic encephalopathy (CTE), herniated disk, National Football League (NFL), high velocity, low amplitude (HVLA) techniques

14.1 Introduction

The intent of this chapter is to introduce the concept of chiropractic as a specialized care that utilizes the belief that a vertebra, when misaligned, can cause nerve pain or dysfunction. It addresses the subjective symptoms that are caused by subluxations of the spine and its contiguous structures. It also emphasizes the significance of the art of both static and motion palpation in detecting subluxation. In addition, this chapter describes frequently encountered disorders seen in the athlete population and describes the most common manipulative and instrument-assisted techniques that are currently used. This chapter also addresses the contraindications for spinal manipulation and the role of the chiropractic physician in the skills of differential diagnosis to rule out other conditions or medical causes not related to spinal misalignments. Spinal manipulation serves as a health care alternative that can be integrated into the medical model of treating an injured athlete and plays a significant role in both prevention and rehabilitation.

14.2 Introduction to Chiropractic

"The doctor of the future will give no medication, but will interest his patients in the care of the human frame, diet and in the cause and prevention of disease."

- Thomas A. Edison

Chiropractic, derived from the Greek words *cheir* and *praktos,* translates as "the practice by hand." Daniel David Palmer, the founder of Palmer College of Chiropractic in Davenport, Iowa in 1895, introduced the world to chiropractic. Through his innovative thoughts and pioneering spirit, chiropractic evolved into a science, art, and philosophy. In its present-day form, chiropractic searches for the cause of the patient's symptom complex rather than simply treating the symptoms. This involves both static and motion palpation of the spine to identify misalignments or subluxations, which is fundamental to the art of chiropractic. The term *subluxation* refers to the altered position of the vertebral segment and its subsequent hypomobility or loss of normal function and biomechanical motion. The practitioner or chiropractor learns palpation skills in chiropractic technique classes and becomes efficient in palpating the vertebral column searching for signs of misalignment including muscle spasm, hypertonicity, weakness, inhibition, anatomical alignment, tenderness, and temperature changes in the surrounding tissues. This chapter will focus on spinal manipulation and the most common chiropractic techniques used, especially as it relates to care of the professional athlete with an emphasis on the National Football League (NFL) players and the concomitant conditions that lead them to seek chiropractic services. This chapter is based on the author's experience from 38 years as the chiropractic physician to the New England Patriots Football team.

14.3 Indications for Spinal Manipulation

14.3.1 Pain

This is the most common symptom prompting an athlete or individual to seek chiropractic care. Due to the most recent opioid epidemic in our country, spinal manipulation offers a natural health care alternative to the utilization of pain medication.

14.3.2 Decreased Range of Motion

Musculoskeletal stiffness or lack of motion in the cervical, thoracic, lumbar, pelvic, sacroiliac, and/or extremities.

14.3.3 Posture

This is associated with mechanical problems such as those encountered with scoliosis or curvature of the spinal column. Postural analysis can include evaluating several factors, including head tilt or forward head carriage, elevated shoulders, scapular positioning, hypo- or hyperlordosis in the cervical and lumbar spine, kyphosis in the thoracic spine, and pelvic imbalance. Postural screenings are usually a component of an examination that can detect muscular imbalances and/or gait disturbances.

14.3.4 Neurological or Nerve Root Entrapment

One of the most commonly encountered problems seen with football players are "burners" or "stingers," in which the player will complain of an electrical sensation radiating into the trapezius muscle or arm. This injury is typically caused by tractioning of nerve roots when the head is hyperflexed or hyperextended from forces seen during collisions or tackling. This is compounded by the weight of the helmet, which can weigh up to 6 to 8 pounds. When a player experiences a transient or temporary loss of motor and sensory function due to blockage of nerve conduction, this is referred to as neuropraxia. The duration of sensation (seconds vs. minutes vs. hours) typically determines the extent of injury to the nerve and the necessary recovery period. Injuries to the brachial plexus, which is formed from the anterior rami of the lower four cervical nerves (C5, C6, C7, C8) and the first thoracic nerve (T1), can affect these nerves exiting the spinal cord. Spinal manipulation can be beneficial in removing nerve interference and alleviating radicular pain in the upper extremities. Another commonly treated condition is sciatica, or inflammation of the sciatic nerve, the longest nerve in the human body. The player will describe this condition as a "hot poker sensation" radiating into the leg or buttock region, which is usually unilateral. These conditions usually occur as a result of low back injuries when a disk can either bulge or herniate, causing the disk material to contact the nerve and create an inflammatory reaction. If symptoms persist without abatement over the course of several weeks, it is advisable to perform magnetic resonance imaging (MRI) to confirm the diagnosis.

Practice Pearl

Another condition that can mimic sciatica is piriformis syndrome. The piriformis muscle is located behind the gluteus maximus in the buttock, and the sciatic nerve is sandwiched between the piriformis layers. When the piriformis muscle spasms, it compresses the sciatic nerve, which can be confused with sciatica from a herniated disk. Piriformis syndrome is considered a "pseudosciatica," or false sciatica. Trigger point therapy applied to the piriformis muscle with either percussive massage or direct acupressure can relax the muscle and alleviate the symptoms.

14.3.5 Sacroiliac (SI) Disorders

Direct impact to the hip, referred to as "hip pointers," occurs from an impact force to the iliac crest or greater trochanter. When the sacroiliac joints misalign, the affected leg will appear shorter when the patient is lying prone on the examination table, since the SI joint most commonly moves posterior and inferior, raising the acetabular region. Chiropractic technique utilizes a leg check test called the Derifield leg length test to determine if the patient has a functional leg length discrepancy caused by misalignment. This should not be confused with an anatomical short leg which can be caused by prior injuries or surgeries to the foot, ankle, or leg or congenital anomalies. When spinal manipulation is used in these functional leg discrepancies, the leg length can be restored to normal.

Practice Pearl

During clinical practice, players with sacroiliac injuries or pelvic disorders often complain of groin pain. Other than initially suspecting and ruling out a sports hernia, one can consider that these symptoms may be emanating from taut ilioinguinal ligaments that become strained during misalignment injuries of the SI joints. After the SI joints are properly manipulated, the ligament can relax and the pain will subside.

14.3.6 Headaches

One of the most studied areas in sports medicine is the effects of concussion injuries and symptoms attributable to post-concussion syndromes. The concussion protocol involves a multidimensional approach to detecting symptoms and allowing the athletes to return to play once they pass a series of tests. The headaches that a chiropractor may treat can be:

- Cervicogenic (resulting from problems in the cervical spine).
- Migraine.
- Vascular.
- Occipital (arising from tension in the occipital fibers).

Since football is a direct contact sport, the likelihood of head and neck injuries is high. Present-day research is focusing on the advent and creation of newly designed helmets that can more accurately dissipate forces and minimize concussion-type injuries. Players are trained with respect to proper tackling skills in attempts to minimize their exposure to these head and neck injuries.

14.3.7 Vertigo, Equilibrium, and Balance Problems

These symptoms can occur from a variety of sources, including inner ear problems, which involve the movement of tiny particles in the ear called otoconia that break loose. These can be repositioned by centrifugal force exercises, but often require more intensive therapy. Most of the dizziness or lightheadedness that chiropractors treat originates from a condition known as benign positional vertigo (BPV). Another common cause of these symptoms in athletes is dehydration. These symptom complexes are also associated with whiplash injuries of the neck, seen in cervical acceleration–deceleration injuries and post-concussion injuries.

Practice Pearls

When a player presents with vertigo and equilibrium problems but has been cleared medically, there is often a relationship between these symptoms and temporomandibular joint (TMJ) dysfunction. The TMJ can be misaligned from face mask injuries, direct contact injuries, or even from grinding the teeth during sleep. When an extremity adjustment is performed to the TMJ, resolution of these symptoms, as well jaw discomfort, headaches, lightheadedness, earaches, clicking or crepitus in the jaw, and even shoulder pain, often occurs.

14.3.8 Whiplash

Commonly occurring as a result of helmet-to-helmet collisions during football or related to motor vehicle crashes (MVCs), these injuries present themselves with cervical spine pain, limited range of motion, and a myriad of secondary symptoms. The player will usually develop tightness or spasms in the trapezius and cervical musculature and may or may not experience radicular complaints. For players who have suffered prior whiplash injuries, neck collars can be fitted to their shoulder pads that prevent the head from hyperextension movements.

14.3.9 Concussion

When a player suffers a concussion, as determined with the appropriate orthopedic and neurological testing, such as the Standardized Concussion Assessment Tool (SCAT), spinal manipulation can help resolve the associated symptoms and allow the player to return to play with diminished physical and cognitive repercussions.

Practice Pearls

Recent developments in the NFL over the last few years have mandated that each of the 32 teams have a board-licensed neurologist present on game day to assess and grade concussions of the injured player(s). Although the medical team and the trainers can share their input, the neurologist has the final responsibility of deciding whether the player can return to active play. With the recent developments and research into chronic traumatic encephalopathy (CTE), this topic of return to play following head injuries is being actively explored to understand the long-term effects of cumulative microtraumas to the brain. Although the CTE diagnosis can only be formally made during postmortem brain studies, new blood tests are being developed to determine if CTE can be identified by markers associated with the tau proteins, which are associated with brain cell death and dementia.

14.3.10 Degenerative Disk Disease (DDD)

This condition is often diagnosed by plain film radiographs or MRI testing. It is associated with diminished interosseous disk space and is usually caused by degenerative changes or desiccation within the disk. Early degenerative disk changes can be seen in athletes who have had cumulative microtrauma to different parts of their spines. Although they are typically asymptomatic and do not require additional intervention, if imaging demonstrates a sequestered or fragmented disk with a free-floating fragment, then these cases should be referred for neurosurgical review and possible surgical intervention.

14.3.11 Degenerative Joint Disease (DJD)

This condition corresponds to degenerative or arthritic changes seen in the spine and its contiguous structures. They are more likely to be seen in athletes who have sustained repetitive stress injuries. There are also genetic predispositions to different forms of arthritis.

14.3.12 Extremity Injuries

Chiropractic physicians trained in extremity adjusting techniques are able to manipulate the TMJ, shoulders, acromioclavicular and sternoclavicular joints, elbows, wrists, fingers, ribs, knees, ankles, feet, and toes. NFL players are constantly misaligning these extremities and joints and feel immediate gratification when the misalignments are corrected.

Practice Pearls

When a player complains of elbow pain and does not respond to treatment, consider the wrist or lower hand. Sometimes the radius and ulna torque can cause pain in the next proximal joint. Likewise, an athlete can complain of knee pain emanating from misalignment of the lower foot involving the tibia and fibula. You must explore other options instead of fixating solely on the area of complaint.

14.3.13 Overall Performance

This is by far the greatest reason that spinal manipulation and chiropractic care have earned their spots in the sports arena. Pain and limited range of motion can distract players as they try to determine the cause of their discomfort. During professional sports, this can alter their response rate by microseconds and affect their optimal performance.

14.3.14 Proactive Care

We have been able to educate professional teams as to the benefit of chiropractic care as a preventative type of health care. Rather than just treat musculoskeletal injuries, chiropractic care attempts to align the spine by removing vertebral subluxations and minimizing nerve interference. In doing so, we can minimize injuries, prolong playing time, and reduce disability associated with injuries. The mindset of seeking care only when pain occurs should not be the norm. The Professional Football Chiropractic Society presently encompasses chiropractors from all 32 NFL teams with the intent of educating other physicians through our annual symposiums about advanced techniques in spinal manipulation and extremity adjusting, concussion forums, and treatment protocols.

14.4 Contraindications for Spinal Manipulation

There are several important contraindications to spinal manipulation that should be considered. These include:

- Any patient who has had a history of prior cerebrovascular hemorrhages or strokes and/or vertebral artery dissection should be considered at high risk for cervical rotational manipulation.
- Fractures.
- Tumors.
- Ankylosing spondylitis.
- History of malignancies or cancers.
- Moderate to severe osteoporosis.
- Cauda equina syndrome.
- Fragmented disk.

Although each case should be individually evaluated, these conditions warrant additional investigative work by the treating physician to determine what care is suitable.

14.5 What is an Adjustment?

An adjustment refers to a spinal manipulation in which a force is applied equal and opposite to the side of misalignment. When a vertebral segment is adjusted, there is usually a sound that is produced, which is referred to as cavitation. The sound has been described by different researchers as carbon dioxide gases released due to a hydrostatic pressure change in the joint surface during the maneuver. One must understand the principles of physics to analyze force vectors, lines of drive, and acceleration. The thrust, or force, is produced by taking the involved vertebral segment to tension or endpoint range and then applying additional pressure, known in the literature as "peak force." Most spinal manipulation performed by chiropractors is referred to as high velocity, low amplitude thrust (HVLA). According to a research study by Nougarou et al, the manipulative force can increase paraspinal electromyography (EMG) activity during both the thrust phase and immediately following the thrust.[1] They concluded that "local mechanical changes induced by spinal manipulation technique may lead to both instantaneous and long-lasting neurophysiological changes at the spinal and supraspinal levels."[2] In another article, Herzog suggests that chiropractic manipulation is a mechanical event.[3] They also determined that spinal manipulation of the cervical spine caused less tension to the vertebral artery than those produced by diagnostic orthopedic testing and passive range of motion.

Chiropractic spinal manipulation is an art, and many research studies have demonstrated a disparity among practitioners in both the pre-load and thrust phases of the adjustment. Some of this can be attributed to different techniques as well as the expertise and clinical experience of the practitioner. In an article by Owens et al, low amplitude chiropractic adjustments can exert peak forces from 100 to 1,400 N at an average thrust rate of 3 N/ms.[4] Their studies also revealed that male practitioners, on average, had higher rates of thrust than their female counterparts.

Prior to performing a spinal manipulation, it is important to take a case history and either do a problem-focused examination or specialized orthopedic and neurological examinations to determine if additional testing or X-rays are required. Imaging can also be helpful in determining hypo- or hyperlordotic cervical and lumbar spines, rotational misalignments (rotational malposition subluxations), and foraminal encroachment or pinched nerves. No examination of the patient is complete without a thorough examination of the spine utilizing both static and motion palpation. If a vertebra is restricted or fixated, motion will be introduced in the form of a chiropractic manipulative thrust. By tracking the patient's subluxation on a weekly basis, we can determine if the patient is responding favorably to chiropractic care. In more chronic cases, the rotation tends to shift from different directions and side to side until the body comes to an equilibrium. Since muscles move bone it can take a period of time, usually 4 to 6 weeks, to retrain the muscles to accept the desired position. The first direction of misalignment in most vertebra(e) is posterior. When the vertebra misaligns, the spinous process comes closer to the surface of the skin and feels sensitive to palpation due to a multitude of sensory nerve fibers that become irritated. The vertebra(e) can then either rotate or laterally flex to one side. The most common chiropractic techniques will be discussed at the end of the chapter.

14.5.1 Practice Pearl

As a chiropractic team physician, you should always consider a broad differential diagnosis. Not all pain is attributable to misalignment. For example, when an athlete complains of headaches, there are other causes that should be considered. Was there a traumatic head or neck injury? Is the player dehydrated? Could it be related to eye strain? Is it cervicogenic in origin from tension in the occipital fibers? Is it related to TMJ disorders? Can it be a side effect from prescribed medications? Understanding referred pain patterns can be helpful in considering other sources of the pain. Severe low back pain, for instance, can result from a kidney stone in the ureter, while pain below the right scapula may be caused by a gallstone. If a player reports numbness in one of the upper extremities, is it caused by brachial radiculitis or can it be of cardiac or circulatory origin? Have you performed a thorough extremity examination to rule out a subluxed shoulder or impingement syndrome? Is there a carpal tunnel syndrome caused by misalignment of the carpal bones that could be affecting the median nerve? Considering these other diagnoses is critical for taking the appropriate next steps in your patient's care.

14.6 The Effects of Spinal Misalignments

When vertebrae misalign, they can cause irritative symptoms, often due to compression of the nerve from the spinal column. We refer to this phenomenon as a somatovisceral response (▶ Fig. 14.1). We can also understand that if an organ becomes irritated it can reflex to the area of the spine that controls its function, known as a viscerosomatic reflex. Understanding the autonomic nervous system helps to visualize how a pathology can develop.[1] The autonomic nervous system controls bodily functions that are not directed by conscious thought, such as breathing, heartbeat, digestion, pupillary response, and urination. It is divided into two systems known as the sympathetic and parasympathetic systems (▶ Fig. 14.2). They act as regulators of each other and maintain homeostasis in the body. For example, if an athlete gets too hot while competing during a game, the autonomic nervous system causes increased blood circulation to the skin, which induces sweat production to cool down the body. A good analogy is to think of the sympathetic nervous system as excitatory since it is involved in the fight or flight response when the body is subjected to extreme stress and the parasympathetic nervous system as inhibitory or lessening the effect. A study published by Welch and Boone found that cervical manipulations result in parasympathetic responses, whereas thoracic manipulations influence sympathetic responses.[5]

CHART OF EFFECTS OF SPINAL MISALIGNMENTS

"The nervous system controls and coordinates all organs and structures of the human body." (*Gray's Anatomy*, 29th Ed., page 4). Misalignments of spinal vertebrae and disks may cause irritation to the nervous system and affect the structures, organs, and functions that may result in the conditions shown below.

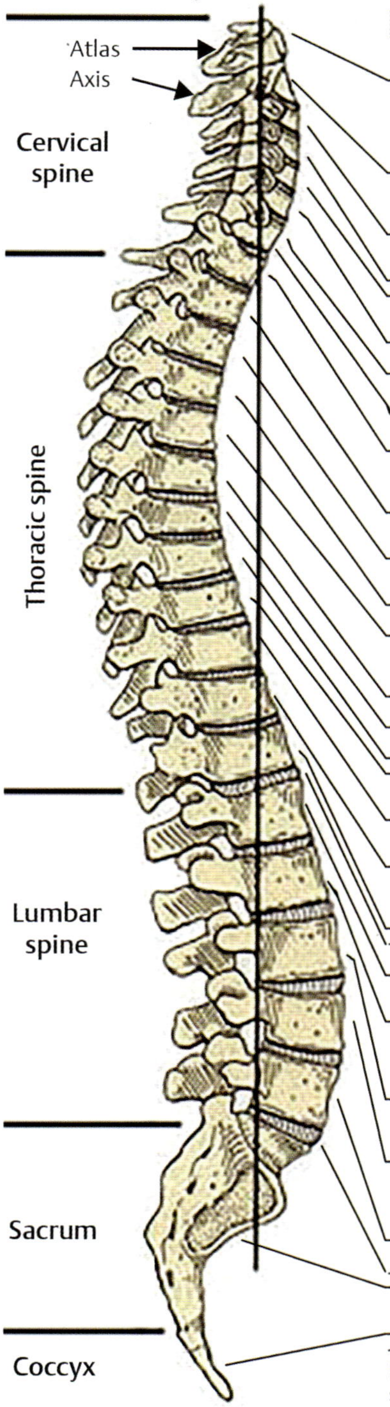

Vertebrae	Areas	Effects
1C	Blood supply to the head, pituitary gland, scalp bones of the face, brain, inner & middle ear, sympathetic nervous system	Headaches, nervousness, insomnia, head colds, high blood pressure, migraine headaches, nervous breakdowns, amnesia,chronic tiredness, dizziness
2C	Eyes, optic nerves, auditory nerves, sinuses, mastoid bones, tongue, forehead	Sinus trouble, allergies, crossed eyes, deafness, eye troubles, earache, fainting spells, certain cases of blindness
3C	Cheeks, outer ear, face bones, teeth, trifacial nerve	Neuralgia, neuritis, acne or pimples, eczema
4C	Nose, lips, mouth, eustachian tube	Hay fever, catarrh, hearing loss, adenoids
5C	Vocal cords, neck glands, pharynx	Laryngitis, hoarseness, throat conditions
6C	Neck muscles, shoulders, tonsils	Stiff neck, pain in upper arms, tonsillitis, whooping cough, croup
7C	Thyroid gland, bursae in shoulder, elbows	Bursitis, colds, thyroid conditions
1T	Arms: elbow down; hands, wrist, fingers; esophagus and trachea	Asthma, cough difficult breathing, shortness of breath, pain in lower arms and hands
2T	Heart: valves and coverings, coronary arteries	Functional heart conditions and certain chest conditions
3T	Lungs, bronchial tubes, pleura, chest, breast	Bronchitis, pleurisy, pneumonia, congestion, influenza
4T	Gall bladder, common duct	Gall bladder conditions, jaundice, shingles
5T	Liver, solar plexus, blood	Liver conditions, fevers, low blood pressure, anemia, poor circulation, arthritis
6T	Stomach	Stomach troubles: nervous stomach, indigestion, heartburn, dyspepsia
7T	Pancreas, duodenum	Ulcers, gastritis
8T	Spleen	Lowered resistance
9T	Adrenal and suprarenal glands	Allergies, hives
10T	Kidneys	Kidney troubles, hardening of the arteries, chronic tiredness, nephritis pyelitis
11T	Kidneys, ureters	Skin conditions: acne, pimples, eczema, or boils
12T	Small intestines, lymph circulation	Rheumatism, gas pains, certain types of sterility
1L	Large intestines, inguinal ring	Constipation, colitis, dysentery, diarrhea, some ruptures or hernias
2L	Appendix, abdomen, upper leg	Cramps, difficult breathing, acidosis, varicose veins
3L	Sex organs, uterus, bladder, knees	Bladder troubles, menstrual troubles: painful or irregular periods, miscarriages, bed wetting, impotency, change in life symptoms, many knee pains
4L	Prostate gland, muscles of lower back, sciatic nerve	Sciatica, lumbago, difficult/painful or too frequent urination, backaches
5L	Lower legs, ankles, feet	Poor circulation in the legs, swollen ankles, weak ankles and arches, cold feet,weakness in the legs, leg cramps
SACRUM	Hip bones, buttocks	Sacroiliac conditions, spinal curvatures
COCCYX	Rectum, anus	Hemorrhoids (piles), pruritis (itching), pain at end of spine on sitting

For further explanation of the conditions shown above and information about those not shown ask your Doctor of Chiropractic.

Fig. 14.1 Depiction of the effects of spinal misalignments.

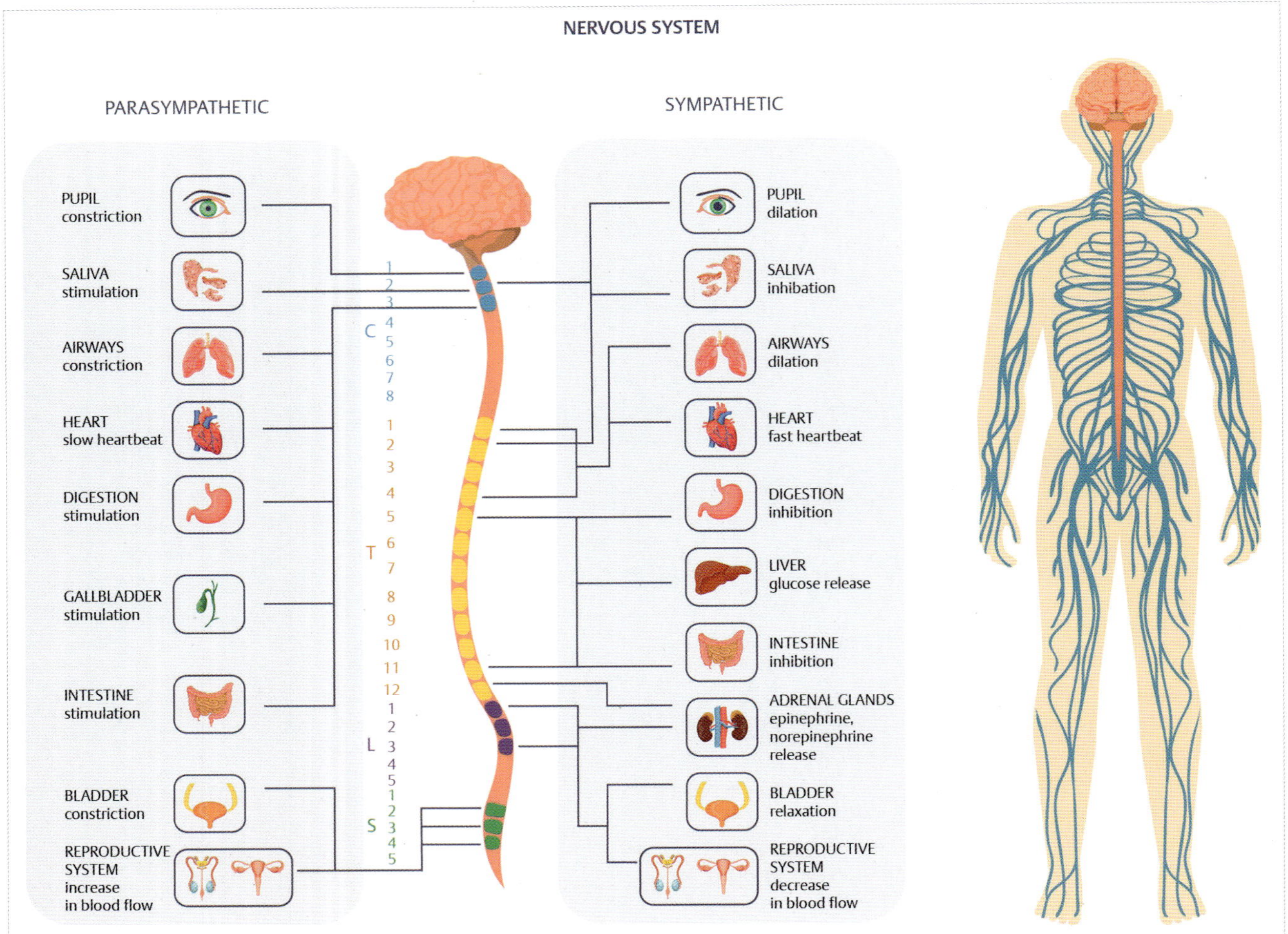

Fig. 14.2 Illustration of the parasympathetic and sympathetic effects in the nervous system.

14.7 Commonly Utilized Chiropractic Techniques[6]

Diversified technique is used by about 90 to 95% of chiropractors in the profession. It is essentially an integration of several techniques that encompass adjustments of the full spine and extremities after identifying subluxations through palpation, X-ray findings, leg length checks, and examination findings. Spinal dysfunction is the tenet of the technique. Some practitioners incorporate postural analysis and gait analysis during evaluation. It is characterized by HVLA thrust. The main objective is to restore joint motion and free the vertebral column from fixation or misalignment.

Extremity adjusting is another specialized skill utilized by approximately 90% of chiropractors. Some of these procedures are taught at chiropractic colleges or as postgraduate training. With many chiropractic sports physicians, this is an essential part of their evaluation protocols.

Gonstead technique is used by 55 to 58% of the chiropractors. Its premise centers around the belief that a vertebra subluxates posteriorly in relationship to the segment below, with the exception of the atlas (the first cervical vertebra). Dr. Gonstead, the inventor of the technique, believed that "subluxation evolved in stages, beginning with fixations, progressing to misalignment and cumulative damage leading to disc disease and finally nerve interference." He also believed that the thrust mechanism of the adjustment would cause the vertebral body to develop a more normal weight-bearing position on the disk. The Gonstead technique uses a specific X-ray analysis to classify the subluxation. Most practitioners take full spine X-rays and use line drawings to determine malposition of the spine. The practitioners may adjust the cervical spine in a seated chair position and the thoracic spine on a knee chest table specifically manufactured for Gonstead technique, which is also an HVLA technique.

Receptor tonus technique, also known as **Nimmo technique** founded by Dr. Raymond Nimmo, is used by approximately 40% of practitioners. It is focused on identifying myofascial trigger points in the musculoskeletal system and uses ischemic compression for 6 to 10 seconds by applying pressure with the examiner's hands into the musculature to release lactic acid deposits and break up adhesions. The pressure applied is directly proportional to the patient's tolerance level. Its philosophy is predicated upon the theory that dysfunctional muscles result in

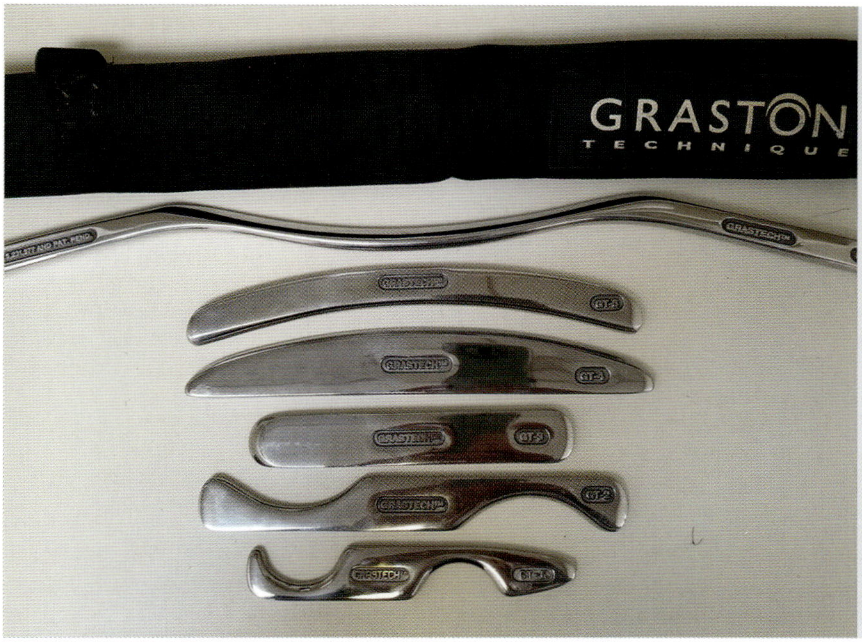

Fig. 14.3 Image of the tools used in the Graston technique.

joint restriction or subluxation as well as creation of abnormal visceral function.

Thompson technique, created by Dr. Clay Thompson, is another commonly practiced technique that uses drop pieces on a chiropractic segmental table to impart forces to the vertebrae with less torque. It also uses leg length analysis to distinguish cervical and pelvic involvement. Like other chiropractic techniques, it is considered an HVLA technique with somewhat lower forces attributable to the spring-loaded drop pieces absorbing some of the thrust.

Palmer package is a subset of techniques taught at Palmer College of Chiropractic and incorporates Diversified, Gonstead, and Thompson techniques. The practitioners can use a combination of different techniques to establish their own method that they feel most comfortable with while adjusting their patients.

Graston technique is referred to as an Instrument Assisted Soft Tissue Mobilization (IASTM) technique designed to break up scar tissue and adhesions in either acute, chronic, or post-surgical conditions. It incorporates specialized stainless-steel instruments that are designed to restore mobility and function and reduce pain. It attempts to break down collagen cross-links found in adhesions and scar tissue. Practitioners must be trained and certified before they are allowed to practice this technique. There are sometimes transient small petechiae, or capillary hemorrhages, that occur as a result of the mechanical rubbing of the instrument against the skin surfaces. Patients who have bleeding disorders or those who are taking blood thinners should be carefully evaluated prior to this technique (► Fig. 14.3).

Active Release Technique (ART) is another soft tissue approach to injury that is often most advantageous as a precursor to spinal manipulation. The technique relies on the palpation skills of the clinician as a stretch is applied to the involved muscles in the direction of venous and lymphatic flow. ART aims to treat muscles through low-compression and high-tension muscle stripping, focusing on antagonist muscles and active motions. By removing fibrous adhesions, biomechanical function is thought to be restored to a normal state.

References

[1] Nougarou F, Dugas C, Deslauriers C, Pagé I, Descarreaux M. Physiological responses to spinal manipulation therapy: investigation of the relationship between electromyographic responses and peak force. J Manipulative Physiol Ther. 2013; 36(9):557–563

[2] Budgell BS. Reflex effects of subluxation: the autonomic nervous system. J Manipulative Physiol Ther. 2000; 23(2):104–106

[3] Herzog W. The biomechanics of spinal manipulation. J Bodyw Mov Ther. 2010; 14(3):280–286

[4] Owens EF, Jr, Hosek RS, Sullivan SGB, Russell BS, Mullin LE, Dever LL. Establishing force and speed training targets for lumbar spine high-velocity, low-amplitude chiropractic adjustments. J Chiropr Educ. 2016; 30(1):7–13

[5] Welch A, Boone R. Sympathetic and parasympathetic responses to specific diversified adjustments to chiropractic vertebral subluxations of the cervical and thoracic spine. J Chiropr Med. 2008; 7(3):86–93

[6] Cooperstein R, Gleberzon B. Technique Systems in Chiropractic. CreateSpace Independent Publishing Platform; 2018

15 Surgery: Anterior Cervical Diskectomy and Fusion

Andrew M. Hersh, Michael D. White, and Nicholas Theodore

Summary

The anterior cervical diskectomy and fusion (ACDF) can be used to treat disk herniations, fractures, and ligamentous hypertrophy contributing to cervical radiculopathy and myelopathy. Athletes tend to have a higher rate of degenerative changes in their spine compared to age-matched controls, owing to excessive forces placed on the spine from athletic movements, and traumatic herniations can also arise from vigorous activity. An ACDF can be used to treat many of these patients by removing the disk and decompressing the spine. Compared to posterior approaches, ACDF has demonstrated reduced blood loss and shorter length of stay. It is typically performed for one- or two-level fusions, with three or more level fusions contraindicated for return to play in athletic populations. This chapter details the surgical technique for ACDF, preoperative workup, and postoperative return to play guidelines.

Keywords: RTP, ACDF, athlete, contact sports, herniation, spondylosis

15.1 Introduction

Fusion, stabilization, and decompression of the spine for treatment of symptomatic radiculopathy or myelopathy can be achieved through both anterior and posterior approaches. The posterior approach is often favored for multilevel fusions, while the anterior approach provides favorable access to the intervertebral disk space and posterior longitudinal ligament (PLL). Consequently, the anterior approach is well-suited for treatment of pathology affecting the anterior segments of the spine, including disk herniations causing ventral compression of the spinal cord or nerve roots, and instability resulting from fractures or diskoligamentous injury. Furthermore, an anterior cervical diskectomy and fusion (ACDF) avoids dissection and splitting of the paraspinous muscles, which can decrease intraoperative blood loss and reduce patients' postoperative pain compared to a posterior fusion.

Clinical trials and meta-analyses have shown similar functional outcomes between patients treated with ACDF and those treated with posterior cervical fusion. However, ACDF typically involves less blood loss, shorter length of stay, and lower risk of infection compared to posterior fusion.[1] Fusion of three or more levels is more commonly performed with posterior approaches. The available literature on three- or four-level ACDF shows improvement in patient-reported outcomes for most patients; however, there is an increased risk of pseudarthrosis and postoperative dysphagia.[2,3,4]

15.2 Preoperative Assessment

Patients can present with a range of symptoms, including back/neck pain refractory to conservative management, upper and lower extremity weakness, numbness, and myelopathy. An athlete may develop symptoms following an acute traumatic injury as a result of acute cervical disk herniations, cervical fractures, or trauma to the cord from instability or preexisting stenosis/narrow spinal canal. Magnetic resonance imaging (MRI) should be obtained to evaluate stenosis of the spinal canal, cord compression, disk herniation, or T2 cord signal change (▶ Fig. 15.1). T2 signal changes within the spinal cord suggest injury to the cord with edema and inflammation and may predict a poorer prognosis. Computed tomography scans are valuable for assessment of the bony anatomy, evaluation of possible fractures, and for operative planning. Finally, flexion-extension X-rays may be ordered for workup of dynamic instability.

15.3 Surgical Technique

15.3.1 Positioning

The patient is positioned supine on the operating table. The patient's head should lay on a well-padded cushion with the head in an extended position. A chinstrap can be used to help pull the chin back and keep the head in an extended position. Alternatively, a Mayfield horseshoe headrest can be used to stabilize

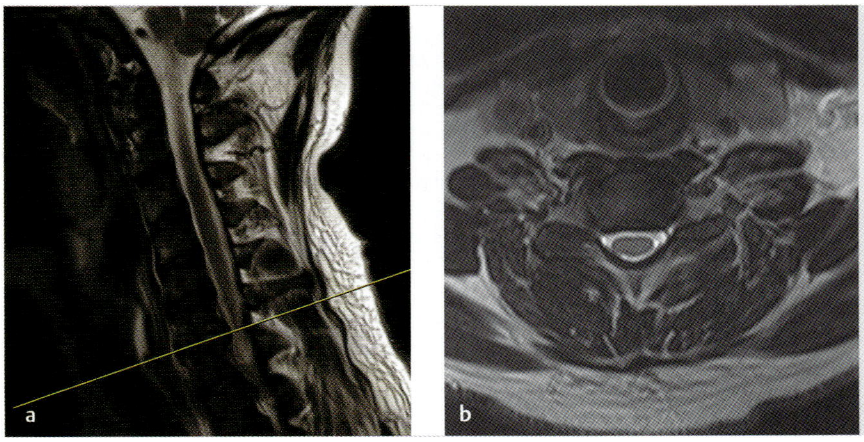

Fig. 15.1 This patient presented with progressively worsening right shoulder pain radiating down the arm. Magnetic resonance imaging (MRI) workup with **(a)** T2-weighted sagittal and **(b)** axial slices illustrating C6–C7 severe right neural foraminal stenosis. Given his debilitating symptoms and slight weakness in the right arm, he underwent a C6–C7 anterior cervical diskectomy and fusion (ACDF).

the head. For cases requiring traction, Gardner-Wells tongs can also be applied. A bump or towel is placed between the scapula to elevate the shoulders and help further open the disk spaces. For cases involving the lower cervical levels where the shoulders may hinder visualization on X-ray, the shoulders can either be taped to the end of the operating room table or wraps can be tied around the arms and pulled down. Care should be taken to ensure there is no excess tension, which can risk injury to the brachial plexus. The surgeon should also ensure monitoring is stable after positioning to avoid excessive extension of the head or tension on the shoulders. The appropriate spinal level should be identified. Anatomical landmarks that aid in identifying the level include the angle of the mandible over the C2 body, the hyoid bone at C3–C4, the thyroid cartilage at C4–C5, and the cricoid cartilage at the C5–C6 space.[5] A metallic skin marker should be placed over the incision site and radiographs obtained to confirm the appropriate spine level. The neck is prepped and draped in the usual fashion.

The anterior spine can be approached either from the patient's right or left side. Often, surgeon's ergonomic preference dictates the side of exposure, with right-handed surgeons preferring to operate on the right side and vice versa. However, the shorter and more oblique course of the right recurrent laryngeal nerve compared to the left nerve has caused some concern for nerve injury and resulting dysphonia.[6] Consequently, some favor a left-sided approach due to the lower risk of nerve injury; however, these concerns are largely historical in nature without significant evidence for any increased incidence of recurrent laryngeal nerve injury from right-sided exposures.[7,8] The location of disk pathology is also a consideration for the side of the approach. The patient's head can be rotated to improve exposure.[9]

15.3.2 Dissection

A transverse incision starting just off midline and extending just medial to the sternocleidomastoid muscle is sufficient for most single- or multilevel diskectomies, although a vertical incision along the sternocleidomastoid may be needed for more extensive procedures.[5] The incision is carried down to the platysma, which is then incised along the length of the incision and elevated, followed by subplatysmal dissection to develop an avascular plane between the carotid sheath laterally and the esophagus and trachea medially. The carotid artery, internal jugular vein, and vagus nerve are contained within the carotid sheath and should be retracted laterally during the procedure. Meticulous hemostasis should be obtained during the dissection and approach to prevent run-down of blood that can obscure visualization during the diskectomy.

Handheld retractors are used to retract the esophagus and trachea medially while the carotid sheath is retracted laterally and can help bluntly dissect down this plane.[5] Once the dissection down to bone is complete, the spinal levels should be confirmed by placing a spinal needle into the disk space or using a hemostat to clamp the prevertebral fascia. Intraoperative fluoroscopy should be used to confirm exposure of the correct level. Once confirmed, the prevertebral fascia is opened to visualize the anterior vertebral column. The longus colli are found overlying the anterior longitudinal ligament and just lateral to the anterior cervical spine. The longus colli should be elevated and retracted laterally to fully expose the anterior vertebral column. Care should be taken not to injure the superficial sympathetic chain which runs over these muscles, by placing the retractors deep to the muscles.[10]

Self-retaining retractors are then secured to the operative field, with medial–lateral retractors sufficient for single-level cases, and rostral–caudal retractors added to multilevel cases. Osteophytes are removed with a rongeur or Kerrison to improve visualization of the intervertebral disk.[9]

15.3.3 Diskectomy and Fusion

The microscope is now brought into the operative field. The annulus is incised with a number 15 blade and pituitary rongeurs and curettes are used to carry out the diskectomy from uncus to uncus. Caspar pins may be placed into the midline of the adjacent vertebral bodies and distracted to further open the disk space. A high-speed drill is used to remove any residual cartilaginous endplate material, square off the endplates, and remove posterior osteophytes. Local bone may be collected for use as morselized autograft. A curved curette can be used to get underneath the PLL and dissect a clear plane between the PLL and the dura. Kerrison rongeurs can also be used to undercut the vertebral bodies to remove posterior osteophytes and release the PLL from its attachments to the bone superiorly and inferiorly until all bony and soft tissue elements compressing the spinal cord have been removed. The vertebral body endplates are then decorticated to promote bony fusion.

Once the disk space has been prepared, distraction can be released and interbody trials of increasing heights can be inserted to determine the appropriate implant size. The appropriate size trial will feel "snug" and will not pull out easily. Care should be taken to not place an implant that is too large as it can damage the endplates during insertion or can over-distract the disk space and cause stretching of the nerve roots. An appropriately sized structural allograft, autograft, or interbody cage is then tapped into place utilizing demineralized bone matrix and/or the patient's own bone for arthrodesis.[10] Once the implants are inserted at all of the operative levels, an appropriate length anterior plate should be placed overlying the anterior spine. The plates are locked into the bone with screws such that each hole of the plate is in excellent apposition with bone. After the screws are tightened flush with the bone, locking mechanisms are deployed for each screw. Final radiographs are obtained to evaluate hardware placement. The wound should then be copiously irrigated with saline solution and hemostasis meticulously obtained. A typical closure for this approach includes using 3–0 vicryl sutures to approximate the platysmas, followed by inverted dermal stitches with 4–0 vicryl or a running 4–0 monocryl. Finally, skin glue can be used superficially over the incision. This approach rarely requires a drain if adequate hemostasis is obtained; however, in patients with higher risk of postoperative bleeding a subfascial drain may be placed.

15.3.4 Postoperative Care

Patients with uncomplicated surgeries can generally go home the same day or be monitored overnight and discharged the following day. Prompt attention to a developing neck hematoma is critical to prevent airway compression and respiratory failure. Early ambulation is encouraged.[10]

15.4 Return to Play after ACDF

The consensus on return to play (RTP) after ACDF is that athletes can generally resume sports activities following single-level ACDF; however, controversy remains for RTP following multilevel ACDF in athletes engaged in contact sports. Patients with preoperative T2 signal cord change or a syrinx may also be at increased risk for poor outcomes following RTP, even after single-level surgery. However, successful RTP after ACDF in patients with signal cord change has been reported in the literature, provided that the athlete completes a full recovery and is asymptomatic when resuming sports.[11]

Several studies have reported successful RTP outcomes after single-level ACDF for athletes participating in contact sports. Watkins et al reviewed outcomes after 27 ACDFs on 26 professional athletes, finding that fusion was achieved in 96% of patients and RTP was achieved in 80% of athletes after an average period of 9.5 months. Their athletic career continued for an average of 3 years after surgery. Two other athletes were still completing rehabilitation and expected to return to their sport.[12] Maroon et al studied 15 professional athletes following single-level ACDF and found an RTP rate of 87% among the athletes.[13] Treatment guidelines and expert panels have also supported RTP after single-level ACDF. For example, the multidisciplinary Spine Trauma Study Group convened a panel in 2010 and provided a strong recommendation in favor of RTP after single-level ACDF, provided that an adequate decompression has been achieved to alleviate stenosis on the spine.[14] A recent systematic review of the literature in 2021 included 349 athletes and found favorable evidence for RTP following ACDF in asymptomatic athletes, noting that the RTP is higher in patients undergoing surgical intervention than conservative management.[15]

Considerably fewer reports have been published of RTP after multilevel ACDF.[15] Increased risk of pseudarthrosis, adjacent level degeneration, hardware failure, and catastrophic neurological sequelae constitute areas of concern for clinicians. A modified Delphi consensus study of the Cervical Spine Research Society found that while 100% of respondents would allow RTP after a one-level ACDF in an asymptomatic football player with no T2 signal changes, the respondents were evenly split for a two-level ACDF. The majority agreed that a three-level ACDF is a contraindication to RTP, suggesting that the major area of controversy concerns the two-level fusion. They also agreed that athletes with persistent T2 signal change following two-level ACDF should not RTP.[16]

Ultimately, the decision to clear an athlete for RTP after ACDF requires consideration of several factors, including the length of fusion, severity of underlying injury, intensity of the sport, and the athlete's position within the sport. A high school athlete not interested in pursuing professional career faces a different calculus than a professional football player whose livelihood is dependent on competing in that sport. Radiographic evidence of stability and fusion are important tools to clear athletes for RTP. All athletes should be counseled on risk of adjacent segment degeneration. Finally, no athlete should be allowed to return to the sport while still symptomatic.

15.5 Clinical Pearls

- Professional athletes have a higher rate of cervical degenerative changes and disk herniations compared to the age-matched population.
- ACDF is an appropriate treatment option for most athletes presenting with cervical radiculopathy or myelopathy.
- Meticulous hemostasis and postoperative monitoring are critical to prevent formation of a hematoma that can rapidly compress the airway.
- A single-level ACDF should not present a barrier to RTP even in contact sports; however, RTP after multilevel ACDF is controversial. Individualized decision-making should be provided for two-level ACDFs.

References

[1] Sattari SA, Ghanavatian M, Feghali J, et al. Anterior cervical discectomy and fusion versus posterior decompression in patients with degenerative cervical myelopathy: a systematic review and meta-analysis. J Neurosurg Spine. 2023; 38(6):1–13

[2] Laratta JL, Reddy HP, Bratcher KR, McGraw KE, Carreon LY, Owens RK, II. Outcomes and revision rates following multilevel anterior cervical discectomy and fusion. J Spine Surg. 2018; 4(3):496–500

[3] De la Garza-Ramos R, Xu R, Ramhmdani S, et al. Long-term clinical outcomes following 3- and 4-level anterior cervical discectomy and fusion. J Neurosurg Spine. 2016; 24(6):885–891

[4] White MD, Farber SH, Pacult MA, et al. Pseudarthrosis after four-level anterior cervical discectomy and fusion without posterior fixation. Neurosurg Focus. 2023; 55(3):E4

[5] Singh K, Vaccaro AR. Pocket Atlas of Spine Surgery. Vol. 1. Thieme; 2012

[6] Thomas AM, Fahim DK, Gemechu JM. Anatomical variations of the recurrent laryngeal nerve and implications for injury prevention during surgical procedures of the neck. Diagnostics (Basel). 2020; 10(9):670

[7] Kilburg C, Sullivan HG, Mathiason MA. Effect of approach side during anterior cervical discectomy and fusion on the incidence of recurrent laryngeal nerve injury. J Neurosurg Spine. 2006; 4(4):273–277

[8] Johnson MD, Matur AV, Asghar F, Nasser R, Cheng JS, Prestigiacomo CJ. Right versus left approach to anterior cervical discectomy and fusion: an anatomic versus historic debate. World Neurosurg. 2020; 135:135–140

[9] Wolfla Christopher E, Resnick Daniel K. Neurosurgical Operative Atlas: Spine and Peripheral Nerves. 2nd ed. Thieme; 2007

[10] Nader R, Berta SC, Gragnaniello C, Sabbagh AJ, Levy ML. Neurosurgery Tricks of the Trade: Spine and Peripheral Nerves. 1st ed. Thieme; 2014

[11] Joaquim AF, Hsu WK, Patel AA. Cervical spine surgery in professional athletes: a systematic review. Neurosurg Focus. 2016; 40(4):E10

[12] Watkins RG, IV, Chang D, Watkins RG, III. Return to play after anterior cervical discectomy and fusion in professional athletes. Orthop J Sports Med. 2018; 6(6):2325967118779672

[13] Maroon JC, Bost JW, Petraglia AL, et al. Outcomes after anterior cervical discectomy and fusion in professional athletes. Neurosurgery. 2013; 73(1):103–112, discussion 112

[14] Dailey A, Harrop JS, France JC. High-energy contact sports and cervical spine neuropraxia injuries: what are the criteria for return to participation? Spine. 2010; 35(21) Suppl:S193–S201

[15] Leider J, Piche JD, Khan M, Aleem I. Return-to-play outcomes in elite athletes after cervical spine surgery: a systematic review. Sports Health. 2021; 13(5):437–445

[16] Schroeder GD, Canseco JA, Patel PD, et al. Updated return-to-play recommendations for collision athletes after cervical spine injury: a modified Delphi consensus study with the Cervical Spine Research Society. Neurosurgery. 2020; 87(4):647–654

16 Surgery: Cervical Arthroplasty

Luis M. Tumialán

Summary

Decompression of the nerve root is indicated in the management of patients with cervical radiculopathy who remain refractory to nonoperative measures. Whenever possible, surgical options that preserve motion should be carefully weighed against those interventions that result in immobilization of a segment. Athletes represent a patient demographic that are typically younger and healthier than the average patient population, and they therefore tend to exhibit less spondylosis. The cause of their cervical radiculopathy is generally a soft disk herniation. In such a patient, motion preservation should be a central consideration for the proposed surgical intervention. The current chapter reviews the rationale, indications, surgical technique, and complication avoidance strategies. When an anterior approach to the cervical spine is needed for management of cervical radiculopathy, cervical arthroplasty accomplishes the goals of decompression and may be associated with a decreased incidence of adjacent segment degeneration.

Keywords: arthrodesis, arthroplasty, cervical, motion preservation, radiculopathy

16.1 Introduction

Immobilization of a segment runs counter to the intuitive hope of patients regarding the surgical management of their cervical spine and counter to the desire of surgeons to preserve the natural motion of the spine. On the other hand, the concept of a surgical option for the management of refractory cervical radiculopathy that preserves motion is alluring to patients and surgeons. In the years since the introduction of cervical arthroplasty, the literature has consistently demonstrated a decreased incidence of adjacent segment degeneration and thereby a decreased need for additional surgery in patients who undergo arthroplasty rather than fusion.[1,2] Motion preservation in the management of cervical radiculopathy, when appropriate, has value in all patients but can be especially valuable in the management of athletes. Arthroplasty forgoes the need to confirm a rigid arthrodesis during the postoperative phase and may expedite return to play. In the military, the use of cervical arthroplasty has demonstrated a decrease in time to return to unrestricted full duty when compared to fusion.[3] This chapter reviews the indications for cervical arthroplasty, the surgical technique, and complication avoidance strategies.

16.2 Preoperative Assessment

Patients with a cervical nerve root compression syndrome that has been refractory to nonoperative measures will typically present with magnetic resonance imaging (MRI) that reveals compression of a cervical nerve root, which may or may not have an element of central stenosis. If, in review of the T2-weighted axial MRI, only unilateral compression of the cervical nerve root is seen without central stenosis, a posterior cervical foraminotomy is a motion-preserving option that should be considered. If the patient has an element of central stenosis in addition to nerve root compression, an anterior approach to the cervical segment may be preferable (▶ Fig. 16.1). Prior to deciding between arthroplasty and arthrodesis, anteroposterior (AP), lateral, flexion, and extension radiographs are essential (▶ Fig. 16.2).

The ideal cervical arthroplasty candidate has minimal spondylosis evident on the lateral radiograph. As a general rule, the symptomatic segment, which may be obvious on the sagittal MRI, should be indistinguishable from any other segment on the lateral radiograph, as seen in ▶ Fig. 16.2a, which shows a patient who is an ideal candidate for cervical arthroplasty. In comparison, the patient in ▶ Fig. 16.2b demonstrates advanced spondylosis at the symptomatic segment.

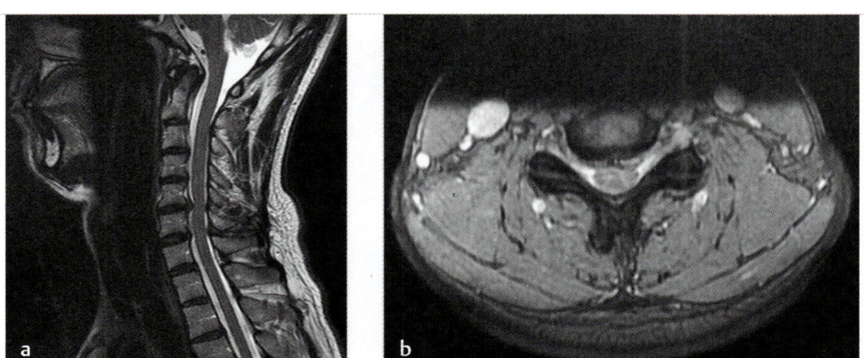

Fig. 16.1 Cervical magnetic resonance imaging (MRI) of a patient with a left C6 radiculopathy. **(a)** Sagittal T2-weighted cervical MRI demonstrating a broad-based disk bulge resulting in central stenosis. **(b)** Axial T2-weighted MRI at the C5–C6 segment. The disk protrusion is in contact with the ventral aspect of the spinal cord, resulting in an element of central stenosis along with foraminal stenosis. A posterior cervical foraminotomy would not accomplish all of the goals of surgery, namely, to decompress the central canal. An anterior approach would be needed for a complete decompression of the segment. Once an anterior approach has been chosen, the question of arthroplasty versus arthrodesis is best decided with review of static and dynamic radiographs. (Used with permissions from Barrow Neurological Institute, Phoenix, Arizona.)

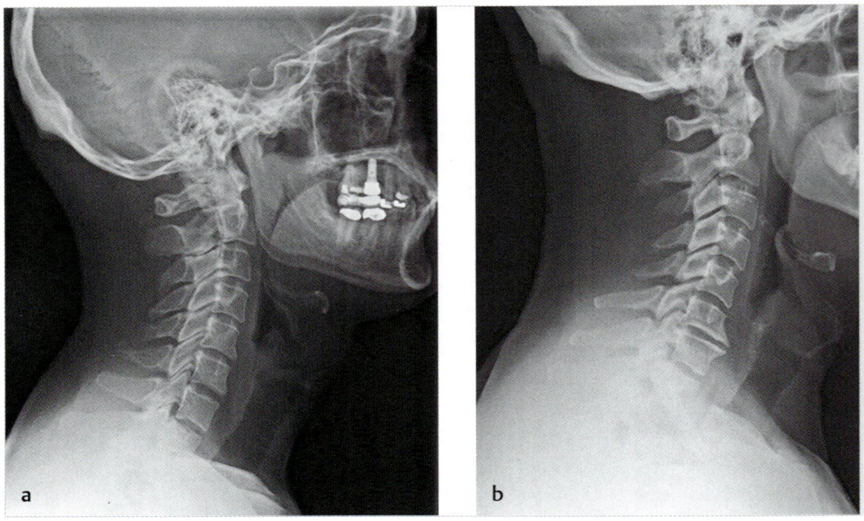

Fig. 16.2 Candidacy for arthroplasty is based on the degree of cervical spondylosis on lateral radiograph. **(a)** Lateral radiograph of the same patient in ▶ Fig. 16.1. No significant cervical spondylosis is identified throughout the cervical spine, namely, at the C5–C6 segment. This patient had normal physiologic motion on flexion and extension views (not shown). **(b)** Lateral radiograph of a different patient who presented with a strong interest in arthroplasty. Although this patient's magnetic resonance imaging (MRI) (not shown) looked similar to ▶ Fig. 16.1, the lateral radiograph demonstrates advanced spondylosis at the symptomatic segment (C6–C7). In this patient, an arthrodesis was recommended in lieu of arthroplasty. (Used with permissions from Barrow Neurological Institute, Phoenix, Arizona.)

16.3 Surgical Technique

16.3.1 Operating Room Setup

The patient is positioned on a standard operating table that is reversed, eliminating the base of the table as a potential barrier to the fluoroscope. It is my preference to use the operating microscope for the decompression, and so the operating microscope is positioned on the side of the incision. The fluoroscope is positioned opposite the microscope.

16.3.2 Positioning

Placement of the arthroplasty implant in the geometric center of the disk space is central to the procedure. Stabilization of the head and neck may aid in the midline placement of the device. Positioning the patient on a Caspar head rest with a chin strap accomplishes several objectives. First, it places the cervical spine into lordosis with a bolster in the back of the cervical spine. Second, it stabilizes the cervical spine in a manner so that, once positioned, there will be very little, if any, movement of the head and neck. Finally, the chin strap serves as a counterforce to taping the shoulders down, which will facilitate visualization of the lower segments of the cervical spine (▶ Fig. 16.3).

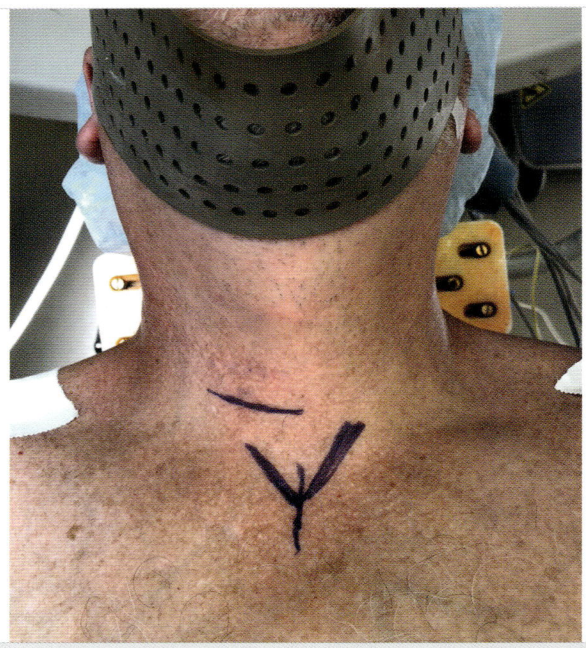

Fig. 16.3 The patient positioned for a C6–C7 artificial disk placement, right-sided approach. In this photograph, the patient is positioned using a Caspar head rest and chin strap to stabilize the spine. The system has a cervical bolster that positions the patient into a cervical lordosis and serves as a counterforce when securing the implant. As seen in this photograph, the sternal notch is marked with a prominent "V" as another marker for the midline. Anteroposterior (AP) and lateral fluoroscopic images are obtained to ensure that the patient is positioned without any element of rotation. (Used with permissions from Barrow Neurological Institute, Phoenix, Arizona.)

Once the patient is positioned with the head secured and shoulders taped down, an AP image parallel to the disk space of the symptomatic segment is obtained to ensure that the patient is positioned without any element of rotation. The uncovertebral joints should be clearly visualized equidistant to the spinous process. If any asymmetry is present, the patient should be adjusted accordingly. Next, a lateral radiograph is obtained to ensure that the target segment can be adequately visualized and the facet joints are perfectly aligned. Acquiring the AP and lateral images prior to even planning the incision is a significant departure from what would be done for a cervical fusion. It underscores the importance of identifying and securing the midline.

The incision is marked immediately over the segment with fluoroscopic guidance, and a standard Smith-Robinson approach is used to access the segment. Once the correct level is confirmed with a lateral fluoroscopic image, the longus colli muscles are mobilized so that a full 22 to 24 mm of the segment can be visualized. Self-retaining retractor blades are placed in a manner that they engage the cuff of the mobilized longus colli. Fluoroscopy guides placement of the Caspar distraction posts, which should be placed completely perpendicular to the back wall of the vertebral body to ensure a lordotic distraction. For keel-based devices, the insertion point is three-quarters rostral to the disk space. For non-keel-based devices, the midpoint of the vertebral body is more than adequate. The segment may be distracted, but not overly so.

16.3.3 Decompression of the Segment

When the retractor blades and the Caspar post distractor are in position, the operating microscope is rolled in. A no. 11 blade is used to create a generous annulotomy, and the disk material is removed. Straight and forward-angled curettes are used to remove the cartilaginous endplate and to begin to expose the cortical endplate. Although it is important not to alter the scalloped configuration of the disk space, it is also important to create an environment conducive to bony ingrowth of the implant. Preparing the endplate in a manner that reveals bleeding cortical bone will allow for bony ingrowth to occur, which is essential for the long-term stability of the implant. It is my preference to refrain from using a drill during arthroplasty procedures. Although using a drill is not a contraindication to arthroplasty, if a drill is needed, careful consideration should be given to whether arthroplasty is the optimal procedure for that particular circumstance.

The exposure should reveal unequivocal visualization of the uncovertebral joints on the left and the right side for a completely symmetric appearance. To confirm the symmetry of the exposure, the operating microscope should be positioned over the top of the segment in a manner to allow for an orthogonal view of the uncovertebral joints and eliminate any parallax. The identification of the midline is another reason to refrain from using a drill for this procedure. Altering the anatomy of the uncovertebral joints will alter the symmetrical view needed for establishing the midline. The midline is marked with cautery on the rostral and caudal vertebral bodies based on the slopes of the uncovertebral joints. An AP image may also be used to confirm the midline; however, that image is less important than the direct visualization of the midline. With retractors in position, visualization of the midline tends to be suboptimal and potentially misleading, whereas nothing should obscure the direct visualization of the uncovertebral joints through the operating microscope.

With the midline marked and confirmed, a complete decompression of the segment may be performed, without the need for a drill in the ideal arthroplasty patient, to include the division of the posterior longitudinal ligament. While resecting this ligament, every effort is made not to alter the anatomy of the scalloped endplate. The dura of the spinal cord is unequivocally visualized, foraminotomies completed, and decompression of the central canal achieved.

16.3.4 Placement of the Arthroplasty Device

Once the decompression is complete, the trials for the type of device selected by the surgeon may be tapped into position. As a general rule, the widest footprint should be considered, because the uncovertebral joints tend to make these larger footprints more self-centering. It is important to recognize the trajectory of insertion to ensure a lordotic position of the implant in the neutral position. The type of U.S. Food and Drug Administration–approved cervical implant is less important than its placement precisely into the geometric midline. Once the trial is tapped into position, the distraction should be removed, and a lateral fluoroscopic image taken. It has been my experience that the majority of implants will be between 5 and 6 mm in height. The trial will have an unmistakable snug fit with the distraction removed. A trial that can be easily moved with the distraction off warrants replacement of the trial with a larger height because a loose-fitting implant may be a recipe for expulsion of the implant. An AP image may be obtained with the trial in position; however, if placement of the implant corresponds with the marking on the vertebral bodies, there is little utility in an AP image, which may be difficult to interpret given the self-retaining retractor and the Caspar post distractor, both of which are still in position.

Placement of the final implant warrants careful attention to the trajectory of the implant into the disk space. Keel-based devices will require the use of a milling bit at this point. It is essential to become familiar with the technique guide for these devices. Once the keel cut is made, the device will pass along the tract that has been milled. If a non-keel-based device is to be used, it may be inserted after the trial. Regardless of the device, it is important that the inserter be held completely parallel to the disk space in the sagittal plane and completely orthogonal to the disk space in the coronal plane. An intermittent fluoroscopic image is worthwhile as the implant is advancing. Although minor adjustments may be made after insertion, nothing is superior to optimal placement of the implant as it enters the disk space from the outset.

Final lateral and AP fluoroscopic images are obtained before removal of the retractors, hemostasis, and closure. Patients are typically discharged on the day of surgery and seen at 30, 90, and 180 days with AP, lateral, flexion, and extension radiographs obtained at each visit (▶ Fig. 16.4). These studies are assessed for incorporation of the device into the endplates, the preservation of motion, and concern for any migration of the implant.

16.4 Complication Avoidance

The similarities in approaches explain the similarities in the complication profile between cervical arthroplasty and cervical arthrodesis. The most common and expected consequence of an anterior approach for this procedure is dysphagia. A recurrent laryngeal nerve palsy is less common but nevertheless a risk of the procedure. Postoperative hematoma is even less common.

The complications unique to arthroplasty are related to the placement of the device. In cervical fusions, midline placement of an interbody graft that will lead to arthrodesis is ideal but not crucial. However, midline placement in arthroplasty is essential for the appropriate distribution of forces on the device and its motion. Ideal placement of the device begins with positioning the patient. Eliminating any rotation of the neck and coronal imbalance will optimize securing the midline. Additionally, wide exposure of the uncovertebral joints for a distance of at least 20 mm and elimination of parallax when marking the midline offer the greatest access to the geometric center of the disk space.

16.5 Return to Play

The literature on return to play in high-performance athletes after cervical arthroplasty is limited, primarily consisting of case reports and small series, but demonstrates successful return to play. I have previously published experience with 12 military patients,

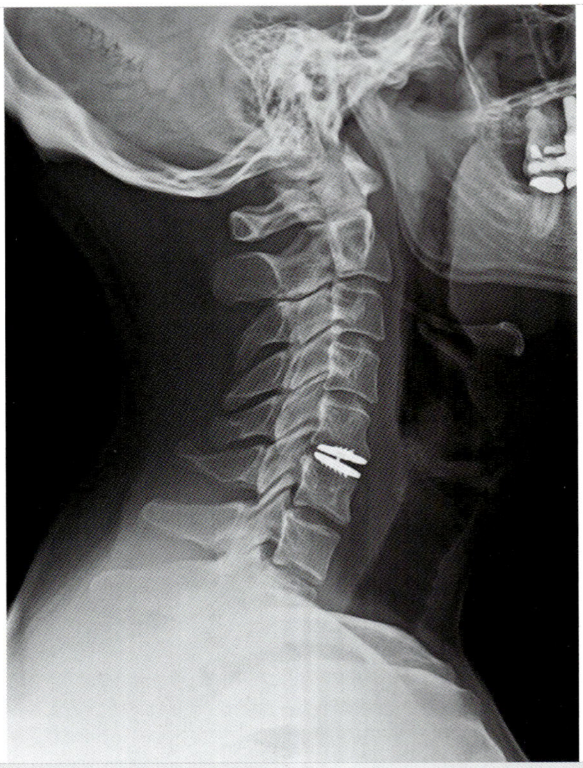

Fig. 16.4 C5–C6 arthroplasty. Lateral radiograph of a patient who has undergone a C5–C6 arthroplasty at 6 months postsurgery. Outcome measures were as follows: Visual Analogue Scale arm was 0 mm (preoperative 77 mm) and Neck Disability Index was 11 (preoperative 42) at 6 months. Lateral radiograph clearly demonstrates the segmental lordosis at the C5–C6 level and improved sagittal balance when compared to the preoperative study in ▶ Fig. 16.2a. Flexion and extension studies (not shown) confirm preservation of motion. (Used with permissions from Barrow Neurological Institute, Phoenix, Arizona.)

all of whom demonstrated the capacity to return to unrestricted full duty earlier with arthroplasty than with arthrodesis.[3] However, it is important to note that the difference was not clinical but rather radiological. Prior to returning a service member to unrestricted full duty, radiographic confirmation of an arthrodesis was needed. The absence of that requirement allowed for service members to return sooner after cervical arthroplasty.[3] Equally important was the absence of device-related complications associated with returning patients to unrestricted full duty. With the notable exception of 1 patient who experienced osteolysis requiring conversion to a fusion 1 year after surgery, the remaining cervical arthroplasty patients remained on unrestricted full duty.[4]

Reinke et al reviewed their experience with cervical arthroplasty in 50 athletes, of whom 2 were professional, 20 were semi-professional, and 24 were hobby athletes. These authors reported the median time to return to play was 4 weeks, and all athletes returned to their preinjured levels of activity.[5]

16.6 Conclusion

In high-performance athletes, motion preservation is a central tenet in the management of a cervical radiculopathy. These patients tend to be younger with less spondylosis than the general population and, as a result, tend to be ideal candidates for either a posterior cervical foraminotomy with diskectomy or cervical arthroplasty. When there is an element of central stenosis and an anterior approach is needed, cervical arthroplasty is a perfectly viable, if not preferable, option.

Although the current literature on return to play in high-performance athletes is limited, the experience in the military has demonstrated the ability to return to unrestricted full duty 3 months after arthroplasty. The published cervical arthroplasty literature for return to play is limited to 2 professional and 20 semi-professional athletes from Germany. The need to explore the experience in American contact sports, specifically in hockey and American football, would be of value to offer guidance to clinicians managing these patients.

16.7 Clinical Pearls

- Assess the degree of cervical spondylosis on AP, lateral, flexion, and extension radiographs to determine whether the patient is an ideal candidate for motion preservation.
- Midline placement of the cervical arthroplasty device begins with positioning the patient. Consider stabilizing the patient's head and bolstering the cervical spine to position the patient in the ideal lordotic configuration.
- Wide exposure of the uncovertebral joints ensures adequate assessment, visualization, and confirmation of the midline.
- In the ideal cervical arthroplasty candidate, there should be little need to alter the bony anatomy.
- When placing the cervical arthroplasty device, particular attention should be paid to the coronal and sagittal trajectories into the disk space.

16.8 Disclosures

LessRay investor (acquired by NuVasive).

Acknowledgments

The author would like to thank the staff of Neuroscience Publications at Barrow Neurological Institute for assistance with manuscript preparation.

References

[1] Lavelle WF, Riew KD, Levi AD, Florman JE. Ten-year outcomes of cervical disc replacement with the BRYAN cervical disc: results from a prospective, randomized, controlled clinical trial. Spine. 2019; 44(9):601–608

[2] Radcliff K, Davis RJ, Hisey MS, et al. Long-term evaluation of cervical disc arthroplasty with the Mobi-C© Cervical Disc: a randomized, prospective, multicenter clinical trial with seven-year follow-up. Int J Spine Surg. 2017; 11(4):31

[3] Tumialán LM, Ponton RP, Garvin A, Gluf WM. Arthroplasty in the military: a preliminary experience with ProDisc-C and ProDisc-L. Neurosurg Focus. 2010; 28(5):E18

[4] Tumialán LM, Gluf WM. Progressive vertebral body osteolysis after cervical disc arthroplasty. Spine. 2011; 36(14):E973–E978

[5] Reinke A, Behr M, Preuss A, Villard J, Meyer B, Ringel F. Return to sports after cervical total disc replacement. World Neurosurg. 2017; 97:241–246

17 Surgery: Posterior Cervical Foraminotomy

Nicholas M. Rabah, S. Harrison Farber, Michael D. White, and Laura A. Snyder

Summary

The authors present posterior cervical foraminotomy as an alternative approach to anterior cervical diskectomy and fusion for the treatment of cervical radiculopathy. This approach requires an intricate understanding of the bony anatomy, paraspinal musculature, and vascular anatomy of the cervical spine, but it spares patients the implant- and fusion-related complications of disk arthroplasty, and it affords patients a faster recovery time and athletes a much sooner return to play.

Keywords: cervical spine, cervical spondylosis, decompression, disk herniation, posterior cervical foraminotomy, radiculopathy

17.1 Introduction

Posterior cervical foraminotomy (PCF) is a well-understood technique originally described in 1951 by Scoville et al[1] and Frykholm[2] for the treatment of cervical radiculopathy. PCF demonstrates similar clinical outcomes compared to the more commonly offered anterior cervical diskectomy and fusion (ACDF) to treat cervical radiculopathy.[3,4] However, PCF offers a unique advantage over ACDF in that patients, particularly young athletes, can return to normal function more quickly because outcomes do not rely on obtaining fusion. Thus, for athletes with unilateral disk herniation or unilateral foraminal stenosis, PCF offers the ability to return to play far sooner than they would after a fusion procedure. Although disk arthroplasty may also be a reasonable option for young athletes with cervical radiculopathy, PCF avoids the risks of implant-related complications. Thus, PCF should be considered routinely as part of the neurosurgeon's armamentarium when treating athletes.

17.2 Indications for PCF

Patients who present with unilateral cervical radiculopathy or symptoms of radiating neck or arm pain along a dermatomal distribution are candidates for PCF. Patients with cervical radiculopathy often experience paresthesia or other sensory abnormalities and possible weakness of the muscle innervated by the affected nerve root.[5] Because patients typically present with one or all of these symptoms, a detailed history should document the location, onset, and triggers of symptoms to define the radiculopathy accurately. Acute radiculopathy typically presents as pain, which may be described as electric or burning, and the location will correspond to the involved nerve root. Typically, this involves only one arm.[6] Notably, sensory disturbances may not reliably follow the classic dermatomal pattern, as normal variations occur among different individuals, and afferent sensory pathways allow for overlap.

The radicular pain experienced by patients can often be reproduced by maneuvers that stretch the nerve root, such as coughing, sneezing, the Valsalva maneuver, and certain cervical movements and positions.[7,8] Clinicians can reproduce radicular symptoms using the Spurling test, which entails maximally extending and rotating the patient's neck toward the involved side while pressing down on the top of the patient's head. This test can also help differentiate true cervical radiculopathy from other etiologies of arm pain.

Cervical radiculopathy results from foraminal compression of the exiting spinal nerve. This compression may arise from disk herniation, diminished disk height due to spondylosis, anterior overgrowth of the uncovertebral joints, or posterior overgrowth of the zygapophyseal joints. In the case of disk herniation, extrusion of disk material through a ruptured annulus fibrosus does not inherently cause pain because the disk does not contain nociceptive fibers. Inflammatory mediators, such as matrix metalloproteinases, prostaglandin E, interleukin-6, and substance P, are released when a disk herniates.[9,10] Pain is felt only when the disk material and inflammatory mediators come into contact with the dura of the nerve root.[11] In the case of cervical spondylosis, disk height is lost, and the ligamentum flavum folds, narrowing the foraminal space. Similar to disk herniation, compression of the nerve root then leads to pain. Anterior overgrowth of the uncovertebral joints or posterior overgrowth of the zygapophyseal joints also causes direct compression of the nerve root, leading to radicular pain down the arm or numbness and weakness in the arm.

Patients with bilateral radiculopathy or bilateral nerve root compression in the foramen are often not good candidates for PCF. The pathology that causes bilateral compression of the nerves is better treated by a procedure that achieves bilateral decompression, such as ACDF or disk arthroplasty, because these procedures allow for bilateral visualization of the nerve roots anteriorly and bilateral decompression of the nerves in the foramen without requiring spinal cord retraction. Bilateral foraminotomies are often not favorable unless the patient has anatomy that makes an anterior approach difficult or dangerous because removal of the bilateral medial facets increases the risk of destabilizing the cervical level.

Patients are not good candidates for PCF if they have considerable neck pain that is not in a radicular or dermatomal distribution or if they have bilateral neck pain or neck pain that occurs with flexion and extension of the neck. These types of pain distributions often indicate cervical instability, cervical spondylosis, degenerative disk disease, or cervical deformity, all of which are often better treated with a stabilization procedure such as anterior or posterior decompression and fusion with fixation.

17.3 Diagnostics

Magnetic resonance imaging (MRI) is considered the gold standard for radiographic evaluation of patients with cervical radiculopathy. MRI correctly identifies 88% of lesions compared to 50% with computed tomography (CT).[12] However, disk herniations are commonly observed in MRIs of asymptomatic individuals.[12,13] Therefore, MRI findings should be carefully correlated with the results of the neurological examination.

CT is also commonly used to evaluate patients with cervical radiculopathy. It offers the distinct advantage of distinguishing neural compression caused by soft tissue from compression related to bony structures, such as facet hypertrophy. CT also has a high spatial resolution, which helps visualize the foraminal region. In addition, CT angiography can be used preoperatively to assess for an anomalous course of the vertebral artery.

A patient with MRI or CT studies that demonstrate unilateral compression of the exiting nerve that correlates with the patient's radicular pain distribution on clinical examination is a good candidate for PCF. For example, a patient is a good candidate for PCF if the patient has C6 nerve compression on the right at the C5–C6 foramen (which houses the C6 nerve root) and complains of pain traveling from the posterior neck down the anterior arm. However, a patient with a midline disk herniation that is causing compression of the nerves either unilaterally or bilaterally is not a good candidate for PCF, because this approach would make it impossible to remove the compressive element without retraction of the spinal cord.

Plain film anteroposterior and lateral radiographs are readily available and inexpensive but offer limited information on the presence and degree of foraminal stenosis. Radiographs may demonstrate whether the patient has a cervical deformity, and if so, standing scoliosis radiographs may enable the surgeon to assess the overall global alignment of the spine before considering surgical intervention. Flexion-extension lateral radiographs can reveal instability that may cause intermittent or positional symptoms. If the patient has cervical instability, or greater than 3 mm of movement of one vertebral body forward or backward on another as seen on the flexion-extension radiographs, the patient is less of a candidate for PCF because this instability may worsen and cause the patient more pain as additional posterior elements are decompressed with PCF.

Electrodiagnostic studies such as electromyography (EMG) and nerve conduction studies can be useful for differentiating the neurological causes of a patient's symptoms. EMG can detect fibrillation potentials and positive sharp waves at rest, which may indicate denervation. Nerve conduction studies can then help rule out peripheral nerve pathology. However, these electrodiagnostic studies can be inaccurate without an imaging adjunct, and they are often unnecessary in patients who have well-defined radiculopathy and good imaging correlation.[14]

17.4 Nonoperative Management

The mainstays of the nonoperative management of radiculopathy are medication and corticosteroid injections because no other therapies have been proven to offer any benefit. For patients with radiculopathy, nonsteroidal anti-inflammatory drugs have been shown in a meta-analysis to be efficacious for treating pain.[15] Anecdotal evidence also suggests that a short course of steroids may help alleviate radicular pain, although no definitive studies have confirmed this anecdotal evidence. Methylprednisolone is often prescribed in a prepackaged dose pack that tapers from 24 mg to 0 mg over 7 days.

Corticosteroid injections are commonly used to treat radiculopathy. Their effect is thought to be multifactorial in nature; they are thought to (1) reduce inflammation through inhibition of prostaglandins; (2) disrupt the input of nociceptive fibers from somatic nerves; and (3) block pain-generating neuropeptide synthesis, among other proposed mechanisms.[15] Much like the medical treatment of cervical radiculopathy, the use of isolated cervical epidural steroid injections for the treatment of cervical radiculopathy lacks definitive supporting data from clinical trials.

Corticosteroid injections may occasionally be both diagnostic and therapeutic for the patient. If a corticosteroid injection is targeted to a given foramen, and the patient receives some pain relief, even for a short period, it may indicate that the foramen that was injected should be the one to be decompressed with PCF. When the steroid injection of a given foramen provides no relief, the provider may consider a trial of an injection of a different foramen to determine if it is the affected level.

17.5 Pertinent Anatomy

Thorough knowledge of the cervical bony anatomy is essential to correct identification of the foramen. The lateral mass of the vertebral body sits at the intersection between the lamina and pedicle. The superior and inferior articular processes project from the lateral mass. A vertebral notch is located on the superior and inferior portions of the pedicle. These notches on neighboring vertebral bodies form the intervertebral foramen, which contains the exiting spinal nerve. Thus, the foramen is bound anteriorly by the intervertebral disk, uncovertebral joints, and vertebral bodies, posteriorly by the facets, and superiorly and inferiorly by the pedicles. The foramen is approximately 8 to 10 mm in the medial–lateral direction, less than 12 mm in cranial–caudal height, and 4 mm in anterior–posterior length, and it sits at a 45° angle from the midsagittal plane (▶ Fig. 17.1).[14]

The cervical nerve roots from C3 to C8 enter the intervertebral foramina at the level of the disk above the pedicle of their respective spinal levels, with C8 exiting above the T1 pedicle. For example, the C7 nerve root exits above the C7 pedicle at the level of the C6–C7 disk space. The most likely point of nerve compression is the medial entry zone of the foramen because it is the smallest segment of the intervertebral foramen; conversely, the largest segment of the nerve root is at the exit from the thecal sac (▶ Fig. 17.2).

17.6 Operative Procedure

For PCF, the patient is brought into the room and anesthetized under general endotracheal anesthesia. Intraoperative neurological monitoring, such as somatosensory evoked potentials and EMG, may be applied. The patient is placed in a three-point Mayfield head clamp to prevent movement of the head. The procedure may be performed with the patient in either prone position or sitting position, with the head slightly flexed. The sitting position allows greater visualization compared to the prone position because it allows the patient's shoulders to fall with gravity; in addition, lateral radiographs of the pertinent anatomy may be more easily obtained. Placing the patient in the sitting position also improves visualization because blood in the surgical field will travel down out of the wound with gravity rather than creating a well of blood in the wound that

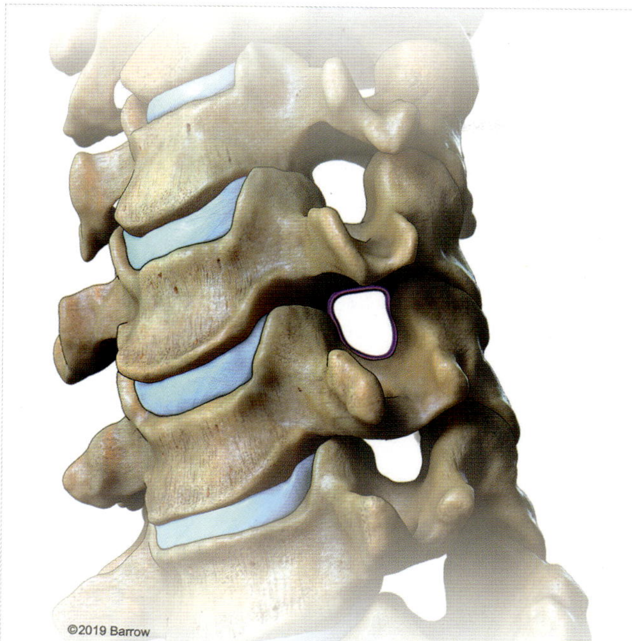

Fig. 17.1 Illustration showing the boundaries of the neural foramen (*purple outline*). (Used with permissions from Barrow Neurological Institute, Phoenix, Arizona.)

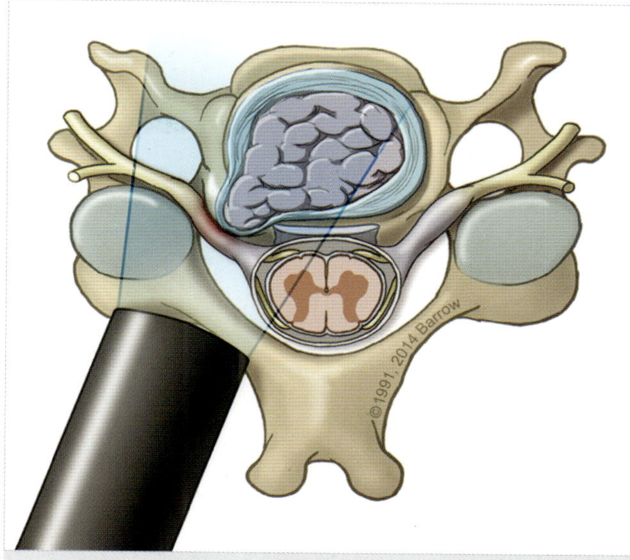

Fig. 17.2 Illustration showing a disk herniation with nerve root compression. The illustration also shows the minimally invasive trajectory to the compressed nerve and associated disk. (Used with permissions from Barrow Neurological Institute, Phoenix, Arizona.)

must be suctioned away, as is the case when the patient is in the prone position. However, air embolisms have been reported with this position because the sitting position increases the risk of air intruding into the venous system. The risk of an air embolism with the patient in the sitting position for PCF varies from 0 to 2.3%.[16]

The patient is then prepared and draped, and a spinal needle is used to mark the spinal level. The incision is typically between 1 and 2 cm in length and is made lateral to the midline at the appropriate foraminal level. The skin incision needs to be just big enough to fit the retractor system, which may be a tubular, microscopic, or endoscopic retractor system, as preferred by the surgeon. Bovie electrocautery is then used to deepen the incision through the posterior fascia. Blunt finger dissection or dissection using Metzenbaum scissors is then used to expose down to the facet. If a tubular retractor system is used, fluoroscopy is used to place sequentially larger retractors until the appropriate size is placed.

Whether visualization is performed using a Weitlaner retractor or a tubular retractor system with an endoscope or a microscope, the retractor should be placed so that the surgeon has visualization of the inferomedial edge of the rostral lateral mass. Dissection is then continued to expose the bony surface of the lateral hemilamina of the level of the affected foramen and the medial facet, including both the superior and inferior lateral mass. Initial dissection begins laterally, where bone can be found, then moves medially, with care taken to identify and avoid entering the interlaminar space.

A small laminotomy, or the removal of a small amount of bone from the inferior lamina of the superior level and the removal of a small amount of bone from the superior lamina of the inferior level, is created using either a 2-mm Kerrison rongeur or a drill to enable visualization of the lateral border of the cervical dura. The rongeur is then used to remove the medial portion of the inferior articular process of the rostral facet and the superior articular process of the caudal facet, thereby exposing the exiting cervical nerve root. Usually, only the medial third of the facet must be removed to decompress the nerve. Frequent dissection with an angled curette should be performed during the bony decompression to facilitate the safe use of the rongeur. If disk material is causing compression on the exiting nerve root, a larger portion of the superior articular process should be removed so that the disk fragment can be visualized. However, no more than 50% of the facet should be removed to prevent destabilization of the level (▶ Fig. 17.3).

At this point, the surgeon must focus on exposing the nerve root. Bipolar coagulation of the venous plexus surrounding the nerve may be required for better visualization. Although the nerve root can be mobilized in a rostral–caudal orientation to allow visualization of the foramen and any osteophytes or disk fragments that may be present, prolonged or frequent retraction of the nerve should be avoided. Free disk fragments can be removed using a nerve hook or a micropituitary rongeur. An angled curette can then be used to tamp down or fracture osteophyte fragments. After the surgeon has determined that the nerve has been decompressed or freed in the foramen, often by both visualizing and feeling with a nerve hook or curette that there is no further compression of the nerve root, the surgeon proceeds to close the wound.

17.7 Complications

Complications after PCF are rare.[17,18] As with any cervical spine surgery, injury to the spinal cord or spinal nerves, cerebrospinal fluid leaks, and infections can occur. Unnecessary traction on the nerve root is best avoided by achieving a

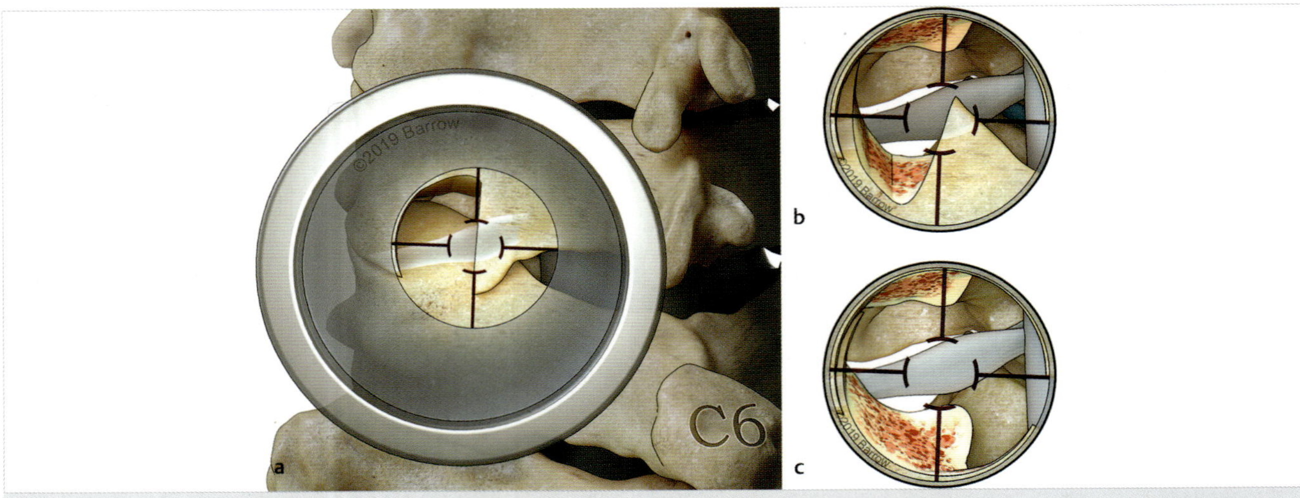

Fig. 17.3 Illustration showing the sequence of drilling the bone in a posterior cervical foraminotomy. **(a)** Drilling should begin at the superolateral aspect of the exposed inferior articular process and rostral lamina, in this case of C5. The position of the nerve root below the bony structures is indicated by the green and white ghosted image. After the superior articular process (SAP) has been identified, the bone work is extended medially over the top of the lamina until the ligamentum flavum can be visualized. At this point, the SAP of C6 will be seen clearly. The symptomatic nerve root can be found immediately behind the C6 SAP. **(b)** Magnified microscopic view showing the next target for drilling is the lateral aspect of the exposure, which is the SAP of the caudal vertebra, which is C6 in this case. **(c)** Magnified microscopic view showing the final parts of the foramen to be drilled are the medial aspect of the rostral SAP and the lamina, which is C6 in this case. (Used with permissions from Barrow Neurological Institute, Phoenix, Arizona.)

thorough and complete bony decompression before any nerve root manipulation.

The incidence of durotomy during PCF has been reported to range from 0 to 9%.[11,19] An unintended durotomy during surgery can be treated using direct visualization and repair with a 6–0 polypropylene suture or by the placement of muscle, fat, or an absorbable gelatin sponge (Gelfoam; Pfizer, Inc., New York, NY) over the tear followed by the application of a dural sealant such as DuraSeal (Confluent Surgical, Inc., Waltham, MA).

The vertebral artery runs immediately anterior to the cervical nerve root and is surrounded by a rich venous plexus. Therefore, when working in this space, the surgeon should be keenly aware of increased venous bleeding, which indicates proximity of the vertebral artery.

17.8 Postoperative Care

Most patients can be discharged home safely on the day of surgery. Incisional pain and neck soreness are expected for 1 to 2 weeks after surgery and can often be managed with a short prescription of a muscle relaxant medication or acetaminophen, or both, or a nonsteroidal anti-inflammatory pain medication. Low-dose narcotics or synthetic narcotics can be used for breakthrough pain. Patients are encouraged to begin ambulation immediately but are advised not to lift more than 10 pounds within the first 2 weeks to promote incisional healing. Most patients can return to work within 2 to 4 weeks. Outpatient physical therapy can be used to improve neck strength and mobility as needed. Athletes are often allowed to return to play after 4 weeks, although, depending on the sport, some surgeons will allow a return to play sooner or later than 4 weeks. Among professional athletes, return-to-play rates have been shown to be as high as 92% after a posterior foraminotomy, with athletes in high-contact sports returning to play at a mean of 238 days after surgery.[20] In contrast, patients who undergo ACDF have a return-to-play rate of 70% at a mean of 366 days after surgery.[20] This earlier return-to-play time frame when compared to that of ACDF procedures, which is often a year, makes PCF the more favorable procedure when it is an option.

17.9 Conclusion

PCF offers safe, reliable treatment of unilateral cervical radiculopathy in athletes and allows faster return to play while avoiding implant-related complications.

17.10 Clinical Pearls

- For athletes with unilateral disk herniation or unilateral foraminal stenosis, PCF offers the ability to return to play far sooner than they would after a fusion procedure.
- Athletes who undergo PCF have demonstrated a higher return-to-play rate and earlier return to play compared to ACDF.
- Patients with bilateral radiculopathy or bilateral nerve root compression in the foramen are not good candidates for PCF.
- The most likely point of nerve compression is the medial entry zone of the foramen because it is the smallest dimension of the intervertebral foramen and because the largest part of the nerve root is at the exit from the thecal sac.
- The vertebral artery runs immediately anterior to the cervical nerve roots and is surrounded by a rich venous plexus. When working in this space, the surgeon should be keenly aware of increased venous bleeding, which indicates proximity of the vertebral artery.
- No more than 50% of the facet should be removed to prevent destabilization of the spinal level.

17.11 Disclosures

The authors have no personal, financial, or institutional interest in any of the drugs, materials, or devices described in this manuscript.

Acknowledgments

We thank the staff of Neuroscience Publications at Barrow Neurological Institute for assistance with manuscript preparation.

References

[1] Scoville WB, Whitcomb BB, McLaurin R. The cervical ruptured disc; report of 115 operative cases. Trans Am Neurol Assoc. 1951; 56(56):222–224

[2] Frykholm R. Lower cervical vertebrae and intervertebral discs; surgical anatomy and pathology. Acta Chir Scand. 1951; 101(5):345–359

[3] Wirth FP, Dowd GC, Sanders HF, Wirth C. Cervical discectomy. A prospective analysis of three operative techniques. Surg Neurol. 2000; 53(4):340–346, discussion 346–348

[4] Ruetten S, Komp M, Merk H, Godolias G. Full-endoscopic interlaminar and transforaminal lumbar discectomy versus conventional microsurgical technique: a prospective, randomized, controlled study. Spine. 2008; 33(9): 931–939

[5] Yoss RE, Corbin KB, MacCarty CS, Love JG. Significance of symptoms and signs in localization of involved root in cervical disk protrusion. Neurology. 1957; 7(10):673–683

[6] Wainner RS, Gill H. Diagnosis and nonoperative management of cervical radiculopathy. J Orthop Sports Phys Ther. 2000; 30(12):728–744

[7] Rubinstein SM, Pool JJ, van Tulder MW, Riphagen II, de Vet HC. A systematic review of the diagnostic accuracy of provocative tests of the neck for diagnosing cervical radiculopathy. Eur Spine J. 2007; 16(3):307–319

[8] Bell GR, Ross JS. Diagnosis of nerve root compression. Myelography, computed tomography, and MRI. Orthop Clin North Am. 1992; 23(3):405–419

[9] Rothman SM, Winkelstein BA. Chemical and mechanical nerve root insults induce differential behavioral sensitivity and glial activation that are enhanced in combination. Brain Res. 2007; 1181:30–43

[10] Rao R. Neck pain, cervical radiculopathy, and cervical myelopathy: pathophysiology, natural history, and clinical evaluation. J Bone Joint Surg Am. 2002; 84(10):1872–1881

[11] Rhee JM, Yoon T, Riew KD. Cervical radiculopathy. J Am Acad Orthop Surg. 2007; 15(8):486–494

[12] Boden SD, McCowin PR, Davis DO, Dina TS, Mark AS, Wiesel S. Abnormal magnetic-resonance scans of the cervical spine in asymptomatic subjects. A prospective investigation. J Bone Joint Surg Am. 1990; 72(8):1178–1184

[13] Caridi JM, Pumberger M, Hughes AP. Cervical radiculopathy: a review. HSS J. 2011; 7(3):265–272

[14] Huntoon MA. Anatomy of the cervical intervertebral foramina: vulnerable arteries and ischemic neurologic injuries after transforaminal epidural injections. Pain. 2005; 117(1–2):104–111

[15] Deyo RA. Drug therapy for back pain. Which drugs help which patients? Spine. 1996; 21(24):2840–2849, discussion 2849–2850

[16] Jadik S, Wissing H, Friedrich K, Beck J, Seifert V, Raabe A. A standardized protocol for the prevention of clinically relevant venous air embolism during neurosurgical interventions in the semisitting position. Neurosurgery. 2009; 64(3):533–538, discussion 538–539

[17] O'Toole JE, Sheikh H, Eichholz KM, Fessler RG, Perez-Cruet MJ. Endoscopic posterior cervical foraminotomy and discectomy. Neurosurg Clin N Am. 2006; 17(4):411–422

[18] O'Toole JE, Eichholz KM, Fessler RG. Surgical site infection rates after minimally invasive spinal surgery. J Neurosurg Spine. 2009; 11(4):471–476

[19] Sampath P, Bendebba M, Davis JD, Ducker T. Outcome in patients with cervical radiculopathy. Prospective, multicenter study with independent clinical review. Spine. 1999; 24(6):591–597

[20] Mai HT, Chun DS, Schneider AD, Hecht AC, Maroon JC, Hsu WK. The difference in clinical outcomes after anterior cervical fusion, disk replacement, and foraminotomy in professional athletes. Clin Spine Surg. 2018; 31(1):E80–E84

18 Surgery: Posterior Lumbar Decompression and Fusion

Luis M. Tumialán

Summary
Posterior lumbar fusions do not preclude a return to play, even in high-performance athletes or active-duty military personnel, who return to high-impact and high-endurance activities postoperatively. Preservation of the midline structures, specifically the spinous processes and the paraspinal musculature, is the central tenet of minimal access approaches to the lumbar spine. A paramedian approach to the lumbar spine provides access to the pedicles for instrumentation, the central canal for decompression, and the disk space for interbody fusion. The objective of the current chapter is to review the rationale, indications, and surgical technique for a minimal access posterior lumbar fusion. Operating room setup along with the various phases of the operation are presented. Complication avoidance strategies and clinical pearls are also presented. Instability of a segment, recurrent disk herniations, and spondylolisthesis in athletes may all be successfully managed with a minimal access posterior lumbar fusion.

Keywords: arthrodesis, interbody fusion, instrumentation, laminectomy, lumbar, pedicle, transforaminal

18.1 Introduction

High-performance athletes may sustain a variety of injuries in their respective sports which may require treatment with a posterior lumbar decompression and/or fusion.[1] The ideal approach for surgical intervention is one which minimizes disruption to the native spine, increasing the likelihood of successful return to play. Clearly defining the surgical target and limiting the exposure reliably achieves that mandate. Exposures that begin in the midline must be considerably larger than the surgical target. Longer incision allows for the appropriate exposure and adequate visualization of the lateral spinal anatomy necessary for instrumentation. The distinct advantage of a minimal access approach is the paramedian trajectory. Placing the surgeon immediately over the requisite anatomy for the procedure forgoes the need for a longer and wider exposure. Instead, a more focused exposure is all that is needed to expose and visualize the requisite spinal anatomy. More importantly, a minimal access approach is less disruptive to the paraspinal musculature and spares the musculature of the midline. Although it has been difficult to quantify the impact of a minimal access approach on returning an athlete back to play, it has been equally difficult to dismiss the importance of midline preservation and safeguarding the multifidus musculature in athletes.[2,3,4,5]

This chapter presents the indications, surgical technique, and complication avoidance strategies for a minimal access posterior lumbar fusion. A case illustration at the end of the chapter provides the context of lumbar fusion in a high-performance triathlete determined to return to competition, whose surgical and postoperative management for spondylolisthesis and a symptomatic radiculopathy are presented.

Although the literature is limited on this topic, ample evidence supports the conclusion that athletes who present with clinical circumstances requiring decompression and stabilization may still return to high levels of performance after a posterior lumbar fusion.[1,6]

18.2 Indications

Lumbar disk herniations, degeneration of the spine, and development of lumbar instability occur frequently in the general population, particularly those with a predominantly sedentary life.[7] Given the degree of impact on the spine associated with several sports, whether sustained as low-impact forces over time such as in marathon running or as sudden high-impact forces such as in football or hockey, it should be no surprise that the lumbar spines of high-performance athletes are prone to lumbar disk injuries and segmental instability. Furthermore, preexisting conditions, such as spondylolysis, may become symptomatic after several seasons of play or after a particularly violent play.

The main indications for a lumbar fusion in an athlete remain the same as in their nonathletic and sedentary counterparts. These indications include a recurrent disk herniation with symptomatic radiculopathy, spondylolisthesis with instability, or advanced degeneration with complete collapse of the disk space. The surgical objectives for the management of these entities include decompression of the neural elements, as well as restoration of the disk height in a lordotic configuration and stabilization of the segment.

18.3 Preoperative Assessment

For the most part, patients rarely present with standard radiographs and instead usually undergo magnetic resonance imaging (MRI) of the lumbar spine. However, plain radiographs, which should include anteroposterior, lateral, flexion, and extension views, are essential for all cases that will require instrumentation. Ideally, the femoral heads and the L1 superior endplate should be included to measure the spinopelvic parameters. It is important to identify any significant disparity between the pelvic incidence and lumbar lordosis. A value greater than 10° should make restoration of lumbar lordosis a priority to mitigate the risk of adjacent segment degeneration.[8] Any significant coronal imbalance or suggestion of scoliosis should prompt a 36-inch scoliosis survey, and decisions should be modified on the basis of the degree and location of the scoliosis.

18.4 Surgical Technique

18.4.1 Operating Room Setup

The patient is positioned on a Jackson table, which serves two purposes. First, a Jackson table optimizes the lordosis of the lumbar spine through positioning. By allowing the abdomen to hang freely, the vertebral bodies of the lumbar spine assume a more lordotic configuration. Additionally, placing the hips into slight hyperextension further optimizes a lordotic position that will be captured by the instrumentation. The second reason is to decrease the intra-abdominal pressure and thereby the central venous pressure. Blood loss tends to be reduced for a patient on a Jackson table compared to a Wilson frame, which places pressure on the abdomen, increasing the central venous pressure and engorging the epidural veins.

For cases where computer-assisted navigation is used, it is important to set up the operating room so that the intraoperative computed tomography unit can enter and exit the operative field unencumbered. If fluoroscopy is to be used, the base of the fluoroscope is positioned opposite to the side of the microscope (▶ Fig. 18.1). The microscope is positioned on the side of the most prominent symptoms. For example, in a patient with a recurrent disk herniation, the microscope is positioned on the side of the radiculopathy. Raynor and colleagues have demonstrated the value of electrophysiological monitoring for confirming placement of pedicle screws without a medial breach.[9] Thus, after positioning of the patient, all connections for pedicle screw stimulation are immediately set up.

18.4.2 Instrumentation of the Spine

With the patient in position, the incisions are planned based on anatomical landmarks. The anterior superior iliac spine, which correlates with the interspinous process space at L4–L5, is palpated, and the interspinous process space is marked in the midline. If the operative segment is L3–L4, the incision is shifted up one segment; if the operative segment is L5–S1, then it is shifted down one segment, and so on. Two paramedian incisions are then planned 4 cm lateral to the midline mark at L4–L5 and L5–S1. Given the intrapedicular distance reported by Panjabi et al,[10] the paramedian incisions at L3–L4 are 3.5 cm lateral to midline. For the rare circumstance of an operation on L1–L2 and L2–L3, the paramedian incisions narrow to 3 cm off the midline.

With the incisions planned, the patient is draped, and spinal needles are passed with a converging trajectory onto the facet joints of the segment to be operated upon to confirm the segment. Fluoroscopy confirms the segment, and the planned incisions are adjusted to optimize an ideal trajectory onto the level. The two incisions are made, and the dissection proceeds simultaneously down to the thoracolumbar fascia. Cautery divides the fascia and a series of dilators of increasing diameters are used to encompass the facet joint of the segment to be operated upon. Minimal access ports are secured over the top of the facet on the left and the right. Cautery exposes the entire facet before opening the minimal access port. If only one surgeon is operating, exposure and instrumentation are completed on one side before proceeding with the contralateral side. If two surgeons are operating, exposures and instrumentation are done simultaneously through both incisions.

One of the criticisms of minimally invasive spinal surgery is the radiation exposure needed for instrumentation of the spine. Percutaneous instrumentation by its very nature mandates some form of additional visualization, whether from fluoroscopy or computer-assisted navigation. Using computer-assisted navigation is one way to neutralize the radiation argument. Another approach is to forego percutaneous technology and directly visualize the pedicle screw entry point. Fluoroscopy at that point is limited to confirming the entry point and establishing a trajectory. Once the junction of the pars interarticularis, midtransverse process, and inferolateral facet is directly visualized for all four pedicles, a drill is placed onto the entry point; a single fluoroscopic image confirms the entry point before the drill creates a breach through the cortical bone overlying the cancellous bone of the pedicle (▶ Fig. 18.2).

A pedicle probe enters the drilled entry point and works its way through cancellous bone of the pedicle and into the vertebral body. There is an unmistakable tactile feel to the tip of the

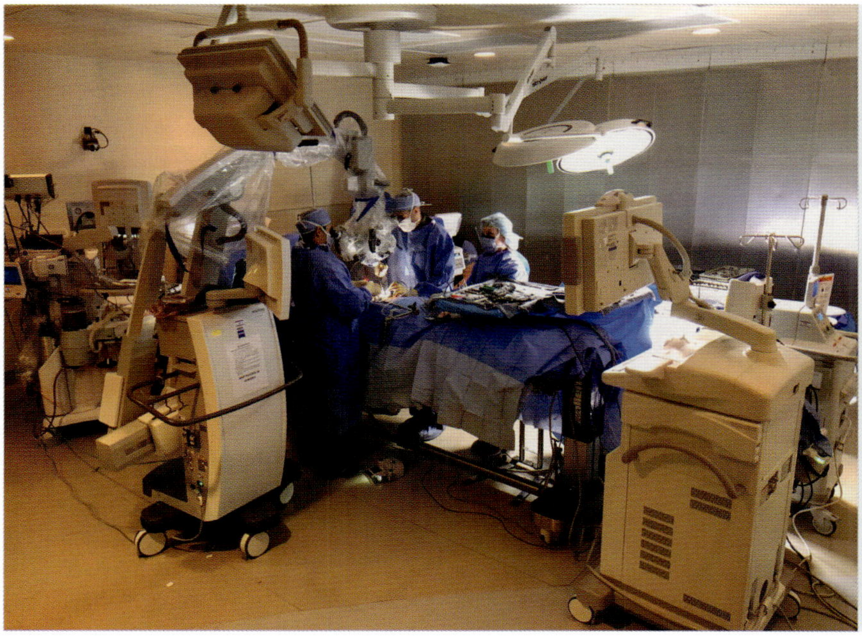

Fig. 18.1 Operating room setup for posterior lumbar fusion. Photograph demonstrating a patient undergoing a left L4–L5 transforaminal lumbar fusion. The patient is positioned on a Jackson table. The base of the fluoroscope is positioned opposite to the microscope, and the tower with the screens of the fluoroscope is at the foot of the bed. At this point in the operation, the pedicle screws have already been placed and the decompression is being performed under the operating microscope. The fluoroscope has been rolled to the head of the bed and will be rolled back into position for the interbody phase of the operation. (Used with permissions from Barrow Neurological Institute, Phoenix, Arizona.)

pedicle probe displacing cancellous bone as it advances through the pedicle. That tactile feel contrasts sharply with the tip encountering cortical bone. If stiff resistance is encountered, the trajectory into the pedicle needs to be adjusted until cancellous bone is once again encountered. Once the probe reaches 30 mm into the pedicle, it is stimulated to 20 mA to rule out a compound motor action potential. If positive, a medial breach may have occurred. The pedicle probe should be removed and a ball-tipped probe used to identify the medial breach. A careful assessment of the entry point and trajectory into the pedicle is warranted. At times, an anteroposterior image may offer further guidance, but should seldom be necessary. The absence of a compound motor action potential at 20 mA should not preclude the use of a ball-tipped probe to confirm the integrity of the pedicle.

A pedicle tap one size smaller than the intended diameter of the pedicle screw is then secured into the pedicle. Again, electrophysiological testing rules out a medial breach before the integrity of the pedicle is confirmed once again with the ball-tipped probe and then the pedicle screw is placed. When two surgeons are operating, simultaneous exposure, probing, tapping, and placement of the pedicle screws decreases the need for fluoroscopy and increases the efficiency of the operation. If only one surgeon is operating, one side is instrumented, and then the surgeon will go to the other side and repeat the process.

18.4.3 Decompression of the Neural Elements

There are three osteotomy cuts that, when completed, offer expansive access to the central canal for decompression of the thecal sac, traversing and exiting nerve roots, and the disk space for interbody fusion (► Fig. 18.2). The first osteotomy cut is a transverse cut through the isthmus of the pars interarticularis just below the rostral pedicle screw. That osteotomy cut extends medially until the confluence of the lamina and spinous process is encountered. The second osteotomy cut is a longitudinal cut at the confluence of the spinous process and lamina. The cut begins at the interlaminar space and extends rostrally until the first osteotomy cut is encountered. Once these two osteotomy cuts are complete, the lamina, pars interarticularis, and the inferior articular process may be removed en bloc. The final osteotomy cut allows for disarticulation of the superior articular process and the superior aspect of the caudal lamina.

Upon completion of the osteotomies, a complete decompression of the segment may be undertaken. Although loupes and headlight provide adequate magnification and illumination for placement of pedicle screws and the osteotomies, it is my preference to complete the decompression under the operating microscope.

The objective of the decompression is a pedicle-to-pedicle decompression of the entire segment. The osteotomies incorporate the insertion points of the ligamentum flavum, and so with the osteotomies complete, the ligamentum flavum may be removed using an en bloc technique. Maintaining the ligamentum flavum over the top of the thecal sac and working at the insertion points minimize the risk of inadvertent injury to the dura. Once the medial and lateral insertion points are released, the entire ligamentum flavum may be removed, and the neural elements are completely decompressed.

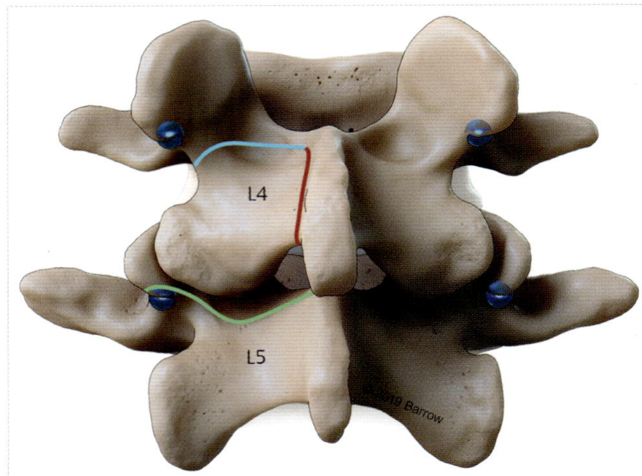

Fig. 18.2 The pedicle screw entry points and osteotomy cuts for an L4–L5 instrumented transforaminal lumbar interbody fusion. The blue fiducial markers in this illustration represent the pedicle screw entry points. Each fiducial is at the junction of the superior aspect of the pars interarticularis, the middle portion of the transverse process, and the inferior and lateral facet. Direct visualization of the pedicle screw entry point limits the role of fluoroscopy to confirm an entry point and establish the trajectory. The osteotomy cuts for the decompression and transforaminal access are denoted in color. The first osteotomy cut (*denoted in light blue*) is a transverse cut across the isthmus of the pars interarticularis to the base of the spinous process. The second cut (denoted in red) is an oblique vertical cut along the base of the spinous process. The third and final cut (*denoted in green*) is the transverse cut across the superior articular process and the caudal lamina. Those cuts encompass the insertions of the ligamentum flavum that will allow for an en bloc resection to decompress the segment. (Used with permissions from Barrow Neurological Institute, Phoenix, Arizona.)

The transforaminal corridor demarcated by the exiting root, the lateral thecal sac, and the traversing root is now in full view (► Fig. 18.3). A common error is referring to the transforaminal corridor as Kambin's triangle, which is a reference to a working triangle *without* removal of the facet, pars interarticularis, and lamina. Given the extensive bony work completed, it would be anatomically inaccurate to refer to the transforaminal corridor by the same name.[11]

The diskectomy is completed through a generous annulotomy from the mid-pedicular line to the lateral aspect of the thecal sac. Large Epstein curettes, straight curettes, and angled curettes are used to remove the cartilaginous endplate and prepare the cortical endplates for arthrodesis. When satisfactory preparation of the endplate is complete, the operating microscope rolls out of the operative field, and the fluoroscope rolls back into its previous position. The surgeon again uses loupes and headlights for the final phase of the operation: placement of the interbody.

18.4.4 Placement of the Interbody

The dimensions of the transforaminal corridor are such that interbody trials may be placed into the disk space without the need for retraction of either the traversing or exiting root. The selection of the interbody height is based on a combination of the first normal disk height among the adjacent segments and the height restored with interbody trials. Trials of increasing heights may be tapped into the disk space until an interbody height that fits securely within the disk space is identified. Morselized autograft and allograft bone is packed into the anterior aspect of the disk space prior to placement of the interbody spacer. It is my preference to use an interbody spacer with a curved geometry (banana shaped) to match the curvature of the disk space and rotate it into the anterior one-third of the disk space. The curved geometry will allow for a second interbody to be nested behind the first. The second interbody increases the stiffness of the segment, creates a larger area for arthrodesis, and maintains greater foraminal height under compression (▶ Fig. 18.4).[12] Once in position, the final rods are placed over the top of the tulip heads of the pedicle screws and the construct is placed under compression to maintain or restore segmental lordosis. If there is a considerable mismatch between the pelvic incidence and the lumbar lordosis, a Smith-Petersen osteotomy contralateral to the transforaminal corridor is instrumental in restoring lordosis. Compression of the pedicle screws on the rods will then accomplish up to 14° of segmental lordosis.[13]

With the rods in place, the expandable minimal access ports are removed and the incision closed in a multilayer fashion. Prior to closure, the skin and muscle are infiltrated with a lidocaine–bupivacaine mixture. Patients are asked to ambulate for approximately 1 hour after recovering from general anesthesia and may be discharged after a 23-hour period of observation or, in some instances, the same day of surgery.

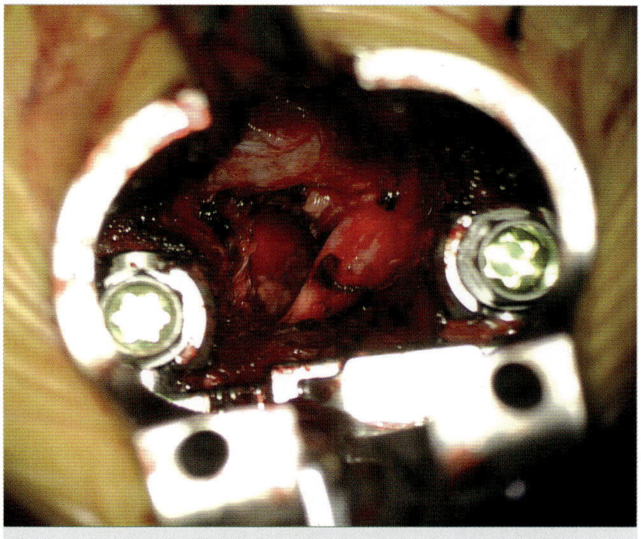

Fig. 18.3 The transforaminal corridor in a right L4–L5 minimally invasive transforaminal lumbar interbody fusion. Intraoperative photograph of an L4–L5 right transforaminal corridor with the diskectomy complete. The exiting L4 nerve root, lateral thecal sac, and traversing nerve root create the transforaminal corridor. (Used with permissions from Barrow Neurological Institute, Phoenix, Arizona.)

18.5 Complication Avoidance

Complications with the minimally invasive transforaminal lumbar interbody fusion may occur either at the time of surgery or in a delayed fashion. The immediate complications are cerebrospinal fluid leak and errant placement of pedicle screws, both of which can occur at the time of surgery. Methodical exposure and unequivocal visualization of the pedicle screw entry points will minimize the risk of a pedicle breach. It is an investment worth the time to meticulously expose the pedicle screw entry point. Ensuring an adequate angle of convergence, depending on the pedicle, will also minimize the risk of a medial or lateral breach. By way of example, at L5 an angle of 25° would be appropriate, but that same angle used at L2, where an angle of 10° to 15° would be more appropriate, would result in a medial breach. Finally, one should not be dismissive of a compound motor action potential under 15 mA with pedicle screw stimulation. Careful assessment of the pedicle is warranted when a threshold of 15 mA triggers a response.

The risk of a cerebrospinal fluid leak may be decreased by maintaining the ligamentum flavum completely intact over the thecal sac until the osteotomy cuts have been completed. Furthermore, removing the entire ligamentum flavum for the entire segment in an en bloc manner will minimize the exposure of the thecal sac to errant passes of an instrument.

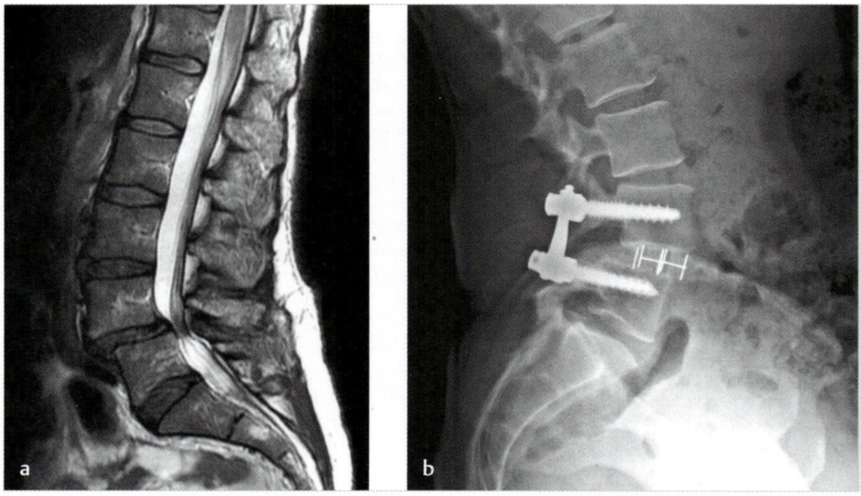

Fig. 18.4 Management of a 42-year-old triathlete who presented with increasing axial back pain and left radicular symptoms. At the completion of each triathlon, she would experience profound dorsiflexion weakness. **(a)** Sagittal T2-weighted magnetic resonance image of the lumbar spine demonstrating a grade I L4–L5 spondylolisthesis. Flexion and extension images (not shown) confirmed 8 mm of translation. The patient underwent a minimally invasive L4–L5 transforaminal lumbar interbody fusion. **(b)** Lateral radiograph demonstrating an instrumented lumbar fusion with nested interbody spacers at 6 months postsurgery. Bridging bone may be seen across the segment. The patient completed an Ironman Triathlon 6 months after surgery. (Used with permissions from Barrow Neurological Institute, Phoenix, Arizona.)

Working beyond the caudal insertion of the ligamentum flavum prevents the action of a Kerrison rongeur in the most constrained aspect of the canal. Therein lies the importance of the third osteotomy cut denoted in green in ▶ Fig. 18.2.

Delayed complications include pseudoarthrosis and adjacent segment degeneration. Meticulous preparation of the cortical endplates and removal of as much disk material as possible are the central tenets of achieving an interbody arthrodesis. Equally important is sizing the appropriate interbody spacer. When using the trials, there should be an unmistakable feel for the ideal interbody height. It should require a slap hammer for removal. An ample amount of bone graft should be placed into the disk space prior to insertion of the interbody. Rotating the interbody into position posterior to the morselized bone graft will help place the graft under a load. As mentioned above, placement of a second graft is a viable option to increase the graft surface area. Placing the entire construct under compression further loads the graft. The combination of these two techniques optimizes the environment for arthrodesis.

The incidence of adjacent segment degeneration may be decreased by limiting the exposure of the rostral facet joint and ensuring that there is no interruption of the facet capsule during the exposure. Second, addressing a significant mismatch between the pelvic incidence and lumbar lordosis will have implications on the development of adjacent segment degeneration.[8]

18.6 Conclusion

High-performance athletes may experience radiculopathy, neurogenic claudication, and axial back pain from either a recurrent lumbar disk herniation, neurogenic claudication secondary to spondylolisthesis, or instability. In certain circumstances, a minimally invasive motion-preserving decompression would not be adequate for the anatomical circumstance, and a more definitive procedure is needed. The need for a lumbar fusion should not be considered the end of an amateur or even a professional athletic career.[14] An instrumented transforaminal lumbar interbody fusion performed through two paraspinal incisions using minimal access ports accomplishes the objectives of decompression, realignment, and stabilization. The preservation of both the midline structures and the multifidus paraspinal musculature prevents the atrophy seen in midline approaches and may optimize the possibility that the athlete may return to play.[1,6]

18.7 Clinical Pearls

- Paraspinal approaches through minimal access ports allow for preservation of the midline structures, namely, the multifidus.
- Complete exposure of the bony anatomy and direct visualization of the pedicle screw entry points decrease the need for fluoroscopy, lower radiation exposure, and prevent errant placement of instrumentation.
- Osteotomy cuts at the levels of the rostral and caudal insertion points allow for removal of the lamina and inferior and superior articular processes in an efficient manner.
- Working only at the insertions of the ligamentum flavum and maintaining the ligamentum flavum intact during the decompression phase protect the thecal sac and potentially decrease the risk of a cerebrospinal fluid leak when compared to piecemeal resection.
- Segmental lordosis may be restored with transforaminal approaches when a Smith-Petersen osteotomy is performed in combination with the transforaminal access.

18.8 Disclosures

LessRay investor (acquired by NuVasive).

Acknowledgments

I thank the staff of Neuroscience Publications at Barrow Neurological Institute for assistance with manuscript preparation.

References

[1] Schroeder GD, McCarthy KJ, Micev AJ, Terry MA, Hsu WK. Performance-based outcomes after nonoperative treatment, discectomy, and/or fusion for a lumbar disc herniation in National Hockey League athletes. Am J Sports Med. 2013; 41(11):2604–2608

[2] Bresnahan L, Fessler RG, Natarajan RN. Evaluation of change in muscle activity as a result of posterior lumbar spine surgery using a dynamic modeling system. Spine. 2010; 35(16):E761–E767

[3] Bresnahan LE, Smith JS, Ogden AT, et al. Assessment of paraspinal muscle cross-sectional area after lumbar decompression: minimally invasive versus open approaches. Clin Spine Surg. 2017; 30(3):E162–E168

[4] Junhui L, Zhengbao P, Wenbin X, et al. Comparison of pedicle fixation by the Wiltse approach and the conventional posterior open approach for thoracolumbar fractures, using MRI, histological and electrophysiological analyses of the multifidus muscle. Eur Spine J. 2017; 26(5):1506–1514

[5] Putzier M, Hartwig T, Hoff EK, Streitparth F, Strube P. Minimally invasive TLIF leads to increased muscle sparing of the multifidus muscle but not the longissimus muscle compared with conventional PLIF—a prospective randomized clinical trial. Spine J. 2016; 16(7):811–819

[6] Tumialán LM, Ponton RP, Riccio AI, Gluf WM. Rate of return to military active duty after single level lumbar interbody fusion: a 5-year retrospective review. Neurosurgery. 2012; 71(2):317–324, discussion 324

[7] Abdu WA, Sacks OA, Tosteson ANA, et al. Long-term results of surgery compared with nonoperative treatment for lumbar degenerative spondylolisthesis in the Spine Patient Outcomes Research Trial (SPORT). Spine. 2018; 43(23):1619–1630

[8] Tempel ZJ, Gandhoke GS, Bolinger BD, et al. The influence of pelvic incidence and lumbar lordosis mismatch on development of symptomatic adjacent level disease following single-level transforaminal lumbar interbody fusion. Neurosurgery. 2017; 80(6):880–886

[9] Raynor BL, Lenke LG, Bridwell KH, Taylor BA, Padberg AM. Correlation between low triggered electromyographic thresholds and lumbar pedicle screw malposition: analysis of 4857 screws. Spine. 2007; 32(24): 2673–2678

[10] Panjabi MM, Goel V, Oxland T, et al. Human lumbar vertebrae. Quantitative three-dimensional anatomy. Spine. 1992; 17(3):299–306

[11] Tumialán LM, Madhavan K, Godzik J, Wang MY. The history of and controversy over Kambin's triangle: a historical analysis of the lumbar transforaminal corridor for endoscopic and surgical approaches. World Neurosurg. 2019; 123:402–408

[12] Soriano-Baron H, Newcomb AG, Malhotra D, et al. Biomechanics of nested transforaminal lumbar interbody cages. Neurosurgery. 2016; 78(2): 297–304

[13] Jagannathan J, Sansur CA, Oskouian RJ, Jr, Fu KM, Shaffrey CI. Radiographic restoration of lumbar alignment after transforaminal lumbar interbody fusion. Neurosurgery. 2009; 64(5):955–963, discussion 963–964

[14] Diaz J. Why Tiger Woods' fans can take heart after his latest surgery. Golf Digest. Published 2017. Accessed January 24, 2019 at: https://www.golfdigest.com/story/why-tiger-woods-fans-can-take-heart-after-his-latest-surgery

19 Surgery: Direct Pars Repair for Spondylolysis

Christina Sarris, Jakub Godzik, and U. Kumar Kakarla

Summary
Spondylolysis afflicts approximately 4% of children by the age of 6 and 7% of adults, but its prevalence can rise to 55% in certain athletic groups. Management of symptomatic athletes remains challenging. Recent years have seen trends toward minimally invasive repairs that decrease hospital stays and accelerate recovery. Direct pars repair is an appealing option which restores local anatomy while preserving normal motion at the involved level. For the properly selected patient who fails conservative management, direct pars repair may provide symptom relief and eventually facilitate resumption of "normal" high-intensity activities.

Keywords: spondylolysis, pars interarticularis, direct pars repair, buck repair, minimally invasive, neuronavigation

19.1 Introduction

Spondylolysis is a defect of the pars interarticularis and is commonly encountered by both the pediatric and adult spine surgeons. It is found in approximately 4% of children by the age of 6 and in 6 to 7% of adults.[1] Its pathogenesis is thought to be either congenital and/or related to chronic microtrauma from rotational and extension movements of the lumbar spine; consequently, it is no surprise that a high percentage of young athletes are afflicted. The prevalence can be as high as 47 to 55% in certain athletes, particularly those participating in sports that involve significant rotational and extension movements, such as gymnastics, soccer, weight lifting, football, bowling, and figure skating.[2,3,4] Although most patients remain asymptomatic,[1] pain and progression can occur which may eventually warrant intervention. Enthusiasm for direct pars repair began in the late 1960s and remains high for these patients, as the procedure restores local anatomy while preserving normal motion at the involved level.[5] In this chapter we will review the presentation, diagnosis, and management of spondylolysis with focus on the different surgical repair options and the trend toward utilization of minimally invasive techniques.

19.2 Spondylolysis

19.2.1 Presentation

Spondylolysis is a common cause of back pain in the pediatric and adolescent population, for those participating in high-intensity sporting activities. A review of 100 adolescent athletes with low back pain by Micheli and Wood found spondylolysis in 47% of the patients.[6] This rate is substantially higher than the adult population in whom only 6% of those with back pain are found to have spondylolysis.[4,6] It has been suggested that this is because the pediatric spine continuously grows and remodels until the mid-twenties when the pars is fully developed, and the pars may be more susceptible to spondylolysis during this remodeling period.[4,7]

Pediatric patients with symptomatic pars defects generally describe a gradual, chronic onset of localized lumbosacral pain with no specific initial injury event associated with symptom onset. Characteristic pain is usually alleviated by rest/recumbency and aggravated by motion.[7] Pain tends to be localized paracentrally, deep below the muscle. Symptoms can also radiate to the hamstrings and buttocks.

The adult presentation of spondylolysis is like that in the adolescent population, with a gradual onset of lumbosacral pain that is worsened with activity. However, in the adult population, where degenerative pathologies including lumbar stenosis, disk herniation, and myofascial pain are more prevalent, the clinician must be able to discern the primary pain generator for the patient.

19.2.2 Diagnosis

Physical Examination

Patients will frequently report tenderness to palpation in the lumbosacral region and may even have muscle spasm (unilateral or bilateral).[7] The practitioner should palpate the entire spine and assess the patient's range of motion. Some patients may have a visibly flattened lumbar lordosis. Typically, extension will renew the patient's pain. A systematic review investigated the diagnostic ability of clinical tests to detect spondylolysis.[8] The one-legged hyperextension test, also known as the "Stork test," is frequently used to help diagnose spondylolysis in the office. The clinician asks the patient to stand on one leg, with the clinician guiding the lumbar spine into extension. A positive result is one that reproduces the patient's painful symptoms. Masci et al reported low sensitivity and specificity for this test in 71 patients with confirmed spondylolysis diagnosed via scintigraphy, while Gregg et al reported 73% sensitivity and 17% specificity.[9,10] Sundell et al investigated the validity of other tests performed by practitioners to detect pars defects, but found that these maneuvers were not able to distinguish spondylolysis from other etiologies for back pain.[11] Rather than discredit these examinations because of the aforementioned studies, astute clinicians must know that these tests are to be interpreted in the context of a detailed history and other physical examination findings.

Radiographs (X-ray)

If the clinician suspects spondylolysis, in those with athletic history and pain worsening with extension, further imaging is warranted. X-ray is the most common first-line study, as it is cost-effective and has a good safety profile in the pediatric and adult populations. The classic radiograph view to detect any pars abnormality is the oblique image—the colloquial "Scottie Dog" image is of an oblique X-ray where a pars fracture appears like the collar around the dog's neck. However, early spondylolysis may not present this view.[4]

The Scoliosis Research Society published a review analyzing the current evidence regarding diagnostic imaging for pediatric spondylolysis.[12] One study conducted by Amato et al reported that radiographs were able to detect 96.5% of pars defects.[13] However, Beck et al found that compared to more advanced imaging, such as computed tomography (CT), magnetic resonance imaging (MRI), or bone scan, radiographs were good for confirmatory examinations due to the low incidence of false-positives but poor screening tests due to a high rate of false-negative results. Interestingly, they also found no difference in sensitivity and specificity between studies that included oblique views versus those that did not, suggesting that there may not be a diagnostic benefit outweighing the additional cost and radiation exposure for additional views.[14]

Given their low cost, decreased radiation, and relative efficacy, two-view plain X-rays are still the recommended first study.

CT Scan

CT scans are widely considered the gold standard in spondylolysis diagnosis.[12] CT scans definitively show the bony anatomy and can assist in diagnosing even the most subtle of fractures through reconstructive images. It can also be very helpful for surgical planning and possibly even in the operating room with CT-navigated technology. However, in particular, for pediatric patients, there is a tradeoff between the radiation dose and the increased diagnostic value of these scans compared to X-rays. Therefore, CT scans should be ordered judiciously in this patient population.

Decreased-dose CT scans of the lumbar spine may be the optimal examination to confirm spondylolysis. The Department of Radiology at Children's Hospital Colorado compared MRI versus low-dose limited CT scans in 42 pediatric patients with low back pain and suspected spondylolysis, finding that agreement and confidence in diagnosis were significantly greater for these CT sequences compared to MRI films.[15]

MRI

MRIs have been reported to have near-perfect detection of spondylolysis while avoiding the radiation exposure of CT scans.[16] However, they have high costs and are not routinely available, and therefore need not be first-line tests. Moreover, an MRI may not be as effective as radiographs or a CT scan in diagnosing other bony abnormalities and causes of pain such as facet fractures.[12]

Other Imaging Techniques

Single photon emission computed tomography (SPECT) has been frequently utilized to diagnose pars defects. The technology allows clinicians to ascertain if the region of interest on the scan is likely causing the patient's pain and can detect changes in the bone prior to pathologic appearance on X-ray.[4,7] This technology can be exceedingly helpful to surgeons, as many patients with low back pain and spondylolysis may be symptomatic from a separate concomitant spinal pathology. Raby and Mathews in the 1990s demonstrated that patients who had pars defects with positive SPECT scans had good results from surgical fixation, whereas those with negative or "cold" SPECT scans did not improve.[17] SPECT continues to be investigated as diagnostic technology for spondylolysis.[12,18,19] SPECT can incur a higher risk of cancer in the pediatric population because of its radiation, and it is not currently viewed as the gold standard.

In addition, MRI and SPECT are highly sensitive for detecting signal changes and edema within the pars. This has led to diagnosis of an entity coined "pars stress reaction," which is associated with image changes within the pars without definitive fracture on CT. This may represent a prelude to spondylolysis, or a separate pathological entity altogether.[20,21]

19.2.3 Management Options

Observation

Most patients with spondylolysis will be asymptomatic. Thus, if pars defects are incidental findings on imaging, or a patient's symptoms of low back pain are not consistent with classic spondylolysis, no intervention should be performed. There are currently no guidelines for the need to re-image or reevaluate those with asymptomatic spondylolysis, although some suggest re-imaging every 6 months during a child's period of rapid growth, or if symptoms begin.[22] Also, some experts advocate for vitamin D supplementation to optimize bone healing.[23]

Activity Restriction

Activity restriction can be essential in the armamentarium of conservative management for spondylolysis for young athletes. Recommendations for rest from sports are variable—ranging anywhere from a few weeks to 6 months. Additionally, the goals of activity restriction differ across providers. Some simply evaluate if patients are pain-free with activity after their rest from sports, without requiring any radiographic follow-up.[3] Others have strong desire to see patients symptom-free with radiographic evidence of bone healing.[22,24] Many studies suggest return to play only after at least 3 months of rest.[4,25,26] El Rassi et al reviewed 57 pediatric soccer players with symptomatic spondylolysis who were recommended stopping sports for at least 3 months, finding that those who complied with the restriction fared better than those who did not.[25] In a subsequent study they demonstrated that those who stopped sports for at least 3 months were 16 × more likely to have an excellent result than those who did not stop sports, and that evidence of bone healing on imaging did not correlate with clinical outcome.[27]

Bracing

Given that the likely pathogenesis for pars defect formation is a combination of extension and rotation forces, an ideal brace would restrict those motions to promote bone healing. Most patients are treated with a hard thoracolumbosacral or lumbosacral orthotic brace in comparison to soft corsets used more commonly in prior decades. Sairyo et al conducted a prospective study in which they evaluated which subtypes of spondylolysis are amenable to bracing and the length of time to achieve bone healing when treated with hard bracing.[28] The defects were classified into three categories based on CT scans, namely, early, progressive, and terminal defects[29]: Hard thoracolumbosacral orthoses (TLSOs) were worn as treatment, and CT scans were obtained every 3 months. Results demonstrated that the bony healing rates were 94% for the early defects and

0% for the terminal defects, illustrating that no terminal defect healed with conservative management. Early defects had a mean time to healing of 3.2 months whereas progressive defects required around 5 months.

As a guide, rigid braces should be worn continuously for 4 to 6 weeks prior to any reassessment by the physician.[23] Physicians can then reassess the patient, and if there is no pain with lumbar hyperextension, patients can wean out of the brace and begin physical therapy on a graduated path toward return to full activity.[23]

Physical Therapy

Physical therapy is directed at strengthening core paraspinal and abdominal muscles, as well as increasing lumbar flexion and extension motions. O'Sullivan et al reported that those whose therapy regimens targeted the hamstrings, lumbar multifidus, and deep abdominal muscles had improved outcomes than those placed on general therapy programs.[30]

Surgery

Prior to any consideration of operative intervention, surgeons must ensure that all other possible pain etiologies have been ruled out as the possible cause. Surgery should not generally be considered unless patients experience unrelenting symptoms despite at least 6 months of conservative therapies. When surgery is discussed for those who have failed nonoperative management, contending options include fixation and fusion across the involved segment versus direct repair.

19.3 Direct Pars Repair

19.3.1 Indications

Direct pars repair remains a favorable alternative to in-situ fusion. Candidates ideally should not have severe disk degeneration or instability, and hence, most of the patients undergoing these repairs are young, healthy patients. By avoiding fusion, it is hoped that these direct pars repairs may preserve mobility at the intervertebral level and ideally spare these patients from accelerated degeneration at adjacent levels.

19.3.2 Techniques

The first reports of attempted pars repair were published in the late 1960s with bone graft used without direct internal fixation.[5] Isolated bone grafts would be placed in the defect, and patients would be put on bedrest in casts postoperatively. Presently, the four traditional options for direct pars repair are (1) Buck repair,[31] (2) Morscher repair,[32] (3) Scott repair,[33] and (4) pedicle screw–based repair.

Buck Repair

The literature has demonstrated that the Buck repair is safe and reliable in carefully selected patients, with high incidence of bone healing. In surgery, the pars defects are exposed and decorticated with a combination of curettage and high-speed drill. The screw entry points are created in the caudal portion of each lamina, approximately 8 to 10 mm lateral to the bottom of the spinous process. To capture the broken pars fragment, the drill is then aimed across the defect angling 30 degrees away from midline toward the pedicle. Cannulated screws are then placed under direct visualization and confirmed with fluoroscopy.[31,34] A lag screw may be used to facilitate bony apposition, with placement of autograft or allograft across the defect to facilitate arthrodesis.

The pooled fusion rate with this technique was 84% in a literature review by Mohammed et al,[35] and it is suspected that accurate screw placement is the most critical factor necessary for fusion across the defect. Compared to pedicle screw placement techniques and conventional fusion procedures, the Buck repair involves less soft tissue/muscle dissection and blood loss. Still, the procedure is challenging and is contingent on the correct capture of the broken pars by correctly aimed screws. Nonunion can occur when the screws do not effectively cross the defects.[36]

Menga et al[37] performed a prospective analysis of 31 patients, 25 of whom were competitive athletes, who underwent repair via the Buck's technique. At mean follow-up of 60 months, pain significantly improved and three-quarters of the patients returned to competitive sports. Using three-dimensional imaging software, they determined the ideal screw placement trajectory to be the path that starts at the caudal edge of the lamina and bisects the pedicle, which provides the largest intracortical width and best bone purchase for fixation.[38] Snyder et al reviewed 16 adolescent patients with symptomatic spondylolysis treated via the Buck repair.[34] Over 90% of patients had complete symptom resolution, with an overall fusion rate of 97%. Importantly, there were eight athletes in the study, and all returned to play following surgical treatment.

Minimally invasive techniques and neuronavigation are being applied to the Buck repair. Higashino et al[39] incorporated the endoscope into the traditional Buck repair with successful subsequent bone healing. Brennan et al,[40] Widi et al,[41] and Nourbakhsh et al[42] all reported use of minimally invasive techniques for pars screw placement with intraoperative navigation. Jia et al[43] reported eight patients treated with minimally invasive approaches (tubular retractors and endoscope), as well as intraoperative O-arm and navigation (Medtronic, Minneapolis, MN). For each patient, a single midline incision was made with subsequent separate fascial incisions on both sides of the spinous process. Tubular retractors were placed on the pars, and using a microendoscopic system the pars was decorticated as in a standard open approach. The O-arm neuronavigation was used in the standard fashion to place screws through the pars defects via percutaneous stab incisions. The patients were kept on bedrest for 4 days postoperatively. The group, however, reported that their mean surgical time and blood loss were not decreased significantly compared to their open approaches, which they attributed to the small number of cases and steep learning curve.

Morscher Repair

In Morscher repairs, screws are inserted into the base of the superior articulating process and then attached to a laminar hook to achieve approximation of the pars defect. Mohammed et al found that this repair was associated with the highest complication rate and the lowest fusion rate, which the authors suspected was secondary to the small area for screw purchase in the base of the superior articular process.[35]

Scott Repair

The repair in a Scott procedure is performed by wrapping a wire around the spinous process and transverse processes in order to fixate across the defect(s) in the pars.[33] First proposed by James Scott of Edinburgh, Scotland, he believed this wiring was not as technically challenging as the Buck repair and that the elimination of screws provided more surface area for bone growth.[44] To perform this procedure, 2-mm holes are drilled at the bases of the transverse processes and a 4-mm hole at the base of the spinous process. Wire is then threaded through the holes in each transverse process and brought out cranially over the transverse process. It is then passed through the hole in the spinous process, effectively creating a figure-of-eight pattern.[44] Criticisms of the procedure are mainly in reference to its larger exposure and muscle dissection which result in greater blood loss, the complication profile with wire breakage/protrusion, and the potential for nerve root damage that can result when the wire crosses under the transverse process.

Pedicle Screw–Based Repair

The pedicle screw–based repairs were popularized in the 1990s by Songer and Rovin.[45] They highlighted that the pedicle screws must be placed in the pedicle superiorly enough to keep the screws out of the pars defect, followed by placement of a 1-mm double cable passed sublaminarly around the spinous process, securing a bone graft in place along the pars defect. Gillet and Petit describe a similar technique but with a V-shaped rod connecting the pedicle screws.[46] Raudenbush et al reported their series of pediatric patients with spondylolysis treated with pedicle screws and laminar hooks, and in their patients nearly 90% returned to preoperative competitive sports activity level.[47]

Noggle et al reported their experience with five pediatric patients undergoing a minimally invasive pedicle screw–based repair.[48] Bilateral pedicle screws and rod and hook constructs were placed via bilateral 2.5-cm skin incisions at L5 under fluoroscopy. Utilizing a minimal-access retractor system, the pars and superior and inferior facets were directly visualized. After identification of the pars defects, the defects were decorticated and pedicle screws were placed using Jamshidi needle wires. The laminar hooks were then placed at L5, and the constructs were compressed and tightened. All patients had evidence of fusion on CT scans obtained 6 months postoperatively.

Reported advantages of the pedicle screw technique are thought to be a larger surface area for bone healing compared to direct pars screws and a more rigid, durable construct than wire techniques.[49] In the experience of the authors, the pedicle screw and hook technique is typically used as a secondary technique if the primary Buck repair is not possible or does not provide adequate apposition.

Other Techniques

Patel et al[50] described the use of laminar screws (akin to those placed for fixation in C2) in a modified fashion for providing fixation across pars defects. Snowden and Sasso,[51] based on the biomechanical hypothesis that pedicle screw–laminar screw constructs would provide rigid fixation with substantial surface area for bone healing across the pars, reported on their use of these combined pedicle screw–lamina screw constructs using image guidance. Pedicle screws were placed in the standard fashion, followed by intralaminar screws. Lastly, if nonunion occurs or neither technique can provide adequate fixation and apposition, fusion may be performed using segmental fixation with bilateral pedicle screw fixation.

19.3.3 Outcomes

A biomechanical study published in 1999[52] compared the Buck, Scott, modified Scott, and pedicle screw–rod–hook fixation in calf cadaveric lumbar spines. The least motion was achieved with the Buck's repair and pedicle screw–rod–hook repair.

In 2003, Mihara et al investigated the biomechanical effects of spondylolysis on adjacent levels of the spine and biomechanical changes from its treatment.[53] Results demonstrated that pars defects at a single level increased the mobility at the vertebral levels above and below the defect. The mobility was stabilized by Buck's repair but increased by the pedicle screw rod fixation technique. The authors suggest that direct pars fixation causes less adjacent level mechanical stress and is therefore preferable.

Mohammed et al conducted systematic review of 46 studies involving 900 patients who underwent direct pars repair.[35] Fusion rates were highest for pedicle screw–based repairs (90%), followed by the Buck repair (83%). The review highlighted complications that appeared to be common with each type of procedure. For example, wire breakage was the most common complication in the Scott repair, along with wire protrusion and transverse process fractures. Nerve root irritation was observed more frequently in the Buck repair. The best functional outcomes were found to be with the Buck repair, with the minimally invasive Buck repair having a better favorable outcome rate than the open Buck repair.

19.3.4 Case Presentation

A 16-year-old female presented with many years of low back pain which she characterized as "stabbing" with associated hip and leg muscle tightness (**Video 19.1**). She had been told by her pediatrician that her symptoms were related to growing pains. On physical examination, she had reproducible pain with extension. Anteroposterior (AP)/lateral X-rays of the lumbosacral spine demonstrated bilateral spondylolysis at L5–S1 with an otherwise healthy disk space and little to no anterolisthesis (▶ Fig. 19.1 and ▶ Fig. 19.2). She was trialed with an lumbosacral orthosis (LSO) brace but the symptoms persisted. She subsequently underwent epidural steroid injections at the location of the pars defects, which was both diagnostic and therapeutic. Direct pars repair via the Buck procedure was recommended.

The patient was brought to the operating room and intubated under general anesthesia. She was positioned prone on the Jackson table. Fluoroscopy was used to plan a midline incision that would allow for exposure of the pars at L5–S1. The soft tissues were dissected from the spinous processes, lamina, and pars to allow visualization of the defects. The defects were decorticated using a combination of curettes and high-speed drilling.

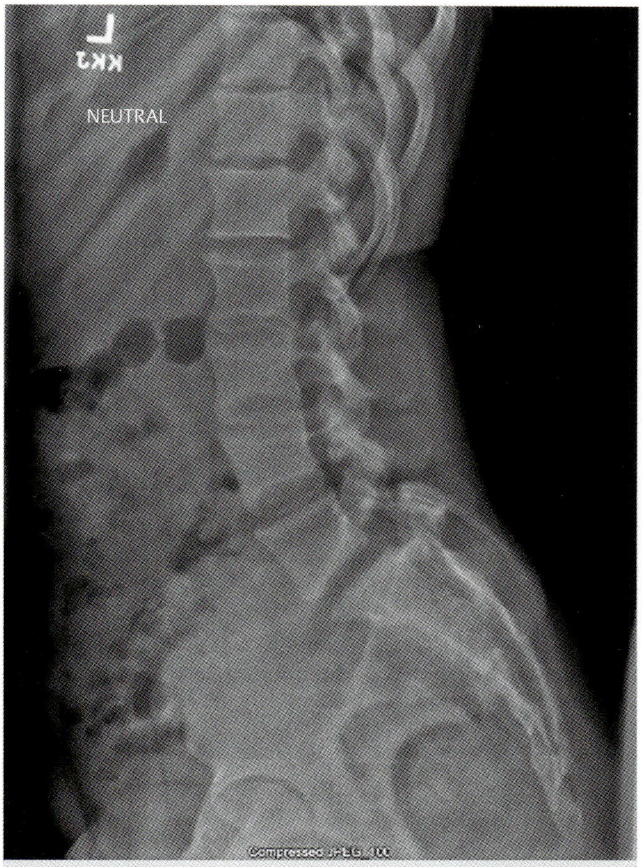

Fig. 19.1 Preoperative lateral X-ray demonstrating pars defect with minimal anterolisthesis at L5–S1 and healthy disk space.

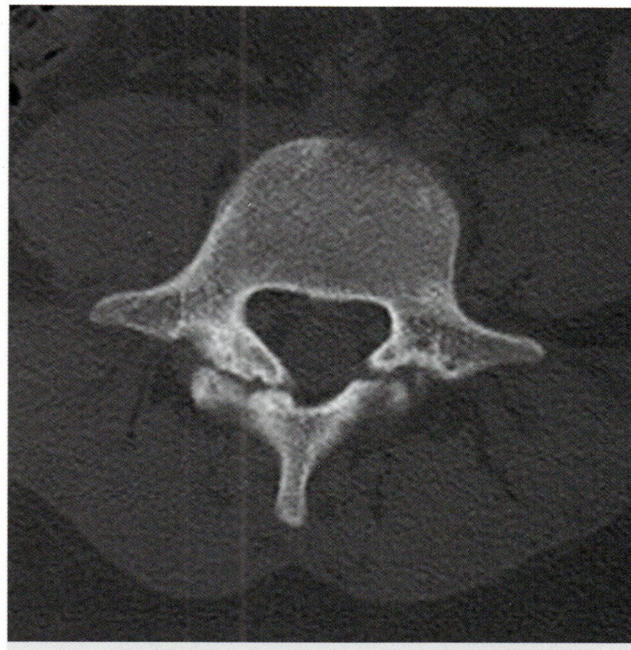

Fig. 19.2 Axial computed tomography (CT) demonstrating bilateral pars defects.

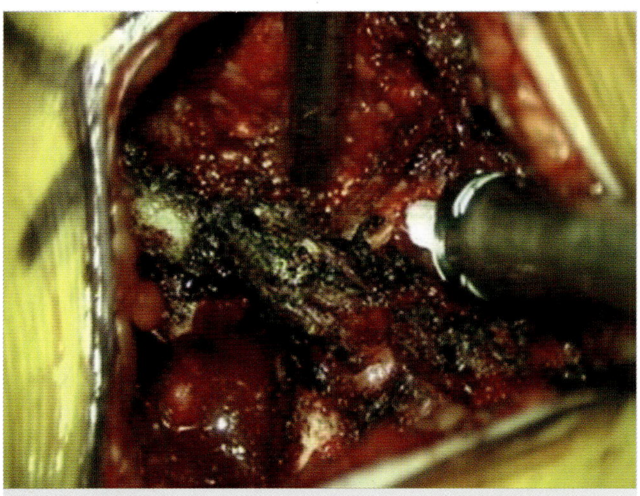

Fig. 19.3 Intraoperative placement of pars screws under direct visualization.

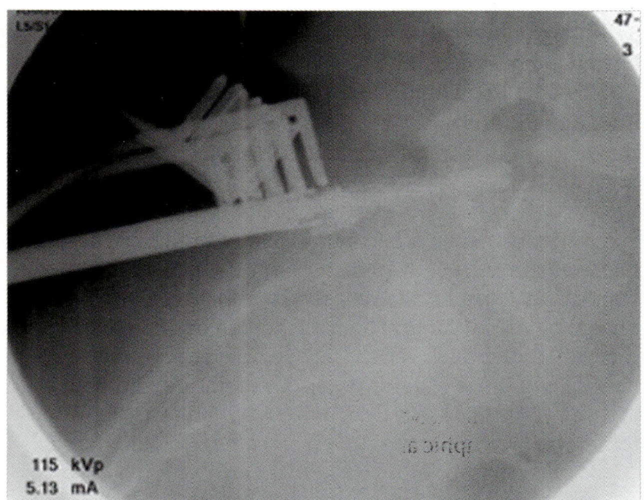

Fig. 19.4 Intraoperative fluoroscopic confirmation of pars screw placement.

Screw entry points were created in the caudal portion of each lamina as described previously and K-wires were inserted across the defects, followed by cannulated screws under direct visualization and lateral fluoroscopy to confirm capture of the fractured pars fragments (▶ Fig. 19.3 and ▶ Fig. 19.4). Autograft, allograft, and bone morphogenetic protein (BMP) were packed within the defect, and standard closure was performed. Estimated blood loss was 30 mL. The patient remained in the hospital for 2 days. She was kept in a custom TLSO. At 2-week follow-up, she had complete resolution of her low back pain and minimal incisional pain (▶ Fig. 19.5).

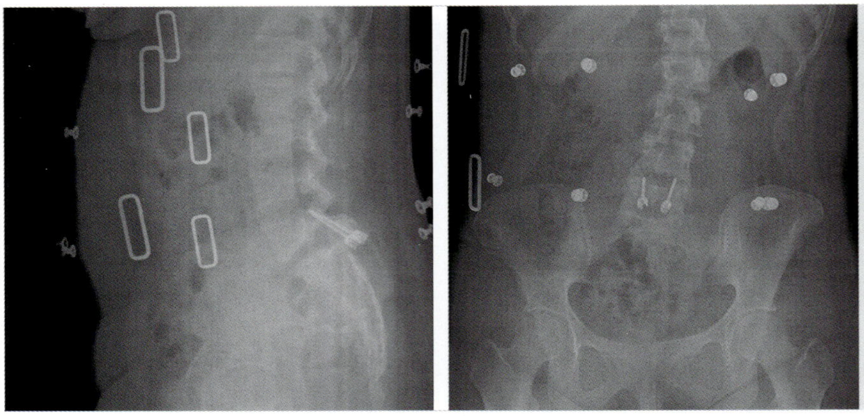

Fig. 19.5 Postoperative anteroposterior (AP)/lateral X-rays demonstrating bilateral pars screws at L5–S1.

19.4 Clinical Pearls

- Spondylolysis affects a high percentage of young athletes, and symptomatic patients who fail conservative therapy can be treated with direct pars repair, which restores local anatomy while preserving normal motion at the involved level.
- There are four traditional options for direct pars repair – (1) Buck repair, (2) Morscher repair, (3) Scott repair, and (4) pedicle screw–based repair. The Buck repair and pedicle screw–based repairs have shown the best outcomes in the literature.
- The Buck repair involves decorticating the pars defects, creating screw entry points in the caudal portion of each lamina, and aiming the drill across the defect angling 30 degrees away from the midline toward the pedicle to capture the broken pars fragment.

19.5 Summary

Spine surgeons should be comfortable with the diagnosis and management of spondylolysis in both the pediatric and adult populations. If patients fail conservative management, there are several successful surgical options that can be offered for symptom relief. The Buck repair and pedicle screw–based repairs have shown the best outcomes in the literature, and both open and minimally invasive techniques have proven successful in terms of radiographic and clinical outcomes.

References

[1] Beutler WJ, Fredrickson BE, Murtland A, Sweeney CA, Grant WD, Baker D. The natural history of spondylolysis and spondylolisthesis: 45-year follow-up evaluation. Spine. 2003; 28(10):1027–1035, discussion 1035

[2] Hardcastle P, Annear P, Foster DH, et al. Spinal abnormalities in young fast bowlers. J Bone Joint Surg Br. 1992; 74(3):421–425

[3] Cassidy RC, Shaffer WO, Johnson DL. Spondylolysis and spondylolisthesis in the athlete. Orthopedics. 2005; 28(11):1331–1333

[4] Lawrence KJ, Elser T, Stromberg R. Lumbar spondylolysis in the adolescent athlete. Phys Ther Sport. 2016; 20:56–60

[5] Kimura M. [My method of filing the lesion with spongy bone in spondylolysis and spondylolistesis] [Article in Japanese]. Seikei Geka. 1968; 19(4):285–296

[6] Micheli LJ, Wood R. Back pain in young athletes. Significant differences from adults in causes and patterns. Arch Pediatr Adolesc Med. 1995; 149(1):15–18

[7] McCleary MD, Congeni JA. Current concepts in the diagnosis and treatment of spondylolysis in young athletes. Curr Sports Med Rep. 2007; 6(1):62–66

[8] Alqarni AM, Schneiders AG, Cook CE, Hendrick PA. Clinical tests to diagnose lumbar spondylolysis and spondylolisthesis: a systematic review. Phys Ther Sport. 2015; 16(3):268–275

[9] Masci L, Pike J, Malara F, Phillips B, Bennell K, Brukner P. Use of the one-legged hyperextension test and magnetic resonance imaging in the diagnosis of active spondylolysis. Br J Sports Med. 2006; 40(11):940–946, discussion 946

[10] Gregg CD, Dean S, Schneiders AG. Variables associated with active spondylolysis. Phys Ther Sport. 2009; 10(4):121–124

[11] Sundell CG, Jonsson H, Ådin L, Larsén KH. Clinical examination, spondylolysis and adolescent athletes. Int J Sports Med. 2013; 34(3):263–267

[12] Ledonio CG, Burton DC, Crawford CH, III, et al. Current evidence regarding diagnostic imaging methods for pediatric lumbar spondylolysis: a report from the Scoliosis Research Society Evidence-Based Medicine Committee. Spine Deform. 2017; 5(2):97–101

[13] Amato M, Totty WG, Gilula LA. Spondylolysis of the lumbar spine: demonstration of defects and laminal fragmentation. Radiology. 1984; 153 (3):627–629

[14] Beck NA, Miller R, Baldwin K, et al. Do oblique views add value in the diagnosis of spondylolysis in adolescents? J Bone Joint Surg Am. 2013; 95 (10):e65

[15] Delavan JA, Stence NV, Mirsky DM, Gralla J, Fadell MF. Confidence in assessment of lumbar spondylolysis using three-dimensional volumetric T2-weighted MRI compared with limited field of view, decreased-dose CT. Sports Health. 2016; 8(4):364–371

[16] Ganiyusufoglu AK, Onat L, Karatoprak O, Enercan M, Hamzaoglu A. Diagnostic accuracy of magnetic resonance imaging versus computed tomography in stress fractures of the lumbar spine. Clin Radiol. 2010; 65(11):902–907

[17] Raby N, Mathews S. Symptomatic spondylolysis: correlation of CT and SPECT with clinical outcome. Clin Radiol. 1993; 48(2):97–99

[18] Gregory PL, Batt ME, Kerslake RW, Webb JK. Single photon emission computerized tomography and reverse gantry computerized tomography findings in patients with back pain investigated for spondylolysis. Clin J Sport Med. 2005; 15(2):79–86

[19] Trout AT, Sharp SE, Anton CG, Gelfand MJ, Mehlman CT. Spondylolysis and beyond: value of SPECT/CT in evaluation of low back pain in children and young adults. Radiographics. 2015; 35(3):819–834

[20] Button JH, Petron DJ. Pedicle stress reaction in a teenage baseball pitcher. Am J Phys Med Rehabil. 2007; 86(11):956

[21] Hollenberg GM, Beattie PF, Meyers SP, Weinberg EP, Adams MJ. Stress reactions of the lumbar pars interarticularis: the development of a new MRI classification system. Spine. 2002; 27(2):181–186

[22] Logroscino G, Mazza O, Aulisa G, Pitta L, Pola E, Aulisa L. Spondylolysis and spondylolisthesis in the pediatric and adolescent population. Childs Nerv Syst. 2001; 17(11):644–655

[23] Berger RG, Doyle SM. Spondylolysis 2019 update. Curr Opin Pediatr. 2019; 31(1):61–68

[24] Sairyo K, Sakai T, Yasui N. Conservative treatment of lumbar spondylolysis in childhood and adolescence: the radiological signs which predict healing. J Bone Joint Surg Br. 2009; 91(2):206–209

[25] El Rassi G, Takemitsu M, Woratanarat P, Shah SA. Lumbar spondylolysis in pediatric and adolescent soccer players. Am J Sports Med. 2005; 33(11): 1688–1693

[26] Standaert CJ, Herring SA. Expert opinion and controversies in sports and musculoskeletal medicine: the diagnosis and treatment of spondylolysis in adolescent athletes. Arch Phys Med Rehabil. 2007; 88(4):537–540

[27] El Rassi G, Takemitsu M, Glutting J, Shah SA. Effect of sports modification on clinical outcome in children and adolescent athletes with symptomatic lumbar spondylolysis. Am J Phys Med Rehabil. 2013; 92(12):1070–1074

[28] Sairyo K, Sakai T, Yasui N, Dezawa A. Conservative treatment for pediatric lumbar spondylolysis to achieve bone healing using a hard brace: what type and how long?: Clinical article. J Neurosurg Spine. 2012; 16(6):610–614

[29] Fujii K, Katoh S, Sairyo K, Ikata T, Yasui N. Union of defects in the pars interarticularis of the lumbar spine in children and adolescents. The radiological outcome after conservative treatment. J Bone Joint Surg Br. 2004; 86(2):225–231

[30] O'Sullivan PB, Phyty GD, Twomey LT, Allison GT. Evaluation of specific stabilizing exercise in the treatment of chronic low back pain with radiologic diagnosis of spondylolysis or spondylolisthesis. Spine. 1997; 22 (24):2959–2967

[31] Buck JE. Direct repair of the defect in spondylolisthesis. Preliminary report. J Bone Joint Surg Br. 1970; 52(3):432–437

[32] Morscher E, Gerber B, Fasel J. Surgical treatment of spondylolisthesis by bone grafting and direct stabilization of spondylolysis by means of a hook screw. Arch Orthop Trauma Surg. 1984; 103(3):175–178

[33] Nicol RO, Scott JH. Lytic spondylolysis. Repair by wiring. Spine. 1986; 11(10): 1027–1030

[34] Snyder LA, Shufflebarger H, O'Brien MF, Thind H, Theodore N, Kakarla UK. Spondylolysis outcomes in adolescents after direct screw repair of the pars interarticularis. J Neurosurg Spine. 2014; 21(3):329–333

[35] Mohammed N, Patra DP, Narayan V, et al. A comparison of the techniques of direct pars interarticularis repairs for spondylolysis and low-grade spondylolisthesis: a meta-analysis. Neurosurg Focus. 2018; 44(1):E10

[36] Songer M. Repair of the pars interarticularis defect with a cable-screw construct. Spine. 1998; 23(2):284

[37] Menga EN, Kebaish KM, Jain A, Carrino JA, Sponseller PD. Clinical results and functional outcomes after direct intralaminar screw repair of spondylolysis. Spine. 2014; 39(1):104–110

[38] Menga EN, Jain A, Kebaish KM, Zimmerman SL, Sponseller PD. Anatomic parameters: direct intralaminar screw repair of spondylolysis. Spine. 2014; 39(3):E153–E158

[39] Higashino K, Sairyo K, Katoh S, Sakai T, Kosaka H, Yasui N. Minimally invasive technique for direct repair of the pars defects in young adults using a spinal endoscope: a technical note. Minim Invasive Neurosurg. 2007; 50(3):182–186

[40] Brennan RP, Smucker PY, Horn EM. Minimally invasive image-guided direct repair of bilateral L-5 pars interarticularis defects. Neurosurg Focus. 2008; 25(2):E13

[41] Widi GA, Williams SK, Levi AD. Minimally invasive direct repair of bilateral lumbar spine pars defects in athletes. Case Rep Med. 2013; 2013:659078

[42] Nourbakhsh A, Preuss F, Hadeed M, Shimer A. Percutaneous direct repair of a pars defect using intraoperative computed tomography scan: a modification of the Buck technique. Spine. 2017; 42(11):E691–E694

[43] Jia M, Wang J, Zhang Z, Zheng W, Zhou Y. Direct repair of lumbar pars interarticularis defects by utilizing intraoperative O-arm-based navigation and microendoscopic techniques. Spine. 2016; 41 Suppl 19:B6–B13

[44] Biswas D, Grauer J, Whang P. Direct repair of the pars interarticularis in the child and adolescent. Tech Orthop. 2009; 24(3):190–195

[45] Songer MN, Rovin R. Repair of the pars interarticularis defect with a cable-screw construct. A preliminary report. Spine. 1998; 23(2):263–269

[46] Gillet P, Petit M. Direct repair of spondylolysis without spondylolisthesis, using a rod-screw construct and bone grafting of the pars defect. Spine. 1999; 24(12):1252–1256

[47] Raudenbush BL, Chambers RC, Silverstein MP, Goodwin RC. Indirect pars repair for pediatric isthmic spondylolysis: a case series. J Spine Surg. 2017; 3(3):387–391

[48] Noggle JC, Sciubba DM, Samdani AF, Anderson DG, Betz RR, Asghar J. Minimally invasive direct repair of lumbar spondylolysis with a pedicle screw and hook construct. Neurosurg Focus. 2008; 25(2):E15

[49] Cheung EV, Herman MJ, Cavalier R, Pizzutillo PD. Spondylolysis and spondylolisthesis in children and adolescents: II. Surgical management. J Am Acad Orthop Surg. 2006; 14(8):488–498

[50] Patel RD, Rosas HG, Steinmetz MP, Anderson PA. Repair of pars interarticularis defect utilizing a pedicle and laminar screw construct: a new technique based on anatomical and biomechanical analysis. J Neurosurg Spine. 2012; 17(1):61–68

[51] Snowden R, Sasso R. Repair of pars interarticularis defect utilizing a pedicle and laminar screw construct: a technique discussion and case series. Tech Orthop. 2021; 36(1):40–44

[52] Deguchi M, Rapoff AJ, Zdeblick TA. Biomechanical comparison of spondylolysis fixation techniques. Spine. 1999; 24(4):328–333

[53] Mihara H, Onari K, Cheng BC, David SM, Zdeblick TA. The biomechanical effects of spondylolysis and its treatment. Spine. 2003; 28(3):235–238

20 Return to Play after Spinal Injury

Melanie Alfonzo Horowitz, Carly Weber-Levine, Andrew M. Hersh, and Nicholas Theodore

Summary

Although athletic events are a common cause for spinal cord injuries (SCIs), there remain unclear guidelines and no consensus on whether athletes can return to play (RTP) after their SCI. This is due to a myriad of reasons, including the low frequency of these incidents, inability to conduct randomized control trials, and discourse among stakeholders, besides the physician and patient. The current gold standard for RTP guidelines was developed by Torg et al and modified by Vaccaro et al. However, these do not apply to all SCIs, leaving many to physician interpretation. Factors to keep in mind while deciding RTP pertain to the type and location of injury, neurological examination findings, imaging results, symptom number and severity, treatment type, and risk of re-injury in the sport. The latest literature focused on RTP based on the segment of spine that was injured, injury type, and surgical operation. Here, we discuss current knowledge and factors to keep in mind when assessing patients with SCI for RTP potential.

Keywords: return to play, spinal cord injury, sports, spine surgery, return to sports

20.1 Introduction

Athletic events are the third most common cause of spinal cord injuries (SCIs), accounting for almost 9% of the annual 125,000 new SCI cases in America.[1] This SCI statistic represents a fraction of all the possible spinal injuries that can occur from sports. The most common sports that lead to spinal injuries are ones that involve contact between players, such as football, hockey, and rugby, and others where athletes have severe falls, such as skiing or equestrian. Spinal injuries sustained from playing sports can range from minor asymptomatic strains to catastrophic SCIs that result in permanent quadriplegia. Regardless of severity, these injuries can have a long-lasting impact on the athlete's health, quality of life, and participation in the professional sport. Although there has been significant debate, there remains a lack of consensus on when, or whether, an injured athlete can return to play (RTP) following a spinal injury.

Currently, there are no universal standardized RTP protocols for athletes following injury to the spine. Decisions regarding RTP are complicated by the amalgamation of social pressures for the athlete's timely return, limited data, and vast amount of medically relevant variables. Current literature and protocols are highly subjective and difficult to employ clinically on a broad scale. Additionally, these protocols are unable to be validated prospectively due to the relatively uncommon nature of spinal injuries. RTP protocols, nonetheless, are important for ensuring athlete's safety, continuation in the sport, and avoiding re-injury. Here, we discuss current RTP guidelines for athletes who sustain spinal injuries.

20.2 Lack of Consensus

There are many factors that contribute to the lack of consensus on RTP following spinal injury.[2] One factor is a provider's experience, such as prior participation as an athlete, years of board certification, or previous clinical work with athletes. If a provider used to participate in higher level athletics, he or she is more likely to allow RTP for sports with maximal impact, as opposed to providers who lacked athletic participation.[3] Another reason for the lack of consensus is the severe, unpredictable, and heterogeneous nature of these injuries, precluding a randomized controlled trial to evaluate optimal RTP time following spinal injury. Most current data come from case reports, literature reviews, and professional opinions. Therefore, there is limited reliable data for athletes, medical providers, and stakeholders in sports to utilize as a guide for making these important decisions. There is also a broad range of injury types (herniated disks, stenosis, fractures, etc.), making it difficult for providers to rely on previously reported cases for insight into RTP decisions.

The current gold standard in RTP guidelines was developed by Torg et al.[4] They divided risk based on stratification of contraindication to RTP: none, relative, and absolute. These guidelines were based on data from 1,200 spinal injury cases provided by the National Football Head and Neck Injury Registry, literature available at the time, an understanding of spinal biomechanics, and Torg's professional experience as a practicing orthopedic surgeon. Expanding on Torg's work, Vaccaro et al provided one of the most comprehensive set of current guidelines with updated criteria to Torg's contraindication classification groupings (▶ Table 20.1).[5]

Although there are standardized RTP protocols for other injuries, such as anterior cruciate ligament (ACL) tear or concussion, there is disagreement surrounding RTP following SCI. This discourse is not just among stakeholders in sports, such as coaches or team managers, but also medical providers as well. In a survey sent out to board-certified spine surgeons, there was a clear lack of agreement among the 62 respondents.[3] For this survey, surgeons were presented with 15 clinical case scenarios of athletes who had sustained various spinal injuries and asked to provide the type of activity (maximal impact, moderate impact, minimal impact, or no sports) and appropriate level of play competitiveness (professional, collegiate, high school, recreational, or none) they would recommend for the injured athlete in the case scenario. Out of the 15 cases 8 had no response option chosen by most respondents. Although the survey was sent to all surgeon members of the Cervical Spine Research Society (CSRS) and the International Society for the Advancement of Spine Surgery (ISASS), only 11% of respondents indicated that their practice had one-third or more of cases being sport-injury related, highlighting the infrequent nature of these injuries and lack of experience to rely upon. Interestingly, these results also revealed limited adherence to the guidelines set forth by Torg et al.[4] Even among professionals with ample experience in treating spinal injuries, there is a lack of consensus in RTP guidelines.

20.3 Considerations for RTP Guidelines

Creating optimal guidelines for RTP following spinal injuries requires the consideration of many different variables, including symptoms, neurological examination findings, and imaging results (▶ Fig. 20.1). Initially, the main factors to consider are the location (cervical, thoracic, or lumbar region) and type of injury to the spine. The presence, severity, time frame, and number of symptomatic episodes within a specified time frame should then be evaluated in the context of the injury. Symptoms can be motor or sensory disturbances, including weakness, paresthesia, dysesthesia, or numbness. Minor symptoms, such as burning or numbness, that last a short duration of time, i.e., a few minutes following injury, usually do not pose contraindications for RTP. Following injury, a neurological examination should be done. Abnormal findings, such as neurological deficits or decreased range of motion at the spinal injury level, would serve as a contraindication for RTP and should be followed up with imaging, preferably magnetic resonance imaging (MRI). In general, athletes should not return to the sport until injury symptoms have resolved.

The chance of injury recurrence is another important factor to keep in mind for RTP decisions. To estimate this, one can take into account the severity of the injury, the age of the individual, the treatment the athlete received, and the risk of the sport. If the sport involves a high chance of substantial axial loading, such as in football or rugby, there is an increased risk of re-injury. A study also found that the use of instrumentation in

Table 20.1 Categorization of different RTP contraindication levels based on Torg and Vaccaro guidelines[4,5]

No contraindication	Relative contraindication	Absolute contraindication
Healed, stable C1 or C2 fracture (treated nonoperatively) with a normal cervical range of motion Torg ratio less than 0.8 in an asymptomatic individual Healed, stable subaxial spine fracture with no sagittal plane kyphotic deformity Cervical fusion that has healed after anterior single level injury Post posterior cervical microlaminoforaminotomy	Previous history of transient quadriplegia or quadriparesthesia A healed, stable two-level anterior or posterior subaxial cervical fusion with or without instrumentation	Presence of cervical spinal cord abnormality noted on MRI More than two previous episodes of transient quadriplegia or quadriparesis Symptomatic disk herniation Three-level cervical spine fusion

Abbreviations: MRI, magnetic resonance imaging; RTP, return to play.

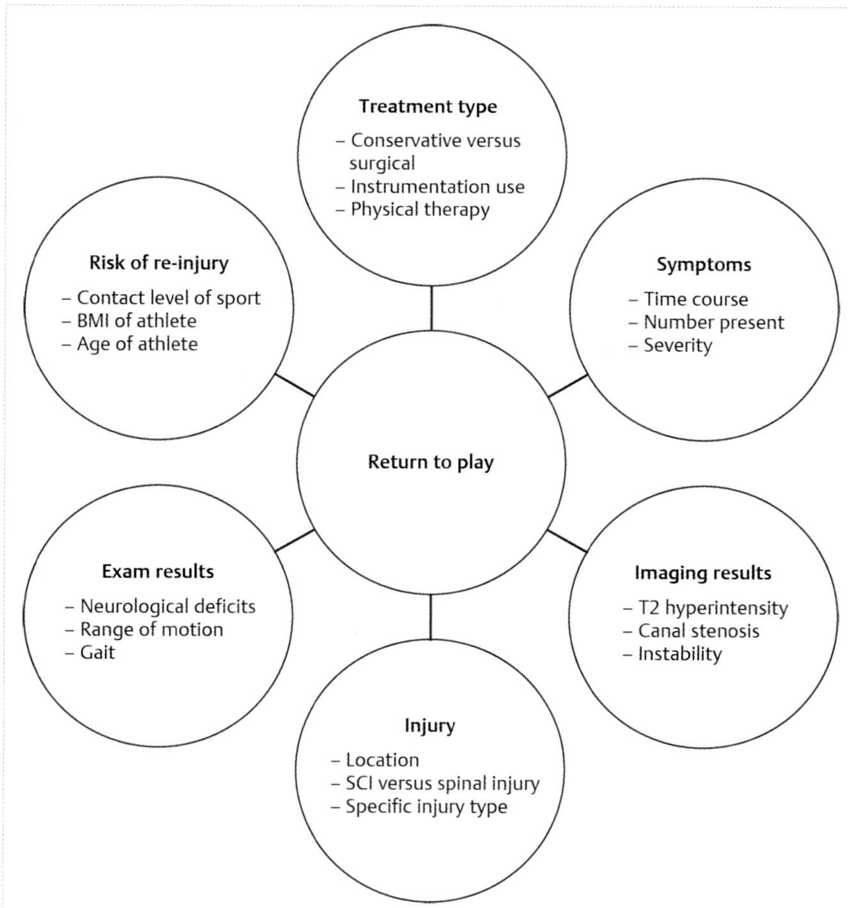

Fig. 20.1 Important factors to consider when determining if and when an athlete should return to play following a spinal injury. BMI, body mass index; SCI, spinal cord injury.

spinal fixation or fusion surgery was highly correlated with faster RTP times when compared to noninstrumented cases that did not involve bone fusion.[6] Therefore, the surgical intervention that the athlete received should be considered when taking RTP decisions.

Additionally, T2-weighted MRI scans should be obtained to evaluate any hyperintensity signal changes in the spinal cord. These changes can reveal anatomic instability in these regions, local edema, or inflammation, which all contribute to an increased risk of future injury.[7] An instability exists when there is greater than 3.5-mm horizontal or 11-degree angular displacement among vertebrae.[8] Another agreed-upon critical factor in RTP decision-making for cervical injuries is the presence of cervical spinal canal stenosis in athletes and its relationship with T2-weighted sequence MRI results.[9] Spinal stenosis is defined as the average spine sagittal diameter being less than 10 mm, with relative stenosis being 13 mm. If a T2-weighted MRI reveals no signal hyperintensity changes and the spinal canal diameter is greater than 10 mm, then RTP is warranted. However, if changes are present on the T2 MRI, then a diameter greater than 13 mm is required for RTP. If the diameter is less than 10 mm, then RTP is contraindicated.

Overall, factors that are favorable to RTP include resolution of symptoms, normal neurologic examination, no evidence of spinal instability on dynamic imaging, absence of T2-weighted MRI hyperintensity signal, full and painless range of motion of the spine, and lack of overall pain. More specific RTP considerations based on the specific injury can be found in the following sections.

20.4 Spine Injury Biomechanics

Axial loading, defined as a force directed through the top of the head and the spine, is one of the main mechanisms leading to cervical spine injury.[10] This is relatively common in impact sports, such as football, gymnastics, and diving, and typically affects the cervical spine. Axial loading occurs when a substantial impact on the top of the head creates a force that is vertically transmitted into the cervical spine. This energy is unable to be dissipated, resulting in disk compression until maximum deformation of the spine is reached. At this point, the athlete may experience fracture, subluxation, or dislocation of the spinal vertebra.

Unlike the cervical spine, the thoracic spine is unlikely to become injured following the impact. This region is relatively immobile compared to its counterparts and is protected by the ribcage.[11] Stenosis is also unlikely to occur in this region due to a large spinal cord to spinal canal diameter ratio. Within the lumbar spine, repetitive axial loading can cause defects in the pars interarticularis, the laminal portion that connects the superior and inferior facets, leading to spondylolysis.[12] There can also be anterior translocation of the facets, causing spondylolisthesis, or herniation, which can lead to lower back pain due to the disk itself or compression of neighboring nerve roots. Therefore, spinal injuries within the cervical and lumbar regions will be the focus of the discussion.

20.5 Cervical Spinal Cord

New algorithms are currently being developed to aid in RTP decision-making following injury to the cervical spine. Bailes et al examined 62 patients with cervical SCI who were treated at the Northwestern University Midwest Regional Spinal Cord Unit.[13] Similar to the Torg's RTP guidelines, the cases were divided into three categories: permanent SCI (type I), transient SCI (type II), and pure radiological abnormality lacking motor or sensory findings (type III). Based on the categorization of SCI, Bailes et al devised an algorithm for whether the patient should return to play or not (▶ Fig. 20.2). Overall, players are advised not to return if they suffer a permanent neurological injury, multiple transient injuries, unstable fracture, or ligamentous instability.

20.5.1 Cervical Disk Herniation

A disk herniation occurs when the nucleus pulposus, the inner part of the disk, protrudes through the annulus fibrosis, the outer portion, potentially compressing nearby nerves or the spinal cord. The levels affected most commonly in the cervical region are C5–C6 and C6–C7. These injuries typically occur in

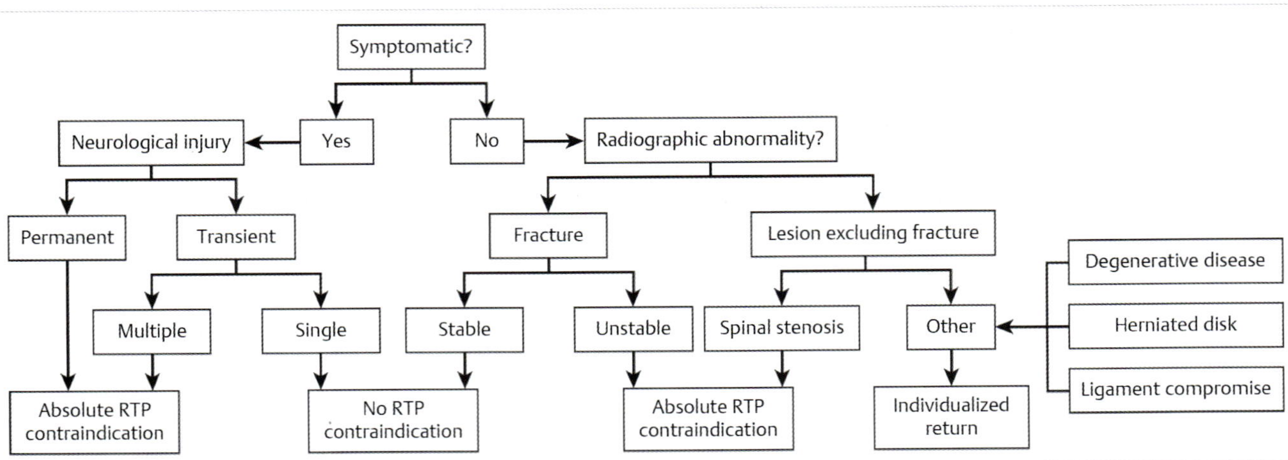

Fig. 20.2 Algorithm devised by Bailes et al for cervical spine return to play (RTP) decisions.[13]

high-contact sports where the cervical spine of the athlete is exposed to repeated stress upon impact, degenerating the shock-absorbent disk, and increasing the likelihood of rupture. Symptoms of a cervical disk herniation include sharp or burning pain, numbness and tingling, or weakness in the upper extremities. Initially, treatment should be conservative and nonsurgical, including noninflammatory pain medications, sports massage, rest, and physical therapy with stretching exercises. Surgery should be considered if the herniation is associated with myelopathy or progressive neurological deficits.[14] In asymptomatic cervical disk herniations, there is no RTP contraindication. However, a symptomatic herniation, potentially leading to spinal stenosis and severe nerve root damage, is an RTP contraindication.[15]

20.5.2 Cervical Cord Neurapraxia

Cervical cord neurapraxia (CCN) is a transient neurological deficit caused by cervical cord trauma that compresses the spinal cord causing a temporary aberration of normal function. It most frequently occurs in football during a tackle, resulting from cervical cord hyperextension.[16] Symptoms can be experienced from 15 minutes to 48 hours and include sensory changes such as burning, numbness, or tingling, and motor changes that range from weakness to paralysis.[16] Treatment is usually supportive care, although surgery can be recommended on an individualized basis based on focal lesions and spine instability found on MRI.[16] If an athlete experiences a single episode of neurapraxia symptoms that lasts less than 24 hours with full resolution of symptoms, there are no RTP contraindications.[17] However, if the symptoms are accompanied by neck discomfort, reduced range of motion, abnormal neurological examination findings, or loss of cerebrospinal fluid (CSF) around the spinal cord, RTP is contraindicated. Likewise, RTP is not advised if athletes suffer multiple episodes or episodes that last longer than 36 hours.[17]

20.6 Lumbar Spine Injuries

20.6.1 Lumbar Disk Herniation

A herniated lumbar disk occurs in athletes who repetitively load their spine and follow with a rotational or bending movement, such as a rebound in basketball. This occurs most often between L4–L5 and L5–S1.[12] A herniated lumbar disk often presents with lower back pain, numbness, and weakness in the lower extremities. Upon injury, athletes should undergo a neurological examination to locate the herniation level with subsequent evaluation of stance and gait and MRI to visualize possible disk degermation.[12] Most athletes respond well to conservative treatment such as rest, nonsteroidal anti-inflammatory drugs (NSAIDs), extension and isometric exercises, and lumbar epidural steroid injections. The extent of injury and chance of recurrence should be considered when determining RTP, including athlete's body mass index (BMI) and sport mechanisms, including tackling or repeated lumbar flexion/hyperextension movements that are common in sports such as football, ice hockey, basketball, and soccer. If conservative management is unsuccessful, surgical management, such as a percutaneous diskectomy, should be consulted and RTP will generally be allowed after 3 months. If multiple recurrences occur, a spinal fusion is recommended for stability, although these athletes are generally not allowed RTP to collegiate or professional level sports.[12]

20.6.2 Spondylolisthesis

Spondylolisthesis occurs when one vertebra is translated anteriorly, most commonly at the lower lumbar region. It occurs in athletes who undergo repetitive lumbar loading, described as excessive extension and rotation, such as in gymnastics, baseball, and football. It can present asymptomatically or with low back pain that often radiates to the buttocks. MRI should be obtained when spondylolisthesis is suspected. Treatment is usually managed conservatively with rest, physical therapy, and NSAIDs. RTP is decided based on the player's symptoms and treatment course. Following successful conservative management, RTP can be granted if full range of spinal motion is obtained, along with the resolution of pain and neurological symptoms. The usual time course is 2 months. Overall, return to full activities in less than 2 months is typically seen in athletes.[12]

20.7 Surgical Considerations

20.7.1 Anterior Cervical Diskectomy and Fusion

Anterior cervical diskectomy and fusion (ACDF) is a surgery to remove a herniated or degenerative disk. A case series was conducted to analyze the postoperative RTP results of 15 professional athletes who underwent ACDF by a single surgeon on various levels of the cervical spine.[18] It was shown that National Football League (NFL) players who had cervical disk herniation and received operative treatment had higher RTP rates and longer careers than those who did not receive operative treatment.[18] Results revealed that RTP for contact sports after a single-level ACDF was allowed if there were no associated neurological deficits or symptoms, and full range of motion was exhibited. If there is risk for an adjacent disk herniation, such as signs of spinal instability, deformity, or nerve root compression, then RTP is contraindicated. An ACDF of three or more levels also serves as a contraindication due to insufficient data on long-term postoperative outcomes.[4]

20.7.2 Percutaneous Nucleotomy

A percutaneous nucleotomy (PN) is conducted to treat disk herniation and consists of removing the nucleus pulposus to reduce disk volume. A study evaluating the postoperative outcomes following different RTP timelines for elite athletes who had undergone PNs for lumbar disk herniation found that there was a significant increase in recurrence of lower back pain and sense of fatigue in athletes who returned to play within 3 months.[19] Also, when matched with nonathletes, athletes experienced worse postoperative complications, most likely due to early resumption of sports participation. Lastly, a greater extent of PN resection was associated with worse athletic outcomes due to the occurrence of lower back pain. Therefore, following a

PN procedure, a longer waiting period of at least 3 months and a less invasive procedure lead to more successful RTP.

20.7.3 Lumbar Diskectomy

A lumbar diskectomy is a surgery to remove a herniated or degenerative disk. After a lumbar diskectomy, it is regarded as the norm for professional athletes to return to their sport, but there is limited information on the timing. After an analysis of 85 athlete patients who suffered a herniated disk and underwent a lumbar diskectomy, researchers found an 89% rate for RTP, with an average RTP time of 5.8 months.[20] The number of patients who successfully returned to sport steadily increased from 50% at 3 months to 72% at 6 months to 77% at 9 months to 84% at 12 months. Importantly, there was no significant change in performance noted between pre- and postoperatively. Therefore, these procedures are relatively safe for professional athletes and lead to good RTP outcomes.

20.8 Clinical Pearls

- RTP guidelines are essential for ensuring a safe return to sport for athletes following a spinal injury.
- There is a lack of consensus regarding RTP protocols following spinal injury.
- RTP considerations should be dependent on location and type of injury, individual case characteristics, and level of contact in the sport.
- Factors that should be considered when determining RTP include symptoms, time course, neurological deficits, range of motion, and imaging.
- The treatment modality the athlete received (conservative vs. operative) should be considered when deciding RTP.

20.9 Disclosures

Melanie Alfonzo Horowitz: None.
Carly Weber-Levine: None.
Andrew M. Hersh: None.
Nicholas Theodore: Royalties from Globus Medical. Stock Ownership in Globus Medical. Consultant for Globus Medical. On Scientific Advisory Board/Other Office for Globus Medical.

References

[1] Huang P, Anissipour A, McGee W, Lemak L. Return-to-play recommendations after cervical, thoracic, and lumbar spine injuries: a comprehensive review. Sports Health. 2016; 8(1):19–25

[2] Morganti C, Sweeney CA, Albanese SA, Burak C, Hosea T, Connolly PJ. Return to play after cervical spine injury. Spine. 2001; 26(10):1131–1136

[3] Ukogu C, Bienstock D, Ferrer C, et al. Physician decision-making in return to play after cervical spine injury: a descriptive analysis of survey data. Clin Spine Surg. 2020; 33(7):E330–E336

[4] Torg JS, Ramsey-Emrhein JA. Cervical spine and brachial plexus injuries: return-to-play recommendations. Phys Sportsmed. 1997; 25(7):61–88

[5] Vaccaro AR, Klein GR, Ciccoti M, et al. Return to play criteria for the athlete with cervical spine injuries resulting in stinger and transient quadriplegia/paresis. Spine J. 2002; 2(5):351–356

[6] Saigal R, Batjer HH, Ellenbogen RG, Berger MS. Return to play for neurosurgical patients. World Neurosurg. 2014; 82(3–4):485–491

[7] Tempel ZJ, Bost JW, Norwig JA, Maroon JC. Significance of T2 hyperintensity on magnetic resonance imaging after cervical cord injury and return to play in professional athletes. Neurosurgery. 2015; 77(1):23–30, discussion 30–31

[8] Meyer PR. Surgery of Spine Trauma. Churchill Livingstone; 1989

[9] Schroeder GD, Canseco JA, Patel PD, et al. Updated return-to-play recommendations for collision athletes after cervical spine injury: a modified Delphi consensus study with the Cervical Spine Research Society. Neurosurgery. 2020; 87(4):647–654

[10] Torg JS. Epidemiology, biomechanics, and prevention of cervical spine trauma resulting from athletics and recreational activities. Oper Tech Sports Med 1993; 1(3):159–168

[11] Burnett MG, Sonntag VKH. Return to contact sports after spinal surgery. Neurosurg Focus. 2006; 21(4):E5

[12] Eck JC, Riley LH, III. Return to play after lumbar spine conditions and surgeries. Clin Sports Med. 2004; 23(3):367–379, viii

[13] Bailes JE, Hadley MN, Quigley MR, Sonntag VKH, Cerullo LJ. Management of athletic injuries of the cervical spine and spinal cord. Neurosurgery. 1991; 29(4):491–497

[14] Zmurko MG, Tannoury TY, Tannoury CA, Anderson DG. Cervical sprains, disc herniations, minor fractures, and other cervical injuries in the athlete. Clin Sports Med. 2003; 22(3):513–521

[15] Kepler CK, Vaccaro AR. Injuries and abnormalities of the cervical spine and return to play criteria. Clin Sports Med. 2012; 31(3):499–508

[16] Clark AJ, Auguste KI, Sun PP. Cervical spinal stenosis and sports-related cervical cord neurapraxia. Neurosurg Focus. 2011; 31(5):E7

[17] Bell GR. Cervical cord neurapraxia and return to play. Contemp Spine Surg. 2003; 4(8):57–64

[18] Hsu WK. Outcomes following nonoperative and operative treatment for cervical disc herniations in National Football League athletes. Spine. 2011; 36(10):800–805

[19] Mochida J, Nishimura K, Okuma M, Nomura T, Toh E. Percutaneous nucleotomy in elite athletes. J Spinal Disord. 2001; 14(2):159–164

[20] Watkins RG, 4th, Hanna R, Chang D, Watkins RG, 3rd. Return-to-play outcomes after microscopic lumbar diskectomy in professional athletes. Am J Sports Med. 2012; 40(11):2530–2535

21 Congenital Spinal Anomalies and Implications for Athletics

Adam Ammar, Andrew M. Hersh, and Alan R. Cohen

Summary

Congenital spinal anomalies in children and adolescents can have implications for athletic participation. Given the benefits of sports participation for the physical, social, and emotional development of children, it is important to understand the specific considerations for various spinal anomalies. Some sports are entirely contraindicated due to the high risk of catastrophic injury in certain patients; however, many patients with spinal anomalies are still able to participate in sports to varying degrees. Patients should be counseled on their individual risks associated with sports participation, and in some instances, adjustments may be able to be made to reduce risk. This chapter will detail the considerations for patients with spina bifida, Klippel-Feil syndrome, Down syndrome, atlanto-occipital and atlanto-axial anomalies, vertebral anomalies, and scoliosis.

Keywords: pediatrics, sports, scoliosis, spina bifida, Klippel-Feil, os odontoideum, hemivertebra, atlanto-occipital fusion, Down syndrome

21.1 Introduction

Pediatric and adolescent athletes are susceptible to acute and traumatic spine injuries, which can be associated with significant limitations on their neurological function and participation in sports activities. The patterns of injury differ from those seen in adults owing to the unique biomechanics of the developing and growing spine. Spondylolysis and fractures of the pars interarticularis are more common in younger athletes. Increased range of motion of the cervical spine combined with a larger head to body size ratio in children renders them more susceptible to traumatic cervical spine injuries. In addition, patients with congenital anomalies of the spine are at increased susceptibility to traumatic injuries and warrant additional considerations when evaluating participation in sports. Some sports are entirely contraindicated due to the high risk of catastrophic injury in certain patients; however, sports participation is overall beneficial to children's physical and emotional well-being, and their participation in sports should be encouraged when safe.

21.2 Spina Bifida

Spina bifida is a congenital malformation of the caudal neural tube that results in a range of structural defects affecting the spine and spinal cord. The four most common types of spina bifida are occulta, meningocele, lipomyelomeningocele, and myelomeningocele (MMC), with MMC being the most common and severe presentation (▶ Fig. 21.1).[1] Symptoms will vary depending on the type and level of the lesion but will often involve motor dysfunction and bowel/bladder incontinence.

When it comes to physical activity, individuals with spina bifida have been shown to have impaired cardiorespiratory endurance, muscle strength, body composition, and flexibility compared to healthy peers. Exercise training has thus been recommended for patients with spina bifida to reduce the risk of cardiovascular disease and obesity.[2] Studies have shown that the proportion of adolescents and young adults with spina bifida who participate in sports is not lower than in those with other physical disabilities, so it is recommended that patients with spina bifida be encouraged to be more physically active and participate in sports.[3]

21.3 Klippel-Feil Syndrome

Klippel-Feil syndrome is the congenital fusion of two or more cervical vertebrae due to the failure of cervical somite segmentation and differentiation during embryogenesis. It has a predilection for females (60–70%). It is subdivided into three types in the Samartzis classification: Type 1 involves a single congenitally fused cervical segment, Type 2 involves multiple, noncontiguous fused cervical segments, and Type 3 involves multiple, contiguous fused cervical segments. The C2–C3 and C5–C6 levels are the most involved. Other congenital abnormalities of the skeletal, pulmonary, cardiovascular, and urogenital systems have been associated with the syndrome but are not necessary for the diagnosis. A high proportion of patients with the disease are asymptomatic and rarely develop neurologic problems or instability; thus, management primarily involves observation. Surgical treatment will vary depending on neurologic signs and symptoms and correction of deformity.[4]

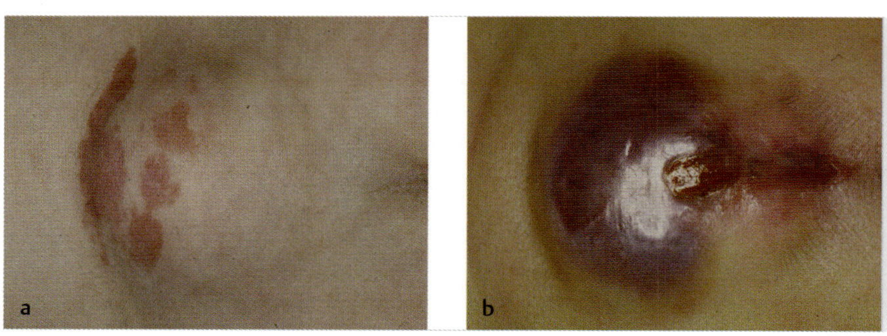

Fig. 21.1 **(a)** A child with lipomyelomeningocele, or fatty mass. This patient has spinal dysraphism covered by skin. **(b)** Photograph depicting an open lumbar myelomeningocele, a more severe phenotype.

Although uncommon, cervical spinal cord injuries (SCIs) during high-impact activities can occur in Klippel-Feil patients. Due to the abnormal mechanics from the fused cervical vertebrae, the adjacent nonfused segments become hypermobile, increasing the risk from contact sports and other high-impact activities.[5] Due to this, sports participation and return to play recommendations in a patient with Klippel-Feil syndrome after SCI is controversial. There are no high-quality evidence-based guidelines in the literature, and whatever recommendations currently exist are expert opinions. Current recommendations are based on the understanding of the altered spinal mechanics predisposing to injury. In general, patients with single-level fusions of the subaxial cervical spine without neurologic symptoms or associated spinal cord abnormalities may be allowed to participate in sports. In mild cases of cervical cord injury that completely resolves and has negative imaging, patients may be cautiously instructed on a return to activity with the knowledge of a heightened risk for future injuries. Any evidence of craniocervical involvement, upper cervical instability, degenerative disk disease, herniated disks, or spinal stenosis on imaging, or previous surgical intervention for Klippel-Feil, should be a contraindication to high-impact activities, however.[4,6] It has also been recommended that the Type 1 lesion be an *absolute contraindication* to participation in contact sports due to the abnormal spinal mechanics and increased instability. In addition, a Type 2 lesion with fusion of multiple noncontiguous segments and associated limited motion and/or associated craniocervical abnormalities, instability, disk disease, or degenerative changes also constitutes an *absolute contraindication* to participation in contact sports. However, Type 2 lesions involving the C3 level and below in an individual with full cervical range of motion and an absence of craniocervical abnormalities, instability, disk disease, or degenerative changes should present *no contraindication*.[7]

21.4 Os Odontoideum

Os odontoideum is a condition in which the dens of the second cervical vertebra is separated from the body of C2; the ossicle is fully corticated, making it a distinct entity from a dens fracture. The etiology is controversial with evidence supporting both traumatic and congenital etiologies. Os odontoideum is classified into two types: orthotopic in which the ossicle moves with C1, and dystopic in which it is fused to the basion and may sublux anterior to the arch of C1. Although it is often an incidental finding, the separation of the odontoid process can lead to atlantoaxial instability (AAI) and has been associated with spinal cord and vertebral artery injuries.[8,9] Symptoms vary based on the biomechanics and neurologic compression. It may present as nondescript pain or occipital–cervical pain, myelopathy, or vertebrobasilar ischemia. Most cases are asymptomatic; those without evidence of instability are typically managed with observation, while the presence of AAI or neurological dysfunction necessitates surgical fixation and fusion.

Although asymptomatic stable os odontoideum can be managed with observation, it may progress to develop AAI either through natural progression or due to acute trauma. The risk of developing a neurological deficit is strongly associated with AAI and narrowing of the spinal canal, and examples of sudden SCI in association with os odontoideum after even minor trauma have been reported.[9,10,11] For this reason, patients should be counseled regarding the risks of participation in contact sports. Any congenital abnormality affecting the normal anatomical structures of the atlantoaxial and atlanto-occipital joints, including odontoid agenesis, odontoid hypoplasia, or os odontoideum, are absolute contraindications to participation in contact or collision sports.[6,7]

21.5 Atlanto-Occipital Fusion

Atlanto-occipital fusion is a rare condition characterized by partial or complete congenital fusion of the atlas to the base of the occiput. It is usually associated with a reduction in the dimensions of the foramen magnum leading to acute or chronic neurovascular compression. Symptoms are typically due to this cord compression and usually occur later in life. This lesion usually progresses insidiously and slowly, but sudden onset or instant death has been reported. Because of this risk, atlanto-occipital fusion as an isolated entity or coexisting with other abnormalities constitutes an *absolute contraindication* to participation in contact activities.[12]

21.6 Atlantoaxial Instability in Down Syndrome

Down syndrome occurs in about 1 in every 700 births and is associated with an increased prevalence of AAI, with 9 to 27% of Down syndrome patients having the abnormality. AAI and cervical spine hypermobility can also be seen in other congenital disorders, such as Ehlers-Danlos syndrome.[13] It is frequently asymptomatic and nonprogressive, with only 1 to 2% of patients eventually developing symptomatic AAI. Symptoms include neck pain, sensory and motor deficits, and loss of bladder control.[14] Nonetheless, patients with AAI are at increased risk for SCI, and extreme movements during sports can worsen the subluxation and induce injury.

Historically, routine radiographs were obtained to evaluate for AAI in patients with Down syndrome; however, studies have shown that these radiographs are poorly predictive of cervical instability and are therefore only recommended for workup of symptomatic patients.[15] Instead, patients should receive a neurological examination before sport participation to rule out symptomatic AAI and be counseled on the risks associated with certain sports, such as gymnastics, diving, and contact sports, which cause hyperextension or place direct pressure on the cervical spine and thereby increase the likelihood of symptomatic AAI.[16] In general, any congenital abnormality affecting the normal anatomical structures of the atlantoaxial and atlanto-occipital joints is an absolute contraindication to participation in contact or collision sports. If there is evidence of craniocervical and upper cervical instability, sports participation should be contraindicated and surgical intervention for instrumentation and fusion should be considered.[6,7] Once instrumented and stabilized, it is reasonable to allow noncontact sport participation and contact sports can be considered when bony fusion has occurred.

21.7 Hemivertebra

Hemivertebra is a congenital spinal abnormality in which only half of the vertebral body forms. The growth plates are typically normal, and so as the asymmetric growth occurs a progressive deformity develops, typically scoliosis (most common), kyphosis, and/or lordosis. Neighboring vertebrae may subsequently undergo asymmetric growth due to the local deformity and asymmetric weight loads. In addition, secondary curves may develop in an attempt to attain equilibration, leading to complex deformities. If untreated, the flexible secondary curves can become structural. Without treatment, 85% of patients with hemivertebra develop severe curves greater than 41 degrees. Although casting and bracing can help delay progression and act as a bridge to surgery in younger children, these are successful on their own in only 5 to 10% of patients. Definitive treatment is surgery for resection of the hemivertebra, correction of any deformity, and instrumentation and fusion.[17] On their own, hemivertebrae are not unstable, and thus considerations for sports participation should follow those of scoliosis patients based on the level of deformity and postoperative considerations for instrumentation and fusion.

21.8 Adolescent Idiopathic Scoliosis

Adolescent idiopathic scoliosis (AIS) refers to excessive lateral curvature of the spine, typically defined as a Cobb angle of at least 10 degrees, and affects about 1 to 3% of children around the age of puberty, with a greater prevalence in females. Curves typically progress over time in the absence of treatment, although there is significant variability in the natural history. Conservative monitoring is recommended for angles < 25 degrees in magnitude, followed by bracing for angles between 25 and 45 degrees, and surgical instrumentation for patients with angles exceeding 45 degrees (► Fig. 21.2).[18] Some studies suggest a higher rate of idiopathic scoliosis in recreational and elite athletes compared to the general population, although the precise cause is unknown. For example, the rate of scoliosis in ballet dancers and gymnasts may exceed the general population by more than 10-fold, potentially reflecting selection bias for the sport, as successful dancers and gymnasts may inherently have increased joint laxity. Other theories point to the repetitive application of asymmetric stresses on the spine, along with weight restriction and delayed menarche, which can produce delays in bone development and abnormal pubertal growth.[19,20]

Patients with AIS are encouraged to participate in athletic activities due to the positive impact on teenagers' development, health, and psychosocial well-being. Indeed, there is evidence showing that participation in sports can protect against curve progression in adolescents with mild forms of AIS.[21] The main consideration for athletes with AIS concerns the return to sports following operative intervention for severe scoliosis. Most surgeons follow a stepwise return to play, with earlier return to low-impact noncontact sports, followed by contact and finally collision sports by 1 year.[22] Improvements in scoliosis surgery and instrumentation have gradually facilitated earlier timing of return to play, and most athletes can return to baseline just a few months after posterior fusion.[23] A 2015 survey by the Spinal Deformity Study Group of 23 experienced deformity surgeons found that surgeons recommended return to running by 3 months following pedicle screw

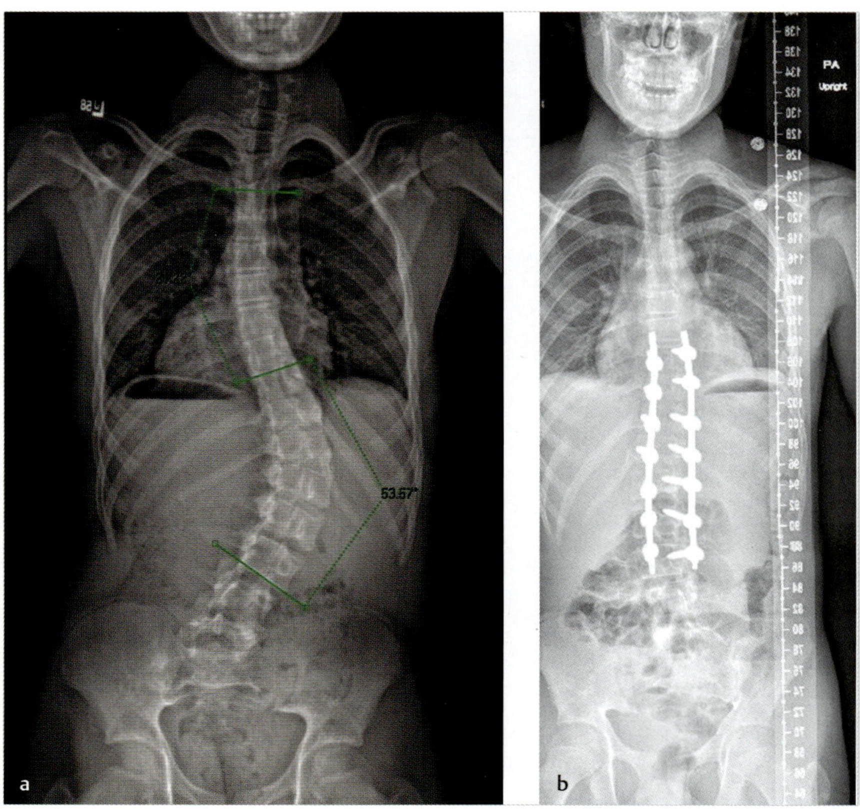

Fig. 21.2 (a) Anteroposterior X-ray of a 15-year-old child with severe scoliosis. The Cobb angle is 54 degrees with a Lenke 5 curve. The patient underwent posterior T9–L3 fusion. **(b)** Postoperative imaging showing instrumentation and improved spinal alignment. The patient was cleared to return to physical activity.

instrumentation, contact sports by 6 months, and collision sports by 1 year. No patients were restricted from noncontact or contact sports, but about 20% of respondents restricted return to collision sports.[24] Some patients will return to athletics but opt for lower impact sports due to reduced spinal flexibility.[25] However, instrumentation surgery should not be viewed as a contraindication to athletics.

One concern that has arisen is whether certain sports are contraindicated due to the risk of progression of AIS. Although some studies have identified a correlation between AIS and specific sports, such as ballet, gymnastics, swimming, and skiing, the causality has been difficult to establish. One study of volleyball players did find progression of scoliosis among athletes over time, attributed to the repetitive rotational movements which induce asymmetric loading of the developing spine. Nonetheless, the curves were typically mild between 10 and 15 degrees and would not warrant intervention.[26]

21.9 Conclusions

The patterns of pediatric spine injuries differ from those seen in adults owing to the unique biomechanics of the developing and growing spine. Patients with congenital anomalies of the spine have additional changes in their biomechanics and development that can increase the risk of injury. These factors warrant additional considerations in evaluating young athletes for participation in sports. Some sports are entirely contraindicated due to the high risk of catastrophic injury in certain patients; however, sports participation is beneficial to children's physical, mental, and emotional well-being, and should be encouraged when safe. Decision-making on sports participation should consider the underlying disease pathology and its natural history, patient's susceptibility to injury, and recovery after treatment. Discussions should include inputs from patients, their family, and sports coach, as well as their team of providers including their pediatrician, surgeon, radiologist, physical therapist, neuropsychologist, and/or sports medicine physician. Patients should be counseled on their individual risks associated with sports participation, and in some instances, adjustments may be made to reduce risk.

21.10 Clinical Pearls

- Athletic activities should be encouraged in children when safe due to the positive impacts on development, health, and psychosocial well-being.
- In general, any congenital abnormality affecting the normal anatomical structures of the atlantoaxial and atlanto-occipital joints is an absolute contraindication to participation in contact or collision sports.
- Instrumentation surgery should not be viewed as a contraindication to athletics. Return to play should be a gradual process with return to contact and collision sports occurring when bony fusion has occurred.

References

[1] Botto LD, Moore CA, Khoury MJ, Erickson JD. Neural-tube defects. N Engl J Med. 1999; 341(20):1509–1519

[2] Oliveira A, Jácome C, Marques A. Physical fitness and exercise training on individuals with spina bifida: a systematic review. Res Dev Disabil. 2014; 35 (5):1119–1136

[3] Buffart LM, van der Ploeg HP, Bauman AE, et al. Sports participation in adolescents and young adults with myelomeningocele and its role in total physical activity behaviour and fitness. J Rehabil Med. 2008; 40(9): 702–708

[4] Litrenta J, Bi AS, Dryer JW. Klippel-Feil syndrome: pathogenesis, diagnosis, and management. J Am Acad Orthop Surg. 2021; 29(22):951–960

[5] Matsumoto K, Wakahara K, Sumi H, Shimizu K. Central cord syndrome in patients with Klippel-Feil syndrome resulting from winter sports: report of 3 cases. Am J Sports Med. 2006; 34(10):1685–1689

[6] Ellis JL, Gottlieb JE. Return-to-play decisions after cervical spine injuries. Curr Sports Med Rep. 2007; 6(1):56–61

[7] Torg JS, Ramsey-Emrhein JA. Suggested management guidelines for participation in collision activities with congenital, developmental, or postinjury lesions involving the cervical spine. Med Sci Sports Exerc. 1997; 29(7) Suppl:S256–S272

[8] Arvin B, Fournier-Gosselin MP, Fehlings MG. Os odontoideum: etiology and surgical management. Neurosurgery. 2010; 66(3) Suppl:22–31

[9] Rozzelle CJ, Aarabi B, Dhall SS, et al. Os odontoideum. Neurosurgery. 2013; 72 Suppl 2:159–169

[10] Hedequist DJ, Mo AZ. Os odontoideum in children. J Am Acad Orthop Surg. 2020; 28(3):e100–e107

[11] Helenius IJ, Bauer JM, Verhofste B, et al. Os odontoideum in children: treatment outcomes and neurological risk factors. J Bone Joint Surg Am. 2019; 101(19):1750–1760

[12] Sharma DK, Sharma D, Sharma V. Atlantooccipital fusion: prevalence and its developmental and clinical correlation. J Clin Diagn Res. 2017; 11(6): AC01–AC03

[13] Mao G, Kopparapu S, Jin Y, et al. Craniocervical instability in patients with Ehlers-Danlos syndrome: controversies in diagnosis and management. Spine J. 2022; 22(12):1944–1952

[14] Caird MS, Wills BPD, Dormans JP. Down syndrome in children: the role of the orthopaedic surgeon. J Am Acad Orthop Surg. 2006; 14(11):610–619

[15] Hengartner AC, Whelan R, Maj R, Wolter-Warmerdam K, Hickey F, Hankinson TC. Evaluation of 2011 AAP cervical spine screening guidelines for children with Down syndrome. Childs Nerv Syst. 2020; 36 (11):2609–2614

[16] Tomlinson C, Campbell A, Hurley A, Fenton E, Heron N. Sport preparticipation screening for asymptomatic atlantoaxial instability in patients with down syndrome. Clin J Sport Med. 2020; 30(4):293–295

[17] Bao B, Yan H, Tang J. A review of the hemivertebrae and hemivertebra resection. Br J Neurosurg. 2022; 36(5):546–554

[18] Weinstein SL, Dolan LA, Cheng JC, Danielsson A, Morcuende JA. Adolescent idiopathic scoliosis. Lancet. 2008; 371(9623):1527–1537

[19] Mousavi L, Seidi F, Minoonejad H, Nikouei F. Prevalence of idiopathic scoliosis in athletes: a systematic review and meta-analysis. BMJ Open Sport Exerc Med. 2022; 8(3):e001312

[20] Tanchev PI, Dzherov AD, Parushev AD, Dikov DM, Todorov MB. Scoliosis in rhythmic gymnasts. Spine. 2000; 25(11):1367–1372

[21] Negrini A, Donzelli S, Vanossi M, et al. Sports participation reduces the progression of idiopathic scoliosis and the need for bracing. An observational study of 511 adolescents with Risser 0–2 maturation stage. Eur J Phys Rehabil Med. 2023; 59(2):222–227

[22] Ho D, Du JY, Erkilinc M, Glotzbecker MP, Mistovich RJ. Getting them back in the game: when can athletes with adolescent idiopathic scoliosis safely return to sports? A mixed-effects study of the Pediatric Orthopaedic Association of North America. J Pediatr Orthop. 2021; 41(9):e717–e721

[23] Tetreault T, Darland H, Vu A, Carry P, Garg S. Adolescent athletes return to sports rapidly after posterior spine fusion for idiopathic scoliosis: a prospective cohort study. Spine Deform. 2023; 11(2):383–390

[24] Lehman RA, Jr, Kang DG, Lenke LG, Sucato DJ, Bevevino AJ, Spinal Deformity Study Group. Return to sports after surgery to correct adolescent idiopathic scoliosis: a survey of the Spinal Deformity Study Group. Spine J. 2015; 15(5): 951–958

[25] Barile F, Ruffilli A, Manzetti M, et al. Resumption of sport after spinal fusion for adolescent idiopathic scoliosis: a review of the current literature. Spine Deform. 2021; 9(5):1247–1251

[26] Modi H, Srinivasalu S, Smehta S, Yang JH, Song HR, Suh SW. Muscle imbalance in volleyball players initiates scoliosis in immature spines: a screening analysis. Asian Spine J. 2008; 2(1):38–43

Part III

Peripheral Nerves

III

22 Anatomy and Physical Examination of the Peripheral Nerves

Jesse Stokum and Allan J. Belzberg

Summary

The purpose of the physical examination is to localize a lesion to a particular point in the central or peripheral nervous system. Although a targeted examination should be made of the area of concern, all patients presenting with a peripheral nerve complaint should be submitted to a full examination, as unanticipated findings may change injury localization and treatment plan. Areas of concern must be examined without clothing, as clothing may mask important signs, such as muscle wasting or scapular winging. In addition to the physical examination, a careful history must be taken, including the time of symptom onset, disease course, exacerbations or alleviating factors, comorbidities, social history, and medical and surgical history.

Sensation should be tested throughout, including light touch and pinprick. Sensory deficits should be marked on the skin with a nontoxic marker, and photographs taken. Reflexes should be elicited with a reflex hammer. Strength testing must be assessed in a systematic manner so as to not skip important muscle groups. Importantly, when examining strength, muscles should be placed in full extension to place the examinee at a mechanical disadvantage so that subtle weakness can be detected.

This chapter presents a systematic physical examination of the extremities, with salient anatomy highlighted. Rather than organize by nerve, sections are organized by joint so that this chapter can serve as a stepwise guide for the examination of the peripheral nervous system.

Keywords: physical examination, peripheral nervous system

22.1 Scapula

Scapular stability and movement are critical for proper shoulder function. Major mediators of scapular movement and stability include the serratus anterior, levator scapulae, rhomboids, and trapezius muscles.[1] The serratus anterior (C5–C7) muscle is innervated by the long thoracic nerve, which originates from the C5–C7 nerve roots. The serratus anterior abducts, upwardly rotates, and stabilizes the scapula during arm movement. Levator scapulae is innervated by branches of the cervical plexus and elevates the scapula. The rhomboid muscles (C5) are innervated by the dorsal scapular nerve, a proximal branch of the C5 nerve root. The rhomboids retract and downwardly rotate the scapula, acting in opposition to serratus anterior. The trapezius, which is innervated by the spinal accessory nerve, stabilizes, elevates, and downwardly rotates the scapula.

When evaluating the scapula, first inspect the patient's unclothed back for wasting. Next, inspect for scapular winging. Winging occurs in the direction opposite to the normal motion of the affected muscle. Serratus anterior weakness results in medial winging, which worsens when the patient reaches forward. Trapezius weakness results in ipsilateral shoulder droop and lateral winging of the scapula, worsened with arm abduction. Rhomboid weakness results in lateral winging of the scapula, worsened during arm extension.

To test strength of scapular muscles, first test serratus anterior. Ask the patient to reach a straightened arm forward to touch a point on the wall, and then push forward against resistance. Scapular winging is worsened with this movement if serratus anterior weakness is present. Patients with serratus anterior weakness may also have difficulty with arm flexion past 120 degrees.[1] Next, test the rhomboids. Ask the patient to place the dorsal surface of the hand against his or her back and push backward against resistance. Finally, test the trapezius, details of which are discussed in the subsequent section.

22.2 Shoulder

Prior to testing upper arm movements, the presence of shoulder subluxation should be palpated for. Upper arm movements include arm abduction and adduction (movement in the plane of the chest), flexion and extension (movement perpendicular to the plane of the chest), and external and internal rotation.

Shoulder abduction is mediated by the supraspinatus, deltoid, and trapezius muscles. The supraspinatus (C5–C6) muscle supports the first 30 degrees of abduction, and is innervated by the suprascapular nerve, which originates from the upper trunk of the brachial plexus and courses posteriorly to pass through the suprascapular notch, a site of potential entrapment. The deltoid (C5–C6) and trapezius muscles support the remaining 30 to 90 degrees of shoulder abduction, and are innervated by the axillary and spinal accessory nerves, respectively. The axillary nerve branches from the posterior cord of the brachial plexus and passes through the quadrangular space to reach the deltoid. The spinal accessory nerve emerges from the jugular foramen and passes under the sternocleidomastoid and across the posterior triangle of the neck to reach the trapezius muscle. To test supraspinatus, ask the patient to first abduct his or her arm against resistance from the side. To test deltoid and trapezius, ask the patient to abduct his or her arm against resistance starting from 30 degrees. Trapezius may also be tested with shoulder shrug.

Shoulder adduction is provided by the teres major, latissimus dorsi, and pectoralis major muscles. The teres major (C5-C6) and latissimus dorsi (C6–C8) are innervated by the lower subscapular nerve and thoracodorsal nerves respectively, both branches of the posterior cord. The pectoralis major, comprised of clavicular (C5, C6) and sternal (C6–T1) heads, is innervated by the lateral and medial pectoral nerves respectively, which are branches from the lateral and medial cords. To test the clavicular head of the pectoralis major, ask the patient to flex the shoulder and elbow 90 degrees, and then sweep the arm toward the midline across the chest against resistance. To test the sternal head of the pectoralis major, ask the patient to abduct the shoulder 30 degrees and flex the elbow 90 degrees, and then adduct the arm against resistance. To test teres major, ask the patient to straighten the elbow and abduct the shoulder 90 degrees, and then adduct the arm against resistance with the palm facing the ground. Finally, to test latissimus dorsi, ask the patient to abduct the shoulder 90 degrees and flex the elbow 90 degrees, and then adduct the arm against resistance.

Shoulder external rotation is supported primarily by the infraspinatus muscle (C5–C6), with some assistance from the teres minor (C5–C6). Infraspinatus, like supraspinatus, is innervated by the suprascapular nerve. Teres minor is innervated by the posterior division of the axillary nerve. To test external shoulder rotation, ask the patient to flex the elbow 90 degrees, and then rotate the forearm outward against resistance.

Shoulder internal rotation is mediated primarily by the subscapularis muscle (C5, C6), which is innervated by the upper subscapular nerve, a branch of the posterior cord. The teres major, latissimus dorsi, and pectoralis major also contribute to internal rotation. To test shoulder inward rotation, ask the patient to flex the elbow 90 degrees, and then rotate the forearm inward against resistance.

Shoulder flexion is mostly mediated by the deltoid muscle. However, when flexing greater than 60 degrees, the serratus anterior muscle will assist. Shoulder extension is mostly mediated by teres major, latissimus dorsi, and pectoralis major.

22.3 Elbow

Elbow function is comprised of flexion and extension. Flexion is supported by the biceps brachii (C5–C6), brachialis (C5–C6), and brachioradialis (C5–C6). The biceps brachii and brachialis are innervated by the musculocutaneous nerve, a terminal branch of the lateral cord. The brachioradialis is innervated by the radial nerve. To test biceps brachii and brachialis, ask the patient to fully extend the elbow with a supinated hand, and then flex against resistance. To test brachioradialis, ask the patient to fully extend the elbow with a halfway supinated hand, and then flex against resistance.

Elbow extension is mediated by the triceps (C6–C8), which are innervated by proximal branches of the radial nerve. To test the triceps, ask the patient to fully flex the elbow, and then extend the elbow against resistance.

22.4 Wrist

Wrist extension is mediated by the extensor carpi radialis longus (C6, C7), extensor carpi radialis brevis (C7, C8), and extensor carpi ulnaris (C7, C8). All wrist extensors are innervated by the radial nerve. To test extensor carpi radialis longus and brevis, ask the patient to extend the wrist in a radial direction against resistance. To test extensor carpi ulnaris, ask the patient to extend the wrist in an ulnar direction against resistance.

Wrist flexion is mediated by the flexor carpi radialis (C6, C7) and flexor carpi ulnaris (C7–T1), which are innervated by the median nerve and ulnar nerves respectively. To test flexor carpi radialis, ask the patient to flex the wrist in a radial direction against resistance. To test flexor carpi ulnaris, ask the patient to flex the wrist in an ulnar direction against resistance.

Wrist pronation is mediated by the pronator teres (C6, C7) and pronator quadratus (C7, C8). Pronator teres is innervated by the median nerve as it traverses the proximal forearm, and the pronator quadratus by the terminal branch of the anterior interosseus nerve. To test pronator teres, ask the patient to fully extend the elbow, and then pronate against resistance. To test pronator quadratus, ask the patient to fully flex the forearm, and then pronate the wrist against resistance.

Wrist supination is mediated by the supinator muscle (C5, C6), which is innervated by the radial nerve as it passes through the arcade of Fröhse. The biceps brachii also contribute to supination with a flexed elbow. To test the supinator, ask the patient to fully extend the elbow, and supinate the wrist against resistance.

22.5 Thumb

Thumb extension can occur at three joints. Extension of the carpometacarpo joint (a movement also referred to as radial thumb abduction) is mediated by the abductor pollicis longus (C7, C8). Extension of the metacarpophalangeal and interphalangeal joints are mediated by the extensor pollicis brevis (C7, C8) and longus (C7, C8) respectively. All three of these muscles are innervated by the radial nerve. To test these muscles, ask the patient to move the thumb away from the index finger in the plane of the hand ("hitchhiker thumb"), and sequentially apply resistance to the thumb metacarpal, proximal phalange, and distal phalange.

Thumb abduction can also occur away from the plane of the hand and is mediated by the abductor pollicis brevis (C8, T1), which is innervated by the thenar motor branch of the median nerve after it passes through the carpal tunnel. To test the abductor pollicis brevis, ask the patient to move the thumb away from the palm of the hand against resistance.

Thumb flexion can occur at either its metacarpophalangeal joint or its interphalangeal joint. Flexor pollicis longus (C8, T1) mediates thumb interphalangeal joint flexion, whereas flexor pollicis brevis (C8, T1) mediates thumb metacarpophalangeal joint flexion. Both muscles are innervated by the median nerve, although the flexor pollicis brevis has dual innervation from the ulnar nerve. To test these muscles, ask the patient to flex the thumb at the metacarpophalangeal or interphalangeal joints against resistance. The anterior interosseus nerve, a branch of the median nerve that innervates both the flexor pollicis longus and flexor digitorum profundus to the second and third digits, can be tested with the "OK" sign.

Thumb opposition is primarily mediated by the opponens pollicis muscle (C8, T1), which is innervated by the median nerve, with additional contribution from adductor pollicis and the thumb flexors. To test opponens pollicis, ask the patient to touch the thumb to the fifth digit against resistance.

Thumb adduction is mediated by the adductor pollicis (C8, T1), innervated by the deep branch of the ulnar nerve. To test adductor pollicis, ask the patient to adduct the thumb against resistance in the plane of the hand.

22.6 Fingers

Finger flexion can occur at three joints: the metacarpophalangeal (MCP) joint, the proximal interphalangeal (PIP) joint, and the distal interphalangeal (DIP) joint. Flexion of the MCP is mediated primarily by the lumbricals (C8, T1), which are innervated by the median nerve (second and third digits) and ulnar nerve (fourth and fifth digits). MCP flexion is assisted by the interossei and the flexor digiti minimi and flexor indicis for the second and fifth fingers. Flexion of the PIP is mediated by the flexor digitorum superficialis (C8, T1), which is innervated by the median nerve in the forearm. Flexion of the DIP is mediated by the flexor digitorum profundus, which is innervated by the median nerve (second and third digits) and ulnar nerve (fourth and fifth digits). To test the lumbricals, hyperextend the MCP, and then ask the patient to extend the PIP against resistance. This is typically performed for the second and fifth fingers to test the median and ulnar lumbricals separately. To test the flexor digitorum superficialis and profundus, ask the patient to lay a supinated hand on the table, and flex the PIP and DIP against resistance, isolating that particular joint. DIP flexion is typically tested for the second and fifth fingers to test the median and ulnar profundus separately.

Finger extension can also occur at three joints: the MCP, PIP, and DIP joints. MCP extension is primarily mediated by extrinsic extensors, including the extensor digitorum communis (C7, C8), extensor digiti minimi (C7, C8), and extensor indicis (C7, C8), which are all innervated by the radial nerve. PIP and DIP extension is mediated by the intrinsic hand muscles: the lumbricals and interossei. To test extensor digitorum communis, ask the patient to extend the finger at the knuckle, applying resistance against the proximal phalanx. Evaluation of the lumbrical and interossi muscles is detailed elsewhere in this section.

Finger abduction is performed by the dorsal interosseus muscles (C8, T1), which move the fingers away from the third finger. Finger adduction is performed by the palmar interosseus muscles (C8, T1), which accomplish the opposite. Both sets of interosseus muscles are innervated by terminal branches of the ulnar nerve. Since all interossei are innervated by the ulnar nerve, only the first dorsal interosseus muscle is tested. Ask the patient to abduct the index finger away from the hand against resistance. The bulk of this muscle should be palpated and noted.

22.7 Hip

Hip adduction (L2–L4) is mediated by the adductor magnus, brevis, and longus, with contributions from the gracilis and the short hip external rotators (superior and inferior gamelli, obturator internus, and quadratus internus). All three adductor muscles and the gracilis are innervated by the obturator nerve, with the adductor magnus receiving dual innervation from the tibial portion of the sciatic nerve. To test hip adduction, have the patient sit with knees bent at 90 degrees, and squeeze the knees together against resistance.

Hip abduction is mediated by the gluteus medius and minimus muscles, the tensor fascia latae, and assisted by the sartorius. The tensor fascia latae, the gluteus medius, and gluteus minimus (all L4–S1) are innervated by the superior gluteal nerve. The sartorius (L2–L4) is innervated by the femoral nerve, and weakly abducts, flexes, and externally rotates the hip. To test the gluteus medius and minimus, ask the patient to stand and attempt to abduct the hip against resistance. To test the tensor fascia latae, ask the patient to sit and attempt to abduct the hip against resistance. To test the sartorius, ask the patient to drag his or her heel up the opposite shin; the muscle can be palpated during this motion.

Hip extension is primarily mediated by the gluteus maximus muscle (L5–S2), innervated by the inferior gluteal nerve. The hamstrings and adductor magnus also contribute to hip extension. To test gluteus maximus, ask the patient to stand, and then extend the hip against resistance with the knee flexed to eliminate hamstring contribution.

Hip flexion is mediated primarily by the iliopsoas muscle (L2–L4), innervated by proximal branches of the femoral nerve near its formation from the lumbar plexus in the psoas muscle. Other minor contributors to hip flexion include the rectus femoris, tensor fascia latae, and sartorius muscles. To test hip flexion, ask the patient to raise the knee against resistance.

Hip external rotation is mediated by the superior and inferior gamelli, obturator internus, and quadratus internus (all L5–S1), with contribution from the gluteus maximus, pectineus, and sartorius. Hip external rotation can be tested by asking the seated patient to resist inward pressure on the ankle while stabilizing the knee. Hip internal rotation is mediated by tensor fascia latae and gluteus medius and minimum with a flexed hip. Hip internal rotation can be tested by asking the seated patient to resist outward pressure on the ankle while stabilizing the knee.

22.8 Knee

Knee extension is mediated by the quadriceps muscles: rectus femoris, vastus lateralis, vastus intermedialis, and vastus medialis, all of which are innervated by the femoral nerve (L2–L4). To test knee extension, ask the patient to kick the lower leg out against resistance. Of note, given the strength of the quadriceps muscles, knee extension should be tested with the knee in full extension or alternatively, the patient can be asked to perform a deep knee bend standing on one leg.

Knee flexion is mediated by the hamstring muscles, including the semitendinous and semimembranous muscles, and the two heads of the biceps femoris (L2–S2). Excepting the short head of the biceps femoris, which is innervated by the common peroneal nerve, the remaining hamstring muscles are innervated by the tibial nerve. To test the hamstrings, ask the patient to flex the knee against resistance.

22.9 Ankle

Ankle plantarflexion is mediated by the gastrocnemius (S1, S2) and soleus (S1, S2) muscles, which are both innervated by the tibial nerve after it passes through the popliteal fossa. To test the gastrocnemius, ask the patient to plantarflex the ankle against resistance with an extended knee. To test the soleus, ask the patient to plantarflex the ankle against resistance with a flexed knee. Given the strength of these muscles, to detect subtle weakness, ask the patient to walk on "tiptoes."

Ankle dorsiflexion is mostly provided by the tibialis anterior (L4–S1), which is innervated by the deep branch of the peroneal nerve. To test the tibialis anterior, ask the patient to dorsiflex the foot against resistance. Similar to above, tibialis anterior can also be tested by asking patients to walk on their heels.

Ankle inversion is mostly mediated by tibialis posterior (L4–L5), which is innervated by the tibial nerve after it passes under the soleus. Inversion is tested by asking the patient to move the sole of the foot medially against resistance. Ankle eversion is mediated by peroneus longus and brevis (L5–S1), which are innervated by the superficial branch of the common peroneal nerve. Ankle eversion is tested by asking the patient to move the sole of the foot laterally against resistance. Importantly, ankle inversion and eversion are critical in differentiating radiculopathic versus peripheral (peroneal) foot drop.[2] Patients with foot drop resulting from L5 radiculopathy may also present with weakness of extensor hallucis longus, diminished L5 reflexes, and weakness of ankle inversion, which are associated with the tibial nerve supply. Patients with a foot drop resulting from common peroneal palsy will also present with weakness of foot eversion.

22.10 Foot

Examination should turn to toe flexion and extension.[3] Extension of hallux and toe is mediated by extensor hallucis longus (L5–S1) and extensor digitorum longus (L5–S1), which are both innervated by the deep peroneal nerve. Toe extension is tested by asking the patient to extend the toes against resistance. Similarly, toe flexion in all of the toe interphalangeal joints is mediated by flexor hallucis longus (S2–S3) and flexor digitorum longus (S2–S3), which are both innervated by the tibial nerve in the posterior compartment of the lower leg. Toe flexion is tested by asking the patient to curl the toes against resistance.

In the volar foot, after passing through the tibial tunnel, the tibial nerve splits into the medial and lateral plantar nerve. The medial plantar nerve innervates the abductor hallucis, flexor digitorum brevis, and flexor hallucis brevis (S1–S2), as well as the first lumbrical (L5–S1). The lateral plantar nerve innervates the quadratus plantae, adductor hallucis, abductor digiti minimi pedis, second to fourth lumbricals, and the dorsal interossei (S1–S3). On the dorsum of the foot, the deep peroneal nerve innervates the extensor digitorum brevis (L5, S1), which extends the toe MCP joint. The intrinsic foot muscles are relatively difficult to isolate and test separately. Foot plantar intrinsic muscles can be tested roughly by asking the patient to cup his or her foot.[4]

22.11 Provocative Tests

Various provocative maneuvers can be performed to identify nerve entrapments. Tinel's sign is a general maneuver that can be elicited by percussing over areas of suspected entrapment. Tinel's sign can also be used to follow the growth cones of regenerating axons. Carpal tunnel syndrome can be evaluated with Durkan's test and Phalen's maneuver.[5] In Durkan's test, the thumb is used to compress the carpal tunnel for 30 seconds. Pain or tingling is considered a positive test result. In Phalen's maneuver, the patient holds the wrist in forced flexion for 30 to 60 seconds. Pain, tingling, or numbness indicates a positive test. Cubital tunnel syndrome can be evaluated with various tests, including the elbow flexion and pressure tests. In the elbow flexion test, the patient holds the elbow in full flexion for 60 seconds. In the pressure test, the patient holds the elbow in 20 degrees of flexion with a supinated forearm, and the examiner presses the cubital tunnel for 60 seconds. Pain, tingling, or numbness indicates positivity. Other useful tests for evaluating the ulnar nerve include Froment's sign and Wartenberg's sign.[6] Thoracic outlet syndrome (TOS) may be tested with the Adson, Eden, and Wright tests.[7] Cervical radiculopathy is aggravated by holding the arm at the side and relieved by tucking the arm behind the head. The opposite occurs in TOS with discomfort being provoked by arm abduction and external rotation. Finally, straight leg raise test and Spurling's test can be used to identify lumbar and cervical radiculopathy, which may be useful in differentiating radiculopathic versus peripheral nerve causes of weakness or pain. Importantly, most provocative tests do not possess sufficient sensitivity and specificity to be diagnostic.[8] However, these tests serve as another technique in the examiner's armamentarium that may help to support a diagnosis.

22.12 Clinical Pearls

- A thorough assessment including motor and sensory testing along with careful history taking is critical to identify peripheral nerve lesions.
- Durkan's test, where the thumb is used to compress the carpal tunnel for 30 seconds, and Phalen's maneuver, where the patient holds the wrist in forced flexion for 30 to 60 seconds, can be used to evaluate for carpal tunnel syndrome.
- The straight leg raise test and Spurling's test can be used to identify lumbar and cervical radiculopathy, respectively, and differentiate between radiculopathy and peripheral nerve problems.

References

[1] Meininger AK, Figuerres BF, Goldberg BA. Scapular winging: an update. J Am Acad Orthop Surg. 2011; 19(8):453–462

[2] Macki M, Lim S, Elmenini J, Fakih M, Chang V. Clinching the cause: a review of foot drop secondary to lumbar degenerative diseases. J Neurol Sci. 2018; 395:126–130

[3] Alazzawi S, Sukeik M, King D, Vemulapalli K. Foot and ankle history and clinical examination: a guide to everyday practice. World J Orthop. 2017; 8 (1):21–29

[4] Russell SM. Examination of Peripheral Nerve Injuries: An Anatomical Approach. Thieme; 2006:xiv, 178

[5] Day CS, Wu WK, Smith CC. Examination of the hand and wrist. N Engl J Med. 2019; 380(12):e15

[6] Goldman SB, Brininger TL, Schrader JW, Koceja DM. A review of clinical tests and signs for the assessment of ulnar neuropathy. J Hand Ther. 2009; 22(3): 209–219, quiz 220

[7] Gillard J, Pérez-Cousin M, Hachulla E, et al. Diagnosing thoracic outlet syndrome: contribution of provocative tests, ultrasonography, electrophysiology, and helical computed tomography in 48 patients. Joint Bone Spine. 2001; 68(5):416–424

[8] Zhang D, Chruscielski CM, Blazar P, Earp BE. Accuracy of provocative tests for carpal tunnel syndrome. J Hand Surg Glob Online. 2020; 2(3):121–125

23 Common Peripheral Nerve Problems in Athletes: Diagnosis and Management

Danielle Golub, Hussam Abou-Al-Shaar, Timothy G. White, and Mark A. Mahan

Summary

Peripheral nerve injuries are a critical but underrecognized cause of sports injury that, when misdiagnosed or undertreated, can cause significant functional deficits or delay in returning to baseline athletic activity. This chapter summarizes the diagnosis and management of the most common peripheral nerve injuries in athletes. The introduction presents an overview of the anatomy-based grading systems used to define peripheral nerve injury, corresponding imaging and electrodiagnostic data, and general principles governing medical and surgical management and prognosis of related injuries. A detailed review of specific peripheral nerve injuries follows, starting with the most common—burner/stinger injuries—followed by other neck (thoracic outlet syndrome), upper extremity (suprascapular nerve, long thoracic nerve, axillary nerve, musculocutaneous nerve, median nerve, ulnar nerve, radial nerve), and lower extremity (sciatic nerve, piriformis syndrome, pudendal nerve, lateral femoral cutaneous nerve, femoral nerve, fibular nerve, tibial nerve, Morton's neuroma) injuries. Discussion of the natural history of recovery and advantages and disadvantages of surgical intervention is included for each nerve injury.

Keywords: peripheral nerve injury, athletic injuries, sports-related nerve injury, burners, thoracic outlet syndrome, carpal tunnel syndrome, piriformis syndrome, Morton's neuroma

23.1 Introduction

Although it is estimated that sports-related injuries contribute to only 6% of all peripheral nerve injuries, delays in athlete reporting and relative clinician inexperience with such injuries tend to significantly delay or even preclude an athlete's safe return to play.[1] Sports-related peripheral nerve injuries are often challenging to diagnose because the presentation can mimic musculoskeletal injuries and the manifestations are often variable. Additionally, it is critical to differentiate acute traumatic injuries from chronic overuse injuries because the underlying biomechanics of peripheral nerve injuries dictate optimal clinical management and rehabilitation strategy.[2] This chapter will provide a broad overview of the diagnosis and management of the most common peripheral nerve injuries seen in sports, including burners and upper and lower extremity pathologies.

The traumatic peripheral nerve injury classification system proposed by Sneddon (1943), which is based on clinical features, and that described by Sunderland (1951), which is a theoretical system based on injury to the neuroanatomical structural layers of nerve, have remained the most widely used since the mid-20th century.[3,4] These classification systems have been more recently corroborated by corresponding imaging and electrodiagnostic criteria (▶ Table 23.1).[5] Seddon defined three grades of injury based on axonal involvement: *Neurapraxia*, which involves focal conduction block but sparing of the axon and typically results in a mild motor and/or sensory deficit with full recovery; *axonotmesis*, which involves the axon but not the nerve's supporting structures (endoneurium, perineurium, and epineurium) and allows the possibility for recovery through slow axonal regeneration; and *neurotmesis*, the most severe form of injury in which there is complete destruction of the nerve (both the axon and its surrounding structures). There is typically no spontaneous recovery of function after neurotmesis, but surgical repair may offer some limited return of function.[3] Similarly, Sunderland described five degrees of injury based on the extent of neuroanatomical involvement: Sunderland's first-degree injuries correspond to Seddon's neurapraxia. His second- through fourth-degree injuries were intended to explain the variable degrees of axonotmesis within Seddon's system by proposing progressive destruction of the internal structural elements of the nerve: disruption of the axon (second degree), injury to the endoneurium (third degree), and then injury to the perineurium (fourth degree), and finally, complete disruption injury (fifth degree, equivalent to Seddon's neurotmesis) through the epineurium.[4] With increasing involvement of the surrounding connective tissue sheath, any regenerating axons are more likely to be misdirected and unable to reinnervate sensory endings or muscle end plates.[6]

Consideration of the type and degree of injury is important to diagnosis and prognosis. Neurapraxia can clinically appear like neurotmesis because there is no distal nerve function; however, electrodiagnostic studies can show that nerve is in continuity in neurapraxic injuries by showing conduction distal to the injury. When conduction is present distal to the injury site (performed at a time when Wallerian degeneration would be complete, approximately 2–3 weeks after injury), good functional recovery is likely. Similarly, when axonotmesis occurs, there is evidence of denervation on needle electromyography (EMG) of the muscle, and atrophy is frequently found on clinical examination. The cause and severity of the axonotmesis can help guide prognosis. Crush or contusion injuries tend to have better recoveries, whereas stretch injuries tend to be worse, with a lower chance of full recovery. The greater the denervation registered on EMG, the less likely that naturally programmed nerve regeneration is going to be successful. Similarly, the types of neurotmetic injuries have different outcomes. Sharp transections that are repaired early, preferably within 3 days, tend to have good outcomes, whereas stretch-induced nerve rupture has the worst outcomes.[7] Indications for surgical nerve repair attempt to weigh the likelihood of natural nerve recovery against the likelihood of recovery from surgical repair.

In addition to anatomical classification of traumatic nerve injuries, the distinction between acute and chronic peripheral nerve injuries is critical. Acute injuries are most often the result of a sudden extrinsic force on the athlete (i.e., a fall or tackle) that leads to instantaneous compression, overstretch, or laceration of the nerve.[8] Chronic peripheral nerve injuries typically represent overuse injuries resulting from repetitive microtrauma or maladaptation due to improper "periodization" of athletic training.[9]

Table 23.1 Peripheral nerve injury classifications

Seddon	Sunderland	Structural injury	Magnetic resonance neurography	Electrodiagnostic studies	Treatment	Prognosis
Neurapraxia	First degree	Myelin	Increased T2 signal intensity of nerve Normal muscle appearance	NCS: Slowing of conduction velocity, conduction block	Medical	Full recovery, days to months
Axonotmesis	Second degree	Axon (+ myelin)	Diffuse nerve enlargement and T2 hyperintensity Enlarged or effaced fascicles from surrounding edema Muscle denervation	NCS: Axon discontinuity conduction block—decreased amplitude of conduction proximal to the lesion NEE: + Fibrillation potentials	Medical	Near-total to full recovery, more proximal lesions with poorer recovery
Axonotmesis	Third degree	Axon (+ myelin) Endoneurium	Same as above (endoneurium not detectable)	NCS: Conduction abnormal Decreased amplitude of conduction at or distal to lesion May also show increased latency due to temporal dispersion of axonal firing NEE: + Fibrillation potentials, reduced MUP recruitment	Medical	Incomplete recovery, proximal lesions associated with poorer recovery
Axonotmesis	Fourth degree	Axon (+ myelin) Endoneurium Perineurium	"Neuroma-in-continuity"—focal fusiform nerve enlargement (internal hemorrhage and fibrosis) Heterogeneous T2 hyperintensity of nerve and fascicles Fascicular discontinuity Muscle denervation	NCS: Conduction failure—decreased amplitude of conduction at, distal, or proximal to lesion, sensory impulses may be not be elicitable NEE: + Fibrillation potentials, significantly reduced or no MUP recruitment	Surgical	Little to no spontaneous recovery, surgical recovery variable
Neurotmesis	Fifth degree	Axon (+ myelin) Endoneurium Perineurium Epineurium	Complete nerve discontinuity with or without hemorrhage and fibrosis in the nerve gap End-bulb neuromas at proximal nerve segment Thickening of epineurium Muscle denervation	NCS: Neither motor nor sensory impulses elicitable NEE: Significant fibrillation potentials, no MUP firing	Surgical	No spontaneous recovery, surgical recovery variable

Abbreviations: NCS, nerve conduction studies; NEE, needle electrode examination; MUP, motor unit potentials.

"Periodization" refers to the cyclical training of athletes involving periods of appropriate overtraining, designated and adequate recovery time, and additional compensatory training (i.e., weight lifting) to develop the proper musculoskeletal support for the primary skills to achieve supercompensation and an improved baseline performance. When athletes overtrain excessively or do not allow for adequate recovery, musculoskeletal maladaptation or repeated microinjury will follow, often resulting in both pain and a functional deficit.[10] The proper identification of chronic injuries therefore requires detailed questioning about the athlete's training strategy, history of injury, and quality of equipment because presentation can vary from a simple inability to perform a repetitive motor task to any combination of pain, weakness, and/or sensory losses. Management may require a significant shift in the athlete's training paradigm in addition to medical or surgical intervention.[2]

Lastly, mononeuropathies that appear suddenly, occur after a bout of intense joint pain (especially in the shoulder), and are associated with muscle atrophy are likely episodes of neuralgic amyotrophy,[11] also known as Parsonage-Turner syndrome. This disorder is an inflammatory condition of peripheral nerves, often associated with prodromal viral illnesses or significant stressors, such as endurance events and surgery. Clinicians should be careful to elucidate the differences between Parsonage-Turner syndrome and its homologs, posterior interosseous nerve and anterior interosseous nerve syndromes, versus more chronic conditions caused by athletic overuse injuries. Greater chronicity and absence of the features described above suggest overuse injuries. Often, electrodiagnostic studies are necessary to identify the pattern of nerve involvement—which are often confusing and do not fit an isolated nerve or nerve root pattern. The patchy involvement on EMG is typical for Parsonage-Turner syndrome.

23.2 Burners and Stingers

Burners (also called stingers) are the most common sports-related nerve injury and are ubiquitous in contact sports, especially in tackle football.[12,13] Burners are a unilateral neurapraxia from traction or compressive injury to the brachial plexus and/or the C5 or C6 nerve roots. They are experienced as transient burning pain that radiates down the arm (with possible concomitant motor deficits).[14] Symptoms usually last for only a few minutes, and therefore most athletes (up to 65% in one study of American football players) will typically not report this type of injury.[15] However, in approximately 10% of cases, paresthesias and weakness of the deltoid, biceps, or spinatus muscles can be prolonged, lasting from days to weeks; a history of repeated burner injuries is common to these refractory cases.[16]

There are three proposed mechanisms for burner injuries: (1) Compression of the nerve root caused by hyperextension of the neck combined with head rotation causing traumatic narrowing of the intervertebral foraminal canal on the side toward which the head and neck are skewed. The foraminal canal is particularly susceptible to mechanical trauma because of the lack of surrounding epineurium and perineurium.[17] This type of "extension–compression" burner is the predominant mechanism of burner injury in older, adult athletes who have predisposing risk factors, including cervical canal stenosis, disk disease, and other degenerative structural changes associated with aging and overuse.[18] Furthermore, "extension–compression" burners are the most likely to result in prolonged injury and become recurrent.[13] (2) Traction of the brachial plexus, typically the upper trunk, from forced distraction of the shoulder from the head and neck (e.g., while being blocked or tackled in American football or landing on the shoulder while the head is being pushed away in wrestling).[15] Unlike "extension–compression" burners, "traction" burners are not typically associated with neck pain, are more common in younger athletes, and are associated with earlier return to play.[13] (3) Direct trauma to the brachial plexus at Erb's point, the point in the supraclavicular region where the brachial plexus is most superficial, often accompanied by clavicular fracture.[14] Injuries to Erb's point in American football have been well characterized and are often a consequence of ill-fitting shoulder pads acting as the blunt object causing injury during player-to-player contact. Other manners of injury include being struck by a hockey or lacrosse stick.[19]

The natural history of transient burner injuries is poorly studied. Most athletes will be able to return to play within minutes to hours of their initial injury, depending on the extent of their symptoms. Athletes with prolonged or chronic burner symptoms can be managed with supportive care including rest, icing, nonsteroidal anti-inflammatory medications, and physical therapy as appropriate.[20] Successful physical therapy regimens take preventative measures against recurrence by focusing on the strengthening of neck muscles.[21] Additional preventative measures, such as the use of a cervical orthosis to limit neck extension and ensuring the use of properly fitted shoulder pads, have been described.[16] Although several criteria for defining safe return to play after burners have been described, the general consensus is that recovery of full motor strength and sensation as well as dissipation of any neuropathic or neck pain is sufficient.[22] Absolute contraindications include radiographic findings of unstable vertebral damage or loss of lordosis, and a relative contraindication is repeated burner injuries within a short period.[23] Although EMG can help localize the injury and is described as a tool in assessing more severe injuries, the use of EMG for predicting adequate recovery in prolonged burners has remained controversial. Significant injuries do not appear on EMG for the first 3 to 5 weeks, and up to 80% of athletes may continue to have an abnormal EMG for more than 4 years after injury—long after musculoskeletal function has normalized.[16] Persistent weakness, however, warrants continued monitoring by EMG and neuroimaging, as well as careful consideration of potential alternate diagnoses, such as cervical cord neurapraxia—especially when symptoms develop bilaterally.[8]

23.3 Upper Extremity Nerve Injuries

23.3.1 Thoracic Outlet Syndrome

Thoracic outlet syndrome (TOS) is a symptom complex of upper extremity pain and paresthesias typically of the lower trunk (C8–T1 spinal nerve or ulnar nerve pattern) resulting from either acute or chronic compression of the neurovascular structures at the thoracic outlet. TOS is typically divided into neurogenic TOS (nTOS), which represents 95% of TOS, and the rarer vascular TOS (vTOS) based on the anatomical cause of compression.[24] Athletes who perform vigorous overhead arm activity are particularly susceptible to both subtypes: sustained or repetitive elevation of the arm can result in scalene muscle strain and inflammation resulting in compression of the brachial plexus nerve roots and nTOS.[25] Throwing athletes, such as baseball pitchers, are particularly susceptible to developing compression of the subclavian artery and limb ischemia because of scapular destabilization from repetitive motion, especially when a bony abnormality, such as a cervical rib, is present.[24,26] Weight lifters and other resistance trainers are most likely to develop venous TOS from acute thrombosis of the subclavian or axillary veins, also known as Paget-Schroetter syndrome, because of overdeveloped trapezius and neck musculature and consequent venous stasis during strenuous lifting.[27]

Diagnosis of TOS is based on thorough neurovascular examination of the upper extremity supplemented by well-described provocative maneuvers, e.g., the Adson maneuver, Wright test, and Roos stress test, as well as imaging to determine the potential cause. The Adson maneuver involves neck extension and turning of the head toward the shoulder in question while the examiner abducts and extends the shoulder and palpates the ipsilateral radial pulse. Loss of the radial pulse or reproduction of paresthesias indicate a positive test. The Wright test similarly looks for diminution of the radial pulse or paresthesias as a result of progressive hyperabduction and extension of the patient's arm. Lastly, the Roos stress test involves the patient repeatedly opening and closing his/her hands over several minutes while his/her shoulders are in abduction and external rotation at 90 degrees and maintaining elbow flexion at 90 degrees. Reproduction of symptoms of pain or weakness or a feeling of heaviness and fatigue is consistent with TOS.[28] Although they are well described, provocative maneuvers for TOS have been historically criticized for high false-positive rates. In a study of these maneuvers on random healthy volunteers, 58% of subjects were found to have at least one positive test result.[29] Requiring multiple positive results across maneuvers may increase the specificity of the physical examination. The use of a pulse oximeter during provocative maneuvers may improve reproducibility and/or objectivity in the examination.[30] Radiologic findings include narrowing of the costoclavicular interval on magnetic resonance imaging (MRI)[31] as well as low-set clavicles on radiographs.[32] We perform the MRI and magnetic resonance angiography (MRA) of the affected brachial plexus in the adducted and abducted shoulder positions to assess for dynamic pathology affecting the brachial plexus neurovascular anatomy.

First-line management of nTOS is conservative, with directed physical therapy supplemented by anti-inflammatory or muscle-relaxant medications or minimally invasive strategies such as transcutaneous electrical stimulation or botulinum injections.[28] Most surgeons agree that if the nTOS does not improve in the first 6 months, surgical management may be pursued.[28] We base our surgical decision on the finding of multiple concordant clinical features: anatomical pathology on MRI or MRA, physical examination with objectively positive provocative maneuvers, denervation or slowing on electrodiagnostic studies consistent with brachial plexus–level lesion, and response to low-volume, ultrasound-guided anesthetic injections (if pain is the primary symptom).

Surgical intervention typically involves a decompression by a combination of scalenectomy, surrounding ligament resection, cervical or first rib resection, and rarely in recurrent cases, neurolysis of the proximal brachial plexus through one of the three approaches: transaxillary, supraclavicular, or posterior.[24] Surgical management is indicated for subclavian vein thrombosis (Paget-Schroetter syndrome) in vTOS and may involve local thrombolysis or embolectomy or arterial reconstruction in an acute arterial ischemic presentation by primary repair, autograft, synthetic prosthesis, or endovascular stenting. Overall success rates in surgical management of TOS range from 70 to 90%, with occupational or sports-related TOS being a factor for poor prognosis.[20]

23.3.2 Other Nerve Injuries about the Shoulder: Suprascapular Nerve, Long Thoracic Nerve, and Axillary Nerve

Similar to TOS, suprascapular nerve injury or entrapment is commonly associated with repetitive overhead motion, as seen in throwing athletes or volleyball players. Although it is a rare presentation overall, suprascapular nerve injury is the most frequently reported injury of the peripheral branch of the brachial plexus in athletes.[33] Suprascapular nerve injury is typically asymptomatic and is often only identifiable by infraspinatus muscle atrophy and subsequent electrodiagnostic testing.[34] Asymptomatic injury or "painless wasting" of the infraspinatus is thought to be associated with an incomplete lesion caused by entrapment at the spinoglenoid notch. In rarer cases involving entrapment at the suprascapular notch, the nerve lesion may be more severe, resulting in atrophy of both the supraspinatus and infraspinatus muscles and symptoms of weakness, activity-related fatigue, and a dull, aching pain or tenderness to palpation in the involved shoulder that is worse in the overhead position. After a compressive lesion, such as a ganglion cyst, is ruled out by imaging, the more severe suprascapular nerve injury with both supraspinatus and infraspinatus atrophy may benefit from surgical decompression. Asymptomatic infraspinatus atrophy can be managed with rest and physical therapy to support recovery.[33]

Long thoracic nerve injury in athletes is typically the result of traction injury and, although rare, can be disabling. It is thought that the length of the long thoracic nerve can be stretched up to twofold between its points of fixation at the scalene medius muscle and the superior aspect of the serratus anterior muscle, but that as little as a 10% stretch can result in neurapraxic injury.[35] Additionally, the long thoracic nerve is uniquely susceptible to acute compressive injury because of its subcutaneous location.[33] Athletes will present with an insidious onset of weakness, particularly when performing overhead activities, accompanied by notable winging of the scapula. The clinical presentation of long thoracic nerve injury must be differentiated from that of spinal accessory nerve injury, which may additionally result in atrophy or paralysis of the trapezius muscle and winging of the scapula with arms in abduction rather than forward elevation.[33] Atraumatic long thoracic nerve injury has a good prognosis for spontaneous recovery within 1 year with appropriate rest and mechanical support by an orthosis to hold the scapula to the chest wall to prevent continued overstretching.[36] Indications for surgical intervention include persistent symptoms beyond 1 to 2 years and lack of improvement on EMG. Surgery most commonly involves muscle transfer, scapulopexy, or scapulothoracic fusion, but these procedures will typically preclude an athlete's return to play.[20]

Axillary nerve injury represents less than 1% of all nerve injuries and is most often seen in athletes as an iatrogenic injury after rotator cuff surgery.[33] More direct trauma from a direct contusion, anterior shoulder dislocation, or proximal humerus fracture is also possible, causing stretching of the nerve across the humeral head.[37] Patients may be asymptomatic or present with deltoid weakness and inefficiencies with arm abduction as well as loss of sensation at the lateral arm. There is generally good prognosis for nerve recovery with nonsurgical management combined with proper management of any accompanying musculoskeletal insult; however, when there is no clinical or electrodiagnostic improvement within 3 to 6 months of rest and rehabilitation, large series suggest that surgical intervention yields the best results, including full recovery, when surgery is performed within 6 months of injury.[38] Surgical approaches may include neurolysis, nerve grafting or transfer, or neurotization.[39]

As previously noted, clinicians should be careful to distinguish isolated mononeuropathies, such as long thoracic palsy, from neuralgic amyotrophy. In our opinion, an isolated long thoracic palsy should be considered inflammatory until proven otherwise, unless there is strong evidence to suggest a mechanical impingement from athletics.

23.3.3 Musculocutaneous Nerve

Musculocutaneous nerve injury results from strenuous or repetitive hyperextension of the elbow, most often seen in weight lifters or players of racket sports, respectively.[8] The musculocutaneous nerve, derived from the lateral cord of the brachial plexus and nerve roots C5–C7, provides innervation to the coracobrachialis, biceps, and brachialis muscles and sensation via the lateral cutaneous nerve of the forearm to the lateral forearm. Most athletes with this type of injury will therefore present with elbow flexion weakness and paresthesias of the forearm that are exacerbated with continued use.[7] In all cases, rest, nonsteroidal anti-inflammatory agents, and an adjustment in training—with specific attention to correcting an overreliance on peripheral arm strength to a more core-based kinetic approach—will be a sufficient treatment paradigm.[8]

If symptoms persist beyond 6 weeks, local injection of steroids or anesthetics is advised, and decompressive surgery may be attempted in more refractory cases.[40]

23.3.4 Median Nerve

The median nerve, derived from both the medial and lateral cords of the brachial plexus from the C5–C8 nerve roots, innervates forearm flexors and some intrinsic hand muscles, particularly in the thenar eminence. Median nerve injury in athletes occurs either proximally along its course, resulting in pronator syndrome, or more distally at the transverse carpal ligament, resulting in the well-described carpal tunnel syndrome.[9]

The pronator syndrome results from proximal medial nerve compression at one of the three susceptible anatomical locations: (1) the lacertus fibrosus at the elbow, (2) between the superficial and deep heads of the pronator teres, and (3) the arch of the flexor digitorum superficialis.[41] Repetitive microtrauma by forceful pronation and supination during pitching or throwing, rowing, weight training, or racket sports has been described as causing pronator syndrome.[42] Additionally, grip-intensive sports, like archery, are known to cause pronator syndrome through compression of the median nerve specifically at the flexor digitorum superficialis of the third and fourth digits (▶ Fig. 23.1).[43] The most common presentation of pronator syndrome is a vague, stinging pain in the volar aspect of the elbow and forearm that worsens with repeated grasping or pronation. The pronator muscle can also present as a firm, inflamed muscle mass with tenderness to palpation.[44] Initial management is nonsurgical and involves rest, immobilization, nonsteroidal anti-inflammatory medications or steroids, and physical therapy. Decompressive surgery is recommended if there is persistent paresis for 3 months and conservative therapies have failed, and surgery has been reported to have a 90% success rate if executed promptly after diagnosis.[44]

Median nerve injury also occurs more distally at the transverse carpal ligament, where compression causes carpal tunnel syndrome, the most common entrapment neuropathy. Carpal tunnel syndrome results from repetitive or prolonged wrist extension (seen in athletes like rowers and bicyclists) that, in turn, generates a local synovitis and nerve compression.[45] Clinical presentation is typical: hand grip weakness and intermittent pain and paresthesias of the wrist and radial 3.5 digits (the median nerve provides sensory innervation to the palmar side of the radial 3.5 digits through its palmar digital branches). A positive Tinel sign and positive Phalen wrist flexion test can both be elicited. Carpal tunnel syndrome also produces characteristic electrodiagnostic findings: evidence of conduction abnormalities with prolonged latency or slowed conduction velocity on nerve conduction studies, with severity indicated by the degree of amplitude reduction of motor and sensory potentials or the presence of fibrillations on needle electrode examination of the abductor pollicis brevis.[46] Wrist splinting to avoid dorsiflexion of the wrist is found to be effective as a first-line treatment in up to 60% of affected patients.[47] Adjunctive conservative management with local corticosteroid injection may also provide temporary relief for up to 1 month.[48] In refractory cases, however, particularly in cases lasting for more than 3 months, surgical decompression is the only definitive treatment with a success rate at achieving a durable response of over 80%.[46,47] Additionally,

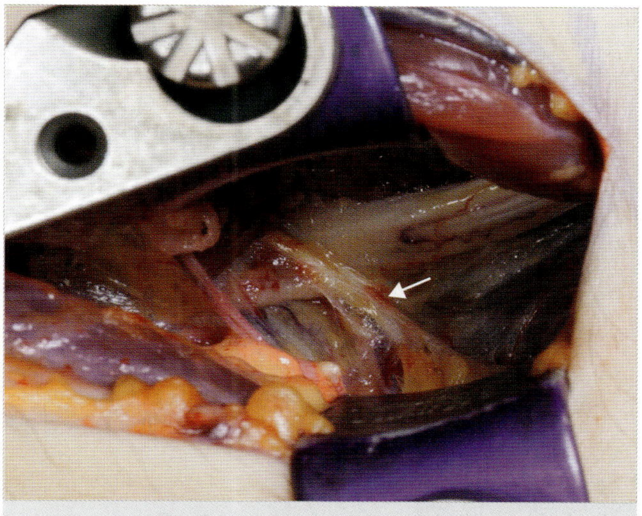

Fig. 23.1 Pronator syndrome in a 58-year-old recreational bicyclist who presented after failed carpal tunnel release. The ligament above the anterior interosseous nerve can be noted just before surgical release (*white arrow*). Note also the loss of vascularity and flow in the nerve due to compression by the ligament. (Used with permission from the Department of Neurosurgery, University of Utah.)

correct localization of the median nerve lesion is critical because the concurrent presence of a more proximal pronator syndrome (or underlying true diagnosis of a more proximal lesion) is a leading cause of failure in surgical carpal tunnel release, as seen in the case presented in ▶ Fig. 23.1.[49]

23.3.5 Ulnar Nerve

The ulnar nerve, derived from the medial cord of the brachial plexus and nerve roots C8–T1, is similarly susceptible to compression injury both proximally at the cubital tunnel and distally from entrapment at Guyon's canal. Proximal ulnar neuropathy is the most common peripheral nerve lesion in baseball players, particularly pitchers.[9] This lesion typically results from repeated microtrauma to the ulnar collateral ligament from excessive elbow valgus forces causing inflammation, calcification, or rupture of the ligament, secondarily causing ulnar nerve stretching or subluxation due to increased nerve mobility in the cubital tunnel.[50] Athletes typically present with paresthesias of the medial palm and the dorsal and palmar surfaces of the fifth and ulnar half of the fourth digits, as well as loss of grip strength. When the injury is severe, there can be an electrodiagnostic picture of axonal loss with the more distal intrinsic hand muscles affected most severely.[9] In a large series of baseball pitchers with ulnar neuropathy, 60% were able to return to competitive play over 2 months with only conservative treatment including rest, training adaptations, and compensatory strengthening exercises. Surgery was required in 33% of patients.[51] Simple decompression is thought to be inadequate for ulnar nerve subluxation, where anterior transposition is typically favored via either submuscular or subcutaneous approach.[52]

In some cases of proximal ulnar neuropathy, athletes may report a snapping or popping sensation—the result of ulnar nerve subluxation followed by the snapping of the medial triceps over the medial epicondyle, also known as snapping triceps syndrome. Anatomical variations such as a prominent medial head of the triceps, hypertrophy of the distal triceps, history of a displaced supracondylar humerus fracture, or hypoplasia of the medial epicondyle can predispose an athlete to snapping triceps syndrome. Snapping triceps is most common in weight-lifter or body-builder athletes. Snapping triceps syndrome is most commonly and most effectively treated with surgery by excising the medial head of the triceps, by transposition of the triceps, or with distal humeral osteotomy.[53]

As in carpal tunnel syndrome, excessive wrist extension and repeated pressure on the wrist can also lead to compressive injury of the ulnar nerve at Guyon's canal. Chronic stress injury is most commonly seen in bicyclists. Fracture of the hook of the hamate can also result in this injury more acutely. Examination will show intrinsic hand and grip weakness, particularly in the hypothenar muscles.[7] The pattern of sensory deficits is distinct between proximal and distal ulnar nerve injuries. In proximal injuries, sensation in both palmar and dorsal hand is affected, along with the digital sensation. In distal injuries, dorsal sensation is uniformly preserved, palmar sensation is variably affected, and digital sensation is always decreased. Electrodiagnostic studies can be used to differentiate a lesion of Guyon's canal from a more proximal ulnar nerve lesion; testing will involve assessing motor latencies from the wrist to the intrinsic hand muscles. Abnormal EMG findings of the flexor carpi ulnaris and the flexor digitorum profundus will indicate a more proximal ulnar lesion.[54] Treatment focuses on conservative management with appropriate rest and adoption of protective equipment like supportive braces or padded gloves for bicyclists.

23.3.6 Radial Nerve

The radial nerve is derived from the posterior cord of the brachial plexus, comprising the C5–C8 nerve roots. Radial nerve injury in sports is generally rare, but when seen, it is most commonly a consequence of a humerus fracture and classically presents with wrist and finger drop as well as sensory loss in the dorsolateral hand.[55] In severe, displaced fractures, complete nerve transection may be seen and require nerve graft repair (▶ Fig. 23.2). Additionally, the posterior interosseous branch of the radial nerve is susceptible to repetitive overuse injury and entrapment at the arcade of Fröhse (the proximal fibrous origin in the supinator muscle) after repetitive pronation and supination. This is particularly common in tennis players. These athletes will present with forearm pain that worsens with supination resistance while the elbow is flexed at 90 degrees, but without sensory loss.[8] Treatment for radial nerve injury involves treating the underlying cause (i.e., humerus fracture) and, particularly in posterior interosseous neuropathy, physical therapy and retraining focused on decreasing forearm dependence in tennis stroke technique. Surgical decompression is rarely used but can be successfully employed in refractory cases.[8] Similarly, isolated posterior interosseous nerve palsy should be carefully distinguished from inflammatory causes.

23.4 Lower Extremity

23.4.1 Sciatic Nerve and Piriformis Syndrome

The sciatic nerve, derived from spinal nerves L4–S3, arises from the sacral plexus and exits the pelvis through the sciatic notch inferior to the piriformis muscle to descend down the posteromedial thigh before splitting into the common fibular nerve and the tibial nerve. In sports, the sciatic nerve is most commonly injured as a consequence of an acute contact/collision causing compression of the nerve against the hip capsule.[7] Athletes with this acute sciatic neuropathy present with hamstring weakness and gluteal paresthesias that typically resolve

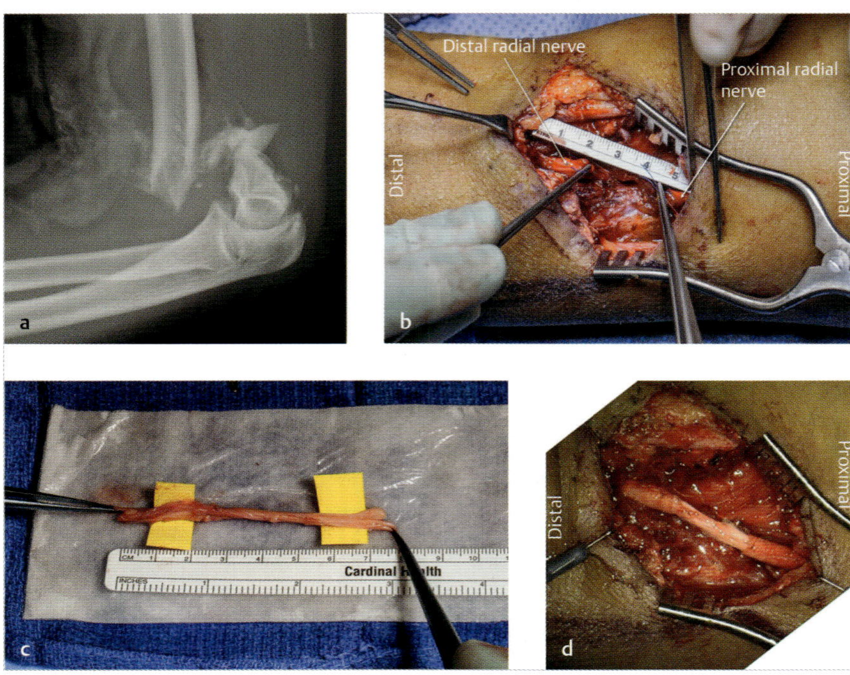

Fig. 23.2 Distal humerus fracture and nerve graft repair in a 14-year-old girl who sustained injury during a horse-riding competition. **(a)** Lateral X-ray showing displaced and multifragmentary distal humerus fracture. **(b)** Anterior exposure of the radial nerve demonstrates complete nerve transection as a consequence of fracture. **(c)** Sural nerve harvested for radial nerve graft. **(d)** Radial nerve after anastomotic repair using sural nerve graft. (Used with permission from the Department of Neurosurgery, University of Utah.)

with conservative management. Electrodiagnostic testing will show decreased compound muscle action potential amplitudes in the fibular and tibial nerves. Notably, EMG of the fibular muscles has been shown to be more sensitive for identifying acute sciatic nerve injury than EMG of the tibial muscles.[56]

A chronic, repetitive overuse sciatic nerve entrapment syndrome called "piriformis syndrome" has also been described. This diagnosis is extremely controversial, as it is frequently used as an explanation for chronic hamstring or vague sciatic pain without focal neurologic signs.[57] The piriformis muscle is innervated by the nerve to the piriformis, originating from spinal nerves S1–S2, but more importantly, it intimately covers the sciatic nerve as it exits the sciatic notch, or may surround the sciatic nerve, known as a split piriformis muscle. Entrapment of the sciatic nerve in this space has been described as due to either piriformis hypertrophy or overuse-related inflammation in athletes, although the frequent lack of accompanying clinical findings of distal sciatica also suggests correlation without causation. Alternatively, entrapment of nearby gluteal nerves or the posterior cutaneous nerve of the thigh may be the cause of chronic pain.[58] Several systematic reviews have established common features of piriformis syndrome for diagnosis, including gluteal pain aggravated by sitting, external tenderness at the sciatic notch, and positive findings with maneuvers that increase piriformis muscle tension. These same studies, however, note that clinical presentation cannot reliably differentiate piriformis syndrome from diskogenic neuropathy, mechanical disorders, or tendinopathies of the hip.[59] First-line management is conservative, but refractory cases may be amenable to decompressive surgery and neurolysis: through blunt dissection of the gluteus maximus and palpation to localize the sciatic nerve, compressive lesions and anatomical variations can be directly addressed, or in cases without obvious abnormality, the piriformis muscle can be divided to reduce potential irritation.[57] Quality outcome studies on the surgical treatment of piriformis syndrome are lacking.

23.4.2 Pudendal Nerve

Pudendal nerve injury is a potential compressive injury, such as those that may occur from prolonged bicycling. The pudendal nerve, with origins in the S2–S4 nerve roots, supplies sensory innervation to the anal and genital regions and some motor and sympathetic innervation for erectile muscles and tissues. Direct compression of the nerve and compression-induced ischemia causing secondary neuropathy are the major causes of pudendal nerve injury in cyclists.[8] Clinical presentation of genital pain, sometimes with sexual or urinary dysfunction, is well characterized. Electrodiagnostic studies will show conduction delay in local somatosensory evoked potentials and, in men, latency of the bulbocavernosus reflex.[60] Treatment focuses on ergonomic modification of the bicycle seat; wider bicycle seats support the ischial tuberosities and thereby distribute pressure away from the perineal area. Physical therapy with pelvic floor strengthening exercises may also be beneficial.[9]

23.4.3 Lateral Femoral Cutaneous Nerve

The lateral femoral cutaneous nerve is a pure sensory nerve that arises from the L2–L3 spinal nerve contributions to the lumbar plexus. It is susceptible to both acute contact/collision injury and chronic overuse injury or entrapment in athletes. After blunt trauma to the inguinal region, athletes may manifest a lateral femoral cutaneous neurapraxia with numbness and paresthesias at the lateral thigh that typically self-resolves within days to weeks.[9] Repetitive overuse injury can be seen in athletes who perform repetitive flexion and extension of the hip, such as gymnasts or other jumping athletes, or as a consequence of chronic compression from ill-fitting gear, such as rock-climbing harnesses.[8] Clinical lesion localization with a unique sensory neuropathy is generally diagnostic. Electrodiagnostic testing tends to be equivocal in these cases.[61] Preventative measures to ensure well-fitting equipment and adequate periodization of training and rest characterize primary management.

23.4.4 Femoral Nerve

The femoral nerve arises from the L2–L4 spinal nerve contributions to the lumbar plexus, and provides motor innervation to the quadriceps and sensory innervation to the medial thigh and anteromedial shin. Although they are rare in athletes, acute femoral nerve injuries from traumatic hyperextension of the hip in gymnastics, dancing, weight training, and contact sports have been described.[8] These neurapraxic injuries present with inguinal pain, sensory loss in the medial thigh, and quadriceps weakness experienced as leg buckling. Provocative maneuvers eliciting pain on hip extension and a diminished knee reflex support the diagnosis. Because femoral neuropathy is typically post-traumatic, MRI of the pelvis is recommended to rule out a concomitant tear or hemorrhage of the iliopsoas muscles, which can require surgical treatment for a psoas compartment syndrome.[62] Treatment is otherwise conservative.

23.4.5 Fibular Nerve

The common fibular nerve is the lateral continuation of the sciatic nerve that courses through the popliteal fossa and runs obliquely around the fibular neck before dividing into superficial and deep branches after passing through the peroneus longus muscle. It is the most commonly injured peripheral nerve of the lower extremity. The fibular nerve can be injured acutely from blunt trauma, as a consequence of traction or destabilizing injury to the knee or ankle, by traction from a lateral knee ligament tear, or by chronic, repetitive stress resulting in either an intrinsic overuse injury or compartment syndrome. In all cases, because of the extensive innervation of the common fibular nerve and its branches, electrodiagnostic studies are essential to localize the site and extent of the lesion and can inform management and prognostication.[9]

The common fibular nerve is most superficial, and therefore most susceptible to external injury, as it crosses the fibular head. Traumatic injury to the nerve resulting in a neurapraxia is common in contact sports, particularly in skiing, soccer, and football.[63] Athletes will present with sudden onset of numbness to the lateral lower leg and dorsum of the foot and a partial-to-complete foot drop that typically self-resolves within days. In refractory cases or those associated with severe pain, imaging is warranted to rule out a concomitant fracture that may require additional fixation. Notably, common fibular nerve injury is also a common complication in the operative treatment of proximal tibial or fibular fracture.[64]

Traction injury to the common fibular nerve with varus knee injuries or to the superficial and deep fibular nerves with lateral ankle sprains is often overlooked. Poor recovery in these injuries is often misattributed to incomplete rehabilitation rather than intrinsic nerve damage.[8] In the knee, particularly after multiple ligament injuries or knee dislocation, the destabilized biomechanics of the knee create increased susceptibility for excessive stretch and subluxation of the common fibular nerve. This type of injury is common with varus knee injuries and can result in a wide degree of injury severities from neurapraxia to axonotmesis (▶ Fig. 23.3). Additionally, clinicians treating ankle sprains should watch for clinical signs of superficial or deep fibular neuropathy, which are known to have a delayed onset in this setting.[65] Conservative management is favored, but surgical management involving neurolysis and nerve decompression is indicated if there is no evidence of functional recovery by 3 to 7 months after the initial injury.[66] Nerve transfers have occasionally been employed for recovery after injury, with variable success in lower quality studies.

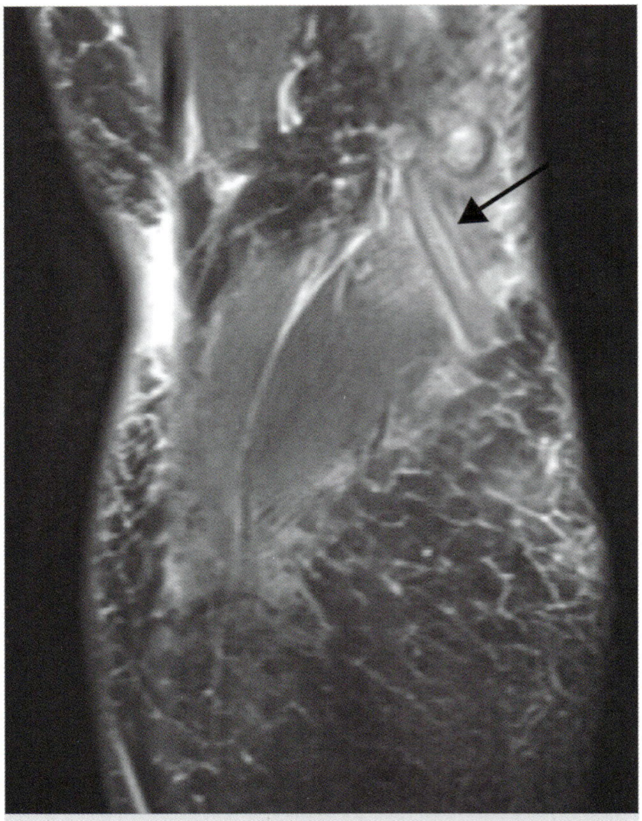

Fig. 23.3 Common fibular nerve traction (stretch) injury in a 42-year-old rock climber secondary to lateral knee distraction injury after an 8-foot fall. Magnetic resonance imaging (MRI) (coronal short tau inversion recovery) depicting fascicular hyperintensity of the common fibular nerve proximal to the fibular head (*black arrow*). Severe axonotmesis was also seen on electromyography (EMG) in this patient. (Used with permission from the Department of Neurosurgery, University of Utah.)

The common fibular nerve is also susceptible to repetitive stress injury, especially in running athletes.[8] With repeated irritation, a tight fascial band can form along the fibular neck where the nerve courses through the peroneus longus muscle, resulting in nerve entrapment. Most affected athletes will be asymptomatic at rest but experience paresthesias and varying degrees of foot drop while running. Although the effectiveness of orthotics or supportive footwear is poorly defined, surgical intervention involving neurolysis or the release of the fascial band has been reported to alleviate symptoms consistently.[8] Running athletes are also more susceptible to ischemic injury to the superficial and deep fibular nerves from chronic exertional compartment syndrome involving either or both of the anterior and lateral lower leg compartments. These athletes will similarly present with pain on exertion, and when compartment syndrome is suspected, clinicians should perform compartment pressure measurements. Treatment typically involves rest, an improved periodization schedule, and possibly changes to the athlete's running technique, but may also involve fasciotomy in more severe cases.[67]

23.4.6 Tibial Nerve

Injury to the tibial nerve, the medial division of the sciatic nerve involving nerve roots L4–S3, is the cause of tarsal tunnel syndrome. Athletes who consistently apply a heavy ankle burden, such as runners, climbers, dancers, and jumpers, are most susceptible to tarsal tunnel syndrome.[68] Because of repetitive overuse, the tibial nerve becomes entrapped between the medial malleolus and the flexor retinaculum. Pain radiating from the medial ankle throughout the foot that worsens with either standing or walking is the predominant symptom. Diagnosis can be difficult because the symptoms of tarsal tunnel syndrome can be explained by a host of other foot and ankle problems. Electrodiagnostic evaluation (including stimulation of the medial and lateral plantar nerves) to identify decreased sensory conduction and subsequent comparison to the unaffected foot supports the diagnosis in over 80% of cases.[69] Symptom control with nonsteroidal anti-inflammatory agents, orthotics, and sometimes corticosteroid injections is the mainstay of treatment. Surgery, mostly commonly involving division of the deep portion of the abductor hallucis fascia and release of the nerve from the flexor retinaculum, is used in refractory cases with only limited reported success.[69]

23.4.7 Morton's Neuroma

Morton's neuroma is a common cause of metatarsalgia, consisting of interdigital nerve disease classically located at the third intermetatarsal space, and is particularly common in ballet dancers and other athletes who recurrently hyperextend their metatarsal arches. Morton's neuroma was first classified by George Morton in 1876 as a pain syndrome of the fourth metatarsophalangeal joint affecting mostly women, and soon after, Hoadley[70] excised the first interdigital neuroma at the third intermetatarsal and redefined the cause of pain. Morton's neuroma has consistently occurred with a higher incidence in women, with a female-to-male ratio of 4:1, and most commonly affects the third intermetatarsal space (66%), followed by the second (32%) and fourth spaces (2%).[71] Patients will present with burning plantar pain radiating to the two involved toes, which is exacerbated by tight footwear or continued stress (i.e., dancing). Mulder's sign, acute intermetatarsal pain, and a palpable clicking sensation induced by applying pressure to the intermetatarsal space while simultaneously tightening the metatarsals with another hand, will be positive with high sensitivity. Lack of pain on the metatarsal heads can differentiate Morton's neuroma from arthritic causes of pain, but X-rays remain essential to rule out other causes when more than one intermetatarsal space is affected or when the clinical picture is unclear.[72]

Although short-term or partial relief can be achieved with conservative management, including plantar orthoses and corticosteroid injections, some have argued that surgical intervention may provide a durable pain response. Surgical neurectomy is the most common treatment, through either a dorsal or plantar approach, while others have recommended decompression.[73] Advocates of the dorsal approach describe its advantages as including easier rehabilitation since the incision is not on a weight-bearing surface, ease of excision of the plantar cutaneous nerves without having to navigate plantar fatty tissue, and lower rates of wound infection, hematoma formation, and other incision-related complications. The plantar approach, however, does not require additional release of the distal metatarsal transverse ligament, which itself has been suggested to be a cause of metatarsalgia. Overall, surgical neurectomy success rates range from 51 to 85% in long-term follow-up.[72] Additional interventions such as percutaneous distal metatarsal transverse ligament release with or without metatarsal osteotomy or dorsal neuroma suspension/transposition surgery have also been described with similar efficacy rates.[74]

23.5 Conclusions

Peripheral nerve injuries remain a critical yet under-reported and under-recognized cause of athletic injury that can significantly delay or preclude an athlete's return to play when not adequately addressed. Clinician's familiarity with the potential causes for such injuries, including differentiating acute traumatic from repetitive overuse injuries, is crucial because etiology intimately informs diagnosis, management, and prognosis. Furthermore, proper diagnosis and management depend on placing the neuropathy in the context of the sport and the athlete's training regimen and periodization strategy. In most cases, initial conservative management is appropriate, especially when the treatment strategy involves a combination of adequate rest, training of compensatory musculature, pain management, and use of preventative measures such as well-fitted equipment or orthoses. Surgical intervention, most commonly nerve decompression, is the mainstay of treatment in refractory cases. However, a critical limitation of the literature on the peripheral nerve in sports-related injury remains the overall relative scarcity of reported cases, series, or trials examining the comparative effectiveness across surgical approaches or even between conservative and surgical management. Furthermore, guidelines informing a strategy or a timeline for an athlete's safe return to play across injury types are inconsistent and, where present, are based on lower levels of evidence.

23.6 Clinical Pearls

- Acute peripheral nerve injuries can be defined by the degree of anatomic nerve disruption according to the classic Seddon criteria: neurapraxia—focal conduction block; axonotmesis—axonal injury without disruption of the nerve; and neurotmesis—complete transection of nerve and surrounding structures.
- Chronic peripheral nerve injury, also known as overuse injury, typically results from repetitive microtrauma or maladaptation of the given nerve due to poor "periodization" of athletic training and will require significant shifts in training paradigms for successful recuperation.
- An important differential diagnosis in the evaluation of acute peripheral nerve injuries includes inflammatory causes, such as neuralgic amyotrophy or Parsonage Turner syndrome. These inflammatory conditions are a common cause of delayed-onset nerve injury after intense sporting events. Oral corticosteroids may be advised in the first 2 weeks after onset.
- "Burners" or "stingers" represent the most common sports-related nerve injury, particularly in contact sports, and, although often overlooked, can lead to prolonged functional deficits in up to 10% of cases. Repeated burner injury is associated with refractory deficits.
- Different sports have common chronic peripheral nerve injuries in the upper extremity, such as pronator syndrome in gripping sports, ulnar neuropathy in throwing sports, or radial nerve trauma in racquet sports.
- In the lower extremity, the common fibular nerve is the lower extremity nerve most susceptible to external traumatic injury given its superficial position as it crosses the fibular head and will result in sudden onset of numbness to the lateral lower leg and dorsal foot with a partial to complete foot drop. Surgical treatment of other diagnoses, such as piriformis syndrome, tarsal tunnel syndrome, and Morton's neuroma, has controversies with regard to appropriate diagnosis and surgical approach.

References

[1] Hirasawa Y, Sakakida K. Sports and peripheral nerve injury. Am J Sports Med. 1983; 11(6):420–426

[2] Hainline B. Peripheral nerve injury in sport: an overview. Handb Clin Neurol. 2018; 158:381–384

[3] Seddon HJ. Three types of nerve injury. Brain. 1943; 66(4):237–288

[4] Sunderland S. A classification of peripheral nerve injuries producing loss of function. Brain. 1951; 74(4):491–516

[5] Wilbourn AJ. The electrodiagnostic examination with peripheral nerve injuries. Clin Plast Surg. 2003; 30(2):139–154

[6] Flores AJ, Lavernia CJ, Owens PW. Anatomy and physiology of peripheral nerve injury and repair. Am J Orthop. 2000; 29(3):167–173

[7] Lorei MP, Hershman EB. Peripheral nerve injuries in athletes. Treatment and prevention. Sports Med. 1993; 16(2):130–147

[8] Hainline BW. Peripheral nerve injury in sports. Continuum (Minneap Minn). 2014; 20 6 Sports Neurology:1605–1628

[9] Lolis AM, Falsone S, Beric A. Common peripheral nerve injuries in sport: diagnosis and management. Handb Clin Neurol. 2018; 158:401–419

[10] Gabbett TJ. The training-injury prevention paradox: should athletes be training smarter and harder? Br J Sports Med. 2016; 50(5):273–280

[11] van Alfen N, van Engelen BG. The clinical spectrum of neuralgic amyotrophy in 246 cases. Brain. 2006; 129(Pt 2):438–450

[12] Krivickas LS, Wilbourn AJ. Peripheral nerve injuries in athletes: a case series of over 200 injuries. Semin Neurol. 2000; 20(2):225–232

[13] Page S, Guy JA. Neurapraxia, "stingers," and spinal stenosis in athletes. South Med J. 2004; 97(8):766–769

[14] Di Benedetto M, Markey K. Electrodiagnostic localization of traumatic upper trunk brachial plexopathy. Arch Phys Med Rehabil. 1984; 65(1):15–17

[15] Sallis RE, Jones K, Knopp W. Burners. Phys Sportsmed. 1992; 20(11):47–55

[16] Speer KP, Bassett FH, III. The prolonged burner syndrome. Am J Sports Med. 1990; 18(6):591–594

[17] Olmarker K. Spinal nerve root compression. Nutrition and function of the porcine cauda equina compressed in vivo. Acta Orthop Scand Suppl. 1991; 242(sup)(242):1–27

[18] Levitz CL, Reilly PJ, Torg JS. The pathomechanics of chronic, recurrent cervical nerve root neurapraxia. The chronic burner syndrome. Am J Sports Med. 1997; 25(1):73–76

[19] Bateman JE. Nerve injuries about the shoulder in sports. J Bone Joint Surg Am. 1967; 49(4):785–792

[20] Safran MR. Nerve injury about the shoulder in athletes, part 2: long thoracic nerve, spinal accessory nerve, burners/stingers, thoracic outlet syndrome. Am J Sports Med. 2004; 32(4):1063–1076

[21] Bland JH. Helping athletes avoid neck injuries. J Musculoskel Med. 1996; 13: 30–38

[22] Bailes JE, Petschauer M, Guskiewicz KM, Marano G. Management of cervical spine injuries in athletes. J Athl Train. 2007; 42(1):126–134

[23] Torg JS, Ramsey-Emrhein JA. Management guidelines for participation in collision activities with congenital, developmental, or postinjury lesions involving the cervical spine. Clin J Sport Med. 1997; 7(4):273–291

[24] Klaassen Z, Sorenson E, Tubbs RS, et al. Thoracic outlet syndrome: a neurological and vascular disorder. Clin Anat. 2014; 27(5):724–732

[25] Chandra V, Little C, Lee JT. Thoracic outlet syndrome in high-performance athletes. J Vasc Surg. 2014; 60(4):1012–1017, discussion 1017–1018

[26] White PW, Fox CJ, Feuerstein IM. Cervical rib causing arterial thoracic outlet syndrome. J Am Coll Surg. 2009; 209(1):148–149

[27] Angle N, Gelabert HA, Farooq MM, et al. Safety and efficacy of early surgical decompression of the thoracic outlet for Paget-Schroetter syndrome. Ann Vasc Surg. 2001; 15(1):37–42

[28] Kuhn JE, Lebus V GF, Bible JE. Thoracic outlet syndrome. J Am Acad Orthop Surg. 2015; 23(4):222–232

[29] Warrens AN, Heaton JM. Thoracic outlet compression syndrome: the lack of reliability of its clinical assessment. Ann R Coll Surg Engl. 1987; 69(5): 203–204

[30] Braun RM, Rechnic M, Shah KN. Pulse oximetry measurements in the evaluation of patients with possible thoracic outlet syndrome. J Hand Surg Am. 2012; 37(12):2564–2569

[31] Demirbag D, Unlu E, Ozdemir F, et al. The relationship between magnetic resonance imaging findings and postural maneuver and physical examination tests in patients with thoracic outlet syndrome: results of a double-blind, controlled study. Arch Phys Med Rehabil. 2007; 88(7):844–851

[32] Cho YJ, Lee HJ, Gong HS, Rhee SH, Park SJ, Baek GH. The radiologic relationship of the shoulder girdle to the thorax as an aid in diagnosing neurogenic thoracic outlet syndrome. J Hand Surg Am. 2012; 37(6):1187–1193

[33] Safran MR. Nerve injury about the shoulder in athletes, part 1: suprascapular nerve and axillary nerve. Am J Sports Med. 2004; 32(3):803–819

[34] Abou-Al-Shaar H, Awad AW, Mahan MA. Bilateral suprascapular nerve injury and novel technique of nerve transfers for restoration of external rotation: case report. Oper Neurosurg (Hagerstown). 2020; 18(4):423–429

[35] Sunderland S. The anatomy and physiology of nerve injury. Muscle Nerve. 1990; 13(9):771–784

[36] Marin R. Scapula winger's brace: a case series on the management of long thoracic nerve palsy. Arch Phys Med Rehabil. 1998; 79(10):1226–1230

[37] Visser CP, Coene LN, Brand R, Tavy DL. Nerve lesions in proximal humeral fractures. J Shoulder Elbow Surg. 2001; 10(5):421–427

[38] Coene LN, Narakas AO. Operative management of lesions of the axillary nerve, isolated or combined with other nerve lesions. Clin Neurol Neurosurg. 1992; 94 Suppl:S64–S66

[39] Petrucci FS, Morelli A, Raimondi PL. Axillary nerve injuries—21 cases treated by nerve graft and neurolysis. J Hand Surg Am. 1982; 7(3):271–278

[40] Bassett FH, III, Nunley JA. Compression of the musculocutaneous nerve at the elbow. J Bone Joint Surg Am. 1982; 64(7):1050–1052

[41] Regan WD, Morrey BF. Entrapment neuropathies about the elbow. In: DeLee J, Drez D, Miller M, eds. Orthopaedic Sports Medicine: Principles and Practice. 2nd ed. Philadelphia: WB Saunders; 2002:1323–1335

[42] McCue FC, Alexander EJ, Baumgarten TE. Median nerve entrapment at the elbow in athletes. Oper Tech Sports Med. 1996; 4(1):21–27

[43] Sicuranza MJ, McCue FC, III. Compressive neuropathies in the upper extremity of athletes. Hand Clin. 1992; 8(2):263–273

[44] Rehak DC. Pronator syndrome. Clin Sports Med. 2001; 20(3):531–540

[45] Collins K, Storey M, Peterson K, Nutter P. Nerve injuries in athletes. Phys Sportsmed. 1988; 16(1):92–100

[46] Arnold WD, Elsheikh BH. Entrapment neuropathies. Neurol Clin. 2013; 31 (2):405–424

[47] Gerritsen AA, de Vet HC, Scholten RJ, Bertelsmann FW, de Krom MC, Bouter LM. Splinting vs surgery in the treatment of carpal tunnel syndrome: a randomized controlled trial. JAMA. 2002; 288(10):1245–1251

[48] Marshall S, Tardif G, Ashworth N. Local corticosteroid injection for carpal tunnel syndrome. Cochrane Database Syst Rev. 2007(2):CD001554

[49] Johnson RK, Spinner M, Shrewsbury MM. Median nerve entrapment syndrome in the proximal forearm. J Hand Surg Am. 1979; 4(1):48–51

[50] Anderson MW, Alford BA. Overhead throwing injuries of the shoulder and elbow. Radiol Clin North Am. 2010; 48(6):1137–1154

[51] Maruyama M, Satake H, Takahara M, et al. Treatment for ulnar neuritis around the elbow in adolescent baseball players: factors associated with poor outcome. Am J Sports Med. 2017; 45(4):803–809

[52] Treihaft MM. Neurologic injuries in baseball players. Semin Neurol. 2000; 20 (2):187–193

[53] Rioux-Forker D, Bridgeman J, Brogan DM. Snapping triceps syndrome. J Hand Surg Am. 2018; 43(1):90.e1–90.e5

[54] Dimberg EL. Electrodiagnostic evaluation of ulnar neuropathy and other upper extremity mononeuropathies. Neurol Clin. 2012; 30(2):479–503

[55] Ljungquist KL, Martineau P, Allan C. Radial nerve injuries. J Hand Surg Am. 2015; 40(1):166–172

[56] Yuen EC, So YT, Olney RK. The electrophysiologic features of sciatic neuropathy in 100 patients. Muscle Nerve. 1995; 18(4):414–420

[57] Durrani Z, Winnie AP. Piriformis muscle syndrome: an underdiagnosed cause of sciatica. J Pain Symptom Manage. 1991; 6(6):374–379

[58] McCrory P, Bell S. Nerve entrapment syndromes as a cause of pain in the hip, groin and buttock. Sports Med. 1999; 27(4):261–274

[59] Hopayian K, Danielyan A. Four symptoms define the piriformis syndrome: an updated systematic review of its clinical features. Eur J Orthop Surg Traumatol. 2018; 28(2):155–164

[60] Ricchiuti VS, Haas CA, Seftel AD, Chelimsky T, Goldstein I. Pudendal nerve injury associated with avid bicycling. J Urol. 1999; 162(6):2099–2100

[61] Sarala PK, Nishihara T, Oh SJ. Meralgia paresthetica: electrophysiologic study. Arch Phys Med Rehabil. 1979; 60(1):30–31

[62] Giuliani G, Poppi M, Acciarri N, Forti A. CT scan and surgical treatment of traumatic iliacus hematoma with femoral neuropathy: case report. J Trauma. 1990; 30(2):229–231

[63] Cho D, Saetia K, Lee S, Kline DG, Kim DH. Peroneal nerve injury associated with sports-related knee injury. Neurosurg Focus. 2011; 31(5):E11

[64] Rausch V, Hackl M, Oppermann J, et al. Peroneal nerve location at the fibular head: an anatomic study using 3D imaging. Arch Orthop Trauma Surg. 2019; 139(7):921–926

[65] Mitsiokapa E, Mavrogenis AF, Drakopoulos D, Mauffrey C, Scarlat M. Peroneal nerve palsy after ankle sprain: an update. Eur J Orthop Surg Traumatol. 2017; 27(1):53–60

[66] Ferraresi S, Garozzo D, Buffatti P. Common peroneal nerve injuries: results with one-stage nerve repair and tendon transfer. Neurosurg Rev. 2003; 26 (3):175–179

[67] Diebal AR, Gregory R, Alitz C, Gerber JP. Effects of forefoot running on chronic exertional compartment syndrome: a case series. Int J Sports Phys Ther. 2011; 6(4):312–321

[68] Kinoshita M, Okuda R, Yasuda T, Abe M. Tarsal tunnel syndrome in athletes. Am J Sports Med. 2006; 34(8):1307–1312

[69] Bailie DS, Kelikian AS. Tarsal tunnel syndrome: diagnosis, surgical technique, and functional outcome. Foot Ankle Int. 1998; 19(2):65–72

[70] Hoadley AE. Six cases of metatarsalgia. Chic Med Rec. 1893; 5:32–37

[71] Kasparek M, Schneider W. Surgical treatment of Morton's neuroma: clinical results after open excision. Int Orthop. 2013; 37(9):1857–1861

[72] Di Caprio F, Meringolo R, Shehab Eddine M, Ponziani L. Morton's interdigital neuroma of the foot: a literature review. Foot Ankle Surg. 2018; 24(2):92–98

[73] Dellon AL. Treatment of Morton's neuroma as a nerve compression. The role for neurolysis. J Am Podiatr Med Assoc. 1992; 82(8):399–402

[74] Song JH, Kang C, Hwang DS, Kang DH, Kim YH. Dorsal suspension for Morton's neuroma: a comparison with neurectomy. Foot Ankle Surg. 2019; 25(6):748–754

Part IV

Sports

IV

24 American Football

Randall W. Porter, Joseph D. DiDomenico, D. Scott Kreiner, Javier Cardenas, and Wayne Kuhl

Summary
This chapter discusses the most common spinal diseases that American football players experience. American football is the most viewed and popular sport across the United States. It accounts for the highest number of high school and college athletic participants, and it exposes these individuals to a high risk of cervical or thoracolumbar injuries. Injuries can vary from simple contusions and strains to life-threatening spinal cord injury. The cervical spine, in particular, is the most common site of injuries to the axial skeleton of American football players, and these injuries are usually associated with flexion and axial load. The most common pathologic conditions associated with football-related cervical injuries are cervical spondylosis, disk herniation, and stenosis. When a player receives a direct blow to a peripheral nerve, most commonly the brachial plexus, the player can experience a stinger, also known as brachial plexus neuropraxia. These injuries are characterized as nondermatomal sudden pain syndromes, with associated paresthesias or dysesthesias, with or without weakness. Thoracolumbar injuries are much less common, are rarely catastrophic, and are often associated with repetitive hyperextension. Disk injuries are most frequently localized to the lumbar spine, and football players have disproportionate rates of degenerative disease. In general, conservative management is the most prudent initial approach when considering an athlete's ability to return to play. However, in cases in which a neurologic deficit or instability is diagnosed, players may require surgical intervention. In all cases, an athlete should return to play only after symptoms have completely resolved, findings from musculoskeletal and neurologic examination are normal, full range of motion has been regained, and soft-tissue injury, bone fracture, or both are completely healed.

Keywords: cervical, disk herniation, football, fracture, neurapraxia, spine, spondylosis, thoracolumbar

24.1 Introduction

American football is one of the most popular sports in the United States, consistently ranking as the most viewed sport on television.[1] Not surprisingly, it has the highest number of participants in high school and college athletics.[2] Despite this popularity, football has come under the spotlight for both concussions and spinal injuries, along with concern for the long-term effects of repetitive injuries. As previously discussed in Part I of this book, mild traumatic brain injuries and concussions in these athletes have been an area of increased focus and extreme attention in the media. Currently, at least three independent neurosurgeons or neurologists attend each National Football League (NFL) game as per the collective bargaining agreement. Spinal injuries, no less important, have received less attention save for the most catastrophic injuries. Evaluation on and off the field and treatment of acute spine injuries in professional football players continue to evolve. Further, no "return-to-play" guidelines have been established. Historically, evaluation was completed on the field by orthopedic surgeons, team doctors, trainers, and now unaffiliated neurotrauma consultants. However, more recently it has become apparent that these injuries should be evaluated and treated more specifically by spine specialists who treat traumatic spinal injuries in their weekly practice. It is no longer appropriate for these players to be evaluated and treated by a neurologist or orthopedic surgeon who does not treat traumatic spine patients as part of his or her regular practice. Ideally, these individuals would, as part of their credentials, cover traumatic spinal injuries at a level I trauma center. Given the sport's high-impact nature, participants are exposed to high risks of cervical and thoracolumbar injuries. The severity of injury can range significantly in the acute stage, from a transient neurapraxia to life-threatening spinal cord injury (SCI). Furthermore, football players, particularly those who play at a high level, are more likely to develop chronic degenerative diseases of the spinal column than nonathletes. These conditions are managed in athletes much like they are in the general population; however, additional consideration is necessary with regard to return-to-play guidelines, decision-making, the time and value lost to injury, and the effect that conservative and surgical interventions may have on performance. This chapter discusses the most common injuries and diseases of the spine affecting American football players.

24.2 Cervical Spine Injuries in Football Players

24.2.1 Epidemiology and Pathogenesis

Contact sports place athletes at higher risk of cervical spine injuries, with 15% of all cervical spine injuries being sports-related.[3,4] American football is one of the greatest contributors to this subset, and the cervical spine is also the most commonly localized site of injury to the axial skeleton of American football players.[3] Athletes at the linebacker, defensive back, running back, or offensive line positions have been reported to have higher rates of cervical pathology than players at other positions.[5,6] In a recent study published on the epidemiology of cervical spine injuries of National Collegiate Athletic Association (NCAA) football players, 7,496 cervical spine injuries were identified.[7] More than 85% were new injuries, occurring at a rate of 2.91 per 10,000 athlete exposures. Of all injuries, the most common were stingers, occurring at a rate of 1.87 per 10,000 athlete exposures, followed by cervical strains at a rate of 0.80 per 10,000 athlete exposures. Injuries were nine times more likely to occur during competition compared with practice settings. Division I athletes were more likely to sustain cervical injuries compared with Division II and III athletes. The primary mechanism of injury was direct contact–related injuries, constituting 90.8% of all injuries sustained. Linebackers and defensive linemen were most likely to sustain injuries. Return to play was common, as 64% of injured players returned to play within 24 hours, and only 3% stayed out for longer than 3 weeks. The severity of the injuries varies widely, but a drop-off in the number of cervical SCI cases occurred after a change in tackling technique in 1976.[8,9] In the 1960s, football players were provided with improvements in helmet design that enabled tacklers to lead with the crown of their head. This correlated with a rise in observed cervical fractures and associated SCI, and ultimately a ban of the "spear" tackling technique.[8] In 2018, helmet-to-helmet hits became a major focus of the NFL Head, Neck, and Spine Committee and the NFL's Commissioner's Office to prevent catastrophic injuries. In 2019, the league added even more scrutiny by giving the NFL's officiating center the power to intervene in egregious hits committed by the players. Most notably, the offensive or defensive player can be flagged for the penalty. The penalty has been most aggressively enforced for the defensive player. As players continue to become stronger and faster, these injuries have become more likely, prompting the NFL to implement stronger penalties and fines. Currently, helmet-to-helmet contact results in a minimum 15-yard penalty. Now, whether intentional or not, when helmet-to-helmet contact occurs, players are frequently ejected from the game. Players may risk suspension for repeated offenses of spearing tackles or dangerous plays deemed to be intentional. Repetitive injuries that involve the axial cervical spine result in early spondylosis, stenosis, disk herniation, or disk–osteophyte complexes that compress the spinal cord.[6]

Acquired and congenital types of cervical stenosis are frequently identified in football players, and the management and return-to-play guidelines for players with these conditions are controversial. Reports on this subject in the medical literature reveal that rates of acute SCI after minor cervical trauma have been demonstrated to be higher for individuals with a midsagittal disk-level spinal canal diameter less than 8 mm, with a positive likelihood ratio of 15.6.[10] However, in a study that followed football players with narrow spinal canals through their professional careers, no incidents of acute SCI were observed.[6] Over time, improper tackling with frequent spearing or helmet-to-helmet technique can also result in the development of stenosis through repetitive axial loading and loss of cervical lordosis. In these instances, the risk of acute SCI is significant.[6,11]

Cervical disk herniation is a common contact-associated injury observed in American football players. In a study of the NFL, these injuries accounted for 6% of all cervical spine pathologies.[12] Linebackers and defensive backs were the most commonly afflicted, correlating with the understanding that tackling mechanisms are most likely to induce an acute herniation. C3–C4, C4–C5, and C5–C6 are the levels most commonly affected.[12]

Injuries to the cervical zygapophyseal joints (Z-joints), or facet joints, are fairly common and under-reported spine injuries in American football athletes. In these athletes, advanced imaging may not be obtained because of the absence of radicular pain, neurologic deficits, or both. These acute injuries often respond to local treatment and are identified as a sprain or strain. A single article identified facet injuries in college football players, demonstrating that 2% of spine injuries are facet related. However, it is known that "whiplash" type injuries are most commonly associated with trauma to the cervical Z-joints,[13,14] and this mechanism mimics some of the high-velocity impacts that can occur on the football field. Imaging of the cervical spine may demonstrate uptake in the Z-joints on fluid-sensitive magnetic resonance images or single-photon emission computed tomography. However, the reliability of imaging modalities in the diagnosis of Z-joint pain is unclear. Diagnostic blocks of the medial branch nerves or Z-joint injections may be required to confirm the diagnosis; however, these procedures are often unnecessary, as most of these injuries result in less than 24 hours of lost time.[7]

Another injury that commonly occurs in football is known as a stinger or burner. Also referred to as brachial plexus neuropraxia (BPN), these injuries have been reported to occur in as many as 50 to 60% of football players. BPN is a sudden acute neurologic constellation of symptoms that is characterized by sudden nondermatomal acute symptoms of paresthesias, dysesthesia, weakness, pain, and numbness, alone or in combination, in a single extremity.[3] These symptoms are usually associated with compression or stretching of the ipsilateral upper trunk of the brachial plexus or exiting cervical nerve root due to a forced neck extension and lateral bending.[15] BPN can be brought on by a mechanism of ipsilateral shoulder depression and contralateral neck bending, resulting in a traction injury of the upper brachial plexus.[16] Over the duration of a player's career, degenerative changes to the neural foramen and associated decreases in the subaxial cervical space also contribute to a syndrome of chronic stingers.[17] The more involved cervical spinal cord neurapraxias, rarely observed in American football, correlate with an associated increase in cervical stenosis and can produce transient quadriplegia or central cord symptoms that involve both upper extremities.[18]

Although cervical fractures and dislocations are relatively rare in the era of modern sports, these injuries can have devastating consequences. Upper cervical injuries involving the atlas and axis occur in less than 5% of football-related cervical injuries.[5] The variable nature of these injuries reflects the great number of combinations of vector forces exerted on the neck and head while tackling or being tackled. Injuries to the posterior tension band, or posterior ligamentous complex, are relatively more common and occur with an axial load and slight flexion, such as the motion of a tackling defender initiating contact with the top of the helmet. The combination of the forces leads to elongation and subsequent disruption of the posterior column.[19] An accompanying shortening of the anterior column may induce a compressive failure known as a teardrop fracture.[3,19] Another compressive injury is that from pure axial load, in which both the anterior and posterior columns shorten. This results in elevated intradiskal pressure and adjacent endplate failure, which can occur anywhere along the spinal axis.[19] The resulting compression deformity, which can also present as a fracture of the articular process (▶ Fig. 24.1), varies in severity. Finally, injuries to the anterior tension band are associated with a posteriorly directed force and lead to failure of the anterior longitudinal ligament and annulus.[3] This can occur when a player's head is hyperextended while being tackled from behind or when anterior helmet contact occurs without sufficient neck stabilization. Although rarely observed in competition, these hyperextension injuries are unstable in nature and can be associated with subluxation, facet disarticulation, or both, and often with spinal canal compromise.

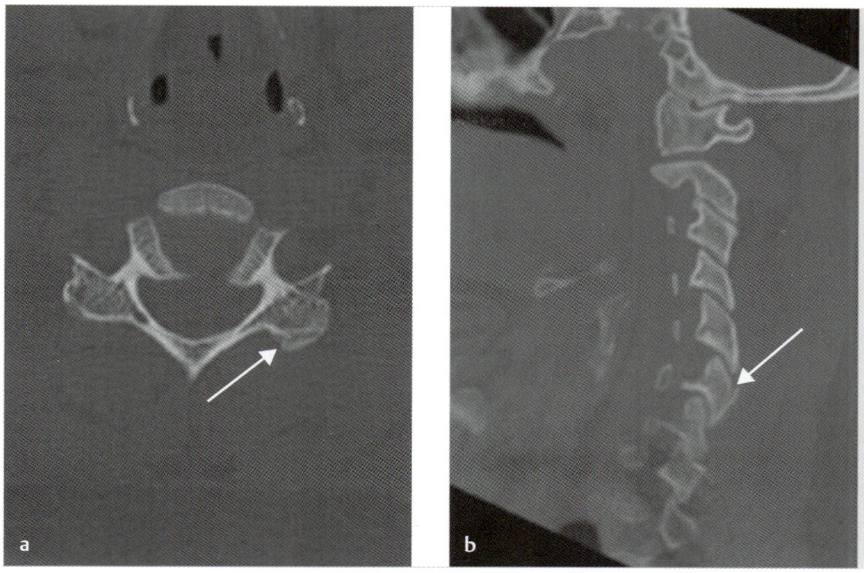

Fig. 24.1 **(a)** Axial and **(b)** sagittal computed tomography images demonstrating an acute left C6 facet fracture through the superior articulating process (*arrows*) in an offensive lineman. The player was held from play for the remainder of the season and was managed conservatively. (Used with permissions from Barrow Neurological Institute, Phoenix, Arizona.)

24.2.2 Diagnosis

Proper diagnosis of cervical spine injuries in American football is of the utmost importance for determining the aggressiveness of management and the appropriateness of return to play. A neurologic examination should be conducted by a specialist with appropriate training on the sidelines or on the field if there is any concern for spinal injury or BPN. If a spinal fracture or SCI is suspected on the field, the player should be immobilized on the field, secured to a back board with the player's helmet in place and facemask removed, and transported to the nearest level I trauma center with SCI certification.

In 1996, a broad classification scheme for cervical spine injuries was proposed focusing on the presence or absence of neurologic deficit and radiologic abnormality.[20] Type I injuries are injuries that produce a permanent SCI and can range from complete paralysis to patterns of incomplete SCI syndromes (e.g., central cord syndrome, Brown-Séquard syndrome, or anterior spinal cord syndrome). Type II injuries encompass injuries resulting in transient neurologic deficits, such as a cervical nerve root or spinal cord neurapraxia, and yield normal findings on radiologic study. Type III injuries are injuries that produce cervical spine abnormalities demonstrated on imaging, without an accompanying deficit, such as cervical stenosis, disk herniation, and fractures without SCI. The incidence and type of neck injury can correlate to head position during tackling. In all cases, obtaining noncontrasted magnetic resonance imaging (MRI) of the cervical spine is necessary to look for intrinsic hyperintense signal within the cervical spinal cord on T2-weighted images. In addition, short tau inversion recovery (STIR) techniques are useful for demonstrating disk or ligamentous injury. Computed tomography (CT) is beneficial for defining bony abnormalities such as fracture characteristics or degenerative disease that may otherwise be undetected on plain films. Dynamic imaging, such as flexion/extension radiography, is particularly effective in assessing risk for type II and III injuries.

24.2.3 Management

The management of cervical spine injuries or BPNs in a football player begins on the field. In the case of a stinger or BPN, players typically become symptomatic immediately after the collision and can walk off the field on their own volition, and they are usually seen shaking their upper extremity, dragging their arm, or holding their shoulder. This type of patient can be safely evaluated on the sidelines. The player who presents with a motor deficit on the field, with or without neck pain, should be immobilized on the field in a cervical collar, taped to a back board, and transported to the nearest level I trauma center with SCI certification. It is imperative that these types of patients are seen, evaluated, and cared for by spine surgeons. Neurologists, neurosurgeons, and orthopedic surgeons who care for the spine in the elective but non-level I trauma setting are not the ideal providers to care for these patients. The care of patients with acute SCIs is very complex, and outcomes are highly dependent on a rapidly responding, highly coordinated team. Including a provider in this setting who does not routinely care for patients with acute spine injuries and who is not used to working in such centers can delay treatment, ultimately impacting the outcome of the injured player.

Because cervical spine injuries may have devastating personal and career implications for the athlete, appropriate selection of management is essential following diagnosis. In addition, because many unstable fractures may occur with minimal neurologic manifestations, it is imperative to immobilize the patient until imaging studies are obtained.

For American football players with sustained traumatic cervical disk herniations (type III injuries), the choice of operative versus nonoperative management has been controversial, and guidelines are not well established. As in the general population, the first consideration is whether a disk herniation is causing substantial spinal canal narrowing or spinal cord compression and whether neurologic deficits are present. For herniations not producing these features, conservative management remains a first-line option (▶ Fig. 24.2). Additional

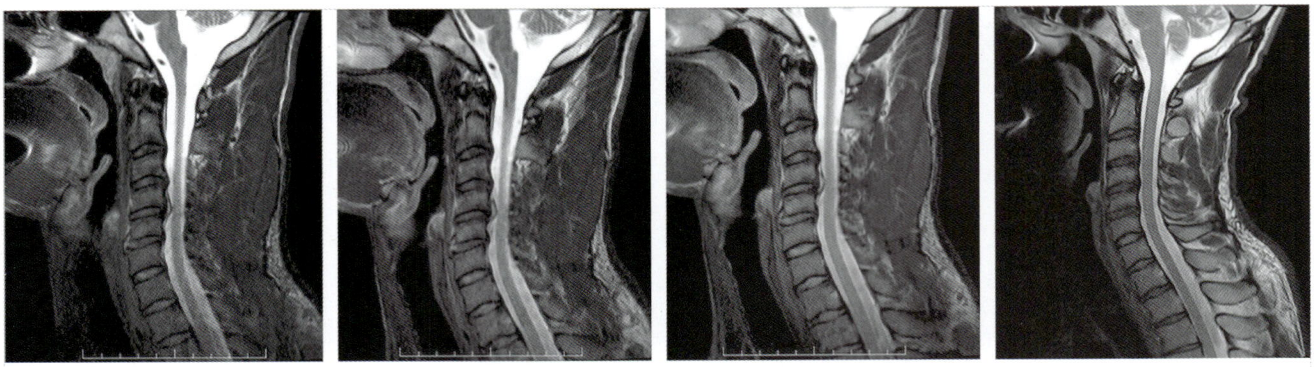

Fig. 24.2 Sagittal T2-weighted magnetic resonance images demonstrating natural progression over time of a cervical disk herniation (C4–C5) in a running back who was managed conservatively and was held from play for more than 12 weeks. (Used with permissions from Barrow Neurological Institute, Phoenix, Arizona.)

treatment considerations unique to American football players are the performance and career implications that the treatment may have. Negative evaluations are unavoidably made on these athletes due to concern of an increased risk for catastrophic injury.[5] A study of players with professional aspirations is representative of this outcome, with players receiving a diagnosis of cervical disk herniation or degenerative disk disease having a lower likelihood of being drafted to the NFL than players without these diagnoses.[6] This disparity occurred in spite of the fact that players with a cervical disk herniation did not differ in the number of years or games played or performance when compared to players without cervical disk herniations.[6] Interestingly, another study has supported surgical intervention of cervical disk herniation in NFL players, in which single-level surgery led to greater success in return to play, a longer career, and no loss of performance compared to nonoperative management.[21] Although prospective data are lacking to direct this decision-making, it appears that these athletes respond favorably to single-level cervical disk surgery, and it is reasonable to intervene to improve symptoms refractory to conservative management or to diminish induced spinal stenosis and the associated risk for SCI. More recently, we have taken the "very aggressive conservative approach" in the management of cervical disk herniations, even in the presence of profound dermatomal muscle weakness. This approach, although it usually results in the player being placed on injured reserve, will allow many of them to return to play the following season without having undergone surgery.

In the setting of a compression–hyperflexion injury with an associated posterior tension band injury or a distraction–extension injury with an associated anterior tension band injury, athletes should undergo surgical stabilization with near uniformity. The injuries can be classified as type I or type III depending on the presence of SCI; however, the instability produced leaves little room for negotiation about performing surgery in the hope of best preserving spinal mechanics and flexibility. Compression or burst fractures differ in management in that players frequently present without neurologic deficit. As a result, players with these injuries are often preferentially treated with conservative management, including a rigid cervical collar. However, if neurologic deficits or concomitant fractures are present, early surgical intervention should be considered.[22] In cases where cervical trauma is treated conservatively without surgical fixation, appropriate dynamic imaging should demonstrate the absence of supraphysiological subluxation or other signs of instability before the athlete is allowed to return to play.

24.3 Thoracolumbar Spine Injuries in Football Players

24.3.1 Epidemiology and Pathogenesis

Although SCIs are a concern with cervical injuries, catastrophic injuries are uncommon at the thoracic or lumbar levels. Thoracic SCIs are especially rare because of the stabilizing capacity of the thoracic cage and the associated oblique, intercostal, serratus anterior, and latissimus dorsi muscles.[23] However, soft-tissue injury, disk herniations, and degeneration in this spinal region are relatively common in American football players and can be a major reason for disability. In a study of axial skeleton injuries in NFL players, thoracic disk herniations led to the greatest amount of time missed from play (▶ Fig. 24.3).[24]

Lumbar injuries, on the other hand, are common in football and are associated with sudden and repetitive hyperextension, rotational injuries, or direct trauma. The etiology of low back pain in football players is also influenced by the age and player position. In adolescent and young adult football players, the most worrisome cause of lumbar pain is spondylolysis, which can be either unilateral or bilateral. It is important that this condition, which occurs most commonly at L5, is recognized early. Early recognition and treatment of a unilateral spondylolysis is likely to result in healing of the fracture and avoidance of isthmic spondylolisthesis. However, if the player develops bilateral pars fractures, the progression to isthmic spondylolisthesis occurs in 40 to 66% of patients by adulthood.[25,26,27] Should this happen, evidence suggests it will have a negative effect on years played, potential draft selection, and career longevity.[28] Although spondylolysis and isthmic spondylolisthesis occur in

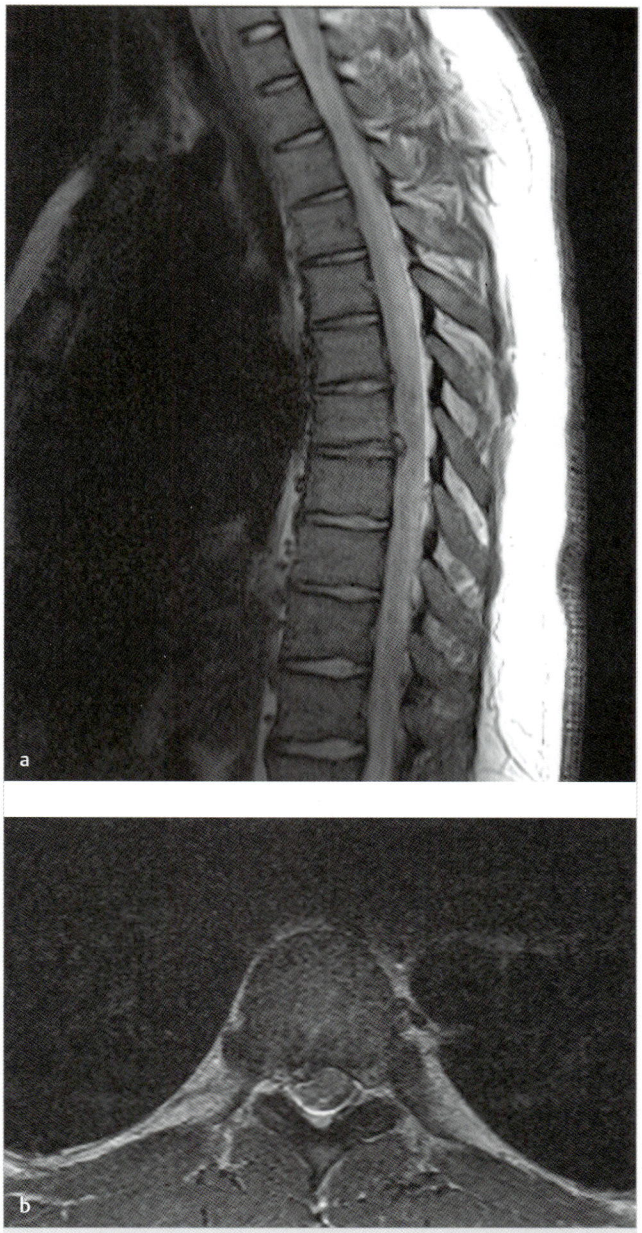

Fig. 24.3 (a) Sagittal and (b) axial T2-weighted magnetic resonance images of an acute thoracic disk herniation in an offensive lineman, requiring the player to be held from play for 8 weeks and to undergo postseason rehabilitation. (Used with permissions from Barrow Neurological Institute, Phoenix, Arizona.)

the general population at a rate of 4 to 8%,[25,26,29,30] the incidence of this condition increases to 15% when incoming college freshman football players are imaged.[31]

As players age and become skeletally mature, the likelihood of developing spondylolysis decreases, and other conditions increase in prevalence. Additionally, as the age of football participants increases, so does the impact velocity and player weight, increasing the forces directed on the spine. Direct trauma in these situations can cause contusions and fractures involving the vertebral body, transverse process, or spinous process. Because of the physical nature and forces generated at impact during a football game, sprains and strains are the most common injuries, accounting for 46% of lumbar spine injuries among NFL players. These injuries are usually short-lived, accounting for a mean loss of 7 to 9 days of playing time.[24]

In addition, football players can experience disk injuries, which increase in frequency with the age of the players. Disk injuries are relatively uncommon in adolescent athletes, but at the professional level, disk injuries or early degeneration is the second most common type of injury and accounts for an average of 51 playing days lost.[24] Of disk injuries occurring in professional football players, more than 75% are localized to the lumbar spine.[12] Within the lumbar spine, the L5–S1 level is most frequently the site of injury, followed by the L4–L5 level.[12] In addition, as a result of the acute injuries and repetitive stress placed on the lumbar spine, these athletes may demonstrate disproportionately higher rates of degenerative diseases of the disk and facets.[32,33] Finally, hyperflexion or extension can occur, resulting in an increased risk of lumbar injuries in offensive players such as running backs and wide receivers, who are frequently in vulnerable positions when being tackled.

24.3.2 Diagnosis

Interestingly, at least one study has suggested that high school and college football players with reported low back pain have a high likelihood of a discoverable radiographic abnormality.[34] As a result, it is advisable to obtain thoracolumbar radiography and MRI for patients with acute or persistent low back pain. The threshold for escalating to a higher resolution MRI study should be low, and such imaging is recommended in all situations in which there is concern for spondylolysis, neurologic deficit, radiculopathy, significant soft-tissue injury, or disk herniation. Dynamic flexion–extension films are advisable to evaluate for instability in these athletes, particularly those with spondylolysis. CT may be useful for the evaluation of spondylolysis and the uncommonly associated thoracolumbar fracture and to observe bony defects.

24.3.3 Management

Although thoracolumbar spine injuries are unlikely to be devastating in football players, they can lead to lost playing time and can affect the player's career aspirations. Preexisting lumbar conditions, including diagnoses of spondylosis, disk herniation, and spondylolysis with or without spondylolisthesis, have not been shown to affect career performance; however, these athletes have been found to play professionally for fewer years and in fewer games, and historically they have been less likely to be drafted.[28]

For football players diagnosed with acute spondylolysis with or without spondylolisthesis, conservative management with rest and lumbosacral orthosis is the preferred treatment modality. The addition of a bone stimulator has shown some limited promise in accelerating healing of these fractures.[35,36,37] Some cases of continued or severe instability may ultimately require surgical fixation and fusion; however, these decisions must take into consideration that a return to contact sports is unlikely after these interventions.[38]

The treatment for lumbar disk herniation in football players includes nonoperative and operative management, similar to treatment in the general population. However, additional attention must be directed at the athlete's daily demands on the spine, a body mass index that is above 35, and the player's interest in returning to peak performance. Reports in the literature have provided conflicting evidence to support equal outcomes or superiority in diskectomy versus nonoperative management.[28,39] Overall, the decision to operate should be determined on a case-by-case basis, with a demonstrated positive response to diskectomy not limiting a return to play for athletes who desire such management, have failed conservative measures, or have significant associated stenosis.

24.4 Return to Play

Overall, return to play following a spinal injury should be determined on a case-by-case basis, as no high-level evidence exists to support a generalized approach. However, in all cases of cervical, thoracic, or lumbar spine injuries, each athlete's return to high-impact competition should include a resolution of symptoms, lack of neurologic deficit, full range of motion, and documented stability of any healing fracture or surgical correction.[40] If all four requirements are not met, return to play is absolutely contraindicated.

Athletes who sustain a stinger during play should be cleared for return after complete resolution of symptoms and demonstration of full strength. Athletes with persistent symptoms of paresthesia, weakness, pain, and numbness should be removed from competition and evaluated by an appropriate medical professional. If onsite imaging is available, cervical spine radiography and/or shoulder imaging should be acquired.

In this chapter, we propose for the first time that return-to-play guidelines be instituted for spine injuries similar to those of the NFL Head, Neck, and Spine Committee's Protocols Regarding Return to Participation Following Concussion (▶ Table 24.1). These guidelines are similar in concept but focus on the player progressing through recovery, starting immediately after the injury. The seven-step progression to return to play has several distinctions that are unique to spine care for NFL injured players. Step 1 starts on the field, rather than 1 day after the concussion, and step 6 is added to allow for moderated graduated contact rather than jumping from football-specific noncontact exercises, such as cone drills, to full contact. This allows the player to experience a trial of contact with sleds and tackle dummies to ascertain if the impact will cause a recurrence of symptoms. If the event leads to persistent or lingering symptoms or deficits, further workup, including evaluation by a qualified physician and undergoing the appropriate imaging, may be required. With respect to return to play for players with stingers, if a player experiences two stingers within the same season, it is recommended that the player be precluded from further game action in that season and undergo workup for possible structural risk factors that place the player at risk for repetitive neuropraxia.[41] In players who display signs of cervical spinal cord neurapraxia, advanced imaging is warranted, and return to play should be based on complete resolution of the transient event and assessment of the severity of any possible stenosis.[16]

For individuals with sustained cervical fractures or disk herniation requiring intervention, in addition to the above features for clearance, these athletes should demonstrate healing or union of their fusion mass and be counseled on the associated risks of reinjury. Generally agreed absolute contraindications, as proposed by Kepler and Vaccaro,[16] include a fusion greater than two levels, atlanto-occipital fusion, continued evidence of atlantoaxial or subaxial instability, trauma-induced sagittal malalignment, acquired canal compromise, or spear tackler's spine. Spear tackler's spine is a syndrome of four features that include loss of cervical lordosis, presence of cervical stenosis, posttraumatic radiographic evidence, and documented spear tackling technique.[42] Documented high rates of type I cervical injuries in these patients have precluded their participation in high-impact competitions.[11]

For thoracic and lumbar injuries, guidelines for returning to play continue to support the above four pillars. Any thoracic fracture with evidence of instability is an absolute contraindication to return to play.[40] After a course of physical therapy and nonsteroidal anti-inflammatory medications, players can expect to return from a lumbar strain after symptoms resolve over a typical period of 1 week.[24] Lumbar disk herniation, regardless of nonoperative or operative management, can be expected to result in a longer loss of playing time. It can be managed with standard conservative therapy and epidural steroid injections and, if deficit and pain persist despite these measures, with operative intervention. A general rule, given the high-impact nature of the sport, is for football players to be held out of play for at least 2 to 6 months for rehabilitation.[43] For cases of spondylolysis with or without spondylolisthesis, management and subsequent return-to-play decisions should depend on the persistence of symptoms, grade of observed slip, and presence of neurologic deficits. In general, asymptomatic low-grade spondylolisthesis should not prevent a player from participating. However, if operative intervention is necessary, the decision on return to play remains controversial and is best managed individually.[40,42] Anecdotal evidence supports abstaining from participation for at least a year,[44] if not permanently. For players with an intention to return to football competition, an installed rehabilitation protocol should emphasize a slow, gradual return to inflicted impact on the injured areas, whether or not instrumentation was included in the management.

24.5 Clinical Pearls

- The high-impact nature of American football makes athletes participating in the sport susceptible to spine injuries.
- Cervical injuries may be catastrophic, both in the physical and economic sense.
- Conservative management of cervical disk herniations is well tolerated.
- Conservative management of stable lumbar spine injuries is reasonable, with surgery warranted on a case-by-case basis.
- Athletes returning to play must demonstrate resolution of symptoms, lack of neurologic deficit, full range of motion, and documented stability of any healing fracture or surgical correction.
- The time has come to develop and refine return-to-play guidelines for spinal injuries and BPN, and a new proposed progression is presented in this chapter.

Table 24.1 Return-to-play guidelines for cervical, thoracic, and lumbar spine injuries with transient neurological deficit, stinger, or soft-tissue injury for injured athlete*,†,‡

Stage	Timing	Activity	Imaging	Objective
Step 1: On field evaluation	Immediately after injury in tent or locker room	Removal from play if stinger, concussion, significant spinal pain, lack of resolution of neurological symptoms within 3 minutes of injury	AP and lateral flexion/ extension films by onsite radiology department	Prevention of further injury
		Immobilization with appropriate orthosis if instability		
Step 2: Rest and recovery	One day after injury	Evaluation by spine specialist# Routine daily activity as tolerated Immobilization with appropriate orthosis if instability Light physical therapy—heat massage, ultrasound, laser (no ROM, stretching or strengthening)	MRI, CT, repeat flexion/ extension films if still symptomatic	Rest and recovery, further definition of injury
Step 3: Light aerobic exercise and physical therapy	After neurological symptoms stabilize and player cleared by specialist radiographically for instability	Light aerobic activity for 20 minutes at < 50% of the targeted heart rate supervised by ATC team Begin light dynamic stretching, range to 50% of maximum Discontinue if symptoms return	Only as symptoms dictate	Cardiovascular challenge to determine if there are any recurrent neurological symptoms
Step 4: Continued aerobic exercise and introduction of strength training	After step 3 is cleared with minimal symptoms	Increase aerobic activity (duration and intensity, introduction of running, sprinting, change of direction exercises, noncontact sport-specific activities, e.g., cone drills) to 50 to 75% of maximum target heart rate Increase as tolerated, stretching, soft-tissue massage, PT modalities Introduction of strength training, 50% of typical weight, excluding injured muscle	Only as symptoms dictate	Progress cardiovascular exercise, add strength training and more complex movements to determine if there are any recurrent neurological or spine-related symptoms
Step 5: Football-specific activities without contact	After step 4 is cleared with minimal symptoms	Participation in all noncontact activities for the typical duration of a full practice and training regimens	Only as symptoms dictate	Increase football-specific demands to determine if there are any recurrent neurological or spine-related symptoms
Step 6: Football activities with moderated contact	After step 5 is cleared	Participation in moderate contact activities, including sleds, dummies, moderate player contact, stressing the symptomatic area, under the supervision of the head athletic trainer	Repeat imaging if symptoms recur	Stress symptomatic area to assess for recurrence of symptoms
Step 7: Full football activity and clearance	When imaging is negative, and player is asymptomatic, and cleared by a spine specialist#	Full participation in practice and contact without restriction	If prior disk herniation, repeat MRI; if prior fracture or suspected instability, repeat CT and flexion/extension plain radiographs	Tolerance of all football activities without any recurrent neurological or soft-tissue symptoms

Abbreviations: AP, anteroposterior; ATC, certified athletic trainer; CT, computed tomography; MRI, magnetic resonance imaging; PT, physical therapy; ROM, range of motion.
Notes: * Adapted from National Football Head, Neck and Spine Committee's Protocols Regarding Return to Participation Following Concussion.
† This table serves as a guideline. There is not a set timeline for return to play, as it is determined by symptoms and signs as determined by team physicians and athletic trainers.
‡ Excludes spinal cord injury.
# A spine specialist is defined as a licensed MD who treats traumatic spine injuries in a level I trauma center and takes spine-specific calls at such a center on a monthly basis.

24.6 Disclosures

The authors have no relevant disclosures.

Acknowledgments

The authors thank the staff of Neuroscience Publications at Barrow Neurological Institute for assistance with preparation of the manuscript and illustrations.

References

[1] Sports. Gallup Historical Trends. Accessed June 13, 2019 at: https://news.gallup.com/poll/4735/sports.aspx
[2] Estimated Probability of Competing in Athletics Beyond the High School Interscholastic Level. NCAA Research. Accessed June 13, 2019 at: https://web.archive.org/web/20140426235239/http://www.ncaa.org/sites/default/files/Probability-of-going-pro-methodology_Update20123.pdf
[3] Schroeder GD, Vaccaro AR. Cervical spine injuries in the athlete. J Am Acad Orthop Surg. 2016; 24(9):e122–e133
[4] Puvanesarajah V, Qureshi R, Cancienne JM, Hassanzadeh H. Traumatic sports-related cervical spine injuries. Clin Spine Surg. 2017; 30(2):50–56
[5] Boden BP, Tacchetti RL, Cantu RC, Knowles SB, Mueller FO. Catastrophic cervical spine injuries in high school and college football players. Am J Sports Med. 2006; 34(8):1223–1232
[6] Schroeder GD, Lynch TS, Gibbs DB, et al. The impact of a cervical spine diagnosis on the careers of National Football League athletes. Spine. 2014; 39(12):947–952
[7] Chung AS, Makovicka JL, Hassebrock JD, et al. Epidemiology of cervical injuries in NCAA football players. Spine. 2019; 44(12):848–854
[8] Bailes JE, Petschauer M, Guskiewicz KM, Maranc G. Management of cervical spine injuries in athletes. J Athl Train. 2007; 42(1):126–134
[9] Torg JS, Truex R, Jr, Quedenfeld TC, Burstein A, Spealman A, Nichols C, III. The National Football Head and Neck Injury Registry. Report and conclusions 1978. JAMA. 1979; 241(14):1477–1479
[10] Aebli N, Rüegg TB, Wicki AG, Petrou N, Krebs J. Predicting the risk and severity of acute spinal cord injury after a minor trauma to the cervical spine. Spine J. 2013; 13(6):597–604
[11] Torg JS, Sennett B, Pavlov H, Leventhal MR, Glasgow SG. Spear tackler's spine. An entity precluding participation in tackle football and collision activities that expose the cervical spine to axial energy inputs. Am J Sports Med. 1993; 21(5):640–649
[12] Gray BL, Buchowski JM, Bumpass DB, Lehman RA, Jr, Mall NA, Matava MJ. Disc herniations in the National Football League. Spine. 2013; 38(22):1934–1938
[13] Bogduk N. On cervical zygapophysial joint pain after whiplash. Spine. 2011; 36(25) Suppl:S194–S199
[14] Schofferman J, Bogduk N, Slosar P. Chronic whiplash and whiplash-associated disorders: an evidence-based approach. J Am Acad Orthop Surg. 2007; 15(10):596–606
[15] Meyer SA, Schulte KR, Callaghan JJ, et al. Cervical spinal stenosis and stingers in collegiate football players. Am J Sports Med. 1994; 22(2):158–166
[16] Kepler CK, Vaccaro AR. Injuries and abnormalities of the cervical spine and return to play criteria. Clin Sports Med. 2012; 31(3):499–508
[17] Levitz CL, Reilly PJ, Torg JS. The pathomechanics of chronic, recurrent cervical nerve root neurapraxia. The chronic burner syndrome. Am J Sports Med. 1997; 25(1):73–76
[18] Torg JS, Pavlov H, Genuario SE, et al. Neurapraxia of the cervical spinal cord with transient quadriplegia. J Bone Joint Surg Am. 1986; 68(9):1354–1370
[19] Banerjee R, Palumbo MA, Fadale PD. Catastrophic cervical spine injuries in the collision sport athlete, part 1: epidemiology, functional anatomy, and diagnosis. Am J Sports Med. 2004; 32(4):1077–1087
[20] Maroon JC, Bailes JE. Athletes with cervical spine injury. Spine. 1996; 21(19): 2294–2299
[21] Hsu WK. Outcomes following nonoperative and operative treatment for cervical disc herniations in National Football League athletes. Spine. 2011; 36(10):800–805
[22] Vaccaro AR, Hulbert RJ, Patel AA, et al. Spine Trauma Study Group. The subaxial cervical spine injury classification system: a novel approach to recognize the importance of morphology, neurology, and integrity of the disco-ligamentous complex. Spine. 2007; 32(21):2365–2374
[23] Kanter AS, Knightly Athletic spinal injuries and return to play. In: Harbaugh RE, Shaffrey C, Couldwell WT, Berger MS, eds. Neurosurgery Knowledge Update: A Comprehensive Review. Thieme; 2015:617–624
[24] Mall NA, Buchowski J, Zebala L, Brophy RH, Wright RW, Matava MJ. Spine and axial skeleton injuries in the National Football League. Am J Sports Med. 2012; 40(8):1755–1761
[25] Fredrickson BE, Baker D, McHolick WJ, Yuan HA, Lubicky JP. The natural history of spondylolysis and spondylolisthesis. J Bone Joint Surg Am. 1984; 66(5):699–707
[26] Beutler WJ, Fredrickson BE, Murtland A, Sweeney CA, Grant WD, Baker D. The natural history of spondylolysis and spondylolisthesis: 45-year follow-up evaluation. Spine. 2003; 28(10):1027–1035, discussion 1035
[27] Fujii K, Katoh S, Sairyo K, Ikata T, Yasui N. Union of defects in the pars interarticularis of the lumbar spine in children and adolescents. The radiological outcome after conservative treatment. J Bone Joint Surg Br. 2004; 86(2):225–231
[28] Schroeder GD, Lynch TS, Gibbs DB, et al. Pre-existing lumbar spine diagnosis as a predictor of outcomes in National Football League athletes. Am J Sports Med. 2015; 43(4):972–978
[29] Kalichman L, Kim DH, Li L, Guermazi A, Berkin V, Hunter DJ. Spondylolysis and spondylolisthesis: prevalence and association with low back pain in the adult community-based population. Spine. 2009; 34(2):199–205
[30] Sakai T, Sairyo K, Takao S, Nishitani H, Yasui N. Incidence of lumbar spondylolysis in the general population in Japan based on multidetector computed tomography scans from two thousand subjects. Spine. 2009; 34 (21):2346–2350
[31] McCarroll JR, Miller JM, Ritter MA. Lumbar spondylolysis and spondylolisthesis in college football players. A prospective study. Am J Sports Med. 1986; 14(5): 404–406
[32] Gerbino PG, d'Hemecourt PA. Does football cause an increase in degenerative disease of the lumbar spine? Curr Sports Med Rep. 2002; 1(1): 47–51
[33] Nagashima M, Abe H, Amaya K, et al. Risk factors for lumbar disc degeneration in high school American football players: a prospective 2-year follow-up study. Am J Sports Med. 2013; 41(9):2059–2064
[34] Iwamoto J, Abe H, Tsukimura Y, Wakano K. Relationship between radiographic abnormalities of lumbar spine and incidence of low back pain in high school and college football players: a prospective study. Am J Sports Med. 2004; 32(3):781–786
[35] Vrable A, Sherman AL. Elite male adolescent gymnast who achieved union of a persistent bilateral pars defect. Am J Phys Med Rehabil. 2009; 88(2): 156–160
[36] Fellander-Tsai L, Micheli LJ. Treatment of spondylolysis with external electrical stimulation and bracing in adolescent athletes: a report of two cases. Clin J Sport Med. 1998; 8(3):232–234
[37] Stasinopoulos D. Treatment of spondylolysis with external electrical stimulation in young athletes: a critical literature review. Br J Sports Med. 2004; 38(3):352–354
[38] Eck JC, Riley LH, III. Return to play after lumbar spine conditions and surgeries. Clin Sports Med. 2004; 23(3):367–379, viii
[39] Weistroffer JK, Hsu WK. Return-to-play rates in National Football League linemen after treatment for lumbar disk herniation. Am J Sports Med. 2011; 39(3):632–636
[40] Rosenthal BD, Boody BS, Hsu WK. Return to play for athletes. Neurosurg Clin N Am. 2017; 28(1):163–171
[41] Cantu RC, Bailes JE, Wilberger JE, Jr. Guidelines for return to contact or collision sport after a cervical spine injury. Clin Sports Med. 1998; 17(1): 137–146
[42] Saigal R, Batjer HH, Ellenbogen RG, Berger MS. Return to play for neurosurgical patients. World Neurosurg. 2014; 82(3–4):485–491
[43] Li Y, Hresko MT. Lumbar spine surgery in athletes: outcomes and return-to-play criteria. Clin Sports Med. 2012; 31(3):487–498
[44] Rubery PT, Bradford DS. Athletic activity after spine surgery in children and adolescents: results of a survey. Spine. 2002; 27(4):423–427

25 Soccer

Vikas Vattipally, Carly Weber-Levine, and Nicholas Theodore

Summary
Soccer is played by millions of athletes across the world, leading to a high prevalence of soccer-related injuries. Specifically, concussions are common after player-to-player contact and can be associated with neurological and psychological impairment. Spinal injuries such as disk herniations or spondylolisthesis have also been noted to occur in soccer, along with injuries to peripheral nerves. Safe play practices, including minimizing risky player-to-player contact, is crucial for the prevention of neurological injuries in soccer. In this chapter, we report the presentation of common injuries to the nervous system that can occur from playing soccer, as well as diagnostic techniques, management, and prevention.

Keywords: soccer, concussion, return to play, spine, peripheral nerve

25.1 Introduction

Soccer, also known as football in countries outside of the United States, is the most-played sport in the world.[1] Soccer has several factors that contribute to a high incidence of neurologic injury, including "headers," in which players use their heads to direct an airborne ball, and collisions with other players.[2] In 2018 alone, nearly 27,000 emergency department visits were related to head injuries caused by soccer play.[3] Although soccer players suffer from spine and peripheral nerve injuries less frequently, there is a larger burden represented by acute brain trauma such as concussion and its sequelae. There is also some evidence to suggest chronic changes in the brain including neuropsychological impairment and neurodegenerative disease. This chapter provides an overview of soccer-related injuries in the brain, spine, and peripheral nerves (▶ Table 25.1, ▶ Fig. 25.1). It also summarizes proposed treatment and prevention strategies and explores some controversies in the literature pertaining to the development of chronic brain pathology in soccer athletes.

25.2 Brain Injury

25.2.1 Concussion

Concussions, which are a mild form of traumatic brain injury (TBI), account for more than 20% of all soccer-related injuries.[4]

Table 25.1 Neurological injuries that may occur in soccer players

Location	Cause	Presentation	Prevention
Brain			
Concussion	Acute head trauma	*Typical:* LOC, memory changes, vomiting, nausea, headache	Avoiding player-to-player collisions, education on safe heading techniques, limiting headers for youth players
Neuropsychological impairment	Chronic repeated head impacts *(disputed)*	*Red Flags:* seizures, anisocoria, severe headache, sensory loss	Using partially deflated soccer balls, replacing ball if wet
CTE	Chronic repeated head impacts *(hypothesized)*	Persistent headaches, impaired memory/attention/concentration, mood changes	Unclear
ICH	Acute head trauma	Progressive early-onset dementia, behavioral changes, LOC, seizures, anisocoria, severe headache, mortality	Avoiding player-to-player and player-to-surface collisions
Spine			
Canal stenosis, spondylosis, spondylolysis, and chronic disk herniation	Chronic repeated head impacts, high-intensity activity	Numbness, weakness, tingling, back pain, instability	Education on proper posturing and technique
SCI	Acute neck or back trauma	Paralysis, anesthesia, mortality	Avoiding player-to-player and player-to-surface collisions
Peripheral Nerve			
Facial nerve palsy	Acute superolateral face trauma *(rarely)*	Ipsilateral facial weakness	Avoiding player-to-player collisions, education on safe heading techniques
Brachial plexus "stingers"	Acute neck or shoulder injury	Transient pain, weakness, numbness, tingling, burning sensation	Avoid impact to neck and shoulders
Fibular nerve palsy	Acute lower leg injury	Impaired dorsiflexion ("foot drop"), impaired anterolateral lower leg sensation	None
Sural nerve palsy	Acute lower leg injury	Impaired heel and lateral ankle sensation	None

Abbreviations: CTE, chronic traumatic encephalopathy; ICH, intracranial hemorrhage; LOC, loss of consciousness; SCI, spinal cord injury.

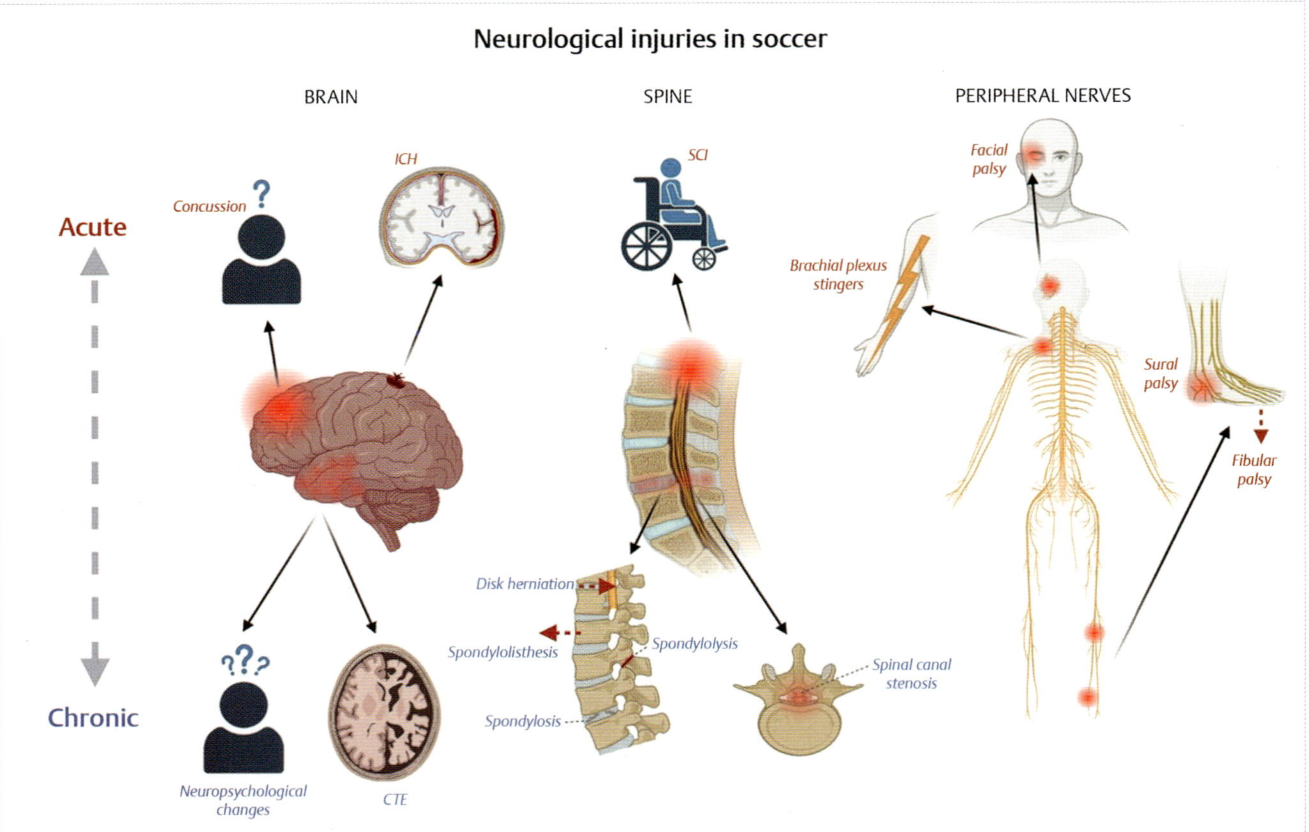

Fig. 25.1 Neurological injuries that may occur in soccer. Acute brain injuries include concussion and intracerebral hemorrhage (ICH), while chronic brain injuries include neuropsychological changes (disputed) and potentially chronic traumatic encephalopathy (CTE). Acute spine injuries include spinal cord injury (SCI), while chronic spine injuries include disk herniation, spondylolysis, spondylolisthesis, spondylosis, and spinal canal stenosis. Peripheral nerve injuries include facial palsy, sural palsy, fibular palsy, and brachial plexus "stingers." (Created with BioRender.com.)

Unfortunately, despite this high and increasing statistic, public awareness of concussions in soccer has been minimal compared to that seen in other sports such as football and boxing.[5,6] This is especially concerning as over 80% of soccer injuries occur in people under the age of 25.[7] Concussions in younger athletes are a more serious concern than in older athletes because disruption to the developing nervous system can result in a longer duration of impairment.[8] The limited public knowledge about soccer-related concussions, as well as social pressure from teammates, coaches, and parents for players to hide symptoms, may contribute to a significant under-reporting of concussions in youth soccer.[5,7,8,9] There may be sex-based differences in the incidence of concussions as well. In a comprehensive review of 64 studies, Mooney et al concluded that concussions are more likely to occur in female soccer players, potentially due to differences in neck muscle strength leading to greater head impact forces. This finding was later corroborated in a review by Dave et al, who specified that female soccer players experience higher rates of concussion than males during heading and goalkeeping.[7,10]

Mechanism of Injury

The most common mechanism of injury, causing an estimated 40 to 80% of soccer-related concussions in adults and youth, is direct contact of a player's head with another player's body, especially elbow-to-head and head-to-head collisions during contested headings.[2,3,11,12,13] There is less evidence to support that heading the ball is a major cause of concussion, especially in young athletes.[12,14] Concussions were also found to be 5.7 times more likely to occur during a regulation match than during a team practice.[7]

Symptoms

Typical symptoms of concussions include a brief loss of consciousness, confusion, impaired memory, behavioral changes, and other executive deficits as well as vomiting, headache, neck pain, nausea, or vertigo. More concerning "red flag symptoms" as defined by the International Federation of Association Football (FIFA) include severe headache, anisocoria, impaired distal sensation, repetitive vomiting, and seizures.[15] FIFA recommends immediately transporting athletes to the hospital for an emergency computed tomography (CT) scan without contrast if they exhibit one or more of these symptoms.[15,16]

Diagnosis

A baseline examination should be conducted for all players using the Sport Concussion Assessment Tool (SCAT5) during the pre-season.[15] If a concussion is suspected, the SCAT5 should be performed by a field examiner and compared to the player's baseline.

If a head injury occurs, FIFA has published an eight-phase approach beginning with observation, on-pitch and off-pitch examinations, and ending in a re-evaluation and eventual return to play if no concussion symptoms are observed within 72 hours of the injury.[15]

Treatment

For soccer players who experience concussions, FIFA recommends withdrawing them from play and employing their Graduated Return-to-Football (Soccer) Program. The athlete should work with the physician, therapist, or trainer through six stages of gradually increasing mental and physical stimulation.[15] Unfortunately, despite the availability of these guidelines and others set by the American Academy of Neurology, only around 50% of concussed soccer players adhere to them, and many continue to play.[4]

Prevention

Prevention of soccer-related concussions is difficult due to players' desire to contest header balls, which can often result in injury from head-to-player or head-to-surface contact. Proposed protective headgear thus far has not been shown to effectively mitigate head collisions and would likely interfere with the play that athletes are accustomed to.[11] Players of all ages should therefore be educated about safe heading techniques to avoid player collisions.[4] Finally, coaches and trainers must be educated about the signs and symptoms of concussions to promote early adherence to treatment guidelines and prevent repeated injuries.[4]

25.2.2 Subconcussive Heading, Neuropsychological Changes and Controversies

In contrast to concussive injuries, subconcussive impacts in soccer do not result in acute brain trauma. Soccer is a unique sport due to players' common, purposeful head contact with the ball. Headings can occur dozens of times per player in a single competitive season and thousands of times in a player's career.[17,18] As discussed above, heading is less likely to cause concussions than player-to-player contact. However, high frequencies of heading among soccer players have potentially been associated with chronic changes in their cognitive functioning. Even still, these findings are not without controversy.

Mechanism of Injury

Regulation soccer balls typically weigh about 1 lb, but can travel at speeds of up to 45 to 55 mph immediately prior to contacting a player's head.[6] The interaction actively diverts the ball toward a target with high velocity, involving a large amount of force imparted onto the skull in a short amount of time.[6] In fact, one experiment with a model head calculated that the acceleration from a soccer ball heading at 40 mph can reach over 30 g, which exceeds typical helmet acceleration in football and hockey.[6,19] Headings occur 6 to 12 times per soccer match per player, potentially contributing to chronic subconcussive brain injury over time.[6]

Symptoms

Repeated exposure to subconcussive heading impacts can present with headaches or dizziness, as well as cognitive impairment in the domains of memory, attention, concentration, and mood.[20,21] Retired former players and players who head the ball more frequently have been shown to experience higher rates of these symptoms or lower scores on neuropsychological testing than current players or those who head the ball less often.[20,21,22] These results suggest that in the long-term, subconcussive heading impacts may contribute to changes in brain functioning without an acute period of impairment.

Despite these findings, more recent prospective and retrospective studies have found no difference in neuropsychological test scores between soccer players who experience purposeful, subconcussive heading impacts and control subjects.[11,13,18,19,23,24] Contemporary authors cite methodological issues in the earlier studies' participant recruitment and study design as potentially leading to falsely positive results.[11,13,16,18,23] Thus, there appears to be conflicting evidence about the role of repeated headings in chronic brain changes.

Treatment

As subconcussive impacts do not cause acute neurological injury, there is no indication for treatment unless contact with the ball produces signs of a concussion or other forms of head trauma. Soccer players with decreasing neuropsychological function not attributable to any other cause should seek medical evaluation and rehabilitation, avoiding headers until medically cleared.

Research supports educating physicians, trainers, and athletes on the difference between repeated concussions, which are strongly associated with chronic cognitive impairment, and repeated subconcussive soccer injuries, which have inconsistent associations with chronic cognitive impairment.[11,16,22]

Prevention

The prevention of subconcussive injury largely centers around optimizing the physical dynamics of ball-to-head contact. Changes in player position at the moment of impact, such as jumping prior to contact and relaxing neck muscles, may reduce stress transmitted to the central nervous system.[6] The ball should be deflated to the lower limit of acceptable play, be made of a hydrophobic material, and should be replaced with a new ball if it accumulates excess water weight from a wet field. These changes maximize the ball's compressibility and limit its mass without significantly affecting play.[6,25] The use of headgear has not been shown to significantly reduce the force of impact and may actually lead to more aggressive headings and player collisions if athletes believe they have a "safety net."[6]

25.2.3 Neurodegenerative Disease and Controversies

Given the strong evidence that football and boxing athletes experience high rates of chronic traumatic encephalopathy (CTE),[26] questions have arisen regarding the long-term neurodegenerative potential of head impacts in soccer. CTE is characterized by neuronal death, behavioral symptoms, and the onset of dementia, and is thought to develop due to repeated concussive or subconcussive head impacts over the course of an athlete's career.[26] Unfortunately, as there is no consistent method to definitively diagnose CTE apart from autopsy examination. Research on living athletes with suspected CTE is limited.[27] As of May 2023, there have only been 14 reported cases of confirmed soccer-related CTE in the literature.[28] Some researchers hypothesize that professional soccer play may potentially increase the risk for CTE, but suggest that genetic and environmental factors may play a role in CTE development.[29] More robust, long-term prospective studies should be conducted before definitively concluding a causal relationship between soccer and CTE.

25.2.4 Intracerebral Hemorrhages

Intracranial hemorrhages (ICHs) are overall rare in soccer but have occurred after head collisions with surfaces or other players. The majority of reported cases were adolescents and recovered after surgical or medical intervention, and some were cleared to return to contact sports.[30,31,32] In a retrospective study summarizing all soccer-related deaths in Australia in the past 30 years, four deaths occurred from a subarachnoid hemorrhage (SAH), three occurred from a subdural hematoma (SDH), and two occurred from an epidural hematoma (EDH). Patients ranged from 15 to 41 years of age, and all bleeds occurred after head collisions with other players or hard surfaces. Only one case report describes an acute SDH after heading the ball alone,[33] and there have been a few cases of chronic SDH that present after soccer ball heading in adolescent players with a history of congenital arachnoid cysts.[34]

Taken together, the risk of developing ICH during soccer play is low. Players should remain cautious about colliding with other players and avoiding head collisions with hard surfaces. Coaches should continue to reinforce these themes and must keep the "red flag" concussion symptoms in mind as potential signals of ICH after players' potential head injury and as indication for transfer to a hospital for imaging and treatment.

25.3 Spine Injury

Fortunately, the incidence of spinal injuries in soccer is low, accounting for only 9 to 14% of soccer injuries.[35] These injuries vary in frequency and severity, from mild degenerative changes to devastating spinal cord lesions resulting in paralysis.

25.3.1 Spinal Degenerative Changes

Although highly acute spinal injuries are rare among soccer athletes, playing the sport for many years has been linked to changes in the spinal column's bony and cartilaginous structures. These include spinal canal stenosis, disk degeneration (spondylosis), spondylolysis, and chronic disk herniations.[35,36] Some studies indicate that playing soccer is associated with higher rates and earlier onset of spinal degenerative changes as compared to nonathletes, with this effect being more prominent in young and adolescent players.[35]

Mechanisms of Injury

Degenerative spinal changes, especially at the cervical levels, have been associated with frequent heading of the ball.[35,36] Although a single heading event is unlikely to cause acute symptoms, multiple heading impacts per match can cause changes in the spine's physiology over time due to repeated cycles of inflammation and repair. Other mechanisms of chronic injury involve the intense biomechanics involved in the sport. In soccer, athletes must sprint constantly, twist to instantaneously shift directions, collide with other players, and put themselves in the way of high-velocity shots. These actions have been theorized to cause microscopic injuries throughout the spinal column, contributing to degenerative change over time.[35]

Symptoms

Stenosis of the spinal canal is a common consequence of degenerative spine changes and can result in numbness, tingling, pain, or paresis in affected dermatomes.[37]

Repetitive strain or trauma can also result in the herniation of intervertebral disks over time, which can contact the spinal cord and cause similar symptoms to the above, or can cause radiculopathy with compression of nerve roots entering and exiting the spinal cord.[35,37] Depending on the nerve roots affected, athletes may experience numbness, weakness, and pain in the distribution of affected nerve roots.

Chronic degeneration of the spine, also known as spondylosis, is another potential complication related to inflammation and aging. Most cases affect the lumbar spine, and its symptoms include low back pain and later instability.[35,38] Similarly, high-force repetitive leg movement such as kicks may contribute to vertebral body stress fractures, including spondylolysis. Spondylolysis is a stress fracture of a vertebral body pars interarticularis and can be complicated by spondylolisthesis when the fracture causes a superior vertebra to translate anteriorly across an inferior vertebra. These commonly occur in the lumbar spine as well, and present with similar symptoms to chronic lumbar disk herniation.[35] Spondylosis and spondylolisthesis can significantly limit players' athletic ability on the field and quality of life off the field.[38]

Treatment

Degenerative spinal changes in soccer players are managed initially with conservative treatment options. These strategies include steroids and anti-inflammatory medications for spondylosis or herniations, and a spine brace for spondylolysis.[35] If these do not manage symptoms adequately, surgical options may be considered when indicated by imaging results. These include vertebral body fusion for spondylosis or spondylolysis and decompression and fusions for disk herniation, especially if the herniated disk causes spinal cord compression.[35] Most soccer players who seek treatment for degenerative spine changes eventually achieve a full recovery and can continue playing with or without modifications.[35]

Prevention

Prevention of degenerative spine changes in soccer is difficult given the high degree of physical stress inherent to the sport.

Coaches and trainers should continue to emphasize proper posture and technique during play. They should also be aware of signs and symptoms related to disk, nerve root, or spinal cord injury to help players seek early intervention.

25.3.2 Spinal Cord Injury

Traumatic spinal cord injury (SCI) involves direct, acute damage to the spinal cord. These cases typically result in significant neurological dysfunction, including paralysis and anesthesia of the trunk and extremities. Reported cases of SCI as a result of soccer play are infrequent—a 2020 review identified only 14 reported cases since 1976.[39] Most cases involved collisions with other players or surfaces, while only three were due to contact with the ball. A vast majority of these injuries affected the cervical spine, likely due to its high mobility and exposed nature.[35,39]

Nearly all the reported cases experienced plegia of two or four extremities. Four patients were able to return to play and two experienced mortality.[39,40]

Patients with soccer-related SCI can be treated conservatively or surgically based on their clinical presentation and prognosis.[39] Given the infrequent nature of SCI in soccer, it is not likely that any preventative measures will change the incidence rate. However, coaches should consistently monitor their players and arrange for urgent intervention if symptoms of SCI arise.

25.4 Peripheral Nerve Injuries

Although instances of soccer-related peripheral nerve injury in the literature are rare, athletes and trainers should familiarize themselves with prototypical peripheral nerve injury syndromes to detect these injuries early and prevent further damage.

25.4.1 Facial Nerve (Cranial Nerve VII) Injury

The facial nerve arises from the ventral pons of the brainstem, courses through the temporal bone, and primarily serves to innervate the muscles of facial expression. Facial fractures from soccer players' collisions with the ball or other players can lead to temporal bone fractures and subsequent facial nerve palsy from direct injury or edema.[41] This palsy is characterized by weakness of ipsilateral facial muscles, which typically resolves. A CT scan should be conducted if a temporal bone fracture is suspected, and appropriate surgical or nonsurgical intervention should be considered as soon as possible to prevent lasting damage.[41]

25.4.2 Brachial Plexus Injury

The brachial plexus arises from the C5–T8 nerve roots and is responsible for most of the sensory and motor functions of the upper extremity. Blunt injury during soccer to the neck and shoulder girdle, where the plexus resides, may cause transient neurological deficits known as "stingers." These are characterized by cervical neuropraxia, a syndrome of transient pain, weakness, numbness, tingling, or burning sensations in the affected arm.[35] As stingers are short-lived, there is no treatment required unless the player experiences them recurrently, in which case further workup is required.[35]

25.4.3 Sciatic Nerve Branches (Fibular Nerve, Sural Nerve) Injury

The fibular nerve branches directly from the sciatic nerve in the posterior thigh and allows for foot dorsiflexion, eversion, and sensation of the anterolateral leg. Given that it runs close to the peroneus longus muscle, injury to this muscle may impair the fibular nerve. Tearing or straining of this muscle during soccer has been rarely shown to cause fibular nerve palsy due to swelling and compartment syndrome. The symptoms of peroneal nerve palsy include impaired dorsiflexion, known as "foot drop," and hypoesthesia in the anterolateral leg. Patients can be treated with peroneus longus fasciotomy, and their symptoms typically resolve.[42,43]

The sural nerve, which branches from both the fibular and tibial nerves, is a purely sensory nerve that runs down the posterior calf to innervate the heel and lateral ankle.[44] Direct trauma to the calf can cause hematoma and impingement of the sural nerve, resulting in loss of sensation in these regions. One case report notes that sural nerve function returned within 2 weeks.[44]

25.5 Conclusions

Given the popularity of playing soccer throughout the world, it is important to increase awareness of the potential neurological injuries that can result from the sport. These injuries range in severity from common but mild concussions to rare but life-threatening spinal cord injuries. Player-to-player or player-to-surface collisions are commonly involved in acute brain injuries such as concussions or intracerebral hemorrhages, while subconcussive ball heading may be associated with CTE or other neuropsychological deficits, although more research should be conducted in these areas. Spinal cord injuries are rare and associated with player collisions, but degenerative spinal changes are more common in soccer players due to headers and high intensity of play. Peripheral nerve injuries in soccer are infrequently reported. Education about avoiding player collisions may help reduce the frequency of acute neurological injuries in soccer. In general, players and coaches should be mindful of the different neurological injuries that occur in soccer so that they may seek early treatment.

25.6 Clinical Pearls

- The most common neurological injuries in soccer occur in the brain, followed by the spine and peripheral nerves.
- Acute neurological soccer injuries are often related to collisions between two players or between one player and a hard surface.
- Prevention of neurological injuries in soccer should focus on emphasizing safe play techniques to minimize player collisions and falls, making efforts to reduce ball stiffness and mass, and educating coaches about early signs of injury.
- Treatment varies by injury type, but many require a withdrawal from play followed by functional therapy and/or medical intervention.
- Concussions are a mild form of acute TBI that is especially common in soccer players, presenting with executive

impairments and other sensory symptoms including dizziness and nausea.
- Repetitive "headers" in soccer may or may not be associated with chronic brain impairment, but are likely related to degenerative changes in the cervical spine.
- Direct injury to the spinal cord is rare in soccer players, but long-term play may accelerate normal degenerative changes to the vertebral bones and disks resulting in neurological symptoms.
- Peripheral nerve injuries are rare in soccer, and athletes typically have a full recovery.

25.7 Disclosures

Vikas Vattipally: None.
Carly Weber-Levine: None.
Nicholas Theodore: Royalties from Globus Medical. Stock Ownership in Globus Medical. Consultant for Globus Medical. On Scientific Advisory Board/Other Office for Globus Medical.

References

[1] Flores G, Giza CC, Bates-Jensen B, Brecht ML, Wiley D. Soccer-related injuries utilization of U.S. emergency departments for concussions, intracranial injuries, and other-injuries in a national representative probability sample: Nationwide Emergency Department Sample, 2010 to 2013. PLoS One. 2021; 16(10):e0258345

[2] Andersen TE, Árnason A, Engebretsen L, Bahr R. Mechanisms of head injuries in elite football. Br J Sports Med. 2004; 38(6):690–696

[3] Agarwal N, Thakkar R, Than K. Sports Related Head Injury. American Association of Neurological Surgeons; 2021

[4] Levy ML, Kasasbeh AS, Baird LC, Amene C, Skeen J, Marshall L. Concussions in soccer: a current understanding. World Neurosurg. 2012; 78(5):535–544

[5] Hubertus V, Marklund N, Vajkoczy P. Management of concussion in soccer. Acta Neurochir (Wien). 2019; 161(3):425–433

[6] Spiotta AM, Bartsch AJ, Benzel EC. Heading in soccer: dangerous play? Neurosurgery. 2012; 70(1):1–11, discussion 11

[7] Mooney J, Self M, ReFaey K, et al. Concussion in soccer: a comprehensive review of the literature. Concussion. 2020; 5(3):CNC76

[8] Chatha K, Pruis T, Peaguda CF, et al. Concussions in soccer: an epidemiological analysis in the pediatric population. Orthop J Sports Med. 2020; 8(10):2325967120951077

[9] Kroshus E, Garnett B, Hawrilenko M, Baugh CM, Calzo JP. Concussion underreporting and pressure from coaches, teammates, fans, and parents. Soc Sci Med. 2015; 134:66–75

[10] Dave U, Kinderknecht J, Cheng J, Santiago K, Jivanelli B, Ling DI. Systematic review and meta-analysis of sex-based differences for concussion incidence in soccer. Phys Sportsmed. 2022; 50(1):11–19

[11] Niedfeldt MW. Head injuries, heading, and the use of headgear in soccer. Curr Sports Med Rep. 2011; 10(6):324–329

[12] Comstock RD, Currie DW, Pierpoint LA, Grubenhoff JA, Fields SK. An evidence-based discussion of heading the ball and concussions in high school soccer. JAMA Pediatr. 2015; 169(9):830–837

[13] McCrory PR. Brain injury and heading in soccer. BMJ. 2003; 327(7411): 351–352

[14] Boden BP, Kirkendall DT, Garrett WE, Jr. Concussion incidence in elite college soccer players. Am J Sports Med. 1998; 26(2):238–241

[15] FIFA Medical Concussion Protocol: Suspect and Protect

[16] Kirkendall DT, Jordan SE, Garrett WE. Heading and head injuries in soccer. Sports Med. 2001; 31(5):369–386

[17] Lipton ML, Kim N, Zimmerman ME, et al. Soccer heading is associated with white matter microstructural and cognitive abnormalities. Radiology. 2013; 268(3):850–857

[18] Rodrigues AC, Lima MDM, de Souza LC, et al. No evidence of association between soccer heading and cognitive performance in professional soccer players: cross-sectional results. Front Neurol. 2019; 10:209

[19] Naunheim RS, Standeven J, Richter C, Lewis LM. Comparison of impact data in hockey, football, and soccer. J Trauma. 2000; 48(5):938–941

[20] Witol AD, Webbe FM. Soccer heading frequency predicts neuropsychological deficits. Arch Clin Neuropsychol. 2003; 18(4):397–417

[21] Tysvaer AT. Head and neck injuries in soccer. Impact of minor trauma. Sports Med. 1992; 14(3):200–213

[22] Matser JT, Kessels AG, Jordan BD, Lezak MD, Troost J. Chronic traumatic brain injury in professional soccer players. Neurology. 1998; 51(3):791–796

[23] Rutherford A, Stephens R, Potter D, Fernie G. Neuropsychological impairment as a consequence of football (soccer) play and football heading: preliminary analyses and report on university footballers. J Clin Exp Neuropsychol. 2005; 27(3):299–319

[24] Guskiewicz KM, Marshall SW, Broglio SP, Cantu RC, Kirkendall DT. No evidence of impaired neurocognitive performance in collegiate soccer players. Am J Sports Med. 2002; 30(2):157–162

[25] Wiles K. Soccer players' head injury risk could be reduced with simple adjustments to the ball, study finds. Purdue University. November 12, 2020. https://www.purdue.edu/newsroom/releases/2020/Q4/soccer-players-head-injury-risk-could-be-reduced-with-simple-adjustments-to-the-ball,-study-finds.html

[26] Stern RA, Riley DO, Daneshvar DH, Nowinski CJ, Cantu RC, McKee AC. Long-term consequences of repetitive brain trauma: chronic traumatic encephalopathy. PM R. 2011; 3(10) Suppl 2:S460–S467

[27] Chronic traumatic encephalopathy. Mayo Clinic. https://www.mayoclinic.org/diseases-conditions/chronic-traumatic-encephalopathy/symptoms-causes/syc-20370921

[28] van Amerongen S, Kamps S, Kaijser KKM, et al. Severe CTE and TDP-43 pathology in a former professional soccer player with dementia: a clinicopathological case report and review of the literature. Acta Neuropathol Commun. 2023; 11(1):77

[29] Ramsay D, Miller A, Baykeens B, Hassan H, Gentleman S. Football (soccer) as a probable cause of long-term neurological impairment and neurodegeneration: a narrative review of the debate. Cureus. 2023; 15(1):e34279

[30] Mummareddy N, Legarreta AD, Yengo-Kahn AM, et al. Sport-related structural brain injury in high school soccer: epidural hemorrhage after a "header.". World Neurosurg. 2019; 127:20–23

[31] Bruzzone E, Cocito L, Pisani R. Intracranial delayed epidural hematoma in a soccer player. A case report. Am J Sports Med. 2000; 28(6):901–903

[32] Ellis MJ, Barnes J, Cordingley DM, Bunge M, McDonald PJ, Ritchie L. Management of an adolescent athlete with sports-related concussion and intraparenchymal hemorrhage. Curr Sports Med Rep. 2018; 17(1):7–9

[33] Lutfi R, Mullett CJ, Nield LS. Acute subdural hematoma: potential soccer injury in an otherwise healthy child. Pediatr Emerg Care. 2009; 25(9): 582–583

[34] Gregori F, Colistra D, Mancarella C, Chiarella V, Marotta N, Domenicucci M. Arachnoid cyst in young soccer players complicated by chronic subdural hematoma: personal experience and review of the literature. Acta Neurol Belg. 2020; 120(2):235–246

[35] Plais N, Salzmann SN, Shue J, Sanchez CD, Urraza FJ, Girardi FP. Spine injuries in soccer. Curr Sports Med Rep. 2019; 18(10):367–373

[36] Kartal A, Yildiran I, Senköylü A, Korkusuz F. Soccer causes degenerative changes in the cervical spine. Eur Spine J. 2004; 13(1):76–82

[37] Raja A, Hoang S, Patel P, Mesfin FB. Spinal Stenosis. Treasure Island, FL: StatPearls Publishing; 2023

[38] Bezuglov E, Lazarev A, Petrov A, et al. Asymptomatic degenerative changes in the lumbar spine among professional soccer players. Spine. 2021; 46(2):122–128

[39] Poudel MK, Sherman AL. Football (soccer)-related spinal cord injury-reported cases from 1976 to 2020. Spinal Cord Ser Cases. 2020; 6(1):106

[40] Kato Y, Koga M, Taguchi T. Chronic spinal cord injury in the cervical spine of a young soccer player. Orthopedics. 2010; 33(5)

[41] Leitch EF, Hanson JR. An unusual case of facial nerve palsy following soccer related minor head injury. Br J Sports Med. 2006; 40(4):e9

[42] Hiramatsu K, Yonetani Y, Kinugasa K, et al. Deep peroneal nerve palsy with isolated lateral compartment syndrome secondary to peroneus longus tear: a report of two cases and a review of the literature. J Orthop Traumatol. 2016; 17(2):181–185

[43] Jellad A, Nouira A, Zrig A, Mnari W, Ben Salah Frih Z. Peroneus longus strain injury associated with common peroneal nerve palsy in a soccer player. Am J Phys Med Rehabil. 2016; 95(5):e77–e78

[44] Babwah T. Sural nerve injury in a footballer related to blunt leg trauma. Res Sports Med. 2012; 20(1):70–73

26 Golf

Corey T. Walker, S. Harrison Farber, D. Scott Kreiner, and Randall W. Porter

Summary

Golf remains one of the most popular sports in the world and is played by people of all ages. There has been a growing focus on back injuries and low back pain, particularly among professional and elite golfers at young ages, which raises concerns that the modern golf swing may contribute to spinal disease. Additionally, many amateur golfers with incidental back pain experience pain during play. In this chapter, we discuss the potential mechanisms by which spinal pathology occurs in golfers and examine how specific elements of the modern golf swing contribute to strain on the low back. We also highlight the key methods of treating low back pain in golfers. These include core strengthening, mobility training, and swing modification. Health care professionals with backgrounds in treating athletes, and particularly golfers, with back pain play a crucial role in appropriately addressing spinal disease in these populations. Spine surgery may be required in some instances, and careful attention should be given to designing a treatment and rehabilitation pathway with the goal of getting the patient back on the golf course.

Keywords: back pain, biomechanics, golf, physical therapy, rehabilitation, repetitive traumatic diskopathy, sports

26.1 Introduction

The game of golf is a commonly played sport that can be enjoyed regardless of age, sex, or socioeconomic status. It is estimated that more than 25 million people in the United States and 6 million people in Europe play golf to some degree each year.[1,2] Golf has been shown to have a multitude of health benefits, especially among the elderly population.[3] However, golf-related low back injuries are common and well described in the literature.[4,5,6] The low back is the most common site of injury in golfers. The prevalence of injuries ranges between 19 and 28% among amateur golfers and between 13 and 54% among professional golfers (▶ Table 26.1).[5,6,7,8,9,10,11,12,13,14,15,16] Injury rates vary by sex, occurring in up to 36% of male golfers and approximately one-quarter of female golfers.[6]

The causes of low back pain and injury in these golfers are likely to be multifactorial. Injuries usually occur as a result of chronic overuse. The golf swing entails a number of biomechanical forces that, over time, may contribute to injury. These forces affecting the spine include compression, torsion, and shear loading. In fact, earlier work has suggested that golfers are at higher risk of various spinal pathologies that include muscle strain, facet arthropathy, spondylolisthesis, disk herniation, and stress fractures of the vertebral body or pars interarticularis.[17] Although the initial management of many of these conditions includes conservative treatments and rest, over time these pathologies may lead to the need for surgical intervention, especially among those who play and practice frequently. This chapter discusses the pathogenesis and treatment of spinal disease relevant to the game of golf.

26.2 Pathogenesis of Spinal Disease in Golf

The etiology of spinal disease among golfers is often difficult to delineate, as degeneration and osteoarthritis are common findings among all elderly human beings, whether they play golf or not. Golfers with spinal disease can be divided into two general

Table 26.1 Summary of the epidemiological literature on the prevalence of low back injuries among amateur and professional golfers

Study	Year	Sample size	Total number of injuries	Portion of total injuries that are low back injuries, %
Amateur golfers				
McCarroll et al[8]	1990	1,144	708	34.5
Batt[9]	1992	193	61	21.3
Burdorf et al[10]	1996	196	62	31.6
Thériault et al[11]	1996	582	198	17.2
Finch et al[12]	1998	34	...	24.0
Gosheger et al[13]	2003	643	527	15.2
McHardy et al[6]	2007	1,634	369	24.9
McHardy et al[5]	2007	588	93	18.3
Mean % (95% confidence interval)				23.4 (18.6–28.1)
Professional golfers				
McCarroll and Gioe[14]	1982	226	393	23.7
Sugaya et al[15]	1998	283	281	54.8
Gosheger et al[13]	2003	60	110	21.8
Mean % (95% confidence interval)				33.4 (12.5–54.4)

Source: Adapted with permission from Cole and Grimshaw.[16]

categories. The first are amateur golfers, who may develop spinal disease and back pain, but because they do not play golf as a career, more traditional protocols may be considered to manage back injuries. These may include time away from the game, physical therapy, and epidural steroid injections, when appropriate. The other distinct category is the group of professional or elite players who develop cervical, thoracic, or lumbar pain. This group presents with more complex issues because of the frequency with which they are swinging the golf club in practice and play, as well as the pressure to get back to playing sooner and the high likelihood of reinjury. Finally, there is also more pressure on health care providers to allow players to return to play sooner because golf is a full-time profession for these individuals.

In the casual amateur player, it is generally unlikely that the player spent enough time practicing or playing to contribute significantly to the disease. Instead, they typically experience spinal disorders due to genetics, wear and tear, and other forces associated with lifestyle choices, occupation, and body mass index, and the golf swing imposes biomechanical strains on a preexisting injured or degenerating back. In comparison, a substantial portion of spinal disorders among professional golfers is associated with their play and is generally thought to be caused directly by destructive swing patterns that are repeated multiple times daily. The diagnosis, evaluation, and treatment of spinal disorders differ somewhat between these two groups of golfers. However, lessons learned from studies involving the latter group can be directly applied to amateur golfers with back pain and disease to help improve their recovery and symptoms.

26.2.1 Repetitive Traumatic Diskopathy

Back injuries seem to be more frequent among the current generation of professional golfers. Although it is difficult to pinpoint an exact reason, and the usual contributors—such as genetics, environment, diet, physical habitus, and daily activity—play a role, it is our belief that the modern golf swing is a major factor. The "modern golf swing," compared with "the classic swing," creates more tension in the lower back. When comparing the current era of golfers with that of legendary greats like Nicklaus, Hogan, and Player, we see a transformation in the biomechanics of the golf swing. The "classic golf swing" employed by the aforementioned players was more fluid, characterized by lifting the left heel off the ground, releasing the tension in the lower back, and involving lateral flexion during the downswing. The modern swing, as taught by current professionals, emphasizes immobilizing the lower body during the backswing as though one is sitting in a chair. This imparts significant torsion on the spine, especially in the lumbar and thoracic segments. The purpose of this change is to create a golf swing that enables the player to hit the ball farther. The popularity of the modern swing, combined with the trend of spending an increasing amount of time in the gym, which includes significant weight training, means that the modern professional golfers expose their joints, disks, and ligaments to greater forces than did golfers of an earlier era. We believe that the modern swing is a major contributor to the increased incidence of back pain and spinal injuries among the newest generation of golfers. Anecdotally, the current head of physical therapy on the Professional Golf Association (PGA) tour has remarked that the top two injuries that are seen on the therapy trucks during tournaments are back and wrist injuries, adding further credence to our observation.

To understand this concept, one needs to have an intricate understanding of the changes that have occurred in the golf swing over the past two decades (▶ Fig. 26.1).[16] The underlying mechanistic change in the golf swing allows for an increased explosiveness during the downswing. Modern golf instruction focuses on creating maximum potential rotational energy during the backswing, akin to winding up a spring. This is achieved by twisting the thorax with a maximal differential between the shoulders and lower torso, a concept originally described by professional Jim McLean and termed the "X-factor" (▶ Fig. 26.2a).[18] McLean's observation was supported by the fact that one of the longest hitters on tour at that time, John Daly, had a differential of 48 degrees, the largest differential of any golfer on the PGA tour. In theory, this torsion of the thorax and shoulders can be unwound in a sequential fashion during the downswing to yield tremendous rotational energy through the clubhead, resulting in increased clubhead speeds. However, it is important to note that there are a number of golfers on the PGA tour who have a much smaller X-factor than Daly.[19] Additionally, players are taught to keep their hands tight into their body during the downswing, driving down with lateral bending of the torso as the hips slide forward and rotate, pulling the body through the follow-through. The lateral flexion on the trail side has been termed the "crunch" (▶ Fig. 26.2b), and it is thought to contribute to large amounts of loading forces on that ipsilateral side of the spine. In fact, we have seen right-handed National Collegiate Athletics Association Division I college golfers with trailing right-sided recurrent herniated disks, presumably attributable to compressive forces (▶ Fig. 26.3).[20] A historic study by Sugaya and colleagues[21] conducted in Japan confirms the observation of increased radiographic asymmetric degeneration of the spine on the trail side of the spine in golfers compared with nongolfer controls.

One of the most interesting observations in the literature is that rotational forces, when combined with asymmetric compressive loading, place tremendous amounts of axial force on the disks, facet joints, and spinal ligaments, making them more likely to fail.[22] With professional and elite golfers swinging hundreds of times per day for multiple years, it is thought that this culminates in lumbar spinal pathology, a disease termed "repetitive traumatic diskopathy."[20] This process aligns with theories of general musculoskeletal injury related to chronic overuse of the axial skeleton.[23] Health care providers in the areas of physical therapy, rehabilitation, interventional spine medicine, and spine surgery are increasingly focusing on this special area of spinal disorders. However, a tremendous amount of research is required to help define this pathology, its pathogenesis, and its treatment.

26.3 Treatment of Spinal Disease in Golf

The treatment of spinal disease in golf follows many of the current standards of care applied to other sports, yet there are also some key distinctions. First, similar to concussion protocols used by the senior author and other neurologists, a baseline evaluation of strength and mobility should be obtained and compared with age-matched norms. When these baseline

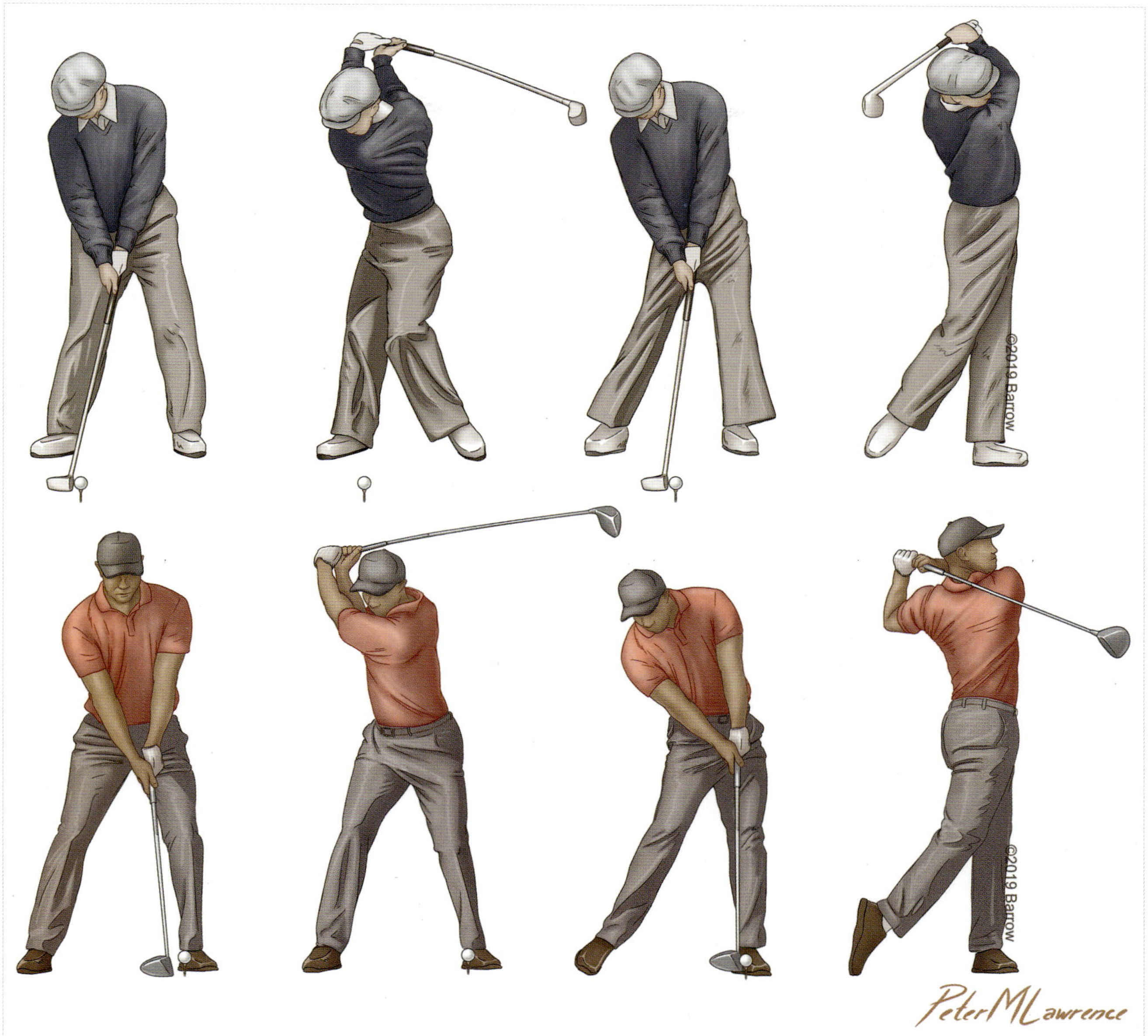

Fig. 26.1 Comparison of the classic (top) and modern (bottom) golf swings. (Used with permissions from Barrow Neurological Institute, Phoenix, Arizona.)

measurements change for the worse in the setting of an acute injury, removal of the athlete from the playing field or the golf course should be seriously considered. Acute low back pain in golf is often related to paraspinal muscle injury or spasm. Similar to the concussion protocol, cessation of participation and rest are the first-line treatment. This treatment includes no physical activity that stresses the injured area. Application of ice, gentle massage, stretching, and adjunctive use of nonsteroidal anti-inflammatory medications and muscle relaxants should be considered. Any refractory symptoms or symptoms associated with radiculopathy may warrant further workup with diagnostic imaging, including magnetic resonance imaging (MRI) and possibly dynamic radiographs, including anteroposterior lateral flexion–extension and lateral bending films, along with full-length standing films. Evaluation by a physician and physical therapists with a special knowledge of golf injuries is highly recommended. It is important to evaluate for structural causes of pain, such as disk herniation, facet syndromes, spondylolysis, spondylolisthesis, stenosis, and severe disk degeneration. Persistent symptoms associated with structural lesions that do not improve with conservative therapies may warrant evaluation by a spine interventionalist and/or spine surgeon. Epidural steroid injections, facet injections, and ablation should be considered in all cases only after appropriate evaluation by a board-certified physical medicine and/or pain physician. In all other circumstances, physical therapy and spine rehabilitation are the best methods for treating back pain. Likewise, many of the same principles may help to prevent further golf-related injury. It is important to identify clinicians with

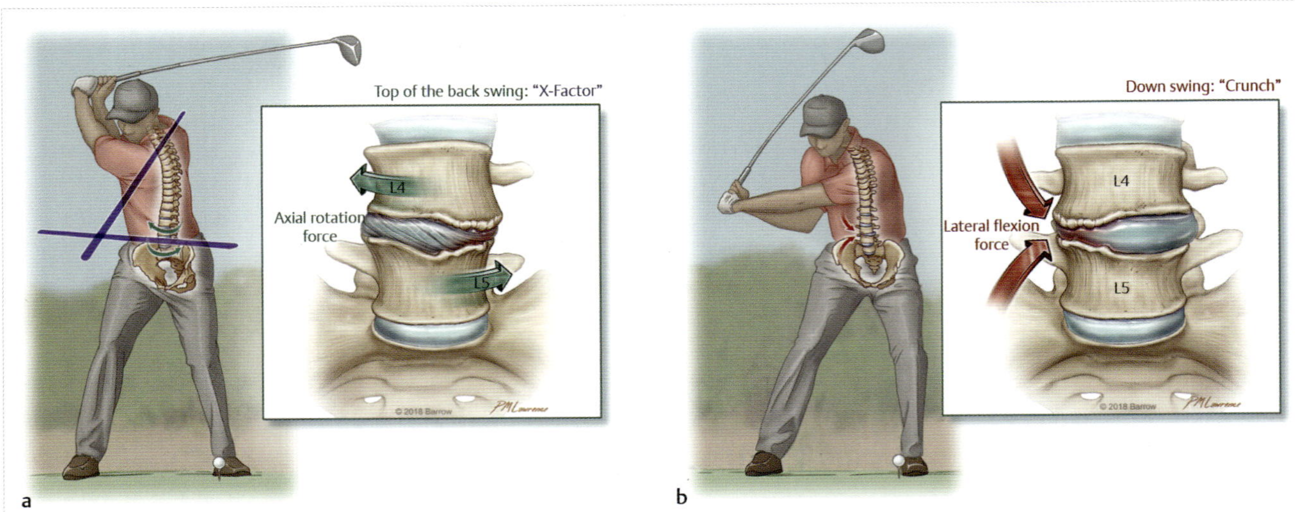

Fig. 26.2 Schematic drawings demonstrating the local effects of the modern golf swing on the lumbar spine (example shown at the L4–L5 level), contributing to repetitive traumatic diskopathy. During the back swing, maximal rotation of the shoulders relative to the hips creates a wound-up potential energy known as the "X-factor,"[18] but it also creates a supramaximal amount of torsional axial rotation of the lumbar spine **(a)**. During this explosive downswing, lateral flexion results in the "crunch" of the trailing side of the spine, asymmetrically loading the disk and facet joints **(b)**. (Used with permissions from Barrow Neurological Institute, Phoenix, Arizona.)

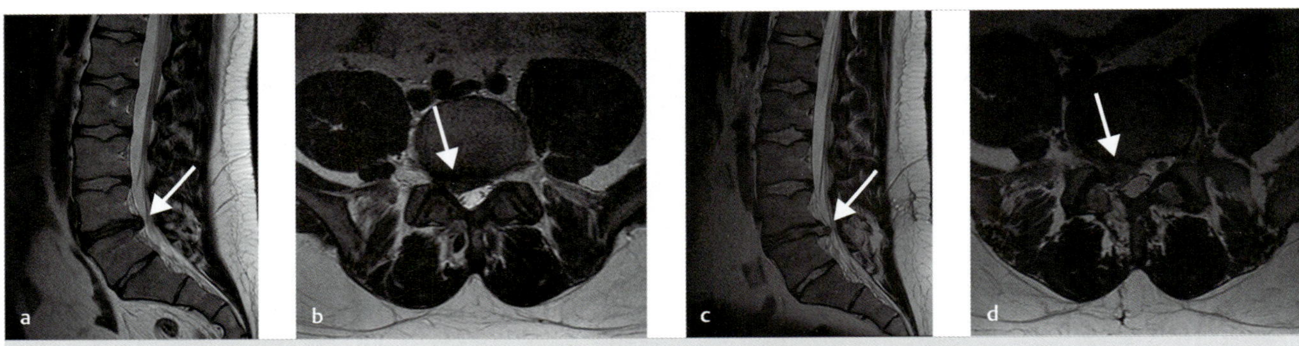

Fig. 26.3 T2-weighted sagittal **(a)** and axial **(b)** magnetic resonance imaging (MRI) of a 22-year-old collegiate elite right-handed golfer presenting with severe disk degeneration at L4–L5 with large disk herniation that caused back pain and severe radiculopathy (*arrows*). The patient underwent a right-sided L4–L5 microdiskectomy procedure. After surgery, he returned to play, but the symptoms recurred 3 years after the operation, at which time T2-weighted sagittal **(c)** and axial **(d)** MRI demonstrated repeated herniation on the right side at the same level (*arrows*). The patient underwent a second microdiskectomy procedure but did not continue with competitive golf. (Reproduced with permission from Walker et al.[20])

a background in treating golfers to maximize and tailor these therapies accordingly.

Return to play should parallel return to play in concussed athletes. First, players should stop all golf-related activity until they are asymptomatic. Second, gradual return to play starting with low-impact short workouts or practice sessions should be trialed with gradient increases in frequency and intensity. No specific guidelines exist, but in our opinion, the establishment of such guidelines is warranted. For example, players could start with chipping and putting, progress to range work, and then play on the course. Initial full swings may start with easy, smooth contact and progress to iron work, where ground contact and creation of a divot may transiently increase instantaneous spinal loads. If symptoms return at any stage, players should return to the prior level that left them asymptomatic. Whether the injured player is an amateur or professional, coordination between the physician, physical therapist, and personal trainer or PGA professional is mandatory.

26.3.1 Physical Therapy and Rehabilitation

Low back pain in golfers requires focused treatment by therapists and trainers familiar with the golf swing biomechanics and preferably with certification in golf-specific therapy from a center such as the Titleist Performance Institute (TPI) in Carlsbad, California. According to the TPI website, the TPI certification program is "designed for golf teaching professionals, medical practitioners and fitness trainers [...] an evidence based, educational pathway designed to teach industry professionals how to increase player performance through a deep understanding of how the body functions during the golf swing."[24] The senior author's practice employs 11 physical therapists, and nearly all have been TPI certified because the practice sees so many golfers. Aggressive treatment has been demonstrated to improve low back pain in many golfers and prevent recurrent symptoms. The main components of these treatments include core muscle strengthening, mobility and stretching exercises, and swing modification, as discussed below. All of these golf-specific interventions change the strains placed on the lumbar disk and facets, potentially abrogating the repetitive forces that are associated with injury.

Core strengthening has been the focus of many therapeutic treatments of low back pain and is well known to help symptoms by improving stabilization of the torso around the spinal elements. Electromyography studies of the golf swing have demonstrated the exquisite sequence of muscular activation involved throughout each step.[25,26] Fatigue, incompetence, or asymmetry of core muscles can result in injuries of the spine or compensatory secondary muscles that step in to maintain trunk stability.

The main muscles targeted in therapy for golf-related low back pain are the multifidi and longissimi posteriorly and the transversus abdominus (TA), external oblique, and internal oblique anteriorly. These muscles have vertebral attachments and are vital stabilizers. The multifidi muscles participate in lumbar extension and protect the spine from torsion and axial rotation during the downswing. Similarly, the TA muscle attaches to the transverse processes, wrapping around the torso and contributing to core and pelvis stabilization during hip and torso rotation. It has been shown that performing exercises centered on strengthening these muscles improves back pain in elite golfers when performed in conjunction with mobility exercises and can result in demonstrable changes in swing kinetics.[27] Additionally, core strengthening requires focus on the other core muscles as well, including the rectus abdominis, erector spinae, quadratus lumborum, and hip abductors, all of which have been implicated in swing analyses and truncal motion control.[28]

Stretching and mobility training is also essential for reducing strain on the back and helping to protect the spine during the golf swing. The golfer should establish a baseline range of motion in all major joints of the body under the supervision of a physical therapist and focus on stretching exercises that address the deficiencies. Limitations of movements in the shoulders, elbows, hips, and knees can all result in increased compensatory strain within the spine. Specifically, deficits in hip range of motion may lead to reduced internal and external rotation that places greater demand on the spinal segments to complete swing rotation.[29] Videographic swing analyses by golf professionals and therapists may help to identify relative deficiencies in mobility and specifically address these limitations during rehabilitation.

26.3.2 Swing Modifications

Extensive swing analysis has been performed to examine differences in swing patterns for patients with and without back pain. Additionally, professional golf instructors have attempted to make changes in golfer's swings to reduce loads on player's spines. Given our hypothesis that repetitive traumatic diskopathy causes trauma to the spine through cumulative damage of repeated spinal microtrauma, small reductions in disk and facet loading may have tremendous long-term benefits. In general, many coaches recommend adopting a swing that mimics that of historic classic styles, rather than the modern technique described above. Although no studies have yet shown that making this change results in decreased back pain, the theory is plausible. That said, there are several specific swing changes that are thought to be beneficial for reducing strain on the spine.

One of the key findings from several studies relates to the golfer's posture and stance at address. It has been suggested that golfers with low back pain tend to be slouched over and less upright, potentially resulting in increased strain on the low back during the downswing. This can also be corrected by standing closer to the ball, allowing for a more upright stance. It is thought that this improves shear stresses on the low back that occur from rotation in a flexed trunk position.[20] Maintenance of lumbar lordosis during rotation likely reduces the intradiskal strains. However, caution must be expressed in applying this recommendation broadly, as facet injuries and pain may actually worsen with extension and rotation. Future focus on the exact source of the injury with respect to the golf swing may allow for more tailored swing modifications based on patient-specific pathology.

Another key focus relates to increasing hip rotation during the backswing and downswing. As stated above, increasing hip mobility and stretching the joints improves this; however, it is important that golfers practice increasing their hip rotation. Some professionals advocate for angling the feet outward at address to assist with this motion. Players need to work on performing appropriate timing of the shoulder and hip rotation that occurs during the critical period of the backswing. Lumbar corsets have been suggested to this end, and they may help to improve extension of the lumbar spine during swinging while simultaneously increasing hip rotation.[30] Additional studies are needed to determine the clinical benefit of wearing lumbar corsets in players with back pain. Similarly, it has been suggested that shortening the backswing may help to decrease trunk muscle activation without significantly decreasing accuracy or clubhead speed. It should be noted that this, in turn, can lead to increased shoulder muscle activation, again highlighting the role of compensatory mechanics in the golf swing. Furthermore, others have suggested swinging while keeping the lumbar and thoracic disks parallel, especially during the downswing.[31]

Altogether, these studies suggest an important role in swing modification for golf rehabilitation in players with back pain. However, a substantial amount of work is still required to improve our understanding of how to best manage these patients. Additionally, it is important that studies focus on both elite and novice golfers, as the goals, alterations, and outcomes may be drastically different between these populations.

26.4 Surgical Management and Return to Play Guidelines

In golfers who require surgical management, we strongly advocate for muscle-sparing, minimally invasive approaches to the spine. It has been well-documented that, with traditional open techniques for lumbar decompression and fusion, extensive paraspinal muscle injury, contraction, and dysfunction occur with midline dissection. Given the integral role of these muscles during the golf swing, we believe that the traditional approach is detrimental and may result in suboptimal outcomes for patients who hope to return to the game. We prefer to perform minimally invasive tubular decompression techniques when possible and to use anterior and lateral retroperitoneal approaches for fusion with percutaneous fixation when required. In fact, in one study, the authors examined the ability to return to play after lumbar fusion among 34 patients.[32] They found that, of the 17 patients who underwent one- or two-level open lumbar fusion, 13 participated in golf with the same or increased frequency after the operation as they had before the operation. They also found that 3 of 5 patients who underwent minimally invasive surgical procedures and 10 of 12 patients who underwent anterior lumbar fusion played the same amount or more often after surgery. The reasons for the differences in return to play were not addressed by the authors; however, we have observed similar results in our clinic. Thus, in the absence of significant instability, obesity, pars defect, or significant scoliosis, we generally recommend minimally invasive anterior or lateral-only approaches for patients who require spinal fusion and are hoping to get back on the golf course. This not only spares the posterior muscles but also, once fusion occurs, allows patients to maintain more mobility, increasing their likelihood of maintaining more range of motion. In fact, most biomechanical studies show that adding posterior instrumentation significantly increases the stiffness of the lumbar spine.[33]

Return after surgical treatment depends on the patient's preoperative health status and postoperative functionality and on the procedure performed. For decompression procedures, including lumbar microdiskectomy and laminectomy, we typically allow for slow reintroduction of play, which usually starts with chipping and putting, 12 weeks after surgery. Once the patient has passed this stage, we encourage playing nine holes and hitting longer shots for no more than 1 to 2 hours per day 3 days per week. If they pass this stage painlessly, patients are approved to play full rounds up to 3 times per week for 2 months. And finally, if they are asymptomatic after 6 months, patients can play without restrictions.

Some surgeons may advocate that players not return to golf after undergoing lumbar fusion because of concerns regarding hardware failure or injury of the fusion construct. In our experience, this is unwarranted, and we have yet to have a patient develop an injury at the site of the fusion attributable to returning to play. On the basis of a survey of spine surgeons from the North American Spine Society members, it is recommended that patients who undergo fusion allow 6 months of recovery time before slowly reintroducing play.[34] This allows sufficient time for bony fusion to take place. In patients with poor bone quality or at high risk for pseudoarthrosis due to comorbidity, it may be worthwhile to wait longer or obtain computed tomography that demonstrates fusion before allowing resumption of play. Although it involved only a small number of patients, a study of golfers who underwent lumbar fusion reported that more than half of patients returned to full play within 1 year of surgery, with approximately three-quarters of those patients playing the same or more golf than before surgery and at a stable or improved handicap.[32] Careful preoperative counseling from health care providers regarding patient expectations and recovery is important, and patients should remain optimistic that they may return to full play even after having lumbar fusion surgery.

26.5 Conclusions

Golf remains one of the most popular recreational sports in the world, but it may cause or exacerbate back pain due to the unique repetitive forces imparted during practice and play. The modern golf swing, along with increased physical strength among players, may result in a greater risk to the lumbar spine, which we have termed repetitive traumatic diskopathy. This may lead to early spinal degeneration and/or herniation in elite golfers as a culmination of subclinical microstrains on the disk annulus and facet joints. This appears to be the result of supraphysiological torsional, compressive, shear, and lateral bending moments that occur. In players with back pain, a multidisciplinary coordination between the physician, swing coach, therapist, and trainer is required to help rehabilitate injuries and prevent future disease progression. Likewise, swing modifications employed in conjunction with professional golf association teachers can be helpful in reducing the repeated stresses on the spinal elements. If conservative therapies cannot be successfully employed, surgical evaluation by a spinal health care provider with a background in treating athletes is necessary. If surgery is required, we advocate anterior and lateral stand-alone techniques to minimize recovery, maximize flexibility, and maximize the chance the golfer will return to play after recovery. Future clinical and biomechanical research is required to augment understanding of spinal disease in golfers so that we can more appropriately guide care pathways, including rehabilitation and surgical intervention.

26.6 Clinical Pearls

- Early diagnosis of diskogenic low back pain and degenerative spinal disease in golfers allows health care providers to identify pathology early in the disease course and treat patients before severe disease develops.
- Focusing on biomechanical changes in the patient's swing can help prevent repetitive damage to the disks and facet joints in the long-term. Players should be referred to professional physiotherapists, trainers, and coaches who can help them with injury prevention.
- When intervention is warranted for spinal pathologies in golfers, minimally invasive, muscle-preserving approaches should be applied to help preserve motion and functionality of the soft-tissue compartment surrounding the spine.

26.7 Disclosures

Randall W. Porter, Owner, Founder, The Medical Memory, Inc.

Acknowledgments

The authors thank the staff of Neuroscience Publications at Barrow Neurological Institute for assistance with manuscript and illustration preparation.

References

[1] Zouzias IC, Hendra J, Stodelle J, Limpisvasti O. Golf injuries: epidemiology, pathophysiology, and treatment. J Am Acad Orthop Surg. 2018; 26(4): 116–123

[2] Farrally MR, Cochran AJ, Crews DJ, et al. Golf science research at the beginning of the twenty-first century. J Sports Sci. 2003; 21(9):753–765

[3] Murray AD, Daines L, Archibald D, et al. The relationships between golf and health: a scoping review. Br J Sports Med. 2017; 51(1):12–19

[4] McHardy A, Pollard H, Luo K. Golf injuries: a review of the literature. Sports Med. 2006; 36(2):171–187

[5] McHardy A, Pollard H, Luo K. One-year follow-up study on golf injuries in Australian amateur golfers. Am J Sports Med. 2007; 35(8):1354–1360

[6] McHardy AJ, Pollard HP, Luo K. Golf-related lower back injuries: an epidemiological survey. J Chiropr Med. 2007; 6(1):20–26

[7] Smith JA, Hawkins A, Grant-Beuttler M, Beuttler R, Lee SP. Risk factors associated with low back pain in golfers: a systematic review and meta-analysis. Sports Health. 2018; 10(6):538–546

[8] McCarroll JR, Rettig AC, Shelbourne KD. Injuries in the amateur golfer. Phys Sportsmed. 1990; 18(3):122–126

[9] Batt ME. A survey of golf injuries in amateur golfers. Br J Sports Med. 1992; 26(1):63–65

[10] Burdorf A, Van Der Steenhoven GA, Tromp-Klaren EG. A one-year prospective study on back pain among novice golfers. Am J Sports Med. 1996; 24(5):659–664

[11] Thériault G, Lacoste E, Gadoury M, Ouellet S, Leblanc C. Golf injury characteristics: a survey from 528 golfers 389. Med Sci Sports Exerc. 1996; 28(5):65

[12] Finch CF, Sherman CA, James T. The epidemiology of golf injuries in Victoria, Australia: evidence from sports medicine clinics and emergency department presentations In: Farrally MR, Cochran AJ, eds. Science and Golf III: Proceedings of the World Scientific Congress of Golf. Champaign: Human Kinetics Publishers; 1998:73–82

[13] Gosheger G, Liem D, Ludwig K, Greshake O, Winkelmann W. Injuries and overuse syndromes in golf. Am J Sports Med. 2003; 31(3):438–443

[14] McCarroll JR, Gioe TJ. Professional golfers and the price they pay. Phys Sportsmed. 1982; 10(7):64–70

[15] Sugaya H, Tsuchiya A, Moriya H. Low back injury in elite and professional golfers: an epidemiologic and radiographic study. In: Farrally MR, Cochran AJ, eds. Science and Golf III: Proceedings of the World Scientific Congress of Golf. Human Kinetics Publishers; 1998:83–91

[16] Cole MH, Grimshaw PN. The biomechanics of the modern golf swing: implications for lower back injuries. Sports Med. 2016; 46(3):339–351

[17] Hosea TM, Gatt CJ, Jr. Back pain in golf. Clin Sports Med. 1996; 15(1):37–53

[18] McLean J, Andrisani J. The X-factor Swing. 1 ed. New York: Harper Collins; 1997

[19] Mann J. Jim McLean's triple-X factor: a critical review. Published 2008. Accessed at: http://perfectgolfswingreview.net/xfactor.htm

[20] Walker CT, Uribe JS, Porter RW. Golf: a contact sport. Repetitive traumatic discopathy may be the driver of early lumbar degeneration in modern-era golfers. J Neurosurg Spine. 2019:1–4. Online ahead of print

[21] Sugaya H, Moriya H, Takahashi K. Asymmetric radiographic findings on the lumbar spine in elite and professional golfers. Orthop Trans. 1997; 21(1): 312–313

[22] Gluck GS, Bendo JA, Spivak JM. The lumbar spine and low back pain in golf: a literature review of swing biomechanics and injury prevention. Spine J. 2008; 8(5):778–788

[23] Kumar S. Theories of musculoskeletal injury causation. Ergonomics. 2001; 44(1):17–47

[24] Yoo IS, Lee SH, Suk S-H. A case of fentanyl intoxication and delayed hypoxic leukoencephalopathy caused by incidental use of fentanyl patch in a healthy elderly man. J Neurocrit Care. 2015; 8(1):35–38

[25] Pink M, Perry J, Jobe FW. Electromyographic analysis of the trunk in golfers. Am J Sports Med. 1993; 21(3):385–388

[26] McHardy A, Pollard H. Muscle activity during the golf swing. Br J Sports Med. 2005; 39(11):799–804, discussion 799–804

[27] Grimshaw PN, Burden AM. Case report: reduction of low back pain in a professional golfer. Med Sci Sports Exerc. 2000; 32(10):1667–1673

[28] Finn C. Rehabilitation of low back pain in golfers: from diagnosis to return to sport. Sports Health. 2013; 5(4):313–319

[29] Vad VB, Bhat AL, Basrai D, Gebeh A, Aspergren DD, Andrews JR. Low back pain in professional golfers: the role of associated hip and low back range-of-motion deficits. Am J Sports Med. 2004; 32(2):494–497

[30] Hashimoto K, Miyamoto K, Yanagawa T, et al. Lumbar corsets can decrease lumbar motion in golf swing. J Sports Sci Med. 2013; 12(1):80–87

[31] Olshock RC. How to Use Biomechanics to Save Your Back and Your Golf Swing: It's All About Posture! Kindle Edition. Bryan Olshock; 2016

[32] Shifflett GD, Hellman MD, Louie PK, Mikhail C, Park KU, Phillips FM. Return to golf after lumbar fusion. Sports Health. 2017; 9(3):280–284

[33] Karahalios DG, Kaibara T, Porter RW, et al. Biomechanics of a lumbar interspinous anchor with anterior lumbar interbody fusion. J Neurosurg Spine. 2010; 12(4):372–380

[34] Abla AA, Maroon JC, Lochhead R, Sonntag VK, Maroon A, Field M. Return to golf after spine surgery. J Neurosurg Spine. 2011; 14(1):23–30

27 Cycling

Carly Weber-Levine, Andrew M. Hersh, and Nicholas Theodore

Summary
Cyclists can be exposed to a variety of neurological injuries through both traumatic, high-speed accidents and chronic use injuries associated with long hours on the bike. In the brain, traumatic brain injury and intracranial hemorrhage can occur in accidents and a medical professional should screen cyclists for any signs of brain injury using the Sport Concussion Assessment Tool. In the spine, injury to the spinal cord most often involves the cervical spine and leads to sprains, fractures, or spinal cord injury. If a spinal injury is suspected, immediate immobilization via a collar is imperative prior to moving the cyclist. In the peripheral nerves, the position of the cyclists can lead to chronic compression injuries of the ulnar, median, and pudendal nerves. If cyclists begin to feel numbness or paresthesias in the distributions of these nerves, changing positions on the bike, modifying the seat and handlebar heights, and resting appropriately are key for preventing further damage. Understanding the identification, treatment, and prevention of these strategies is imperative for keeping riders safe and allowing them to participate in the sport as long as possible.

Keywords: cycling, neurological injuries, peripheral nerve injuries, sports medicine

27.1 Introduction

Cycling is a low-impact form of cardiovascular exercise that has grown significantly in popularity, both recreationally and competitively.[1] Competitive cycling can be a hazardous sport, with hundreds of riders cycling near one another at speeds as high as 80 km/hr.[2,3] Unfortunately, neurological injuries can occur to the brain, spine, and peripheral nerves (▶ Fig. 27.1). Acute traumatic events, such as collisions resulting in falls, can cause devastating injuries. Chronic use of bicycles and the position adopted by bikers for hours on end can predispose cyclists to peripheral nerve injuries, specifically in the median, ulnar, and pudendal nerves. This chapter discusses the common neurological injuries seen in cyclists and provides prevention and treatment strategies (▶ Table 27.1).

27.2 Brain

Brain injuries are the leading cause of cycling-related mortality and commonly occur because of acute traumatic events, predominantly collisions with other cyclists or motor vehicles.[10] Abrupt changes in the weather or road conditions can increase the risk of cyclists falling from their vehicles. Brain injuries common in cyclists include traumatic brain injury (TBI) and intracranial hemorrhage (ICH), typically involving the cerebral cortex.[11] Concussions, a milder form of TBI, account for as much as 9% of cycling-specific injuries.[12] Other types of injuries, such as diffuse axonal injury, are comparatively rarer after a crash, likely due to the lower crash speeds seen in cycling as compared to those in car accidents.[13]

After a crash, medical trainers should screen cyclists for severe or increasing headache, confusion, loss of consciousness, vomiting, dizziness, change in vision, balance problems, inability to speak or swallow, or overt head trauma.[4,6,12] These symptoms are deemed red flags by the governing body of professional cycling, Union Cycliste Internationale (UCI), and require immediate withdrawal from the competition.[12] UCI also recommends the routine use of the Sport Concussion Assessment Tool (SCAT) in competitions to evaluate suspected concussions.[4,14,15] If the cyclist does not exhibit any concussive symptoms, he or she can return to the race, but SCAT testing should be repeated after the race and the day after.[12]

Following a collision, the rider's face, neck, and helmet should be inspected for any signs of life-threatening events. Assessment of an acute traumatic event should always begin with evaluation of the airway and breathing. The patient's Glasgow Coma Score (GCS) and overall respiratory status should be considered for the need for intubation (GCS ≤ 8).[6] Following assessment of the patient's hemodynamic status and performance of any required stabilization, a neurological examination with imaging can be performed. Most importantly a noncontrast computed tomography (CT) should be performed as soon as possible.[6]

If an ICH occurs, decompressive surgery may be needed to evacuate the hematoma and reduce pressure on the brain parenchyma.[6] Following a head injury, cyclists should take appropriate amount of rest to recover, ranging anywhere from one week to several months, depending on the severity of the injury, followed by a gradual return.[4] UCI recommends waiting at least 1 week after all symptoms have resolved.[12] For patients with more severe injuries, consulting a neurologist or neurosurgeon before return is important to prevent worsening injury.

Helmets are the most important prevention tool and reduce the risk of head injuries by over 70%, with a decline in mortality of 44%.[10,11] A meta-analysis of 55 studies investigating the effect of bicycle helmets on preventing head injury found that helmets reduce any head injury, severe head injury, fatal head injury, and TBI by 48, 60, 71, and 53%, respectively.[16] Accordingly, competitive cycling governing bodies, like USA Cycling, require helmets that meet either the U.S. Department of Transportation or the Consumer Product Safety Commission standards in all competitions.[1,17]

27.3 Spine

Although head injuries are significantly more common than spinal injuries, the latter can also occur following traumatic accidents.[7] Spinal injuries include musculoskeletal sprains, fractures, and spinal cord injury (SCI). They typically involve the cervical spine.[11] A study in Norway found an incidence of cervical spinal injuries of 1.7 per 100,000 person-years among cyclists.[18] Between 2000 and 2015, the incidence of cervical fractures in cycling increased significantly from 0.67 to 2.7 per million.[19] In a study of 26,380 patients with neck sprains and

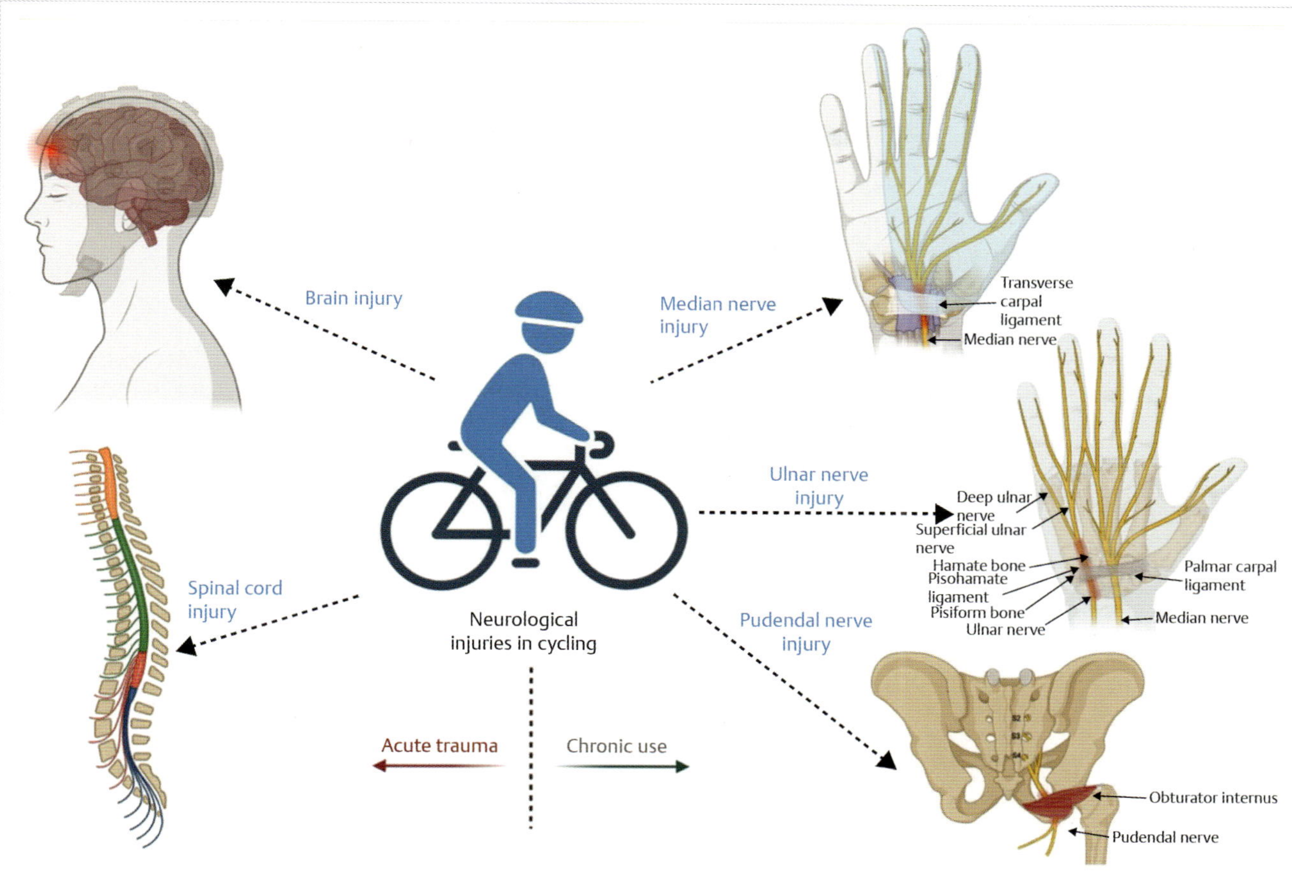

Fig. 27.1 Neurological injuries in cycling include those caused by acute trauma or chronic use. Acute trauma can lead to traumatic brain injury (TBI) or intracranial hemorrhage (ICH) in the brain and fractures or spinal cord injury (SCI) in the spine, and chronic use can lead to problems in the median, ulnar, and pudendal nerves. (Created with BioRender.com.)

Table 27.1 Neurological injuries common in cycling

Location	Cause	Presentation	Prevention
Brain			
TBI	Acute trauma	Confusion, headache, change in vision, nausea, vomiting, loss of consciousness, dizziness, memory loss[4,5]	Helmets
ICH	Acute trauma	Confusion, headache, change in vision, nausea, vomiting, loss of consciousness, dizziness, seizure, lethargy, altered mental status[5,6]	Helmets
Spine			
Cervical fractures	Acute trauma	Neck pain, stiffness, tenderness[7]	None
SCI	Acute trauma	Neck pain with decreased sensation, muscle weakness, paralysis, or difficulty breathing[7]	Immediate immobilization of the spine following injury
Cervical radiculopathy	Chronic use	Pain radiating to the upper extremities, numbness, and paresthesia	Elevation of the stem or handlebars
Peripheral Nerve			
Ulnar	Chronic use, compression at Guyon's canal[8]	Grip weakness, paresthesias, and numbness in half of the fourth and full fifth digits	Padded gloves, padded handlebars, frequent changes in hand position, correctly positioned seat[9]
Median	Chronic use, compression at carpal tunnel[8]	Paresthesias and pain in the first through half of the fourth digits	Padded gloves, padded handlebars, frequent changes in hand position, correctly positioned seat[9]
Pudendal	Chronic use, compression of the perineum[8]	Genital numbness, paresthesias, and sexual dysfunction[8]	Tilt nose of saddle down, align height of seat with handlebar, hard saddle

Abbreviations: ICH, intracranial hemorrhage; SCI, spinal cord injury; TBI, traumatic brain injury.

1,166 patients with neck fractures, cycling was the third most common cause of neck sprains and the most common cause of cervical fractures.[19] Musculoskeletal and SCIs are often concomitant, with approximately 12% of cyclists with cervical fractures also having an SCI.[18] More severe spinal injuries are often the result of cyclists being thrown over the handlebars.[20]

Common symptoms that suggest a cervical spinal fracture include neck pain, stiffness, or point tenderness. SCI should be suspected if any of these symptoms occur alongside evidence of neurological injury, such as loss of sensation or motor weakness.[21] Initial evaluation should begin with stabilizing the spine and minimizing any additional neck movement. Imaging should be done either with an X-ray or a CT scan to assess for injuries to the bony spine. Magnetic resonance imaging (MRI) is not the first-line imaging but can be performed for evaluation of the spinal canal and cord if neurological deficits are present and other imaging is normal.[21]

External immobilization via a collar can treat minor cervical fractures without neurological deficits. If the injury is unstable, surgical fixation via fusion may be necessary. In the event of SCI, surgical decompression via laminectomy may be necessary to reduce pressure on the spinal cord.[21]

There are limited prevention strategies for spinal injuries. Some studies have suggested that helmets may help prevent cervical spinal injuries, but other studies have shown no effect or even an increased risk.[18] Immediate immobilization is the most important strategy for mitigating further damage.

Chronic injury to the spine can also occur. The aerodynamic positioning of the cervical spine in extension and protraction may lead to cervical radiculopathy or spinal stenosis.[1] This typically presents with pain radiating to the upper extremities, numbness, and paresthesias. Repositioning the bike to avoid cervical extensions, such as elevating the stem or handlebars, may help alleviate symptoms.

27.4 Peripheral Nerves

Peripheral nerve injuries (PNIs) are more commonly linked to long-term, chronic compression injuries and are the most common neurological injuries associated with cycling. In a study of 551,612 patients presenting to emergency departments for PNI across the US from 2009 to 2018, cycling was the second most common cause with 7,211 affected patients.[22] The cycling position can put significant pressure on several nerves, including the ulnar, median, and pudendal nerves.

27.4.1 Ulnar Nerve

The ulnar nerve is derived from the medial cord (C8 and T1 roots) of the brachial plexus and is the most commonly affected nerve in cycling.[11] In cyclists, it is most typically compressed in Guyon's canal, formed by the pisiform bone in the ulnar border, the hamate bone in the radial border, the palmar carpal ligament on the roof, and the pisohamate ligament on the floor.[23] The Guyon's canal measures about 4 cm and can be divided into several zones. Zone 1 is proximal to the division of the ulnar nerve into the deep motor and superficial sensory branches, which form Zone 2 and Zone 3, respectively.[23] Grip pressure on the handlebars with the wrists in hyperextension can cause compression of the ulnar nerve at any point in the Guyon canal.[24]

Ulnar nerve injury commonly presents with numbness, paresthesias, and weakness in the hand, specifically in the ulnar half of the fourth and fifth digits, commonly referred to as "cyclist's palsy" or "handlebar neuropathy."[8,25] Sensory symptoms often occur first due to compression of the superficial sensory branch against the hamate in hyperextension.[23,26] In a study of 25 cyclists riding 600 km over 4 days, 70% of the riders developed motor and sensory symptoms in the hands, such as reduced grip strength or numbness.[9]

In most cases, ulnar compression is a clinical diagnosis, but electrophysiological testing can measure sensory or motor changes in the nerve.[27] For example, after a 420-mile bike ride over 6 days, cyclists had a significant increase in motor latency in the deep branch of the ulnar nerve.[28]

Most cases resolve spontaneously with rest. In rare cases, patients may require surgical decompression to release sites of compression, such as the fascia or aponeurosis of the hypothenar muscle.[24] Prevention includes the use of padded gloves and handlebars and frequent adjustments in hand position.[11] Relative to tops and hood position, drops position is associated with the greatest hypothenar pressure, greater wrist extension, and lower percentage of body weight supported by the saddle, indicating that the tops or hoods positions may be more protective of the ulnar nerve.[26]

27.4.2 Median Nerve

The median nerve is derived from the C6–T1 roots of the brachial plexus. It is commonly compressed in the carpal tunnel, which is bounded by the transverse carpal ligament and bones of the hand, leading to carpal tunnel syndrome.[11] Cyclists may present with paresthesias or pain in a median nerve distribution, i.e., the thumb and first two and a half fingers, after prolonged positioning of the wrists in extension or direct pressure on the wrist from the handlebars. Carpal tunnel syndrome is also a clinical diagnosis based on symptoms. Provocative maneuvers, including Phalen and Tinel tests, can aid in the diagnosis.[29] If the diagnosis remains unclear, nerve conduction studies can be used. Imaging is generally not helpful unless there is a structural abnormality that may be causing the compression.

Similar to ulnar compression, carpal tunnel syndrome commonly resolves through rest.[11] A neutral angle hand splint may help avoid further nerve compression, especially while sleeping.[29] In recurrent cases, patients can receive cortisone injections or undergo surgical intervention to release the carpal tunnel.[30] Prevention of this injury is the same as in the ulnar nerve: padded gloves, frequent adjustments in hand position, and appropriate bike fit.

27.4.3 Pudendal Nerve

The pudendal nerve is derived from the S2–S4 roots of the sacral plexus. The nose of the seat may compress the pudendal nerve, where it exits the bony pelvis in the perineum.[11] It may also be compressed as it passes through Alcock's canal, a space formed by the obturator internus and ischial bone.[8]

Pudendal nerve compression typically presents with genital numbness, paresthesias, and sexual dysfunction, deemed as "bicycle seat neuropathy."[1,8] In a study of 160 male cyclists riding 540 km in 1 day, 35 (22%) reported symptoms related to the pudendal nerve, including genital numbness ($n=33$) and impotence ($n=21$).[31] Following the event, many symptoms continued for days or weeks. Genital numbness was reported by 10 participants, which lasted for over a week, and 3 participants reported that the impotence continued for over a month.[31]

Pudendal nerve injury is a clinical diagnosis based on presenting symptoms. Pain should occur along the pudendal nerve distribution while the patient is in a sitting position. Electrophysiological testing can aid in diagnosis.[32] Although most cases resolve with rest, refractory cases can be treated with pudendal nerve blocks, pulsed radiofrequency ablation, or surgical decompression of the nerve at Alcock's canal.[1,32]

Saddles that distribute weight bearing across the buttocks and ischial tuberosities, rather than predominantly on the perineum, may help prevent injury.[11] Additionally, having the nose of the saddle tilt downward and aligning the seat's height with the handlebar help reduce pressure on the perineum.[11] In a study of 132 cyclists riding 500 miles over 8 days, symptoms related to the pudendal nerve were significantly more common in people using a padded saddle; 30/75 with padded saddle versus 7/37 with hard seats reported buttock symptoms ($p=0.004$).[25] Therefore, cyclists should opt for a hard saddle.

27.5 Conclusions

With the growing popularity of cycling, clinicians should be aware of the presentation and treatment of common neurological injuries associated with the sport (▶ Fig. 27.1). Accidents, in the form of riders falling from their bikes or colliding with others, can lead to brain and spinal cord injuries. Helmets are essential for reducing the severity of these injuries. Chronic use injuries include cervical radiculopathy and PNIs in the ulnar, median, and pudendal nerves. Cyclists typically use a forward riding position, in which the upper body is flexed and leaned over the handlebars.[24,30] Several points bear a significant proportion of the body's weight during cycling, including the hands and ischial tuberosities.[31] Bicycle adjustments, including low handlebars, high saddle, and nose of the saddle titled down, can help create the optimal position biomechanics and avoid injuries to these nerves. Treatment strategies ultimately aim at getting riders back on the road as quickly and safely as possible.

27.6 Clinical Pearls

- The most common brain injuries in cycling are TBI and ICH.
- "Red-flag" symptoms for head injury include severe or increasing headache, confusion, loss of consciousness, vomiting, dizziness, change in vision, balance problems, inability to speak or swallow, or overt head trauma, and are indications for immediate removal from the race.
- The most common spinal injuries in cycling are cervical spinal fracture and cervical SCI.
- External immobilization following spinal injury is key to preventing additional injury.
- The most common peripheral nerve injuries include damage to the ulnar, median, and pudendal nerves.
- Injury to peripheral nerves can be prevented by using padded gloves and handlebars, frequently adjusting one's position on the bike, and having an appropriate bike fit.

27.7 Disclosures

Carly Weber-Levine: None.
Andrew M. Hersh: None.
Nicholas Theodore: Royalties from Globus Medical. Stock Ownership in Globus Medical. Consultant for Globus Medical. On Scientific Advisory Board/Other Office for Globus Medical.

References

[1] Kotler DH, Babu AN, Robidoux G. Prevention, evaluation, and rehabilitation of cycling-related injury. Curr Sports Med Rep. 2016; 15(3):199–206

[2] Greve MW, Modabber MR. An epidemic of traumatic brain injury in professional cycling: a call to action. Clin J Sport Med. 2012; 22(2): 81–82

[3] Decock M, De Wilde L, Vanden Bossche L, Steyaert A, Van Tongel A. Incidence and aetiology of acute injuries during competitive road cycling. Br J Sports Med. 2016; 50(11):669–672

[4] Rice S, Iaccarino MA, Bhatnagar S, Robidoux G, Zafonte R, Kotler DH. Reporting of concussion-like symptoms after cycling crashes: a survey of competitive and recreational cyclists. J Athl Train. 2020; 55(1):11–16

[5] Ahmed BZ, Benton AH, Serra-Jovenich M, Toldi JP. Postconcussion symptoms and neuropsychological performance in athletes: a literature review. Curr Sports Med Rep. 2023; 22(1):19–23

[6] Tenny S, Thorell W. Intracranial Hemorrhage. In: StatPearls [Internet]. StatPearls Publishing; 2022

[7] Agarwal N, Thakkar R, Khoi T. Sports-related Neck Injury—Statistics, Symptoms and Treatments. American Association of Neurological Surgeons. Accessed January 12, 2023 at: https://www.aans.org/Patients/Neurosurgical-Conditions-and-Treatments/Sports-related-Neck-Injury

[8] Toth C, McNeil S, Feasby T. Peripheral nervous system injuries in sport and recreation: a systematic review. Sports Med. 2005; 35(8):717–738

[9] Patterson JMM, Jaggars MM, Boyer MI. Ulnar and median nerve palsy in long-distance cyclists. A prospective study. Am J Sports Med. 2003; 31(4): 585–589

[10] Joseph B, Azim A, Haider AA, et al. Bicycle helmets work when it matters the most. Am J Surg. 2017; 213(2):413–417

[11] Kennedy J. Neurologic injuries in cycling and bike riding. Phys Med Rehabil Clin N Am. 2009; 20(1):241–248, xi

[12] Swart J, Bigard X, Fladischer T, et al. Cycling-Specific Sport Related Concussion. Union Cycliste Internationale. Accessed January 2023 at: https://assets.ctfassets.net/761l7gh5x5an/2GrX7plDBf6jDiznMr3fcU/3732e5536a721a98af407705502e9110/HARROGATE_CONSENSUS_AGREEMENT_CYCLING-SPECIFIC_SPORT_RELATED_CONCUSSION.pdf

[13] Olivier J, Creighton P. Bicycle injuries and helmet use: a systematic review and meta-analysis. Int J Epidemiol. 2017; 46(1):278–292

[14] Union Cycliste Internationale. UCI Cycling Regulations E0115 Medical Rules 1 Part 13 Medical Rules. Accessed in January 2023 at: https://assets.ctfassets.net/761l7gh5x5an/4dfXPdgyPYHuFUwsEpXO5v/2611cc440358c188af2746d6195659f2/part-xiii—medical-rules—01.03.2020.pdf

[15] Sport concussion assessment tool—5th edition. Br J Sports Med. 2017; 51 (11):851–858

[16] Høye A. Bicycle helmets—to wear or not to wear? A meta-analyses of the effects of bicycle helmets on injuries. Accid Anal Prev. 2018; 117:85–97

[17] Policy I. Helmets. USA Cycling. Accessed January 31, 2023 at: https://usacycling.org/about-us/governance/policy-i

[18] Eng SF, Næss I, Linnerud H, et al. Bicycle-related cervical spine injuries. N Am Spine Soc J. 2022; 10:100119

[19] DePasse JM, Durand W, Palumbo MA, Daniels AH. Sex- and sport-specific epidemiology of cervical spine injuries sustained during sporting activities. World Neurosurg. 2019; 122:e540–e545

[20] McGoldrick NP, Green C, Burke N, Synnott K. Acute traumatic spinal injury following bicycle accidents: a report of three cases. Acta Orthop Belg. 2012; 78(3):409–413

[21] Torlincasi AM, Waseem M. Cervical Injury. StatPearls. Published online August 22, 2022. Accessed January 12, 2023 at: https://www.ncbi.nlm.nih.gov/books/NBK448146/

[22] Li NY, Onor GI, Lemme NJ, Gil JA. Epidemiology of peripheral nerve injuries in sports, exercise, and recreation in the United States, 2009–2018. Phys Sportsmed. 2021; 49(3):355–362

[23] Rauch A, Teixeira PAG, Gillet R, et al. Analysis of the position of the branches of the ulnar nerve in Guyon's canal using high-resolution MRI in positions adopted by cyclists. Surg Radiol Anat. 2016; 38(7):793–799

[24] Brubacher JW, Leversedge FJ. Ulnar neuropathy in cyclists. Hand Clin. 2017; 33(1):199–205

[25] Weiss BD. Nontraumatic injuries in amateur long distance bicyclists. Am J Sports Med. 1985; 13(3):187–192

[26] Slane J, Timmerman M, Ploeg HL, Thelen DG. The influence of glove and hand position on pressure over the ulnar nerve during cycling. Clin Biomech (Bristol, Avon). 2011; 26(6):642–648

[27] Capitani D, Beer S. Handlebar palsy—a compression syndrome of the deep terminal (motor) branch of the ulnar nerve in biking. J Neurol. 2002; 249 (10):1441–1445

[28] Akuthota V, Plastaras C, Lindberg K, Tobey J, Press J, Garvan C. The effect of long-distance bicycling on ulnar and median nerves: an electrophysiologic evaluation of cyclist palsy. Am J Sports Med. 2005; 33(8):1224–1230

[29] Bland JDP. Carpal tunnel syndrome. BMJ. 2007; 335(7615):343–346

[30] Sirisena DC, Sim SHS, Lim I, Rajaratnam V. Median and ulnar nerve injuries in cyclists: a narrative review. Biomedicine (Taipei). 2021; 11(4):1–12

[31] Andersen KV, Bovim G. Impotence and nerve entrapment in long distance amateur cyclists. Acta Neurol Scand. 1997; 95(4):233–240

[32] Kaur J, Leslie SW, Singh P. Pudendal Nerve Entrapment Syndrome. In: StatPearls [Internet]. Treasure Island, FL: StatPearls Publishing; 2023

28 Rowing

A. Karim Ahmed, John Theodore, and Nicholas Theodore

Summary

Owing to the lean body type required, rowers are classically prone to lumbar overuse injuries. The rowing stroke consists of four key parts, namely, the catch, drive, finish, and recovery. Rowers may generate up to 848 Newtons of force in a single stroke, or 4.6 times that of their body weight, causing injuries with lumbar intervertebral disk, pars, or stress injuries being the most common. This chapter outlines the overall pattern of injuries, prevalence, and biomechanical factors for rowers with spinal injuries.

Keywords: lumbar spine, rowing, spondylolysis

28.1 Basic Technique

Rowing is a popular sport that dates back to the Doggett's Coat and Badge Race, first held on the Thames River in England in 1715. The modern sport of rowing, however, truly began with the Oxford-Cambridge race of 1829 and the Henley Royal Regatta in 1839, also held on the Thames River. Competitive rowing was included in the first modern Olympic Games of 1896, held in Athens, Greece.[1] The first heavyweight men's Olympic rowing regatta occurred in 1900, but heavyweight rowing did not become an Olympic sport for women until 1976. The enactment of Title IV in 1972 led to a significant increase in the number of intercollegiate rowing programs. Lightweight rowing for both men and women joined the Olympic ranks in 1996.[2]

Rowers traditionally have a tall, lean body habitus, with high respiratory tidal volumes. Rowers with a large build are preferred as the resistance to forward motion is proportional to two-thirds of the combined power of the boat and crew.[3,4] Rowing performance is highly related to anaerobic threshold, as races require 70% aerobic and 30% anaerobic activity.

Rowers may use a single oar (called a sweep), or one oar per hand, which is known as sculling. Sweep may be performed with two, four, or eight rowers in a boat. Sculling may be performed with one, two, or four rowers in a boat. Rowers are seated facing opposite the direction of motion, on a sliding seat, with their feet fixed in place. With the oar secured to the boat, acting as a fulcrum, each motion exerted on the oar handle corresponds to an opposite motion in the oar's blade. As such, anterior motion of the oar handle brings the blade posterior, and upward motion of the oar handle drops the oar blade into the water.[2]

The rowing stroke consists of the *catch, drive, finish,* and *recovery.* The *catch* is the entry of the oar into water, with the arms extended and knees flexed (▶ Fig. 28.1). The *drive* involves powerful leg extension, hip extension, and elbow flexion with the oar handle brought to the torso. During the drive, there is acceleration peaking at the midpoint. Ergometric studies demonstrate that the peak shear load during this period reaches up to 848 Newtons for males and 717 Newtons for females.[2,5] Even more impressive than the shear force, the peak compressive force in the lumbar spine during the drive was found to be 4.6 times the body weight of the rower.[5] The *finish* consists of *feathering* the oar—wherein the wrist extension places the oar in a horizontal position to be removed from the water. The *recovery* is the return for the following *catch* phase—ending the stroke to reset for the subsequent stroke.

Although the legs provide the majority of force during the *drive*, back extension from 30 degrees of flexion at the *catch* to 30 degrees of extension at the *finish* provides additional force.[2] Myoelectric studies by Hosea et al[2,6] demonstrate substantial paraspinal muscle involvement from T7 to L3 throughout the *drive*, with the rectus femoris providing power and the thoracic paraspinal muscles stabilizing the spine during the *drive* phase.[2] The increase in shear and compressive force at the lumbar spine

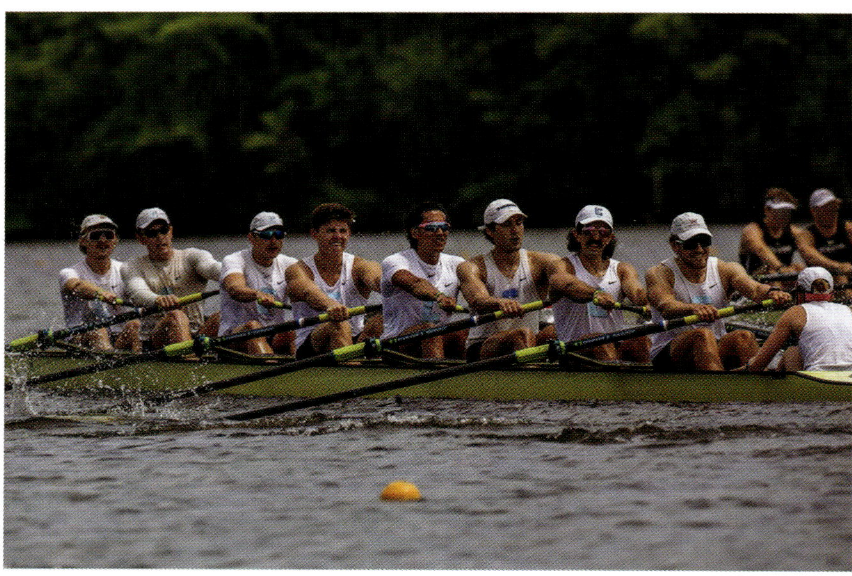

Fig. 28.1 Image of a varsity collegiate rowing team demonstrating the posture and position of the athletes during the *catch* phase of the rowing stroke.

may account for the substantial incidence of low back pain seen in competitive rowers.

28.2 Common Spinal Injuries

Most rowing injuries occur from repetitive insult due to muscle overuse and poor form.[2] In a study of female rowers by Howell,[7] the incidence of low back pain was 82% compared to 20 to 30% in the general population matched by age and sex. This study also found a significant correlation between hyperflexion motion in the lumbar spine, demonstrated in 75% of the cohort, and the incidence of low back pain. There was also a negative correlation between regular stretching and the incidence of low back pain.

One of the largest studies is an analysis of injuries in 180 collegiate rowers at Harvard and Rutgers University over a 3-year period.[8] Injuries were directly related to the time and intensity of training during the fall and winter months leading up to the racing season, peaking in February and March. In order of increasing incidence, the most common sites of injury were the ribcage (16/180), upper extremity (25/180), foot/ankle (25/180), spinal column (39/180), and knee (52/180). Of the spinal injuries, mechanical pain was the most common condition (29/39), followed by intervertebral disk herniation (5/39), and spondylolysis (5/39).[8]

Upper extremity injuries in rowers include extensor tenosynovitis of the wrist due to *feathering*. In *feathering*, the abductor pollicis longus, extensor pollicis brevis, and extensor carpi radialis longus/brevis are utilized during wrist extension to bring the blade of the oar from a submerged vertical position to a horizontal position at the end of the stroke. Rowing knee injuries most commonly consist of chondromalacia patella and iliotibial band friction syndrome due to constant loading of the knee under flexion and extension.[2]

Several studies demonstrate that back injuries and back pain are increasingly among the most common injuries in rowers, which may relate to high-pressure training techniques and schedules along with an evolution in rowing technique, which places increased strain on the back.[9] In a 2009 study of 398 elite junior rowers at the Junior World Rowing Championships in Beijing, Smoljanovic et al reported back pain as the most common injury, followed by knee and forearm/wrist injury.[10] Low back injuries accounted for 37 out of 103 traumatic injuries and 90 out of 290 overuse injuries in these rowers. Chest/thoracic spine injuries were 3 out of 103 traumatic injuries and 15 out of 290 overuse injuries. Neck/cervical spine injuries constituted 1 out of 103 traumatic injuries and 3 out of 290 overuse injuries. Overall, spinal injuries comprised 37% (149/398) of all injuries.[10] Injuries were more common in female than male rowers and in less experienced rowers compared to more experienced rowers. Acute-onset low back injury was seen in athletes rowing sweep that changed rowing side during a season (i.e., port to starboard or vice versa). Spondylolysis in rowers, often caused by hyperextension, may clinically manifest as pain lateral to the midline, in the absence of sciatica or neurologic symptoms.

Even when asymptomatic, elite young rowers have a significantly higher prevalence of lumbar spine imaging abnormalities than their nonathletic counterparts. In a study of 22 asymptomatic adolescent male rowers and 22 matched controls 12 to 17 years of age, 9 rowers (41%) had at least one magnetic resonance imaging (MRI) abnormality in the lumbar spine compared to 2 control subjects (9.1%).[11] Interestingly, in the group of 9 rowers, 7 had structural changes in the intervertebral disks (4 degeneration, 2 herniation, 1 bulging disk) and 6 had pars abnormalities (5 stress reactions, 1 spondylolysis). In contrast, among control subjects, no pars defects were observed. Similarly, Soler and Calderón observed spondylolysis in 17% of elite rowers.[12]

In a 12-month prospective study of 20 international rowers with 44 injuries, the greatest number of injuries was seen in the lumbar spine (32%), followed by the knee (16%), and the cervical spine (11%).[13] Lumbar spine injuries were significantly associated with high-volume ergometer training. This study did not find a significant difference in spine injuries based on rowing technique, such as sweep versus sculling, as had been suggested by others.[14] Furthermore, another group did not observe trunk muscle asymmetries in the oarside versus non-oarside cross-sectional areas of sweep rowers.[15]

Not surprisingly, a study of 1,829 intercollegiate rowers showed that rowers with a history of preexisting back pain developed back pain during their collegiate rowing career more often than those without a history of back pain (57% vs. 37%). Of note, however, disability from pain was more significant for those intercollegiate rowers who had not experienced prior back pain. Among the cohort with preexisting back pain, 55% had to miss practice due to pain and 8% had to end their intercollegiate rowing career. For rowers who did not have preexisting back pain, 62% had to miss practice from pain and 17% had to end their career.[16]

28.3 Imaging

Intervertebral disk changes (i.e., desiccation, bulge, herniation) and abnormalities in the pars interarticularis are the most common findings in the lumbar spine of rowers.[11] Disk changes are best seen on T2-weighted MRI, where the loss of water content in degenerated disks makes them appear darker than normal disks. Stress reactions may also be seen on MRI as increased short tau inversion recovery (STIR) or T2-weighted signal intensity at the pars interarticularis. For conditions such as a pars fracture (spondylolysis), with or without spondylolisthesis, the simplest and most diagnostic imaging modality may be an X-ray of the lumbar spine. Bony structures are also well appreciated on computed tomography (CT) imaging. It is important for clinicians to follow evidence-based guidelines when ordering imaging for all patients, including elite athletes.[17]

28.4 Prevention and Treatment

Given the prevalence of spine injuries among rowers, good training regimens should emphasize injury prevention. In a study of 1,632 former intercollegiate rowers, Teitz et al showed that age, a history of rowing before the age of 16, the use of a hatchet oar blade, college height/weight, and ergometer training sessions exceeding 30 minutes were significantly associated with back pain and injury during competitive intercollegiate rowing.[18] Stretching and teaching good technique can substantially decrease the risk of lower back injuries among rowers.[17]

Physiotherapy aimed at core muscle development and training of muscles surrounding the spine has the potential to provide stability following lower lumbar injuries in rowers. In a study by O'Sullivan et al, 44 patients with symptomatic and radiologic spondylosis or spondylolisthesis were randomly assigned to either a 10-week specific exercise or control group.[19] The exercise group participated in specific training of the deep abdominal muscles, with co-activation of the lumbar multifidus proximal to the site of the pars defects. The control group had traditional treatment by their health care provider. The exercise group demonstrated a significant reduction in pain intensity and improved function, which was maintained even at the 30-month follow-up.

Finally, erector spinae muscle fatigue drastically increases the amount of lumbar flexion and can promote injury in rowers.[20] The incorporation of stretching, warming up, and reduction in activity after the onset of trunk muscle fatigue is not only an integral part of prevention but can contribute to accelerated rehabilitation in rowers with lumbar spinal injuries.[21]

28.5 Clinical Pearls

- During the rowing stroke, the lumbar spine can experience peak compressive forces up to 4.6 times the body weight of the rower.
- Spinal injuries seen in rowers are typically a result of repetitive insult, muscle overuse, or poor form.
- Mechanical pain is the most common form of injury, followed by intervertebral disk herniation and spondylolysis.
- MRI and CT scans are most useful to identify intervertebral disk changes and spondylolysis, respectively.
- Teaching proper technique, incorporating stretching, shortening ergometer training sessions, and strengthening core muscles are critical for preventing the development of spinal injuries.

References

[1] BBC. Oxford Culture—History of Rowing and Henley. 2014. Accessed at: http://www.bbc.co.uk/oxford/culture/2004/02/henley_museum/history_rowing.shtml

[2] Hosea TM, Hannafin JA. Rowing injuries. Sports Health. 2012; 4(3):236–245

[3] Shephard RJ. Science and medicine of rowing: a review. J Sports Sci. 1998; 16(7):603–620

[4] Secher NH. Rowing. In: Reilly T, Secher N, Snell P, Williams C, eds. Physiology of Sports. London: E & FN Spon; 1990:259–286

[5] Morris FL, Smith RM, Payne WR, Galloway MA, Wark JD. Compressive and shear force generated in the lumbar spine of female rowers. Int J Sports Med. 2000; 21(7):518–523

[6] Hannafin J, Hosea T. Oar sports. In: Garret WE, Kirkendall DT, Squire DL, eds. Principles and Practice of Primary Care Sports Medicine. Philadelphia, PA: Lippincott, Williams & Wilkins; 2001:531–540

[7] Howell DW. Musculoskeletal profile and incidence of musculoskeletal injuries in lightweight women rowers. Am J Sports Med. 1984; 12(4): 278–282

[8] Hosea TM, Boland A, McCarthy K, Kennedy T. Rowing injuries. Postgrad Adv Sports Med. 1984; 3(9):1

[9] Stallard MC. Backache in oarsmen. Br J Sports Med. 1980; 14(2–3):105–108

[10] Smoljanovic T, Bojanic I, Hannafin JA, Hren D, Delimar D, Pecina M. Traumatic and overuse injuries among international elite junior rowers. Am J Sports Med. 2009; 37(6):1193–1199

[11] Maurer M, Soder RB, Baldisserotto M. Spine abnormalities depicted by magnetic resonance imaging in adolescent rowers. Am J Sports Med. 2011; 39(2):392–397

[12] Soler T, Calderón C. The prevalence of spondylolysis in the Spanish elite athlete. Am J Sports Med. 2000; 28(1):57–62

[13] Wilson F, Gissane C, Gormley J, Simms C. A 12-month prospective cohort study of injury in international rowers. Br J Sports Med. 2010; 44(3): 207–214

[14] Perich D, Burnett A, O'Sullivan P. Low back pain and the factors associated with it: examination of adolescent female rowers. In: Schwameder H, Stutzenberger G, Fastenbauer V, et al, eds. XXIV Symposium of the International Society of Biomechanics in Sports. Konstanz, Germany: University of Konstanz; 2006:355–358

[15] McGregor AH, Anderton L, Gedroyc WM. The trunk muscles of elite oarsmen. Br J Sports Med. 2002; 36(3):214–217

[16] O'Kane JW, Teitz CC, Lind BK. Effect of preexisting back pain on the incidence and severity of back pain in intercollegiate rowers. Am J Sports Med. 2003; 31(1):80–82

[17] Purcell L, Micheli L. Low back pain in young athletes. Sports Health. 2009; 1 (3):212–222

[18] Teitz CC, O'Kane J, Lind BK, Hannafin JA. Back pain in intercollegiate rowers. Am J Sports Med. 2002; 30(5):674–679

[19] O'Sullivan PB, Phyty GD, Twomey LT, Allison GT. Evaluation of specific stabilizing exercise in the treatment of chronic low back pain with radiologic diagnosis of spondylolysis or spondylolisthesis. Spine (Phila pA 1976). 1997; 22(24):2959–2967

[20] Adams MA, Green TP, Dolan P. The strength in anterior bending of lumbar intervertebral discs. Spine. 1994; 19(19):2197–2203

[21] Reid DA, McNair PJ. Factors contributing to low back pain in rowers. Br J Sports Med. 2000; 34(5):321–322

29 Professional Motorsport Racing

Arjun K. Menta, Carly Weber-Levine, Andrew M. Hersh, and Nicholas Theodore

Summary

This chapter explores the spectrum of neurological trauma in motorsport racing, underscoring the incidence and management of brain, spinal cord, and peripheral nerve injuries. Innovations like the HANS device and the halo-type cockpit have played a critical role in decreasing the prevalence of severe injuries, including craniovertebral dissociation, traumatic brain injuries, and cervical spine injuries—notably during high-velocity collisions. Despite these advancements, the distinct high-speed and high-impact nature of motorsport racing poses specific challenges, such as an elevated risk of sciatic and peroneal neuropathy due to the constrained cockpit space, and brachial plexus injuries resulting from limited movement. The chapter highlights the essential role of advanced safety devices, explores the different influences of the racing environment, and emphasizes preventive strategies. Nevertheless, existing gaps in literature signal an urgent need for additional research. Bridging these gaps through systematic investigation will not only improve care and safety for motorsport drivers but also propel the field of motorsport medicine forward.

Keywords: neurosurgery, neurological trauma, motorsport racing, safety devices, spinal cord injury, peripheral nerve injury, traumatic brain injury

29.1 Introduction

Motorsport racing, a sport marked by high-speed turns and dangerous crashes, encompasses a diverse array of competition formats—such as off-road, sprint, and endurance—on tracks across the globe. Tracing its origins back to 1895, the sport has witnessed growing popularity, a trend recently fueled by mainstream media attention, including Netflix's series, *Drive to Survive*.[1,2,3]

While comprehensive demographic data across all forms of motorsport racing are limited, there are observable trends. Predominantly comprised of male athletes, motorsport racing attracts a wide age range of participants, with an average age of around 30 years and decreasing each year.[4,5] The sport attracts drivers from across the world, often hailing from higher socioeconomic backgrounds due to the financial demands intrinsic to entry-level participation. Age variation is substantial across the sport's disciplines, as seen in the contrast between Formula 1 and National Association for Stock Car Auto Racing (NASCAR) demographics.[6]

Motorsport drivers grapple with an array of physical forces, including the intense acceleration and deceleration associated with high-speed maneuvers and abrupt stops, the gravitational forces or "g-forces" during races, the impact forces from crashes, and the chronic strain of vehicle vibrations. These drivers are subject to significant physical stress, under which they must execute precise muscular movements for vehicle control, necessitating both gross and fine motor adjustments. These cumulative forces represent a substantial physical burden on drivers. Postrace analysis of 137 auto racing drivers revealed that 26% reported lumbar pain, 20% reported shoulder pain, and 18% reported neck pain; posture and seat comfort were identified as key factors in mitigating the impact forces experienced during races.[7]

Injury rates appear to be influenced by multiple factors, including the type of racing, competitive level, and adherence to safety standards. A study conducted by Minoyama and Tsuchida, investigating injuries in professional motor car racing at a competitive circuit in Japan from 1996 to 2000, reported an injury rate of 1.2 per 1,000 competitors.[8] These injuries primarily encompassed bruising, cervical spine injury, and concussions. Given the advances in safety technology and changes in regulations over the last two decades, these numbers likely have improved today. However, it is crucial to continually monitor and analyze these data to inform best practices for injury prevention and management in this high-impact sport.

Interestingly, the emergence of motorsport racing coincides with the dawn of modern neurosurgery. Neurosurgery has been instrumental in driving the evolution of safety standards and equipment integral to today's motorsport racing.[9] However, with the breadth of different racing subtypes and lack of comprehensive data tracking injuries, there is a lack of information summarizing the types of neurological injuries prevalent across motorsport racing. This deficiency represents a significant gap in the sport's clinical literature and the health care provided to its participants. In this chapter, we explore the most prevalent types of neurological injuries surrounding motorsport racing, along with diagnostic and treatment modalities.

29.2 Different Types of Neurological Injury

29.2.1 Brain Injury

Among all sports, motorsport has one of the highest incidences of concussion, a mild form of traumatic brain injury (TBI).[10] Despite the increased incidence, significant knowledge gaps exist with variable screening protocols and underreporting of injury. A 2020 survey of 209 motorsport medical personnel revealed that 87% had encountered concussed drivers and 34% reported experiencing pressure to prematurely clear drivers following a concussion.[11] The need for rigorous education and training in trackside concussion assessment is therefore paramount, particularly when deciding whether a driver can safely return to the race.

Concussions in motorsport can result from both nonimpact forces, such as abrupt stops and g-forces, and impact forces leading to head injury.[10,12] Despite featuring a wide range of neurological symptoms, concussions commonly present as confusion, nausea, photophobia, dizziness, memory loss, and head pain.[13] Recommendations for diagnosing concussions trackside include the comprehensive Sports Concussion Assessment Tool (SCAT5).[14] In a hospital setting, SCAT5 and Immediate Post-Concussion Assessment and Cognitive Test (ImPACT) can assess cognitive function, visio-vestibular system tests can evaluate oculomotor function, and the Balance Error Scoring System (BESS) can measure balance.[14,15] If an intracranial injury is suspected, a head computed tomography (CT) scan without contrast should be performed.

Management is primarily observational, with rest as the key intervention, and recovery timelines unique to each patient.[16] The guidelines for returning to play after a concussion are not well studied in the specific context of motorsport. General concussion guidelines recommend that drivers should be symptom-free for at least 5 days before considering a return to racing, with some guidelines suggesting a longer symptom-free period of 14 to 21 days.[10,17] Postconcussion syndrome, typically presenting as a headache and postural vertigo within 72 hours of a head injury or concussion, should also be assessed.[18] Protective equipment, such as helmets, head and neck support (HANS) devices, and headrests, is crucial in concussion prevention; however, robust data supporting their use in motorsport settings to specifically prevent concussions remain insufficient.

More severe TBI beyond concussions contributes significantly to morbidity in motorsport racing. TBI is typically sustained through high-speed motor vehicle crashes resulting in impact forces or penetrating objects leading to neuronal injury. Following the introduction of compulsory helmet use, the majority of cranial trauma is now closed head injuries.[19] A study reported that cranial trauma accounted for 29% of all injuries in professional auto racing, with open head injuries constituting a mere 5%.[20] Injuries from impact forces are predominantly axonal damage, with intracranial hemorrhages being relatively rare.[21]

Athletes also regularly contend with substantial vertical and axial g-forces, which can exceed 4 g, or four times the force of gravity, during races. The physical demand of resisting these forces, particularly during high-speed turns, is considerable.[22] During crashes, the magnitude of g-forces can amplify dramatically. A 2006 study analyzing 374 crashes in the IndyCar Racing League found that drivers face impact forces exceeding 150 g. When g-forces reach or surpass 50, there is a concern for TBI.[23]

Drivers with TBI may present with a range of symptoms including loss of consciousness, headaches, motor dysfunction, balance changes, sensory alterations, photophobia, confusion, disorientation, and speech abnormalities.[24] Immediate on-site evaluation includes the Glasgow Coma Scale (GCS) assessment with concurrent stabilization and hospital transfer. In the interim, spinal fractures should be assumed until ruled out, necessitating spinal immobilization precautions. Furthermore, hemodynamic and respiratory parameters should be stabilized to a systolic blood pressure > 90 to 100 mmHg, pulse oximetry value > 90 to 95%, and end-tidal CO_2 between 35 and 40 mm Hg.[25,26] If a patient presents with signs of cerebral herniation, hyperventilation therapy can be utilized. Patients should undergo noncontrast CT imaging for neurological damage assessment.[27,28] Prevention strategies against TBI parallel those used for concussion mitigation. These include helmets, HANS devices, and padded headrests, even though studies substantiating their use in auto racing to reduce TBI incidence remain limited. Given the contact nature of the sport, any of the following presentations are contraindications to return to play: neurologic or pain-producing abnormalities around the foramen magnum, permanent central neurologic effects, hydrocephalus, subarachnoid hemorrhage, and persistent postconcussion symptoms.[29] For athletes who endure life-threatening head injuries, the recovery period often extends beyond one year, potentially preventing their return to the sport.

29.2.2 Spinal Cord Injury

While injuries to the back and torso are some of the most common types of injuries in motor racing, spinal cord injury (SCI) is one of the most devastating outcomes a driver may encounter.[30] While data surrounding SCI are scarce, it has become the focal point of substantial investigation by the Fédération Internationale de l'Automobile (FIA).[31] A study conducted in 1990 suggested that spinal injuries accounted for approximately 20% of all reported injuries among motorsport drivers.[32] These injuries are commonly seen in incidents such as vehicular rollovers, further underscoring the need for enhanced safety measures and SCI research in motorsport racing.

The chronic effects of whole-body vibrations have also been scrutinized as contributing to SCI, though with conflicting evidence. Although these vibrations constitute a persistent impact force, current safety equipment, comfort considerations, and standard postrace recovery periods may alleviate their effects. In an investigation of the long-term impacts of rally driving—a subtype of closed-wheel racing that occurs "off-road"—there was no lumbar degenerative findings on magnetic resonance imaging (MRI) among 18 experienced drivers.[33] While postrace discomfort due to chronic vibrations is common, these studies suggest that chronic vibrations may not lead to neurological injury.

Seat posture is another critical risk factor for SCI in drivers. Fundamentally, motorsport racing can be split into two types: open-wheel and closed-wheel racing (▶ Fig. 29.1). Open-wheel racing series involve events such as IndyCar and Formula 1, while closed-wheel racing series involve events such as the World Rally Championship and NASCAR. While safety standards differ across subtypes, a critical aspect between the two larger categories is seat positioning in the car. Open-wheel race car drivers sit in a narrow, shallow cockpit in a reclined "near-supine" fashion. On the other hand, closed-wheel race car drivers sit upright, cramped against the dash and steering wheel.

A 2016 study simulating the kinematics of reclined occupants akin to those encountered by open-wheel race car drivers revealed that seatbelt usage in such positions may result in unfavorable force distribution during frontal collisions. Particularly, if the recline angle is less than 60 degrees from the vertical, a collision could precipitate excessive spinal flexion and body rotation, heightening the risk of spinal injury.[34] Additionally, a 2006 study using a pedestrian model suggested that even low-speed crashes could predispose reclined occupants to SCI.[35] While both these studies were conducted outside of a motorsport racing context and utilized simulated models, their findings might have implications for the safety of open-wheel race car drivers. This notion is corroborated by injury data from open-wheel IndyCar drivers, who are traditionally seated in a reclined position. An analysis revealed that spinal fractures accounted for a significant 18.7% of all racing injuries sustained between 1996 and 2005.[36] Therefore, the data suggest the need for further research and potential modifications to safety measures in this high-risk sporting environment.

Ultimately, most spinal injuries or fractures in auto racing can be attributed to the substantial compressive loads or excessive

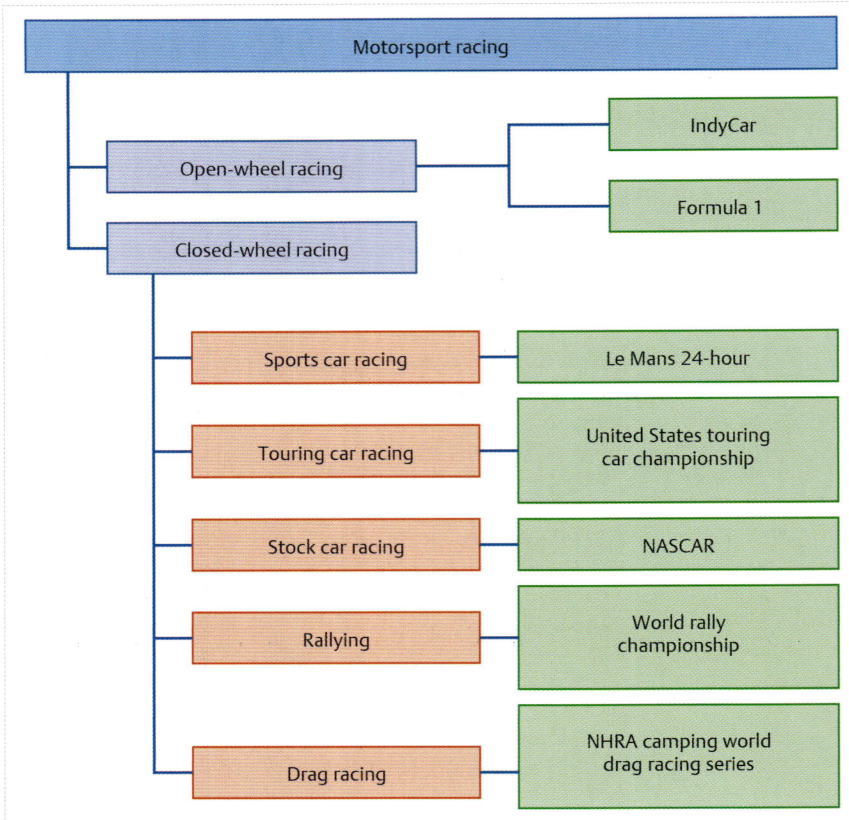

Fig. 29.1 Breakdown of motorsport racing into open- and closed-wheel racing along with examples of the major competitions that represent the different types of racing.

flexion experienced by drivers. Symptoms include pain at rest or during movement, extremity weakness, and potential loss of motor, sensory, and/or autonomic function. It is essential to note that SCIs in auto racing can present with a highly variable clinical presentation, from something as subtle as neck pain to more obvious deformities, underscoring the need for further imaging if suspicion for injury arises.[37] Initial on-scene treatment involves the rapid stabilization of the patient and full immobilization of the patient's spine to mitigate secondary injury.[38] Even minimal symptomatology warrants immediate transport to the nearest hospital for advanced imaging, including CT or MRI.[39,40,41] MRI imaging is better for assessing soft-tissue injury but CT provides faster insight—unfortunately, there does not appear to be clear guidelines on which imaging is mandatory in this setting.[42,43,44,45]

Upon arrival at the hospital, it is critical that the patient is evaluated by a multidisciplinary team specializing in acute spinal trauma, ideally encompassing trauma surgery, neurosurgery, and orthopaedics, to develop a comprehensive and personalized treatment plan.[46] Prevention strategies should include ensuring properly fitted seating and optimal posture.

29.2.3 Peripheral Nerve Injury

Though less common, peripheral nerve injuries do occur in motorsport racing. While existing data on incidence rates and management approaches are limited, Trammell and Olvey provide a preliminary examination of various mechanisms leading to peripheral nerve injury.[32] The narrow confines of the racing car's cockpit, combined with the requirement for awkward leg placement, increase the risk of sciatic and peroneal neuropathy. Similarly, securing the arms to the HANS device and helmet, along with limited maneuverability for hand placement, might elevate the risk of brachial plexus injuries in drivers. The suggested course of treatment and prevention for these types of neuropathy primarily consists of the use of excess padding, analgesics, and physical therapy.[47]

Carpal tunnel syndrome (CTS) is among the most extensively documented peripheral nerve injuries specific to racing environments. The syndrome commonly arises due to the intense grip on the steering wheel combined with the cumulative trauma induced by vibrations, complex maneuvers, and collisions typical in racing. Symptoms predominantly include numbness, paresthesias, and decreased grip strength. Diagnosing CTS requires a comprehensive approach involving an exploration of medical and surgical history as well as a physical examination assessing for the common CTS symptoms. Joint mobility, including range of motion and palpation of the joints, as well as electrophysiological response should be evaluated bilaterally for the upper extremities. Phalen's maneuver, the Kirk Watson test, and the Reagan shuck test are recommended adjunctive tools.[48]

Typically, patients demonstrate favorable responses to nonsurgical management strategies,[49] chiefly comprising rest, wrist splinting,[50,51] and glucocorticoid injections. Glucocorticoid injections are often the preferred intervention for those requiring rapid relief or for individuals not compliant with wrist splinting. For patients with severe, refractory symptoms, surgical intervention involving division of the flexor retinaculum and antebrachial fascia may be considered. However, it is worth noting that post-operative patients often report diminished grip strength, potentially impacting their racing performance.[52] Moreover, to ensure recovery and avert irreversible worsening of the condition, it is advised to abstain from the inciting activity until symptom resolution. For prevention, padded gloves or wrist padding have been reported to alleviate symptoms.[48]

29.3 Safety Equipment for the Prevention of Neurological Injury

Prevention of neurological injuries in motorsport racing is primarily through car-embedded safety measures, such as the halo cockpit and seat/head padding, and driver-integrated safeguards, including the HANS device, helmets, and accelerometers.[53,54]

Noteworthy safety features integrated into race cars include the halo-type cockpit, which became mandatory for many open-wheel race cars, including being deployed in Formula 1 starting in the 2018 season.[55] The halo has the potential to prevent TBI and cervical spine injury during high-speed collisions. Despite initial adaptation challenges associated with visibility and navigation, studies indicate that the halo has neither increased fatigue nor significantly altered head position for drivers.[56] Headrest and seat padding can also attenuate the strain on drivers' necks and spines when subjected to high g-forces.[10] Restraint belts also play a crucial role in preventing spinal and peripheral nerve injuries by minimizing abnormal flexion, rotation, or extension during impacts when combined with the padded seat.[57]

Safety gear worn by drivers is individualized for maximum protection. While the driver's seatbelt secures the chest, abdomen, and pelvis, the head and neck remain vulnerable to dangerous frontal loads and axial forces. Introduced in 1980, the HANS device mitigates craniovertebral dissociation injuries—previously the leading cause of death in motorsport racing—by redistributing weight from the head to the shoulders.[58] Biomechanical impact tests and a single retrospective study suggest a benefit of the device in preventing flexion-distraction injury during impact.[59,60] Since the implementation of the HANS device, which is now mandatory across most competitive auto racing events, there has not been a single fatal craniovertebral junction injury reported.[61] Helmets further enhance safety by extending the deceleration distance through cushioning and reducing overall impact force.[62]

In the wake of limited data on neurological injuries in this context, there has been a push to assess the forces drivers face. This has led to the integration of accelerometers within helmets and other driver equipment, thereby allowing a better understanding of standard racing forces and their relation to neurological injury presentation.[63] These devices also assess the effects of various safety interventions in the racing world. Other experimental devices, such as instrumented mouthpiece kinematics sensors, are also being tested on racing drivers to provide more detailed force information, aiming to enhance injury assessment and improve safety.[64]

29.4 Conclusion

Neurological trauma in motorsport racing presents a unique spectrum, encompassing brain, spinal cord, and peripheral nerve injuries. Advancements in safety measures have played a significant role in mitigating these risks. However, the high-speed, high-impact nature of the sport necessitates a deeper understanding of injury mechanisms and their management. Going forward, a systematic approach to documenting and analyzing these injuries will be crucial. This could lead to more effective preventive measures and targeted treatment plans, enhancing the care and safety of motorsport drivers in this rapidly evolving field.

29.5 Clinical Pearls

- Helmets, HANS devices, and padded headrests can prevent concussions and more severe TBI, highlighting the importance of these safety measures.
- Concussions in motorsports can stem from both nonimpact forces, such as abrupt stops and g-forces, and impact forces leading to head injury.
- The comprehensive SCAT5 is highly recommended for on-site concussion diagnosis.
- Spinal injuries or fractures in auto racing often result from the considerable compressive loads or excessive flexion experienced by drivers.
- The HANS device and halo-type cockpit both mitigate craniovertebral dissociation injuries and have the potential to prevent TBI and cervical spine injury during high-speed collisions.
- Ensuring properly fitted seating and maintaining optimal posture serve as key preventive strategies against spinal injuries.
- The narrow confines of the racing car's cockpit, combined with the requirement for awkward leg placement, can increase the risk of sciatic and peroneal neuropathy.
- The practice of securing the arms to the HANS device and helmet, alongside restricted hand placement, may increase the risk of brachial plexus injuries in drivers.

References

[1] Netflix. Formula 1: drive to survive. Accessed August 17, 2023 at: https://www.netflix.com/title/80204890

[2] Global Industry Analysts, Inc. Motorsports - global strategic business report. Accessed August 17, 2023 at: https://www.researchandmarkets.com/report/motorsport

[3] Britannica. Automobile racing. Accessed August 17, 2023 at: https://www.britannica.com/sports/automobile-racing

[4] Motorsport.com. Average driver age differs in auto racing series across the world. Accessed August 17, 2023 at: https://us.motorsport.com/general/news/average-driver-age-differs-in-auto-racing-series-across-the-world/1804838/

[5] F1 Chronicle. Why are Formula 1 drivers so young? Accessed August 17, 2023 at: https://f1chronicle.com/why-are-formula-1-drivers-so-young/ (2023)

[6] Swanson H. How hybrid technology advances speed & performance in Formula 1 racing. Accessed August 17, 2023 at: https://www.apcela.com/blog/formula-1-hybrid-technology/

[7] Koutras C, Buecking B, Jaeger M, Ruchholtz S, Heep H. Musculoskeletal injuries in auto racing: a retrospective study of 137 drivers. Phys Sportsmed. 2014; 42(4):80–86

[8] Minoyama O, Tsuchida H. Injuries in professional motor car racing drivers at a racing circuit between 1996 and 2000. Br J Sports Med. 2004; 38(5): 613–616

[9] Matur AV, Ngwenya LB, Prestigiacomo CJ. The surgical history of head injury in motor vehicle collision. J Neurosurg. 2020; 135:1–7

[10] Deakin ND, Hutchinson PJ. Concussion in motorsport: incidence, awareness and future directions. Concussion. 2017; 2(3):CNC43

[11] Adams SA, Turner AP, Richards H, Hutchinson PJ. Concussion in motorsport? Experience, knowledge, attitudes, and priorities of medical personnel and drivers. Clin J Sport Med. 2020; 30(6):568–577

[12] Deakin N, Cronin T, Trafford P, et al. Concussion in motor sport: a medical literature review and engineering perspective. J Concussion. 2017; 1. DOI: 10.1177/2059700217733916

[13] Luo TD, Clarke MJ, Zimmerman AK, Quinn M, Daniels DJ, McIntosh AL. Concussion symptoms in youth motocross riders: a prospective, observational study. J Neurosurg Pediatr. 2015; 15(3):255–260

[14] Sport concussion assessment tool—5th edition. Br J Sports Med. 2017; 51 (11):851–858

[15] Cohen A, King D, Pearce AJ. Impact monitoring and King-Devick ocular testing provide a relatively simple process for objectively identifying and managing concussion in sports participants. Br J Sports Med. 2017; 51: A81

[16] Cantu RC. Clinical report—sport-related concussion in children and adolescents. Year Book Sports Med. 2011; 2011:15

[17] Grilley B. Revising the common rule: changes to the federal policy protecting human subjects. Mol Ther. 2016; 24:S282

[18] Ramos-Zúñiga R, González-de la Torre M, Jiménez-Maldonado M, et al. Postconcussion syndrome and mild head injury: the role of early diagnosis using neuropsychological tests and functional magnetic resonance/spectroscopy. World Neurosurg. 2014; 82(5):828–835

[19] Fernandes FA, de Sousa RJA. Head injury predictors in sports trauma–a state-of-the-art review. Proc Inst Mech Eng H. 2015; 229(8):592–608

[20] Toth C, McNeil S, Feasby T. Central nervous system injuries in sport and recreation: a systematic review. Sports Med. 2005; 35(8):685–715

[21] Gennarelli TA. Cerebral concussion and diffuse brain injuries. Head Injury 1987:108–124

[22] Norton C. Formula One drivers feel the G-force. The Telegraph. May 10, 2010. https://www.telegraph.co.uk/motoring/motorsport/7681665/Formula-One-drivers-feel-the-G-force.html

[23] Weaver CS, Sloan BK, Brizendine EJ, Bock H. An analysis of maximum vehicle G forces and brain injury in motorsports crashes. Med Sci Sports Exerc. 2006; 38(2):246–249

[24] Agarwal N, Thakkar R, Than K. A neurosurgeon's guide to sports-related head injury. Accessed August 17, 2023 at: https://www.aans.org/Patients/Neurosurgical-Conditions-and-Treatments/Sports-related-Head-Injury

[25] Campbell JE. Brady International Trauma Life Support for Prehospital Care Providers. Pearson; 2008

[26] Badjatia N, Carney N, Crocco TJ, et al. Guidelines for prehospital management of traumatic brain injury 2nd edition. Prehosp Emerg Care 2008;12(suppl 1): S1–S52

[27] McHugh GS, Engel DC, Butcher I, et al. Prognostic value of secondary insults in traumatic brain injury: results from the IMPACT study. J Neurotrauma. 2007; 24(2):287–293

[28] Stocchetti N, Furlan A, Volta F. Hypoxemia and arterial hypotension at the accident scene in head injury. J Trauma. 1996; 40(5):764–767

[29] Cantu RC. Return to play guidelines after a head injury. Clin Sports Med. 1998; 17(1):45–60

[30] Ebben WP, Suchomel TJ. Physical demands, injuries, and conditioning practices of stock car drivers. J Strength Cond Res. 2012; 26(5):1188–1198

[31] Trafford P, Henderson M, Trammell T. Spinal injuries and motor sport. Auto + Med. 2014:30–41

[32] Trammell TR, Olvey SE. Crash and injury statistics from Indy-car racing 1985–89. Presented at: Proceedings of the Association for the Advancement of Automotive Medicine Annual Conference. 1990; 34:329–335

[33] Videman T, Simonen R, Usenius J, Österman K, Battié M. The long-term effects of rally driving on spinal pathology. Clin Biomech (Bristol, Avon). 2000; 15(2):83–86

[34] Ji P, Huang Y, Zhou Q. Mechanisms of using knee bolster to control kinematical motion of occupant in reclined posture for lowering injury risk. Int J Crashworthiness. 2017; 22:415–424

[35] Richards D, Carhart M, Raasch C, Pierce J, Steffey D, Ostarello A. Incidence of thoracic and lumbar spine injuries for restrained occupants in frontal collisions. Annu Proc Assoc Adv Automot Med. 2006; 50:125–139

[36] Trammell TR, Weaver CS, Bock H. Spine fractures in open cockpit open wheel race car drivers. Paper presented at: Motorsports Engineering Conference & Exposition; December 5, 2006; Dearborn, Michigan

[37] Gorove L. Motorsport injuries, current trends and concepts. In: Doral M, ed. Sports Injuries: Prevention, Diagnosis, Treatment, and Rehabilitation. Berlin, Heidelberg: Springer; 2012:1113–1119

[38] Deasy C, Cameron P. Routine application of cervical collars–what is the evidence? Injury. 2011; 42(9):841–842

[39] Kreinest M, Scholz M, Trafford P. On-scene treatment of spinal injuries in motor sports. Eur J Trauma Emerg Surg. 2017; 43(2):191–200

[40] Cantu RC, Li YM, Abdulhamid M, Chin LS. Return to play after cervical spine injury in sports. Curr Sports Med Rep. 2013; 12(1):14–17

[41] Huang P, Anissipour A, McGee W, Lemak L. Return-to-play recommendations after cervical, thoracic, and lumbar spine injuries: a comprehensive review. Sports Health. 2016; 8(1):19–25

[42] Fernando F, Biffi A, Borra F, De Carli F, Monetti G, Sirico F. Formula 1 World Championship. In: Canata GL, Jones H, eds. Epidemiology of Injuries in Sports. Springer; 2022:95–106

[43] Levitt MA, Flanders AE. Diagnostic capabilities of magnetic resonance imaging and computed tomography in acute cervical spinal column injury. Am J Emerg Med. 1991; 9(2):131–135

[44] Selden NR, Quint DJ, Patel N, d'Arcy HS, Papadopoulos SM. Emergency magnetic resonance imaging of cervical spinal cord injuries: clinical correlation and prognosis. Neurosurgery. 1999; 44(4):785–792, discussion 792–793

[45] Matsumura A, Meguro K, Tsurushima H, Kikuchi Y, Wada M, Nakata Y. Magnetic resonance imaging of spinal cord injury without radiologic abnormality. Surg Neurol. 1990; 33(4):281–283

[46] Macias CA, Rosengart MR, Puyana JC, et al. The effects of trauma center care, admission volume, and surgical volume on paralysis after traumatic spinal cord injury. Ann Surg. 2009; 249(1):10–17

[47] Torg JS, Shephard RJ. Current Therapy in Sports Medicine. Mosby; 1995

[48] Masmejean EH, Chavane H, Chantegret A, Issermann JJ, Alnot JY. The wrist of the formula 1 driver. Br J Sports Med. 1999; 33(4):270–273

[49] Kaplan SJ, Glickel SZ, Eaton RG. Predictive factors in the non-surgical treatment of carpal tunnel syndrome. J Hand Surg [Br]. 1990; 15(1):106–108

[50] Page MJ, Massy-Westropp N, O'Connor D, Pitt V. Splinting for carpal tunnel syndrome. Cochrane Database Syst Rev. 2012; 2012(7):CD010003

[51] Gerritsen AAM, Korthals-de Bos IB, Laboyrie PM, de Vet HC, Scholten RJ, Bouter LM. Splinting for carpal tunnel syndrome: prognostic indicators of success. J Neurol Neurosurg Psychiatry. 2003; 74(9):1342–1344

[52] Hui ACF, Wong S, Leung CH, et al. A randomized controlled trial of surgery vs steroid injection for carpal tunnel syndrome. Neurology. 2005; 64(12): 2074–2078

[53] Russell JK, Melvin J. Developments in Modern Racecar Driver Crash Protection and Safety-Engineering beyond Performance. SAE International; 2013

[54] Patalak JP. Lessons from the track: crash safety principles and practices from the world of motorsports. Accessed August 17, 2023 at: https://www.jasp-online.org/asjournal/spring-2021/lessons-from-the-track-crash-safety-principles-and-practices-from-the-world-of-motorsports/

[55] Duxbury A. History of safety devices in Formula 1: the halo, barriers & more. Accessed August 17, 2023 at: https://www.autosport.com/f1/news/history-of-safety-devices-in-formula-1-the-halo-barriers-more-4982360/4982360/?deployment=overlay&device=mobile&segments=

[56] Rosalie SM, Malone JM. Effect of a halo-type structure on neck muscle activation of an open-cockpit race car driver training under qualifying conditions. BMJ Case Rep. 2018; 2018:bcr2017224013

[57] Patalak J, Gideon T, Melvin JW, Rains M. Improved seat belt restraint geometry for frontal, frontal oblique and rollover incidents. SAE Int J Transp Saf. 2015; 3:93–109

[58] Hubbard RP, Begeman PC. Biomechanical performance of a new head and neck support. Paper presented at: 34th Stapp Car Crash Conference; October 1, 1990; Orlando, Florida

[59] Trammell TR, Hubbard RP. Medical and technical outcomes of HANS® use in cart. Paper presented at: 2002 SAE Motorsports Engineering Conference and Exhibition; December 2, 2002; Indianapolis, Indiana

[60] Newman JA, Withnall C, Wonnacott M. An integrated helmet and neck support (iHANS) for racing car drivers: a biomechanical feasibility study. Paper presented at: 56th Stapp Car Crash Conference; October 29, 2012; Savannah, Georgia

[61] Kaul A, Abbas A, Smith G, Manjila S, Pace J, Steinmetz M. A revolution in preventing fatal craniovertebral junction injuries: lessons learned from the Head and Neck Support device in professional auto racing. J Neurosurg Spine. 2016; 25(6):756–761

[62] Barth JT, Freeman JR, Broshek DK, Varney RN. Acceleration-deceleration sport-related concussion: the gravity of it all. J Athl Train. 2001; 36(3):253–256

[63] Olvey SE, Knox T, Cohn KA. The development of a method to measure head acceleration and motion in high-impact crashes. Neurosurgery. 2004; 54(3): 672–677, discussion 677

[64] Filben TM, Pritchard NS, Oravec CS, et al. Pilot characterization of head kinematics in grassroots dirt track racing. Traffic Inj Prev. 2022; 23 suppl 1: S38–S43

30 Gymnastics

Carly Weber-Levine, Kelly Jiang, and Nicholas Theodore

Summary
Gymnasts regularly perform gravity-defying maneuvers that involve significant strength, flexibility, and coordination. Gymnastics requires an early introduction to the sport and time-intensive training regimens, which predispose athletes to many chronic injuries. While acute traumatic injuries in the form of concussions can occur when gymnasts fall and make contact with the mat, chronic injuries to the lumbar spine develop over years and are unfortunately common. These spinal injuries include spondylolysis, degenerative disc disease, spondylolisthesis, and disc herniation. Imaging, including computed tomography or magnetic resonance imaging, should be used to diagnose these conditions, followed by appropriate rest and rehabilitation exercises for recovery. Ultimately, recognizing, treating, and preventing these injuries is imperative for keeping gymnasts safe and aiding them in continuing their passion as long as possible.

Keywords: gymnastics, neurological injuries, sports medicine, return to play, sports injuries

30.1 Introduction

Gymnastics has grown significantly in popularity over the past several decades, likely due to publicity through collegiate athletics and the Olympic Games.[1,2] Female gymnastic competitions consist of four events: vault, uneven bars, beam, and floor. Male gymnastic competitions include six events: floor, pommel, rings, vault, parallel bars, and horizontal bar.[3] With the time-intensive training regimens and dangerous movements, gymnasts are at significant risk of injury. It is estimated that 72,542 gymnastics-related injuries occur nationally each year in 7- to 17-years-old gymnasts.[4] According to the National Collegiate Athletic Association, gymnastics has one of the highest injury rates of all collegiate sports, comparable to that of wrestling and football.[2] To achieve the highest level of the sport, athletes must start at a young age, typically younger than 8 years old.[4] In 2019, of 4.8 million gymnasts, 49% were 6 to 12 years old.[4] This leads to a significant duration of time during which traumatic accidents can occur and chronic injuries can develop.[5] While musculoskeletal injuries of the upper and lower extremities are the most common, injuries to the brain and spine can cause significant morbidity.[4] In this chapter, we will present the most common neurological injuries in gymnasts, along with treatment and prevention strategies.

30.2 Brain Injuries

The most common head injury in gymnastics is concussion.[6] Concussions are a form of mild traumatic brain injury that account for about 8% of the most common injuries in gymnasts.[4] In a study of 418 injuries reported in collegiate women gymnasts, Kerr et al reported lower rates of concussions, with 12 concussions documented.[2] Other studies of male gymnasts have found similar rates of 7 to 9.1%.[6,7]

30.2.1 Mechanism of Injury

Concussions are typically caused by impact of the head, face, neck, or body with the mat or floor during a fall and occur most frequently for female gymnasts during uneven bars (40%), floor exercise (40%), and balance beam (20%).[2] A whiplash effect can also cause concussions, in which the head moves forward and backward due to impact of the body elsewhere.

30.2.2 Symptoms

Common concussion symptoms include headache, balance problems, nausea, vomiting, drowsiness, dizziness, blurred vision, sensitivity to light or noise, fatigue, irritability, neck pain, confusion, and concentration or memory difficulties. Symptoms that may indicate an injury more severe than a concussion, deemed "Red Flags," include double vision, severe or worsening headache, weakness or numbness in arms or legs, seizure, loss of consciousness, and a deteriorating mental state. If these more severe symptoms are present, it is imperative to call an ambulance immediately and for the athlete to remain still until medical professionals arrive.[8,9]

30.2.3 Diagnosis

The Fédération Internationale de Gymnastique (FIG) recommends that a concussion be suspected in any gymnast that sustains impact to the head, face, neck, or body and demonstrates signs or reports any symptoms of a concussion, as specified above. A health care professional can evaluate the athlete with the Sports Concussion Assessment Tool 5 (SCAT5).[10] While a concussion is a clinical diagnosis, imaging, such as noncontrast computed tomography (CT), may be used to rule out more severe brain injury, such as an intracranial hemorrhage.[8,9]

30.2.4 Treatment

If a possible concussion has occurred, the athlete should be removed immediately from practice or competition and evaluated by a medical professional. The athlete should rest until all symptoms have resolved, which takes an average of 2 to 4 weeks for children and 7 to 10 days for adults. Following symptom resolution, athletes should undergo a stepwise return to the sport, outlined by the Gymnastics-Specific Return-to-Sport Strategy.[8] FIG recommends that gymnasts start with light aerobic activity, such as stationary bike, and progress to nondynamic inversions, dynamic stretching, and gymnastics strengthening. Afterward, gymnasts can reintroduce flipping and twisting, followed by a gradual return to advanced skills and full training. Along each step of the recovery process, the athlete should be monitored for the return of any concussion symptoms. If any symptoms do return, the athlete should return to the previous stage and wait a minimum of 24 hours for symptoms to resolve fully. A medical professional should determine when it is safe for the athlete to return to full sports activities.[8,9]

30.3 Spine Injuries

Spinal injuries account for 17.2% of injuries in Olympic gymnasts and most commonly involve the lumbar spine (▶ Fig. 30.1).[11] Injuries are typically characterized by degenerative changes associated with the chronic, high-impact use required by the sport. Gymnasts frequently report the lower back as a source of pain, affecting as many as 25% of gymnasts.[12] One study of 163 injuries in 84 male gymnasts found that the lower spine is the third most common region affected by acute (9%) injuries and the most frequently affected by chronic use injuries (19.6%).[6]

30.3.1 Spondylolysis

Spondylolysis, defined as a stress fracture in the pars interarticularis of the neural arch, affects approximately 11% of female gymnasts. While typically caused by age-related chronic wear, it occurs in gymnasts almost four times as frequently as in the general population and most often involves the fifth lumbar vertebra.[11,13,14] In a study of 24 German national team gymnasts, 6 had bilateral spondylolysis at L5 by the end of their careers.[15]

Mechanism of Injury

Spondylolysis is likely due to the high, repeated impact forces, twisting maneuvers, and lumbar hyperextension in gymnastics.[13] Maximum lumbar extension occurs during front and back walkovers, front and back handsprings, and the handspring vault.[16] Of all the maneuvers, the handspring vault produces the greatest vertical and lateral impact forces during landing, as measured by a force plate.[16] Meanwhile, front and back walkovers and back handsprings produce the greatest lumbar hyperextension.[16] This hyperextension can result in stress shifting posteriorly and the shear force on the spine increasing.[16] Studies estimate that the average landing shear force at L5–S1 can be as high as 2.2 times the body weight, while compressive forces can be as high as 14.8 times the body weight.[17] This force ultimately leads to spondylolysis due to the development of stress fractures in the pars interarticularis.[11]

Symptoms

Spondylolysis typically presents with pain in the lumbar region that worsens with extension and improves with rest and flexion.[11] While this pain can be associated with paresthesias and radiation to the buttocks and thighs, patients generally do not have nerve root signs or muscle weakness.[11,18]

Diagnosis

Any back pain that persists longer than 2 weeks should be further examined.[19] Upon physical examination, the gymnasts may demonstrate excessive hyperlordosis.[11] Imaging is critical to the diagnosis. While plain radiographs may be initially used, CT or single-photon emission computed tomography scans are highly sensitive and specific for identifying the stress fractures.[14,20]

Treatment

Initial treatment should focus on rest and rehabilitation exercises, including thoracic, core, and hip extension stretching exercises.[19] Generally, it takes approximately 3 months of rest

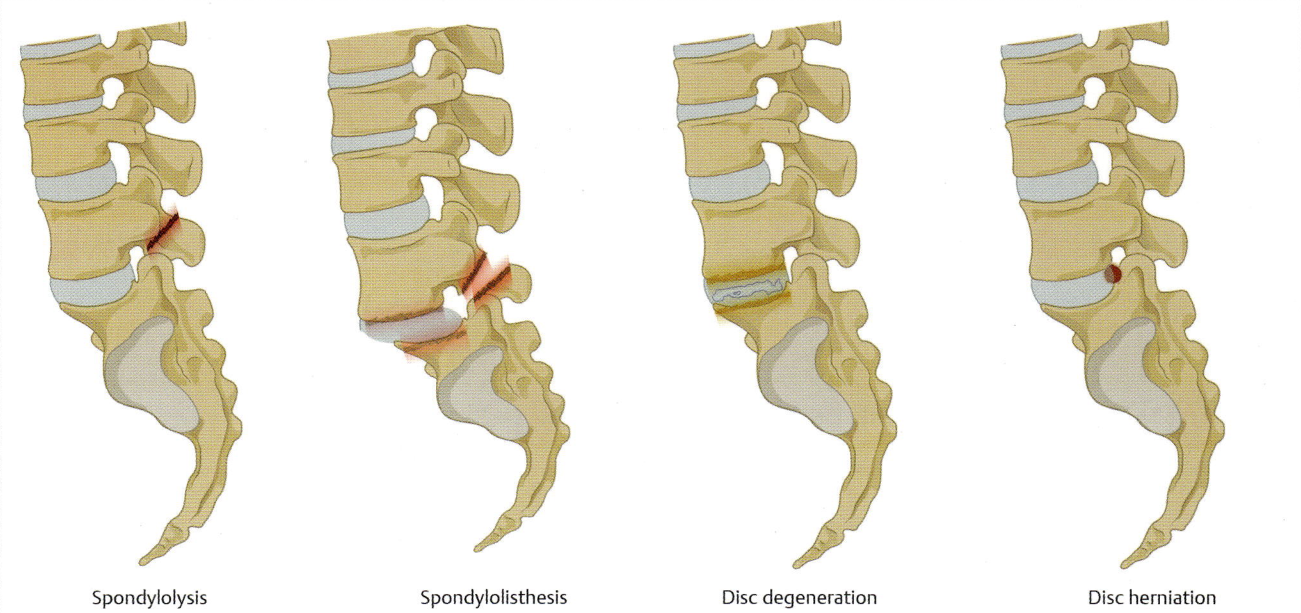

Fig. 30.1 Depiction of the most common spinal injuries seen in gymnastics. (Created with BioRender.com.)

to achieve bony healing. If the patient remains symptomatic after 2 to 4 weeks of rest, lumbosacral bracing can be used to further reduce spinal motion further. A follow-up CT scan at 12 weeks can be used to assess bony healing before return to play.[14] If symptoms continue for greater than 6 months following conservative treatment, surgical treatment can be performed to repair the pars defect directly.[20]

30.3.2 Degenerative Disc Disease

Degenerative disc disease is also one of the most common spinal injuries in gymnasts. In the general population, this disease affects 40% of people by the age of 40 years, but higher rates are seen in gymnasts well before adulthood.[21] Bennett et al studied 19 Olympic-level female gymnasts aged 12 to 21 and found that 12 (63.2%) had degenerative disc disease.[22] Swärd et al examined 24 elite male gymnasts under the age of 30 years and identified 18 (75.0%) as having disc degeneration.[23] Koyama et al studied 104 Japanese collegiate gymnasts competing at levels ranging from pre-elite to Olympic levels and detected lumbar disc degeneration in 42 (40.4%) participants.[24] Gymnasts competing below the elite level may have lower frequencies of disc degeneration. For example, in a study of 35 gymnasts mainly competing at district and national levels, only 3 (8.6%) were detected to have evidence of disc degeneration on magnetic resonance imaging (MRI).[25] This lower frequency may be explained by differences in the amount and intensity of training required for different levels of gymnastics.

Mechanism of Injury

Excessive compression, flexion, and rotational stress on the spine can lead to traumatic intraosseous herniation, gradual loss of hydration in the disc, and subsequent degeneration.[25,26]

Symptoms

Disc degeneration typically presents with low back pain.[25]

Diagnosis

Degenerative disc disease is diagnosed via a decreased signal in the nucleus pulposus on T2-weighted MRI.[26,27] MRI can also detect osteophyte formation, Schmorl's nodes, and disc space narrowing, which commonly occur in degenerative disc disease.[22,25]

Treatment

Management should first be conservative with rest and nonsteroidal anti-inflammatory drugs. Epidural injections can also help with controlling pain. Once pain is reduced, rehabilitation and plyometric exercises should be incorporated to strengthen the lumbar extensor and abdominal muscles. Athletes can return to play once full, painless range of motion is achieved. Athletes should focus on maintaining a neutral spine position as much as possible and continuing their rehabilitation exercises. Surgical treatment via disc replacement or lumbar fusion may be pursued if symptoms do not resolve with conservative management.[20]

30.3.3 Other Spinal Injuries

Spondylolisthesis and disc herniation may also occur in gymnasts. Spondylolisthesis is defined as the anterior slippage of a superior vertebral body over the inferior one and can sometimes result from the progression of spondylolysis.[17,22] It typically presents with back pain and can be diagnosed through plain radiographs or a CT scan.[17,27] Studies have shown that an L5–S1 spondylolisthesis may be associated with a greater pelvic incidence and sacral slope in gymnasts.[28] Disc herniation is typically caused by repetitive flexion and compression, presents with radicular pain, and can be diagnosed with MRI.[29] In the study of 19 Olympic-level female gymnasts, Bennett et al identified spondylolisthesis and disc herniation in 3 and 4 gymnasts, respectively.[22] Similarly, in a study of 24 German national team gymnasts, spondylolisthesis was detected in 3 athletes using lumbar radiographs.[15] While most cases of spondylolisthesis and disc herniation can be treated conservatively with rest and rehabilitation exercises, if symptoms continue to worsen or if the spondylolisthesis is greater than > 50%, fusion or discectomy surgery may be required.[29]

Other spinal injuries that cause significant morbidity in other sports, such as spinal cord injury, remain infrequent in gymnastics.[27] These traumatic accidents typically involve the cervical spinal cord and account for less than 1% of injuries.[2,30] For example, between 1975 and 1987, only 5 out of 3,200 patients presenting with spinal injuries were related to gymnastics.[30] A severe spinal injury should be suspected in gymnasts presenting with neck pain alongside neurological symptoms, such as weakness, numbness, or paresthesias in the arms or legs. If this occurs, it is imperative to call an ambulance, keep the athlete still, and immobilize the spine as quickly as possible.[8,9] Patients will generally undergo CT or other imaging to determine if surgery, most commonly fusion, is indicated.[30]

30.4 Prevention of Injury

Preventing injury is critical for gymnasts to partake in the sport longer and avoid life-long injuries. Most injuries, approximately 85%, occur during practice, while a minority occur during competitions (15%). The competition injury rate, however, is significantly higher than the practice injury rate (11.94/1,000 vs 8.69/1,000, respectively).[2] Moreover, injuries most commonly occur from contact with the mat or through overuse. The floor and uneven bars are associated with the greatest number of injuries in women, and the floor and vault in men.[2,6,7] Accordingly, injury prevention strategies include using spotters to help prevent acute traumatic accidents and equipment to reduce forces exerted on the body during takeoffs and landings. These include foam rubber landing mats, tumbling mats, crash pads, landing pits, and twisting belts.[1] Thicker mats, for example, have been shown to reduce mechanical loading on the spine.[31] Finally, formal instruction on how to fall can also help gymnasts avoid more severe fall-related injuries. Unfortunately, gymnasts' injuries often remain symptomatic following the discontinuation of the sport. Lower back injuries can especially be long-term, causing extended pain, stiffness, and weakness.[32] Therefore, introducing these prevention strategies can improve gymnasts' experiences while they are practicing the sport and for the duration of their lives.

Table 30.1 Summary of the most common brain and spine injuries in gymnasts

Location	Mechanism of injury	Symptoms	Diagnosis	Treatment
Brain				
Concussion	Impact with mat or floor, whiplash effect	Headache, balance problems, nausea, vomiting, drowsiness, dizziness, blurred vision, sensitivity to light or noise, fatigue, irritability, neck pain, confusion, and concentration or memory difficulties	Clinical, SCAT5	Rest until all symptoms have resolved (typically 2–4 wk in children and 7–10 d in adults), gymnastics-specific return-to-sport strategy
Spine				
Spondylolysis	Impact forces, twisting, lumbar hyperextension	Lumbar pain	SPECT, CT	Rest, rehabilitation exercises, lumbosacral bracing
Spondylolisthesis	Lumbar hyperextension, anterior slippage of the superior vertebral body	Lumbar pain	CT, plain radiographs	Rest, rehabilitation exercises, fusion surgery if > 50%
Disc degeneration	Compression, flexion, rotation, loss of hydration in the disc	Lumbar pain	T2 MRI	Rest, NSAIDs, epidural injections, rehabilitation exercises, fusion surgery
Disc herniation	Repetitive flexion and compression	Radicular pain	MRI	Rest, rehabilitation exercises, discectomy surgery

Abbreviations: CT, computed tomography; MRI, magnetic resonance imaging; NSAID, nonsteroidal anti-inflammatory drug; SCAT5, Sports Concussion Assessment Tool 5; SPECT, single-photon emission computed tomography.

30.5 Conclusions

Gymnastics is filled with captivating, gravity-defying maneuvers that can expose athletes to significant injury risk. While musculoskeletal injuries of the extremities make up the majority of gymnastics-related injuries, brain and spine injuries are also common and can cause considerable morbidity. In this chapter, we introduced the most frequent brain and spinal injuries and discussed the mechanisms, symptoms, diagnosis, and treatment of these conditions (▶ Table 30.1). Acute injuries to the brain include concussions, while chronic use injuries to the spine include spondylolysis, degenerative disc disease, spondylolisthesis, and disc herniation. Ultimately, treatment and prevention strategies aim to protect gymnasts from these injuries and aid them in continuing their passion as long as possible.

30.6 Clinical Pearls

- The most common brain injury in gymnastics is concussion, a mild form of traumatic brain injury.
- The SCAT5 can be used to evaluate concussion.
- The most common spinal injuries in gymnastics include spondylolysis, degenerative disc disease, spondylolisthesis, and disc herniation.
- Immobilization of the spine following injury is key to preventing further damage.
- Injury prevention includes equipment to reduce forces on the body during takeoff and landing and formal instruction on how to fall.

30.7 Disclosures

Carly Weber-Levine: none.
Kelly Jiang: none.
Nicholas Theodore: Royalties from Globus Medical. Stock Ownership in Globus Medical. Consultant for Globus Medical. On Scientific Advisory Board/Other Office for Globus Medical.

References

[1] Daly RM, Bass SL, Finch CF. Balancing the risk of injury to gymnasts: how effective are the counter measures? Br J Sports Med. 2001; 35(1):8–18, quiz 19

[2] Kerr ZY, Hayden R, Barr M, Klossner DA, Dompier TP. Epidemiology of National Collegiate Athletic Association women's gymnastics injuries, 2009–2010 through 2013–2014. J Athl Train. 2015; 50(8):870–878

[3] Campbell RA, Bradshaw EJ, Ball NB, Pease DL, Spratford W. Injury epidemiology and risk factors in competitive artistic gymnasts: a systematic review. Br J Sports Med. 2019; 53(17):1056–1069

[4] Tisano B, Zynda AJ, Ellis HB, Wilson PL. Epidemiology of pediatric gymnastics injuries reported in US emergency departments: sex- and age-based injury patterns. Orthop J Sports Med. 2022; 10(6):23259671221102478

[5] Snook GA. Injuries in women's gymnastics. A 5-year study. Am J Sports Med. 1979; 7(4):242–244

[6] Ahmad B, LaBella CR, Wolf SF. Boys gymnastics injuries: a 9-year retrospective review. Phys Sportsmed. 2022; 50(4):311–315

[7] Kruse DW, Nobe AS, Billimek J. Injury incidence and characteristics for elite, male, artistic USA gymnastics competitions from 2008 to 2018. Br J Sports Med. 2021; 55(3):163–168

[8] Fédération Internationale de Gymnastique. FIG-concussion guidelines. Accessed January 2023 at: https://www.gymnastics.sport/site/pages/medical/Medical_FIG_Concussion%20Overview.pdf

[9] USA Gymnastics. Sports concussion guidelines. Accessed January 22, 2023 at: https://nfhslearn.com/courses/concussion-in-sports-2

[10] Sport concussion assessment tool - 5th edition. Br J Sports Med. 2017; 51 (11):851–858

[11] Mohriak R, Vargas Silva PD, Trandafilov M, Jr, et al. Spondylolysis and spondylolisthesis in young gymnasts. Rev Bras Ortop. 2015; 45(1):79–83

[12] Sastre-Munar A, Pades-Jiménez A, García-Coll N, Molina-Mula J, Romero-Franco N. Injuries, pain, and catastrophizing level in gymnasts: a retrospective analysis of a cohort of Spanish athletes. Healthcare (Basel). 2022; 10(5):890

[13] McAuley E, Hudash G, Shields K, et al. Injuries in women's gymnastics. The state of the art. Am J Sports Med. 1987; 15(6):558–565

[14] Standaert CJ. Spondylolysis in the adolescent athlete. Clin J Sport Med. 2002; 12(2):119–122

[15] Konermann W, Sell S. The spine–a problem area in high performance artistic gymnastics. A retrospective analysis of 24 former artistic gymnasts of the German A team [in German]. Sportverletz Sportschaden. 1992; 6(4):156–160
[16] Hall SJ. Mechanical contribution to lumbar stress injuries in female gymnasts. Med Sci Sports Exerc. 1986; 18(6):599–602
[17] Urushibara M, Kawasaki T, Aihara T, Kojima A. Association of lumbar spondylolytic spondylolisthesis with the incidence and prognosis of anterior ring apophyseal abnormalities of the vertebrae in young gymnasts. Orthop J Sports Med. 2023; 11(1):23259671221142560
[18] Weber MD, Woodall WR. Spondylogenic disorders in gymnasts. J Orthop Sports Phys Ther. 1991; 14(1):6–13
[19] Sands WA, McNeal JR, Penitente G, et al. Stretching the spines of gymnasts: a review. Sports Med. 2016; 46(3):315–327
[20] Burgmeier RJ, Hsu WK. Spine surgery in athletes with low back pain-considerations for management and treatment. Asian J Sports Med. 2014; 5(4):e24284
[21] Secretariat MA, Medical Advisory Secretariat. Artificial discs for lumbar and cervical degenerative disc disease -update: an evidence-based analysis. Ont Health Technol Assess Ser. 2006; 6(10):1–98
[22] Bennett DL, Nassar L, DeLano MC. Lumbar spine MRI in the elite-level female gymnast with low back pain. Skeletal Radiol. 2006; 35(7):503–509
[23] Swärd L, Hellström M, Jacobsson B, Nyman R, Peterson L. Disc degeneration and associated abnormalities of the spine in elite gymnasts. A magnetic resonance imaging study. Spine. 1991; 16(4):437–443
[24] Koyama K, Nakazato K, Min S, et al. Radiological abnormalities and low back pain in gymnasts. Int J Sports Med. 2013; 34(3):218–222
[25] Tertti M, Paajanen H, Kujala UM, Alanen A, Salmi TT, Kormano M. Disc degeneration in young gymnasts. A magnetic resonance imaging study. Am J Sports Med. 1990; 18(2):206–208
[26] Hasz MW. Diagnostic testing for degenerative disc disease. Adv Orthop. 2012; 2012:413913
[27] Kruse D, Lemmen B. Spine injuries in the sport of gymnastics. Curr Sports Med Rep. 2009; 8(1):20–28
[28] Toueg CW, Mac-Thiong JM, Grimard G, Poitras B, Parent S, Labelle H. Spondylolisthesis, sacro-pelvic morphology, and orientation in young gymnasts. J Spinal Disord Tech. 2015; 28(6):E358–E364
[29] Ball JR, Harris CB, Lee J, Vives MJ. Lumbar spine injuries in sports: review of the literature and current treatment recommendations. Sports Med Open. 2019; 5(1):26
[30] Bailes JE, Hadley MN, Quigley MR, Sonntag VK, Cerullo LJ. Management of athletic injuries of the cervical spine and spinal cord. Neurosurgery. 1991; 29 (4):491–497
[31] Goldstein JD, Berger PE, Windler GE, Jackson DW. Spine injuries in gymnasts and swimmers. An epidemiologic investigation. Am J Sports Med. 1991; 19(5):463–468
[32] Wadley GH, Albright JP. Women's intercollegiate gymnastics. Injury patterns and "permanent" medical disability. Am J Sports Med. 1993; 21 (2):314–320

31 Equestrian

Meghana Bhimreddy, Andrew M. Hersh, and Nicholas Theodore

Summary
Equestrian sports, with their ancient roots and modern popularity, pose significant risks of neurological injuries due to the unpredictable behavior of horses and the high speeds involved. These injuries typically result from a fall and include concussions, vertebral column fractures, and spinal cord injury, with factors such as gender, age, rider experience, and horse temperament influencing the severity. By promoting safety measures such as helmet use and rider education, the equestrian community can minimize the incidence of neurological injuries and foster a safer environment for riders of all levels.

Keywords: equestrian, horseback riding, neurological injury

31.1 Introduction

Equestrian sports have an ancient history, with horseback riding dating back to the second millennium BCE.[1] Since then, equestrianism has progressed from a means of transport to a highly popular sport that draws nearly 30 million riders annually in the United States alone.[2] Currently, equestrian sports encompass a wide range of activities that are performed both competitively and for leisure, including dressage, polo, show jumping, and vaulting, among many more.[3]

Due to the unpredictable behavior and large size of horses, as well as the high speeds and height involved in horseback riding, equestrian riders face serious risk of neurologic injuries.[4] While some injuries are benign, many cause catastrophic brain and spinal injuries that require immediate neurosurgical intervention and can result in permanent damage or death.[5] In fact, equestrian sports have been reported as the greatest contributors to sports-related traumatic brain injury (TBI) and sports-related spinal injuries, with rates of severe injury higher than automobile racing, motorcycle racing, rugby, skiing, and American football combined.[6,7] This chapter discusses the mechanism, risk factors, symptoms, diagnosis, and treatment of the most common neurological injuries caused by equestrian sports, followed by several prevention strategies.

31.2 Mechanism of Injury

Equestrian injuries can be sustained regardless of the rider being mounted or unmounted. When in the mounted position, riders can experience a fall during dismount, due to a horse fall, while riding, or as a result of being bucked.[8] When in the unmounted position, riders are in danger of neurologic injuries caused by a kick, crush, drag, or bite from the horse when in close proximity.[8] Unmounted injuries can occur for multiple reasons including a spooked, untrained, or bad temperament horse.[9]

Typically, falls can result in concussions, intracranial hemorrhages and hematomas, and severe TBI.[7] One of the factors influencing the likelihood of concussion is the surface upon which the rider lands. Hard asphalt had a slightly higher probability (33.4%) of causing a concussive episode than grass/dirt surfaces (26.5%) or indoor riding arena floor surfacing (20.8%).[10] Spinal injuries due to falls are less common than head injuries and result in mostly transverse process fractures.[11] The direction of a fall also determines the type of spinal injury sustained. Landing on the head, for instance, is more likely to result in hyperflexion injuries to the cervical spine, while landing on the buttocks results in thoracolumbar junction injuries.[12] Analysis of equestrian spinal cord injuries (SCIs) from South Wales during the late 1900s indicates that acute SCIs due to falls are more common among leisure and occupational rides, not competitive ones.[13]

Falls are the most common mechanism of neurologic injury. Data from the University of Kentucky Trauma Registry revealed that 54% of equestrian injuries occur due to falls, with kicks following at 22%.[14] Though less common than falls, horse kicks are just as dangerous and transfer more than 10,000 N of force.[15] Compared with mounted riders, unmounted riders are more likely to sustain catastrophic head injuries and require intensive care or surgical intervention.[14]

31.3 Risk Factors

Young, amateur female riders and older, professional male riders are at the highest risk of neurologic injuries due to a fall or crush.[16] Analysis of the National Pediatric Trauma Registry, for example, identified a female majority among the patients brought to the emergency department for equestrian-related concussions.[17] Data from the National Electronic Injury Surveillance System from 1987 to 1988 also reveals that injury rates were highest among 5- to 24-year-old females. Once the age of riders increased to 44 + years, however, men began to outnumber women in terms of injuries.[16] This gender and age disparity is due to the demographics of equestrian sports, which are popular among young female participants.[18] Professional equestrian riders may suffer from more severe injuries than amateurs due to the increased rigor of their training, faster riding speeds, higher obstacle heights, and propensity for working with more unpredictable horses.[2]

Similar to professional experience with horse riding, a lack of familiarity with equestrian sports increases risk of injuries to riders.[16] Riding a young horse is another contributing risk.[16] Analysis of a detailed questionnaire sent to patients with major equestrian injuries found that the average age of their horses was 7 years.[9] Horses older than 15 years are the safest mounts for riders when compared with those < 5 or between 5 and 14 years of age.[19]

31.4 Brain Injuries

After extremity injuries, head injuries are the most common effect of equestrian trauma. These injuries typically result in TBIs, which range from mild TBI with no imaging findings and concussions to more severe structural impairment, which can include pathologies such as hematomas and hemorrhage, cerebral contusions, and fractures of the skull, especially involving the cranial vault.[7,11] Around 10% to 15% of all equestrian injuries that present at the hospital are concussions, making them the most common form of TBI among riders.[7] Typically, these concussive episodes are accompanied by loss of consciousness and cause jockeys to lose around 43 riding days annually during their career.[20]

Signs of concussion vary based on the extent of the head trauma, and symptoms should be classified as mandatory or discretionary visible signs to guide treatment. Examples of mandatory symptoms include loss of consciousness, immobility greater than 5 seconds, disorientation, amnesia, a vacant look, uncoordinated motor movement, tonic posture, seizures, and ataxia. Examples of discretionary visible signs include head clutching, slow standing, and possible facial fracture.[21] Presence of a lump or swelling will indicate a potential skull fracture. Other signs include but are not limited to pain at a localized spot on the skull, cerebrospinal fluid leaking from the nose or ears, difficulty swallowing, bruising, and bleeding from the head.[22]

Based on the Berlin Consensus Statement on Concussion in Sport, any rider displaying the aforementioned signs of TBI should immediately be removed from the arena for neurologic evaluation by a physician.[21] A qualified medical professional should assess the rider using the Concussion Recognition Tool 5 and the Sports Concussion Assessment Tool 5. Riders should also be evaluated for possible cervical spine, maxillofacial, and airway injuries through inspection of the head and neck.[23] A pupillary dilation test should be conducted. If a skull fracture is suspected, an X-ray radiograph or ultrasound can be used to confirm the diagnosis. After stabilization of the patient, computed tomography (CT) imaging should immediately be ordered in patients with suspected skull fractures or heavy trauma to screen for pathologies such as intracranial hematomas, hemorrhage, edema, and contusions.[24] For patients with impaired consciousness, a Glasgow Coma Scale (GCS) score should be calculated. Patients that have low presenting GCS scores may benefit from placement of an intracranial pressure monitor, which will reveal if high pressures are present and need alleviation.[25]

Presently, most equestrian organizations do not have formal return-to-play policies, but the United States Eventing Association does recommend clearance by a physician before resuming riding.[2] If no concussion is diagnosed, riders may return to their sport but should receive regular reassessments over the next 2 days to account for delayed symptoms.

Return-to-play should occur on a graded basis dependent on the extent of the concussive episode. Riders diagnosed with mild concussions should be restricted from riding until they complete a 24-hour break after full recovery of consciousness and a normal mental state.[16] If headaches are present, riders should not return until symptoms resolve. Most concussions will resolve with rest after a period of ~3 weeks for pediatric patients and ~1.5 weeks for adult patients. For moderate concussions, riders should recover for 1 week after injury.[16] Severe concussions will require extensive evaluation by a physician who can provide approval for resumption of equestrian activities.

In cases with high intracranial pressures that may cause secondary brain injury, surgical management can include a decompressive craniotomy or ventriculostomy.[26] Either can be supplemented with an external ventricular drain.[27] A craniotomy can also be performed for evacuation of a subdural hemorrhage or washout and elevation of a depressed skull fracture.[11] If a craniotomy is risky, a smaller burr hole can be used for similar purposes.[28] While some patients will recover quickly, others may experience functional impairment months after discharge and can benefit from the services of a rehabilitation center.[9]

31.5 Spine Injuries

Although not as common as head injuries, traumatic spine injuries can occur from equestrian causes. Riders are elevated 2 to 3 meters off the ground when mounted on a horse, putting them at risk of spinal trauma from a fall. Between 2% and 14% of equestrian-related injuries have a spinal component, with the lumbar region being the most common (51%), followed by thoracic (32%) and cervical spine (17%) regions. Spinal injuries usually consist of vertebral column fractures and SCI, with the latter being less common.[29]

31.5.1 Vertebral Column Fractures

During a fall that results in the head/neck pointing toward the ground, a rider may suffer from a hyperextension or flexion injury. Flexion injuries have a compressive presentation, resulting in damage to the anterior cervical spine. This involves wedging and vertebral body chip fractures, with very rare instances of dislocation. Flexion injuries also result in ligament rupture on the dorsal side of the spine. Extension injuries, such as the ones caused by whiplash, result in compression among the posterior aspects of the cervical region, resulting in damage to the spinous processes and facets.[5] A fall may also result in burst fractures, which occur when the vertebral column encounters a vertical trauma. The force is transmitted along the stacked vertebrae, causing end-plate fractures and disc rupture.[30] For riders that fall backward and land on their buttocks, thoracolumbar fractures in the T11–L2 area are more common.[31]

Vertebral column fractures will have varied symptoms based on the exact location of injury, angle of contact, and amount of force transferred. Some signs include muscle spasm, back pain, decreased flexibility/mobility in the spine, paralysis, bowel/bladder incontinence, neck pain, tingling, and numbness.[32] Once the patient is stable, they should be assessed using the American Spinal Injury Association (ASIA) scale and screened for SCI. For bony fractures, a CT scan is recommended, though other imaging modalities can be added if needed. For instance, magnetic resonance imaging (MRI) scans can indicate if a ligamentous injury is also present. A vertebral fracture assessment can also be conducted.[32]

Appropriate treatment for spinal fractures will vary. Some fractures can heal over a short period of 4 weeks with simple rest. This process involves wearing a back brace, which secures the spine in alignment and ensures proper healing.[33] For more severe fractures, instrumentation and fusion procedures are a viable option. Some surgeons may perform vertebroplasty or kyphoplasty to strengthen vertebral fractures and realign the spine.[34] Referral to physical and occupational therapy is imperative to prevent bone loss and reduce the risk of future spinal fractures.

31.5.2 Spinal Cord Injury

According to the U.S. National SCI Statistical Center database, neurologic function after equestrian-related SCI is most likely to be preserved in the following regions: C4–C6, T12, and L1. Riders with SCI have a variety of outcomes, including incomplete tetraplegia (41%), complete paraplegia (24%), incomplete paraplegia (20%) and complete tetraplegia (8.3%).[35]

Signs of SCI include bowel/bladder urgency or incontinence, impaired breathing, loss of sensation, tingling, weakness or loss of motor control, difficulty with balance, or extreme pain/pressure at a specific location on the spine. SCI is accompanied by an increased risk for cardiovascular dysfunction, such as a stroke, heart attack, abnormal blood pressure, arrhythmia, or variable heart rate.[36]

SCI should be diagnosed through a thorough examination of the patient after they are stabilized and classified according to the ASIA scale. Assessing the patient for typical symptoms of SCI will provide insight into the region of the cord that may be affected. Complete transection of the cord, for instance, is likely to be accompanied by complete bilateral loss of function, proprioception, nociception, and tactile sensation below the site of injury. Anterior cord damage, on the other hand, will lead to bilateral loss of nociception and temperature sensation, but vibration, proprioception, and tactile sensation will remain intact.[36] Imaging is imperative to confirm any suspicions. An MRI scan should be ordered immediately to pinpoint the location of the SCI. Other imaging modalities, such as X-ray radiographs or CT scans, can supplement the MRI if needed.

All patients with suspected neurologic injury should be handled with spinal precautions in place. Spinal immobilization should be utilized in cases with severe trauma or symptoms. Maintain airway, breathing, and hemodynamic ability in accordance with the Advanced Trauma and Life Support protocols. If SCI is confirmed, surgical decompression can be indicated to alleviate deformity, remove a blood clot, or lessen compression against a herniated disc.[37] The patient should be monitored in the intensive care unit. Prescribe high-dose steroids for acute treatment. After their inpatient stay, patients with severe SCIs will likely experience lifelong functional deficits, including headaches, psychosocial challenges, difficulties with balance, limited mobility, and chronic pain. For patients with these deficits, rehabilitation therapy should be provided. Rehabilitation teams are responsible for assisting patients with regaining independence, mobility, and sense of safety. Injured riders work alongside therapists to practice and strengthen their activities of daily living before returning home.[9]

31.6 Prevention and Protective Measures

Despite its function as protective gear, helmet use in equestrian sports is low. Equestrian helmets consist of foam surrounded by a hard plastic or resin coating, giving them greater flexibility than their American football counterparts.[7] When a force is applied, the elastic nature of the helmet causes deformation and absorbs energy. Helmets halve the risk for TBI, but only 9% to 25% of riders wear them.[38] The usage of helmets decreases with age, with adults and teens utilizing them at lower rates than young children. Pads and protective waistcoats can be additional buffers for falls and trauma, but their usefulness is not as well characterized. Body protectors do not shield riders from spinal rotation or compression injuries, but are useful for nonneurologic injuries such as rib fractures and soft-tissue injuries.[39]

Experience and knowledge of equestrianism act as a protective factor against head and spine injuries. Riders can be divided into four categories based on familiarity with equestrian sports: novice, intermediates, advanced, and professional. Novice riders have 3 to 8 times the risk of injuries compared with the remaining groups. All riders should aim for a minimum of 100 hours of experience to lower their risk of neurologic injuries.[40] Furthermore, nearly 65% of riders are unsure of concussion guidelines, with 13% having no knowledge whatsoever. Many riders believe that dizziness and disorientation after a fall are innocuous symptoms (33%), while others would return to play on the same day as a concussive episode (30%).[41] Educating equestrian riders on detection and treatment of potential head and spine injuries will help mitigate this misinformation.

31.7 Conclusion

Equestrianism is among the most dangerous sports, with high rates of neurologic injuries compared with other athletic activities (▶ Fig. 31.1). Due to the high speeds, elevation, and sometimes volatile horse–rider relationship, many opportunities emerge for head and spinal injuries to occur (▶ Table 31.1). Despite awareness of this heightened risk, riders of all ages and experience levels enjoy the sport for competitive, occupational, and leisure purposes. As a result, prevention strategies should focus on increasing awareness of protective gear use, increasing rider experience to at least 100 hours, and providing education on recommended guidelines for concussion management.

31.8 Clinical Pearls

- Due to the high speeds, height, and unpredictable behavior of horses, equestrianism has a high risk for neurological injury and is the greatest contributor to sports-related TBI and spinal injuries.
- Young, amateur female riders and older, professional male riders are at highest risk of neurological injuries due to a fall or crush.
- Experience and knowledge of equestrianism are protective factors against injury. Education about neurological injury symptoms and the importance of helmet use may prevent injuries.

31.9 Disclosures

Meghana Bhimreddy: none.
Andrew M. Hersh: none.
Nicholas Theodore: Royalties from Globus Medical. Stock Ownership in Globus Medical. Consultant for Globus Medical. On Scientific Advisory Board/Other Office for Globus Medical.

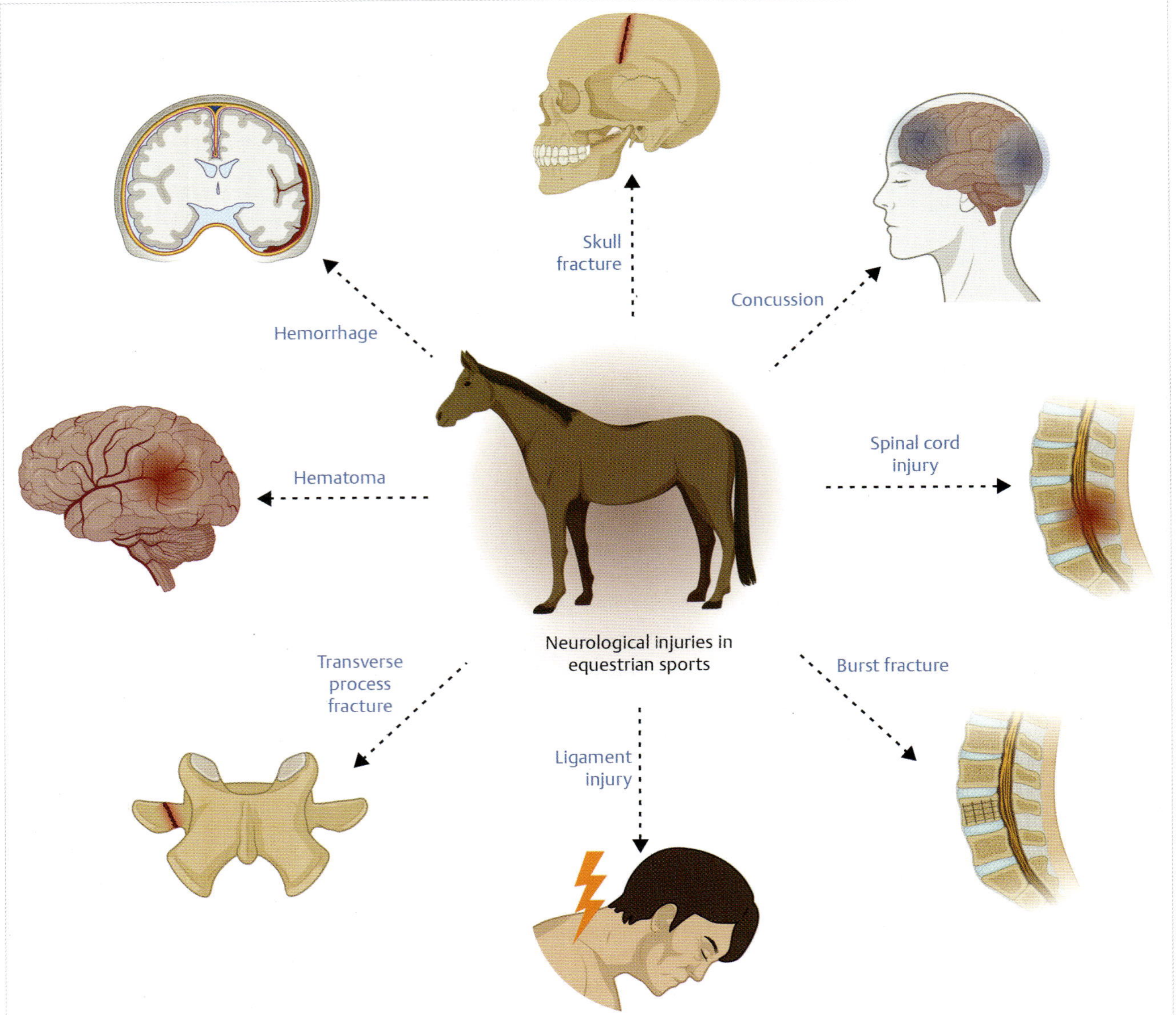

Fig. 31.1 Depiction of the most common head and spinal injuries seen among equestrian riders. (Created with BioRender.com.)

Table 31.1 Summary of the most common brain and spine injuries in equestrian sports

Location	Mechanism	Symptoms	Diagnosis	Treatment
Brain				
Concussion	Impact with floor, whiplash, horse kick	Loss of consciousness, immobility greater than 5 s, disorientation, amnesia, a vacant look, uncoordinated motor movement, tonic posture, seizures, ataxia, etc.	Clinical, SCAT5, CRT5. CT scan if bleeding suspected	Removal from play, rest until normal. Period for return to play will vary based on extent of concussion
Skull fracture	Impact with floor, horse kick, crush, or bite	Presence of lump, pain at a localized spot on the skull, CSF leaking from the nose or ears, difficulty swallowing, bruising and bleeding from the head, etc.	SCAT5, CRT5, CT scan	Removal from play. Craniotomy or burr hole for washout and elevation of a depressed skull fracture
Spine				
Spinal cord injury	Fall from mounted position	Bowel/bladder urgency or incontinency, impaired breathing, loss of sensation, tingling, weakness or loss of motor control, difficulty with balance, extreme pain/pressure at a specific location on the spine, etc.	MRI	Surgical decompression, steroids, rehabilitation therapy
Burst fracture	Vertical fall from mount	Muscle spasm, back pain, decreased flexibility/mobility in the spine, paralysis, bowel/bladder incontinence, neck pain, tingling, numbness, etc.	CT scan, vertebral fracture assessment	Back brace, instrumentation, and fusion
Transverse process fracture	Hyperextension injury	Muscle spasm, back pain, decreased flexibility/mobility in the spine, paralysis, bowel/bladder incontinence, neck pain, tingling, numbness, etc.	CT scan, vertebral fracture assessment	Back splint/cast, instrumentation, and fusion
Disc herniation	Vertical fall from mount	Burning or stinging pain, radicular pain, limited flexion, pain exacerbation with straining, coughing, sneezing, etc.	MRI	NSAIDs, exercise and heat, stretching, steroid injection, discectomy
Ligamentous injury	Flexion injury during fall	Worsening pain with neck movement, neck stiffness, headaches, pain between shoulder blades, etc.	MRI	Pain relief medications, massage, heat/ice. Cervical collar if needed

Abbreviations: CRT5, Concussion Recognition Tool 5; CSF, cerebrospinal fluid; CT, computed tomography; MRI, magnetic resonance imaging; NSAID, nonsteroidal anti-inflammatory drug; SCAT5, Sports Concussion Assessment Tool 5.

References

[1] McMiken DF. Ancient origins of horsemanship. Equine Vet J. 1990; 22(2):73–78

[2] Havlik HS. Equestrian sport-related injuries: a review of current literature. Curr Sports Med Rep. 2010; 9(5):299–302

[3] Holmes TQ, Brown AF. Champing at the bit for improvements: a review of equine welfare in equestrian sports in the United Kingdom. Animals (Basel). 2022; 12(9):1186

[4] Gates JK, Lin CY. Head and spinal injuries in equestrian sports: update on epidemiology, clinical outcomes, and injury prevention. Curr Sports Med Rep. 2020; 19(1):17–23

[5] Wolff CS, Cantu RC, Kucera KL. Catastrophic neurologic injuries in sport. Handb Clin Neurol. 2018; 158:25–37

[6] Bernstorff MA, Adler C, Schumann N, et al. Traumatic spinal cord injuries in sports: a 22-year analysis performed by a specialized trauma centre [in German]. Sportverletz Sportschaden. 2023; 37(2):87–95

[7] Zuckerman SL, Morgan CD, Burks S, et al. Functional and structural traumatic brain injury in equestrian sports: a review of the literature. World Neurosurg. 2015; 83(6):1098–1113

[8] Van Balen PJ, Barten DG, Janssen L, Fiddelers AAA, Brink PR, Janzing HMJ. Beware of the force of the horse: mechanisms and severity of equestrian-related injuries. Eur J Emerg Med. 2019; 26(2):133–138

[9] Ball JE, Ball CG, Mulloy RH, Datta I, Kirkpatrick AW. Ten years of major equestrian injury: are we addressing functional outcomes? J Trauma Manag Outcomes. 2009; 3:2

[10] Meredith L, Ekman R, Thomson R. Horse-related incidents and factors for predicting injuries to the head. BMJ Open Sport Exerc Med. 2018; 4(1): e000398

[11] Srinivasan V, Pierre C, Plog B, Srinivasan K, Petraglia AL, Huang JH. Straight from the horse's mouth: neurological injury in equestrian sports. Neurol Res. 2014; 36(10):873–877

[12] Silver JR. Spinal injuries resulting from horse riding accidents. Spinal Cord. 2002; 40(6):264–271

[13] Roe JP, Taylor TK, Edmunds IA, et al. Spinal and spinal cord injuries in horse riding: the New South Wales experience 1976–1996. ANZ J Surg. 2003; 73 (5):331–334

[14] Carmichael SP, II, Davenport DL, Kearney PA, Bernard AC. On and off the horse: mechanisms and patterns of injury in mounted and unmounted equestrians. Injury. 2014; 45(9):1479–1483

[15] Stier R, Tavassol F, Dupke C, et al. Retrospective analysis of 15 years of horse-related maxillofacial fracture data at a major German trauma center. Eur J Trauma Emerg Surg. 2022; 48(4):2539–2546

[16] Bixby-Hammett D, Brooks WH. Common injuries in horseback riding. A review. Sports Med. 1990; 9(1):36–47

[17] Ghosh A, Di Scala C, Drew C, Lessin M, Feins N. Horse-related injuries in pediatric patients. J Pediatr Surg. 2000; 35(12):1766–1770

[18] Burbage J, Cameron LJ. An investigation of bra concerns and barriers to participation in horse riding. Comp Exerc Physiol. 2018; 14:1–10

[19] Hasler RM, Gyssler L, Benneker L, et al. Protective and risk factors in amateur equestrians and description of injury patterns: a retrospective data analysis and a case - control survey. J Trauma Manag Outcomes. 2011; 5:4

[20] Press JM, Davis PD, Wiesner SL, Heinemann A, Semik P, Addison RG. The national jockey injury study: an analysis of injuries to professional horse-racing jockeys. Clin J Sport Med. 1995; 5(4):236–240

[21] Patricios JS, Ardern CL, Hislop MD, et al. Implementation of the 2017 Berlin Concussion in Sport Group Consensus Statement in contact and collision

sports: a joint position statement from 11 national and international sports organisations. Br J Sports Med. 2018; 52(10):635–641

[22] Arneitz C, Sinzig M, Fasching G. Diagnostic and clinical management of skull fractures in children. J Clin Imaging Sci. 2016; 6:47

[23] Silverberg ND, Iaccarino MA, Panenka WJ, et al. American Congress of Rehabilitation Medicine Brain Injury Interdisciplinary Special Interest Group Mild TBI Task Force. Management of concussion and mild traumatic brain injury: a synthesis of practice guidelines. Arch Phys Med Rehabil. 2020; 101 (2):382–393

[24] Diaconis JN, Rao KC. CT in head trauma: a review. J Comput Tomogr. 1980; 4 (4):261–270

[25] Castaño-Leon AM, Gomez PA, Jimenez-Roldan L, et al. Intracranial pressure monitoring in patients with severe traumatic brain injury: extension of the recommendations and the effect on outcome by propensity score matching. Neurosurgery. 2022; 91(3):437–449

[26] Kriss TC, Kriss VM. Equine-related neurosurgical trauma: a prospective series of 30 patients. J Trauma. 1997; 43(1):97–99

[27] Muralidharan R. External ventricular drains: management and complications. Surg Neurol Int. 2015; 6 Suppl 6:S271–S274

[28] Natarajan M, Asok Kumar N, Jawahar G. Usefulness of exploratory burr holes in the management of severe head injury. J Indian Med Assoc. 1989; 87(11): 256–258

[29] Schicho A, Einwag D, Eickhoff A, Richter PH, Riepl C. Impact of spinal fractures in horseback riding [in German]. Sportverletz Sportschaden. 2015; 29(4):231–235

[30] Gill SS, Boden BP. The epidemiology of catastrophic spine injuries in high school and college football. Sports Med Arthrosc Rev. 2008; 16(1):2–6

[31] Siebenga J, Segers MJ, Elzinga MJ, Bakker FC, Haarman HJ, Patka P. Spine fractures caused by horse riding. Eur Spine J. 2006; 15(4):465–471

[32] Kendler DL, Bauer DC, Davison KS, et al. Vertebral fractures: clinical importance and management. Am J Med. 2016; 129(2):221.e1–221.e10

[33] Chang V, Holly LT. Bracing for thoracolumbar fractures. Neurosurg Focus. 2014; 37(1):E3

[34] McCall T, Cole C, Dailey A. Vertebroplasty and kyphoplasty: a comparative review of efficacy and adverse events. Curr Rev Musculoskelet Med. 2008; 1 (1):17–23

[35] Lin CY, Wright J, Bushnik T, Shem K. Traumatic spinal cord injuries in horseback riding: a 35-year review. Am J Sports Med. 2011; 39(11):2441–2446

[36] Bennett J, Das JM, Emmady PD. Spinal cord injuries. In: StatPearls. Treasure Island, FL: StatPearls Publishing; 2022

[37] Li Y, Walker CL, Zhang YP, Shields CB, Xu XM. Surgical decompression in acute spinal cord injury: a review of clinical evidence, animal model studies, and potential future directions of investigation. Front Biol (Beijing). 2014; 9 (2):127–136

[38] Bier G, Bongers MN, Othman A, et al. Impact of helmet use in equestrian-related traumatic brain injury: a matched-pairs analysis. Br J Neurosurg. 2018; 32(1):37–43

[39] McCrory P, Turner M, LeMasson B, Bodere C, Allemandou A. An analysis of injuries resulting from professional horse racing in France during 1991–2001: a comparison with injuries resulting from professional horse racing in Great Britain during 1992–2001. Br J Sports Med. 2006; 40(7):614–618

[40] Mayberry JC, Pearson TE, Wiger KJ, Diggs BS, Mullins RJ. Equestrian injury prevention efforts need more attention to novice riders. J Trauma. 2007; 62 (3):735–739

[41] Kuhl HN, Ritchie D, Taveira-Dick AC, Hoefling KA, Russo SA. Concussion history and knowledge base in competitive equestrian athletes. Sports Health. 2014; 6(2):136–138

32 Baseball

Zoe Soulé, Denis Routkevitch, and Nicholas Theodore

Summary
This chapter discusses the most common central nervous system injuries experienced by baseball players. Back and core injuries account for 12% of all major league injuries, and baseball players experience disproportionate rates of low back pain and disc degeneration. The lumbar spine is a critical link in transferring energy from the lower to upper extremities during baseball-related movements. Factors that increase the likelihood of injury include improper timing of these motions, strength deficits in the spine and core, and restricted range of motion about the thoracolumbar spine. The repetitive lumbar extension and rotation in pitching and batting predisposes athletes to lumbar injuries such as spondylolysis, disc herniations, and annular tears. Other common injuries include muscular strains, facet joint pain, sacroiliac pain, and stenosis. Conservative treatment is usually warranted initially, but surgical treatments can improve players' return to play when warranted in cases of refractory or debilitating pain or myelopathic deficits.

Keywords: baseball, low back pain, kinematics, lumbar, injury, spine, spondylolysis, peripheral nerve injury, catastrophic injury, disc degeneration

32.1 Introduction

Baseball, commonly referred to as America's "national pastime," first reached North America in the 1830s, although historians report that the first game of baseball ever to be recorded took place in Surrey in 1749.[1] Currently, there are approximately 19 million student-athletes and adults playing in organized baseball in the United States, with an estimated 65 million people in over 140 countries worldwide.[2] Spinal injuries in baseball can lead to lost time playing and early career terminations. David Wright, seven-time all-star and beloved third baseman for the New York Mets, was diagnosed with spinal stenosis in 2015, a narrowing of the spinal canal that can cause nerve compression and pain. Despite an extensive physical therapy and workout routine, Wright was unable to return to play without pain, and after 3 years of rehab, he retired in 2018. At only 35 years of age, this was an early ending to one of the greatest careers in Mets history.

32.2 Biomechanics and Basic Technique

The type and prevalence of baseball-associated neurological injuries reflect the unique biomechanics of the sport, which involves two major categories of motion: pitching/throwing and batting. The biomechanics of each are detailed in the following.

32.2.1 Pitching

Major League Baseball (MLB) pitchers have twice the rates of injury compared with players in other positions.[3] The pitching motion is a particularly complex throwing movement that requires dynamic control and coordination of multiple muscle segments in the body. The six phases of pitching include the windup, early cocking, late cocking, acceleration, deceleration, and follow-through.[4] Spinal flexion and extension are integral to the pitching motion and feature significant degrees of trunk rotation and angular acceleration.[5] The substantial compressive and rotational forces placed on the spine render lumbar and core strength critical for preventing injury. Indeed, poor lumbopelvic control has been shown to be a predictor of injury occurrence and severity in MLB pitchers,[6] and data suggest that 15% of all pitchers will ultimately experience low back pain (LBP).[7]

The most common injuries in pitchers involve the upper extremities.[8] Injuries to the spine and core constituted around 12% of MLB injuries from 2006 to 2008.[6] The pitching motion requires strength, mobility, and proper kinematic sequencing to efficiently transfer force. Improper timing of this kinematic sequence and failure to maintain proper strength and range of motion are all factors that increase the risk of injury.[9]

32.2.2 Batting

The baseball swing also involves high-velocity sequencing of multiple muscle segments to transfer energy from the lower to upper extremities. The rotational motion of the trunk is the primary source of power generation for the swing.[5] Studies have reported that this repetitive trunk axial rotation places up to 4,800 N of force on the L4–L5 disc.[10] The repeated flexion/extension of the spine and axial rotation of the trunk involved in baseball batting likely accounts for the high levels of LBP in both professional and adolescent players.

Common injuries experienced by batters involve the spine, trunk, pelvis and surrounding core musculature. These include stress fractures, disc herniations, and paravertebral muscle strains.[11] ▶ Fig. 32.1 summarizes the common locations and modes of spinal injuries in baseball.

32.3 Catastrophic Injuries in Baseball

Catastrophic injuries are severe sports injuries that can be further categorized as fatal, nonfatal, and serious. Many of these injuries involve the brain and spinal cord and include fracture, paralysis, and neurological damage, with one study analyzing injuries between 1981 and 2002 noting that head injuries accounted for over half of the catastrophic injuries, followed by cervical fractures and ligament injuries representing nearly 20% of cases. The most common mechanism of injury resulted from a collision between two players (42%), a pitcher hit by a batted ball (34%), and a fielder (nonpitcher) hit by a batted ball. Indeed, baseball has a relatively high rate of catastrophic injuries compared with other sports, with almost two catastrophic injuries per year, despite being a noncontact sport.[12]

A preventable cause of catastrophic injury is the headfirst slide, as it can result in axial compression of the spine, with

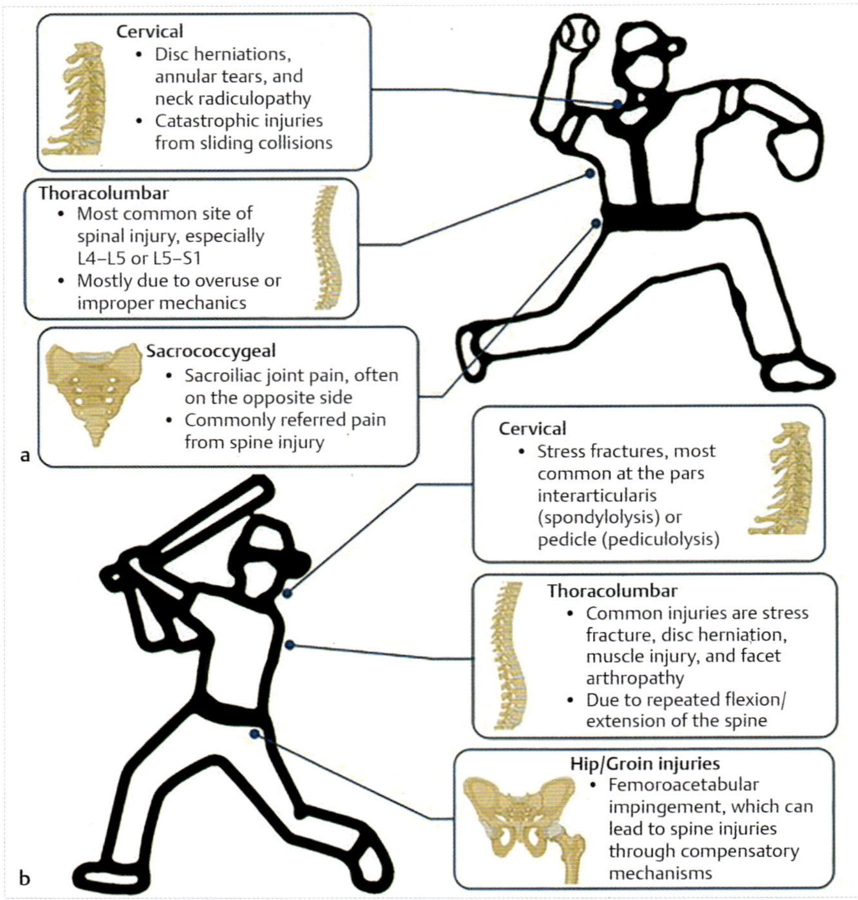

Fig. 32.1 Common injuries in baseball pitchers and batters. **(a)** The pitching motion requires extreme coordination and control through spinal flexion and extension that predisposes pitchers to spinal injuries. These injuries can lead to symptoms such as neck radiculopathy, lower back pain, and hip pain as a result of spinal pathology. **(b)** Batters also experience similarly high torsional forces and overuse injuries due to the explosive nature of the swing. Common injuries of the spine, core musculature, and hip can result in lower back pain as well as neurological symptomology. (Created with BioRender.com.)

possible fracture, subluxation, or dislocation with spinal cord injury. Headfirst sliding is not allowed in Little League Baseball, and many investigations recommend that headfirst sliding should be banned in both the high school and college levels, as it has not been shown to be faster than feet-first sliding and it presents considerable risk to the brain and spine.[13,14]

32.4 Noncatastrophic Spine Injuries

Professional baseball athletes are also predisposed to noncatastrophic spinal injuries due to the inherent repetition of high-velocity motions such as batting and pitching. Compared with other sports, athletes who played baseball were significantly more likely to experience LBP and disc degeneration.[15] Recently, epidemiologic reports of injuries in the MLB have reported that around 12% of these injuries related to the spine, predominantly the lumbar, followed by cervical spine.[3] These injuries included disc herniations, sciatica, lumbar nerve root impingement, and cervical radiculopathy.[3] Compared with cervical injuries, lumbar injuries led to more days missed on average and accounted for more season-ending injuries. Notably, this suggests that the lumbar injuries suffered by baseball players are more severe than cervical injuries.

Lumbar issues are particularly common among baseball players, likely due to the excessive lumbar rotation involved in both the bat swing and the repetitive flexion and extension of the lumbar spine in pitching. Common lumbar injuries include stress fractures, annular tears with or without disc herniation, facet or sacroiliac (SI) joint pain, and stenosis.[6] The distribution of injuries also varies by age, with the most common cause of LBP in adolescent athletes attributable to spondylolysis. Baseball has been noted to have a higher incidence of lumbar spondylolysis compared with many other sports, specifically at the L5 level.[16] Older players had higher rates of discogenic pain, lumbar disc herniation, and facet joint arthritis.[17]

One of the common etiologies experienced by baseball players is SI joint pain, particularly in their nondominant side, especially when resuming pitching after a break.[18] This stems from the abrupt reintroduction of torsional strain to the facet joint and intervertebral discs. The SI joint and posterior iliac spine pain are also the most common areas for referred pain from the lower back.[18]

32.4.1 Disc Herniation

The unique set of repetitive forces exerted on the lumbar spine from axial rotation make baseball pitchers and batters predisposed to annular tears and disc herniations.[6] The majority of disc degenerations occur at the L4–L5 and L5–S1 intervertebral levels.[19] Annular tears generally present with severe LBP accompanied by spasms and pain radiating into the lower extremities, with progressive losses in sensation and strength.[6] Pitchers are also prone to cervical disc herniations, presenting as neck radiculopathy with shooting pains in the shoulder and arm, often accompanied by numbness and weakness that can progressively worsen.[19]

Cervical disc surgery can lead to neck stiffness and altered spine mechanics that can impact performance-based outcomes.[20] Therefore, conservative treatment is recommended in most cases and includes epidural steroid injections, physical therapy, and activity modification.[20] Surgical indications include failing conservative treatment, presenting with symptoms that drastically impact play ability, or imaging that shows larger herniations, significant nerve compression, or other spinal cord pathologies.[21] Surgical treatment of a cervical disc herniation often involves a single-level anterior cervical discectomy and fusion or cervical disc replacement. Similar considerations apply to lumbar herniations, which can be treated with lumbar microdiscectomy and laminotomy/foraminotomy.

Return to Play

Overall rates of return-to-play are high for athletes with disc herniations. A study of 11 MLB pitchers with cervical disc herniations found that 73% returned to play after around 12 months. Returning pitchers overall pitched fewer innings per season; however, there was no observable change in performance as measured by earned run average, innings pitched, walks, and hits allowed per inning.[21] Conclusions are limited, however, by the small sample size and lack of further studies. A larger study of 69 MLB players treated for lumbar disc herniations found an overall return-to-play rate of 97% and that baseball players had the longest average career length after lumbar discectomy (4.8 years) compared with other sports. However, pitchers and batters treated operatively demonstrated significantly worse performance following surgery compared with those treated nonoperatively.[22] Although the authors attempted standardization of injury severity between the groups, it is possible that the players who underwent surgery initially had more severe injuries.

32.4.2 Lumbar Spondylolysis

Presentation

Untreated spondylolysis can progress to more severe conditions such as spondylolisthesis. Spondylolysis is common in sports involving repetitive lumbar extension and rotation and is present in up to one-third of athletes with LBP.[6] Specific to the batter, incorrect timing of a swing can lead to significant lumbar strain alongside high compressive forces. The majority of spondylolysis cases occur at L5, followed by L4 and then combined L4–L5 involvement.[23]

Due to the progression of spondylolysis to spondylolisthesis, early diagnosis of spondylolysis is critical. Patients usually present with LBP in the lumbar region exacerbated by extension or twisting of the spine. Neurological signs are rare, but there may also be restricted lumbar flexion and extension.[23] Key diagnostic tests of both spondylolysis and spondylolisthesis include palpation of the lumbar spinous process, lateral trunk flexion–extension, and double-leg raising.[24] These results can be confirmed with magnetic resonance imaging (MRI), computed tomography (CT), and bone scans to visualize edema surrounding the pedicle.[25]

Treatment

Initial treatment of spondylolysis involves rest and immobilization, followed by progressive physical therapy and a 4- to 6-week period of return-to-sport.[23] Choi et al reported success using a conservative spondylolysis treatment algorithm consisting of sports activity cessation, a custom thoracolumbosacral orthosis brace, and a bone stimulator for 3 months, followed by a structured physical therapy program. Of their 201 patients, of which baseball/softball players were the second most common, 197 (98%) returned to similar sporting activities and 49.8% showed bony healing on CT scans.[26] This shows the majority of athletes with pars defects are treated nonoperatively with excellent outcomes. Surgery may be required for particularly traumatic cases; however, the guidelines regarding return-to-sport after fusion of spondylolysis are highly variable, and a survey found that 27% to 36% of surgeons allowed patients to return to collision sports 1 year postoperatively.[27,28] Direct pars repair as a surgical treatment option is detailed earlier in the book.

Return to Play

A study of 272 MLB players with LBP that underwent spinal imaging diagnosed 75 (27%) with a pars defect, with more than one-third of these cases demonstrating spondylolisthesis.[29] All these athletes except for one returned to professional baseball with an average return-to-play time of 51 days, and over 89.3% of these athletes returned with the same level of performance. These results are similar to those of another study done by Iwamoto et al, in which 88% of 104 amateur athletes with symptomatic spondylolysis returned to their original level of competition following nonoperative treatment.[30]

32.5 Traumatic Brain Injuries

Baseball has a relatively low rate of injuries to the head compared with other sports.[31] However, when these injuries do occur, they can be extremely severe, ranging from a mild concussion to sudden death.[32] The two most common mechanisms for traumatic brain injury (TBI) involve being struck with either a bat or a ball and player-to-player collisions. Catchers are at a significantly increased risk of concussion and accounted for 40% of diagnosed concussions in the 2011–2012 MLB season.[33]

Despite symptom resolution, MLB players perform significantly worse after returning from a concussion.[34] Neurological deficits such as balance, concentration, and tracking ability may remain compromised even after physical symptoms seem to have returned to baseline.[34] Increased attention to athlete performance postconcussion and a delayed return-to-play protocol warrants consideration.

The MLB has taken steps to decrease the risk of concussions. In 2013, rule changes regulated home plate collisions and significantly reduced the number of concussions caused by collisions at home plate and those incurred by catchers in general.[35,36] However, studies have pointed to the existence of high rates of underreporting and pressures for athletes to play through concussive symptoms.[37,38] Therefore, preventative measures should focus on education for athletes, parents, and coaches about TBI as well as enforcement of rules and protective equipment at all levels.

32.6 Peripheral Nerve Injuries

32.6.1 Suprascapular Neuropathy

Baseball pitchers are at an increased risk of peripheral nerve injuries due to the repetitive forces experienced by the elbow and shoulders during the pitch. These accumulated microtraumas lead to injuries such as suprascapular neuropathy, quadrilateral space syndrome, and cubital tunnel syndrome. These nerve injuries are relatively rare and often diagnosed alongside other common shoulder injuries in the overhead-throwing athlete.[9]

Suprascapular neuropathy generally presents with posterior shoulder pain and weakness, often accompanied by isolated infraspinatus muscle atrophy.[9,36] The suprascapular nerve innervates the supraspinatus and infraspinatus muscles, two of the four rotator cuff muscles that are responsible for stabilizing the shoulder as it rotates and accelerates forward. The pitching motion places the shoulder in extreme abduction and external rotation, which causes the muscles to compress the motor branches of the nerve.[36] While there is no consensus on the dominant cause of suprascapular nerve injuries, patients with a suspected injury should confirm the diagnosis with MRI and electrodiagnostic studies.[36] After diagnosis, nonoperative treatment involves stopping throwing activity, increasing flexibility, and strengthening surrounding muscles once nerve impingement symptoms have subsided.[9] If operative treatment is needed, surgical decompression is done to release the spinoglenoid ligament and has good results for pain resolution and return of muscular strength.[9]

32.6.2 Ulnar Neuropathy

The repeated valgus stress placed on the nerve during the throwing motion makes pitchers prone to ulnar neuropathies, the most common of which is cubital tunnel syndrome. The pathophysiology behind this injury is the extreme valgus forces placed on the medial side of the elbow through extension.[9] In addition to the traction placed on the nerve during throwing, pitchers may also have hypertrophied flexor muscles that can compress the ulnar nerve.[39] The ulnar nerve innervates most of the intrinsic muscles of the hand, and patients will generally present with digital numbness and hand weakness with point tenderness to the medial aspect of the elbow and pain that is exacerbated by prolonged elbow flexion.[38] MRI, ultrasound, radiographic imaging, and nerve conduction studies should be done to confirm the morphological changes in the nerve.

Initial nonoperative treatment involves cessation of aggravating activities, splinting, and nonsteroidal anti-inflammatory medication. After symptoms have subsided, athletes can begin a strengthening program focused on elbow stabilization and then slowly progress back to throwing. If nonoperative treatment is not successful in alleviating symptoms, common surgical procedures include decompression or anterior transposition, both of which have been shown to be equally effective in treating cubital tunnel syndrome.[40]

Surgeries involving the ulnar collateral ligament have good outcomes for pitchers. Most pitchers are able to return to the same level of performance after ulnar decompression/transposition.[41] Similarly, a majority of pitchers who underwent ulnar collateral ligament reconstruction were able to return to competitive play, with only 32% displaying symptoms of ulnar neuritis.[42]

32.7 Prevention of Injuries

The high prevalence of spinal injury and LBP in baseball players indicates the need for training programs geared toward injury prevention. As many of the injuries occur during rotation when the back is extended, deep core strength and lumbar control are important for stabilizing the spine and preventing increased amounts of hyperextension.[22] Range of motion in the hip is also critical, as Camp et al found that hip internal rotation deficits were predictive of back and abdominal injuries.[43]

In youth baseball, overuse remains the leading cause of injury, so prevention should focus on load management as much as implementing proper stretching and strengths programs.[44] A study done by Nakase et al analyzed 97 high school pitchers and found that deficits in the range of motion of the throwing shoulder was a significant independent risk factor for lower back pain and that an improvement in this range of motion by 13.8 degrees decreased injury risk by 68%.[45] The study proposes the mechanism that decreased shoulder horizontal adduction may lead to excessive use of the trunk for force transfer and highlights the importance of shoulder range of motion in injury prevention. Interestingly, for professional players, overuse has not been proven to be a risk factor for injury.[44] Despite this fact, pitchers at all levels should perform multimodal arm care programs that are tailored to fit the current demands of their schedule to reduce the risk of throwing-related injury.[35,37]

A comprehensive understanding of the biomechanics behind baseball motions is essential to understanding injuries and developing prevention protocols. Additionally, knowledge of the game can help inform studies to design interventions and assess rule changes that can improve the safety of the sport.

32.8 Disclosures

Zoe Soulé: none.
Denis Routkevitch: none.
Nicholas Theodore: Royalties from Globus Medical. Stock Ownership in Globus Medical. Consultant for Globus Medical. On Scientific Advisory Board/Other Office for Globus Medical.

References

[1] Sulat N. Why isn't baseball more popular in the UK? BBC News. July 26, 2013. Accessed March 8, 2023 at: https://www.bbc.com/news/magazine-23425907

[2] World Baseball Softball Confederation. Report: baseball/softball top list as most participated team sport in U.S. Accessed March 8, 2023 at: http://www.wbsc.org/en/news/report-baseballsoftball-top-list-as-most-participated-team-sport-in-u-s

[3] Makhni MC, Curriero FC, Yeung CM, et al. Epidemiology of spine-related neurologic injuries in professional baseball players. Spine. 2022; 47(6): E265–E271

[4] Anderson MW, Alford BA. Overhead throwing injuries of the shoulder and elbow. Radiol Clin North Am. 2010; 48(6):1137–1154

[5] Fleisig GS, Hsu WK, Fortenbaugh D, Cordover A, Press JM. Trunk axial rotation in baseball pitching and batting. Sports Biomech. 2013; 12(4): 324–333

[6] Camp CL, Conti MS, Sgroi T, Cammisa FP, Dines JS. Epidemiology, treatment, and prevention of lumbar spine injuries in Major League Baseball players. Am J Orthop. 2016; 45(3):137–143

[7] Singh H, Lee M, Solomito MJ, Merrill C, Nissen C. Lumbar hyperextension in baseball pitching: a potential cause of spondylolysis. J Appl Biomech. 2018; 34(6):429–434

[8] Camp CL, Dines JS, van der List JP, et al. Summative report on time out of play for major and minor league baseball: an analysis of 49,955 injuries from 2011 through 2016. Am J Sports Med. 2018; 46(7):1727–1732

[9] Cummins CA, Schneider DS. Peripheral nerve injuries in baseball players. Neurol Clin. 2008; 26(1):195–215, x

[10] McGill SM, Hoodless K. Measured and modelled static and dynamic axial trunk torsion during twisting in males and females. J Biomed Eng. 1990; 12 (5):403–409

[11] Daniels SP, Greditzer HG, 4th, Mintz DN, Dines JS, Bogner EA. Swinging injuries in competitive baseball players. Skeletal Radiol. 2023; 52(7):1277–1292

[12] Bode BP, Prior C. Catastrophic spine injuries in sports. Curr Sports Med Rep. 2005; 4(1):45–49

[13] Kane SM, House HO, Overgaard KA. Head-first versus feet-first sliding: a comparison of speed from base to base. Am J Sports Med. 2002; 30(6): 834–836

[14] Boden BP, Tacchetti R, Mueller FO. Catastrophic injuries in high school and college baseball players. Am J Sports Med. 2004; 32(5):1189–1196

[15] Hangai M, Kaneoka K, Hinotsu S, et al. Lumbar intervertebral disk degeneration in athletes. Am J Sports Med. 2009; 37(1):149–155

[16] Kato K, Otoshi K, Kobayashi K, Kaneko Y, Nakazawa S, Konno SI. Clinical characteristics of early-stage lumbar spondylolysis detected by magnetic resonance imaging in male adolescent baseball players. J Orthop Sci. 2024; 29(1):35–41

[17] Morimoto M, Okada R, Sugiura K, et al. Low back pain and lumbar degeneration in japanese professional baseball players. Orthop J Sports Med. 2022; 10(10):23259671221125513

[18] Watkins RG, IV, Chang D, Watkins RG, III. Spinal injuries in the overhead athlete. Curr Rev Musculoskelet Med. 2022; 15(6):521–534

[19] Wasser JG, Zaremski JL, Herman DC, Vincent HK. Prevalence and proposed mechanisms of chronic low back pain in baseball: part i. Res Sports Med. 2017; 25(2):219–230

[20] Hsu WK. Outcomes following nonoperative and operative treatment for cervical disc herniations in National Football League athletes. Spine. 2011; 36(10):800–805

[21] Roberts DW, Roc GJ, Hsu WK. Outcomes of cervical and lumbar disk herniations in Major League Baseball pitchers. Orthopedics. 2011; 34(8): 602–609

[22] Earhart JS, Roberts D, Roc G, Gryzlo S, Hsu W. Effects of lumbar disk herniation on the careers of professional baseball players. Orthopedics. 2012; 35(1):43–49

[23] Tawfik S, Phan K, Mobbs RJ, Rao PJ. The incidence of pars interarticularis defects in athletes. Global Spine J. 2020; 10(1):89–101

[24] Wasser JG, Zaremski JL, Herman DC, Vincent HK. Assessment and rehabilitation of chronic low back pain in baseball: part II. Res Sports Med. 2017; 25(2):231–243

[25] Tatsumura M, Gamada H, Ishimoto R, et al. Prevalence of curable and pseudoarthrosis stages of adolescent lumbar spondylolysis. J Rural Med. 2018; 13(2):105–109

[26] Choi JH, Ochoa JK, Lubinus A, Timon S, Lee YP, Bhatia NN. Management of lumbar spondylolysis in the adolescent athlete: a review of over 200 cases. Spine J. 2022; 22(10):1628–1633

[27] Huang P, Anissipour A, McGee W, Lemak L. Return-to-play recommendations after cervical, thoracic, and lumbar spine injuries: a comprehensive review. Sports Health. 2016; 8(1):19–25

[28] Rubery PT, Bradford DS. Athletic activity after spine surgery in children and adolescents: results of a survey. Spine. 2002; 27(4):423–427

[29] Gould HP, Winkelman RD, Tanenbaum JE, et al. Epidemiology, treatment, and performance-based outcomes in american professional baseball players with symptomatic spondylolysis and isthmic spondylolisthesis. Am J Sports Med. 2020; 48(11):2765–2773

[30] Iwamoto J, Takeda T, Wakano K. Returning athletes with severe low back pain and spondylolysis to original sporting activities with conservative treatment. Scand J Med Sci Sports. 2004; 14(6):346–351

[31] Kerr ZY, Roos KG, Djoko A, et al. Epidemiologic measures for quantifying the incidence of concussion in national collegiate athletic association sports. J Athl Train. 2017; 52(3):167–174

[32] Lyman S, Fleisig GS. Baseball injuries. Med Sport Sci. 2005; 49:9–30

[33] Green GA, Pollack KM, D'Angelo J, et al. Mild traumatic brain injury in Major and Minor League Baseball players. Am J Sports Med. 2015; 43(5):1118–1126

[34] Wasserman EB, Abar B, Shah MN, Wasserman D, Bazarian JJ. Concussions are associated with decreased batting performance among Major League Baseball players. Am J Sports Med. 2015; 43(5):1127–1133

[35] Green G, D'Angelo J, Coyles J, Penny I, Golfinos JG, Valadka A. Association between a rule change to reduce home plate collisions and mild traumatic brain injury and other injuries in professional baseball players. Am J Sports Med. 2019; 47(11):2704–2708

[36] Madani A, Creteur V. Nerves around the shoulder: what the radiologist should know? J Belg Soc Radiol.; 101 Suppl 2:9

[37] Yard E, Comstock D. Compliance with return to play guidelines following concussion in US high school athletes, 2005–2008. Brain Inj. 2019; 23(11): 888–898

[38] Assmus H, Antoniadis G, Bischoff C, et al. Cubital tunnel syndrome - a review and management guidelines. Cent Eur Neurosurg. 2011; 72(2):90–98

[39] Norkus SA, Meyers MC. Ulnar neuropathy of the elbow. Sports Med. 1994; 17(3):189–199

[40] Caliandro P, La Torre G, Padua R, Giannini F, Padua L. Treatment for ulnar neuropathy at the elbow. Cochrane Database Syst Rev. 2016; 11(11): CD006839

[41] Erickson BJ, Chalmers PN, D'Angelo J, Ma K, Romeo AA. Performance and return to sport after ulnar nerve decompression/transposition among professional baseball players. Am J Sports Med. 2019; 47(5):1124–1129

[42] Rao S, D'Amore T, Willier DP, III, et al. Return-to-play rates and clinical outcomes of baseball players after concomitant ulnar collateral ligament reconstruction and selective ulnar nerve transposition. Orthop J Sports Med. 2021; 9(11):23259671211055428

[43] Camp CL, Spiker AM, Zajac JM, et al. Decreased hip internal rotation increases the risk of back and abdominal muscle injuries in professional baseball players: analysis of 258 player-seasons. J Am Acad Orthop Surg. 2018; 26(9):e198–e206

[44] Melugin HP, Leafblad ND, Camp CL, Conte S. Injury prevention in baseball: from youth to the pros. Curr Rev Musculoskelet Med. 2018; 11(1):26–34

[45] Nakase K, Shitara H, Tajika T, et al. An analysis of pre-season risk factors for low back injury in high-school baseball pitchers: a prospective study. Sci Rep. 2021; 11(1):11415

33 Skiing

Nicholas Kats, Denis Routkevitch, and Nicholas Theodore

Summary

The rising popularity of skiing as both a professional and recreational sport has brought about concerns regarding proper instruction of beginner athletes, management of ski resorts, and treatment of skiers involved in accidents. In particular, the association of skiing-related falls with spinal injuries has resulted in a need to further study skiing biomechanics and develop more robust safety guidelines. The thoracolumbar region is the most common site of spinal injury in skiers, with burst and compression fractures accounting for most high-risk accidents. The cervical spine, though injured less frequently, carries the highest risk for neurologic damage via injury to the spinal cord. Skiers may return to the sport only when radiographic and neurological examinations are normal and after completing appropriate physical therapy. Safety mechanisms and procedures designed to reduce the frequency and severity of accidents at ski resorts should be consistently re-evaluated to ensure they are up to date.

Keywords: falling, fracture, sport safety, skiing, ski resort management, spinal cord, spine, subluxation

33.1 Introduction

Skiing is one of the most popular winter sports worldwide, with a rich recreational and professional history dating back over a century.[1] For the 2021–2022 season alone, the National Ski Areas Association reported 61 million visits to ski resorts, the highest number ever recorded since tracking began in 1978.[2] Therefore, even as the safety precautions taken by ski resorts have expanded, the popularity of the sport results in a high risk for accidents and injuries due to overcrowding, decreased risk awareness, and attempts at technically challenging maneuvers at high speeds.[3] The most common accidents experienced among skiers admitted into hospital emergency rooms are those involving traumatic brain injury (TBI), followed by injuries affecting the spine.[4] Notably, spinal trauma is often accompanied with injuries to other regions of the body. While the overall rate of injury among skiers and snowboarders has steadily declined in recent years, the rate of spinal injury has actually plateaued or increased according to most accounts.[5,6]

This chapter will focus on spinal injuries in skiers. We will discuss current literature on the epidemiology and describe biomechanics, diagnostic techniques, medical interventions, preventative techniques, and policies available to medical providers and ski resorts. Since skiing and snowboarding are similar sports from an accident-awareness perspective, some comparisons between the two will be made. Additionally, we will note subtle differences among various disciplines of skiing, including freestyle and alpine, to provide a more nuanced analysis of available epidemiological and biomechanical data.

33.2 Spinal Injuries in Skiing

33.2.1 Epidemiology, Nature of Injury, and Biomechanics

Dynamic maneuvers and risk of collisions put skiers at enhanced risk for spinal injuries. A 9-year retrospective study at one California resort found that between 1983 and 1992, the incidence rate of cervical spine injuries increased from 0.02 to 0.04 injuries per 1,000 skier days.[5] Skier days serve as the literature and industry standard for measuring resort attendance; one skier day represents one ticket sold at a ski resort. Injury incidence rates for the back in general increased from 0.05 to 0.09 injuries per 1,000 skier days over the same time period. Though studies on the epidemiology of skiing injuries tend to focus on a small area, often a particular ski resort or hospital, there is significant concurrence across retrospective studies of injury incidence, type, and outcome. An analysis of patients admitted to a tertiary trauma center in Bern, Switzerland, for snow sports–related injuries found that among the 728 patients studied, 140 (20%) exhibited a spinal injury.[7] Severe spinal injuries were found in 73 patients (10%), including spinal fractures, subluxations, dislocations, and concomitant injuries to the spinal cord.

The literature is divided on whether skiers and snowboarders suffer asymmetric rates of spinal injuries. One study of patients admitted to an emergency room in Banff, Canada, between 1988 and 1990 found that 12% of snowboarders presented with spinal injuries compared with 4% of skiers.[8] In contrast, a study of patients in Denver, Colorado, from 1987 to 1994 found that skeletal injuries to the spine were more common among skiers (24% of patients studied) than snowboarders (5% of patients studied).[9] Given the variability in the epidemiology of spinal injuries among athletes of common winter sports, the high incidence of spinal injuries should take precedence over minute differences between snow sports.[10]

Another important consideration for skiing- and snowboarding-related injuries is patient skill level. One study compared injury incidence among beginner snowboarders and skiers. Investigators showed that nearly 80% of injuries are sustained by participants classified as beginner snowboarders, often without instruction from professional trainers. Similar data on training in skiers were not provided, so it may be beneficial to conduct more studies on the relationships between the type of instruction beginner skiers receive—whether from peers, professional instructors, or none at all—and the incidence of injury. Such data could be helpful in informing safety policies at ski resorts or perhaps ensuring that beginner skiers receive adequate training on how to correctly fall, avoid obstacles, etc., prior to hitting the slopes.

Nature of Common Spinal Injuries

Most severe spinal injuries suffered by skiers are fractures, including burst and compression fractures, which can be particularly debilitating.[11] The next most common spinal injuries studied in a report by Tarazi et al were compression fractures, in which small cracks form along the vertebrae causing weakening of the vertebral body.[12] The commonality of burst fractures among skiers is concerning, particularly because such injuries tend to be more severe than compression or subluxation injuries. The severity of burst fractures stems from the danger of these injuries sending bone fragments in all directions from the impact site, potentially causing lacerations and other damage to the spinal cord.[11] Spatially, the thoracolumbar spine is typically the most common site of injury, with T12 and L1 accounting for an estimated 50% of all skier fractures.

These sports are also associated with a high rate of spinal cord injuries. One study found that 24% of skiing and 9% of snowboarding-related spinal fractures were accompanied by neurologic damage, mostly correlated with cervical injuries.[13] Injuries to the thoracic and lumbar spine were less likely to lead to neurologic deficits. However, a review of over 13,000 cases at Sumi Memorial Hospital found no significant differences between the location of spinal injuries in skiers and snowboarders, although the type of injuries sustained between both sports differed.[13] Across both sports, anterior compression fractures were more common than transverse process fractures, but snowboarding-related transverse process fractures were significantly more common than similar injuries in ski accidents.

A summary of the common injury locations and their general causes is provided in ▶ Fig. 33.1.

Biomechanics of Common Spinal Injuries

Some differences in injury type can be ascribed to biomechanical considerations regarding the athlete's position on skis versus on a snowboard. The riding position of snowboarders puts their center of mass farther back than skiers, resulting in a greater risk of falling backward and consequentially incurring axial-loading injuries.[14] These types of injuries are less common among skiers as they tend to fall forward, instead leading to cervical spine hyperextension and an increased incidence of cervical spine injuries in skiers compared with snowboarders.[3,14]

Another difference involves the circumstances of injury. Skiers tend to suffer more collisions than snowboarders, whether with other skiers or with obstacles such as trees.[10] In the former case, skier-versus-skier injuries resulted in 50% of all cervical injuries reported by Levy and Smith.[10] Since such injuries are more commonly associated with neurologic damage, it is relatively unsurprising that the highest incidence of postinjury neurologic deficits came from injuries resulting from two skiers colliding with one another. Interestingly, when the authors looked at similar injuries among snowboarders, none of the patients analyzed suffered neurologic deficits after being treated and released. The review ascribed the younger age of snowboarders in general, and the lack of degenerative diseases present among them, to account for their superior postinjury neurologic outcomes. Additionally, it should be noted that snowboarder-versus-snowboarder collisions were rare in this study, accounting for only five patients examined.

Conversely, in the sport of snowboarding, jumps seem to account for injuries to a greater extent than in skiing. Spinal injuries of all varieties arising from falls after jumps were sustained in 16% of snowboarders versus only 9% of skiers in one review of data from St. Anthony Central Hospital in Denver, Colorado.[10] In a study by Yamakawa et al, around 90% of all patients sustaining spinal injuries were snowboarders.[13] Among all falls from failed jump attempts, thoracic and lumbar fractures were most common for both skiers and snowboarders—although the distribution of thoracic to lumbar injury was more uniform for snowboarders (50%-50%) compared with skiers (56%-31%).[10]

It should be noted, however, that the above-mentioned differences highlighted are focused on alpine skiing. Freestyle skiing, in which athletes undertake jumps and maneuvers more similar to those found in snowboarding, is growing in popularity, but the distinction has not been made in the literature. As a result, more discipline-specific studies will be warranted to determine the types of injuries these athletes experience.

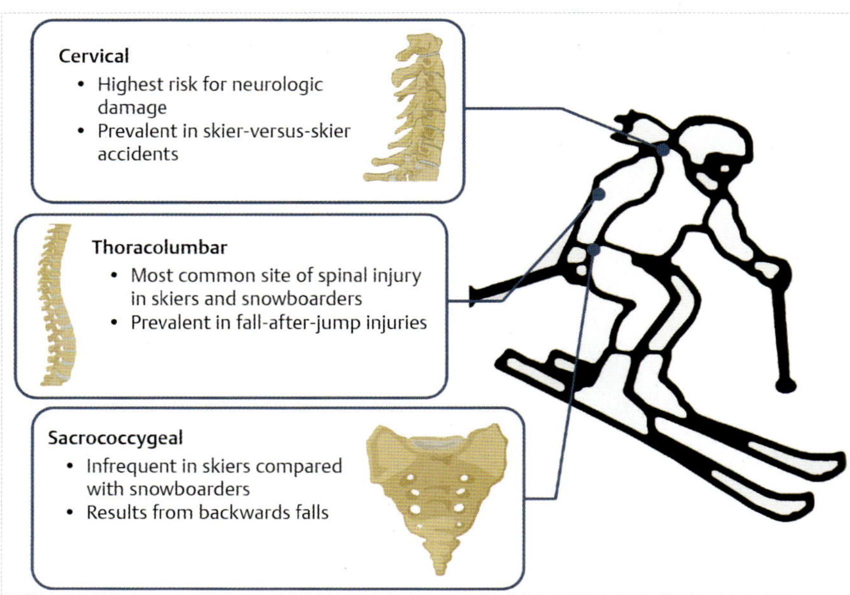

Fig. 33.1 Most common types of spinal injuries among skiers organized by anatomical location, associated concerns, and brief mechanisms of injury. (Created with BioRender.com.)

Additional rare injuries can arise from falls from chairlifts or be caused by natural catastrophes such as avalanches. Tarazi et al noted approximately 15% of spinal fractures in skiers originating from chairlift falls.[12] Other studies have reported similar numbers, although a pediatric trauma center in Utah found that falls from chairlifts tended to result in more injuries to lower extremities and may cause femur fractures.[15] Generally, musculoskeletal injuries are of greatest concern in these accidents. Further studies into chairlift safety and design, as well as improved educational initiatives, are warranted in order to limit incidence rates.

With cross-country and backcountry skiing rising in popularity, avalanche risk is also an important consideration and cause of injury. In this injury mechanism, however, spinal trauma is often not the primary concern. Rather, asphyxiation resulting from partial or complete burial under snow is the most frequent pathology and cause of death in avalanche-related accidents.[16] A study of avalanche victims from one Austrian hospital found that fractures to extremities were among the most common presentations and were found in 19% of victims, of whom 74% were skiers. Following these injuries, chest trauma was the second most common presentation of avalanche victims, though the study notes that some of the chest injuries occurred as the result of attempted resuscitation in patients exhibiting cardiac arrest at the time of discovery.

33.2.2 Diagnosis

All diagnostic evaluations of suspected acute injuries in skiers should begin with a recount of accident history by the patient or, if the patient is unresponsive or unable to give a recount, by a reliable bystander who witnessed the accident.[6,17,18] At the accident site, extra care must be taken to protect the spine if the extent of injury cannot be immediately deduced.[17,18]

Given the frequency of multiple injuries originating from skiing and snowboarding trauma, a thorough physical and neurologic examination is necessary once the patient has been transported to and stabilized in the emergency room. Initial diagnostic imaging should consist of radiographic evaluations such as X-rays, which are necessary to determine the areas of the spine affected by the potential injury.[6] Images offering multiple anatomical views, in particular visualizations of bony structures along the anterior–posterior, lateral, and oblique directions, are useful for accurately identifying the presence and extent of the vertebral fractures discussed earlier. In addition to radiography, computed tomography (CT) scans can aid in identifying the spatial anatomy of spinal fractures and therefore assist in the diagnosis and management decision-making process. Furthermore, magnetic resonance imaging (MRI) is useful for evaluating the extent of damage to soft tissue. In particular, the spinal cord, nerve roots, and intervertebral discs can be visualized to a high level of precision using MRI scans, making the imaging technique imperative in patients with suspected neurologic trauma.

33.2.3 Treatment, Management, and Rehabilitation

Perhaps, the most important step during injury management for patients with actual or suspected spinal trauma is immediate transport to a high-level trauma center where treatment protocols can be initiated. Emergency facilities located at ski resorts are largely unequipped to deal with spinal injuries, especially spinal cord trauma, which can require prompt decompressive laminectomy, followed by maintenance of mean arterial pressure and strict monitoring of neurological function in the intensive care unit.[6,19,20,21] As the patient recovers, physical therapy and rehabilitation can be initiated. Other experimental treatments are currently being explored for spinal cord injury, but none have proven particularly effective in improving outcomes.

33.2.4 Prevention

Policies for the prevention of skiing-related injuries should be implemented using a two-pronged approach that emphasizes (1) reducing the frequency of accidents and (2) lessening the severity of accidents should they occur. Ski resorts should prioritize strategies and initiatives that educate attendees, particularly novice skiers and snowboarders, on risk-taking behaviors and how to reduce them. However, as with all such initiatives, effective implementation is difficult at large scale. Potentially fruitful strategies would focus specifically on educating skiers of spinal injury risks associated with the sport and factors that serve to heighten these risks, such as fatigue, alcohol and drug consumption, and attempting to ski routes or in conditions beyond a skier's current abilities, especially without proper professional instruction.

Moreover, the proper fitting of ski equipment is also paramount to reducing injury. If skiers are renting equipment, resort staff should take extra care when measuring attendees, and ski resorts should invest in high-quality equipment that fits a wide range of potential participants. Certain less commonly used tools, such as spine protectors, could be considered by attendees who elect to rent equipment.[6] Wearing helmets should always be required, especially among children and adolescents, which can significantly reduce the risks of TBI.[21]

The preparation and maintenance of ski slopes is also critical to reducing both the frequency and severity of spinal injuries and should therefore be a priority for all ski resorts. Proper grooming of slopes includes ensuring that frequent maintenance by professional employees is performed to identify and remove foreign obstacles that are not intended to be on routes. Padding obstacles on more advanced routes and ensuring that they are properly visible are also effective strategies to increasing attendees' awareness of potential dangers. Additionally, ensuring that runs are monitored for overcrowding and limiting the number of skiers and snowboarders that can be on a run simultaneously is necessary for augmenting safety, particularly among inexperienced participants.[6] Finally, the design and installation of terrain parks dedicated to practicing jumping techniques in a safe and controlled manner could be beneficial in decreasing spinal injury incidence among skiers and snowboarders. Having professional coaching staff at these terrain parks further enhances participant safety and aids in promoting correct techniques and risk-informed behaviors.

Other equipment used by ski resort attendees such as chairlifts should also be frequently maintained, professionally staffed, and modernized. Studies into chairlift technologies that best optimize ease of use and safety are important to the goal of advancing their safety. Lap bars, for example, are installed on most modern chairlifts but had a compliance rate of only 41% at one New England ski resort.[22] Therefore, mandating the use of existing safety technology is a reasonably simple and effective way to reduce chairlift-related accidents and should be taken into consideration by all ski resorts.

References

[1] Sood S. Where did skiing come from? BBC. Accessed March 10, 2024 at: https://www.bbc.com/travel/article/20101221-travelwise-where-did-skiing-come-from

[2] Isaac A. The State of the Ski Industry: NSAA Reports Record Visitation in the 2021–22 Season. National Ski Areas Association

[3] Bigdon SF, Gewiess J, Hoppe S, et al. Spinal injury in alpine winter sports: a review. Scand J Trauma Resusc Emerg Med. 2019; 27(1):69

[4] Corra S, Girardi P, de Giorgi F, Braggion M. Severe and polytraumatic injuries among recreational skiers and snowboarders: incidence, demographics and injury patterns in South Tyrol. Eur J Emerg Med. 2012; 19(2):69–72

[5] Davidson TM, Laliotis AT. Alpine skiing injuries. A nine-year study. West J Med. 1996; 164(4):310–314

[6] Kary JM. Acute spine injuries in skiers and snowboarders. Curr Sports Med Rep. 2008; 7(1):35–38

[7] Franz T, Hasler RM, Benneker L, Zimmermann H, Siebenrock KA, Exadaktylos AK. Severe spinal injuries in alpine skiing and snowboarding: a 6-year review of a tertiary trauma centre for the Bernese Alps ski resorts, Switzerland. Br J Sports Med. 2008; 42(1):55–58

[8] Abu-Laban RB. Snowboarding injuries: an analysis and comparison with alpine skiing injuries. CMAJ. 1991; 145(9):1097–1103

[9] Prall JA, Winston KR, Brennan R. Severe snowboarding injuries. Injury. 1995; 26(8):539–542

[10] Levy AS, Smith RH. Neurologic injuries in skiers and snowboarders. Semin Neurol. 2000; 20(2):233–245

[11] Ceders-Sinai. Burst fracture. Accessed March 9, 2023 at: https://www.cedars-sinai.org/health-library/diseases-and-conditions/b/burst-fracture.html#:~:text=If%20a%20vertebra%20is%20crushed,may%20damage%20the%20spinal%20cord

[12] Tarazi F, Dvorak MFS, Wing PC. Spinal Injuries in Skiers and Snowboarders. Am J Sports Med. 1999; 27(2):177–180

[13] Yamakawa H, Murase S, Sakai H, et al. Spinal injuries in snowboarders: risk of jumping as an integral part of snowboarding. J Trauma. 2001; 50(6):1101–1105

[14] Nakaguchi H, Fujimaki T, Ueki K, Takahashi M, Yoshida H, Kirino T. Snowboard head injury: prospective study in Chino, Nagano, for two seasons from 1995 to 1997. J Trauma. 1999; 46(6):1066–1069

[15] Glissmeyer EW, Metzger RR, Bolte R. Chair lift falls and injuries in children. Pediatr Emerg Care. 2018; 34(2):106–108

[16] Hohlrieder M, Brugger H, Schubert HM, Pavlic M, Ellerton J, Mair P. Pattern and severity of injury in avalanche victims. High Alt Med Biol. 2007; 8(1):56–61

[17] Banerjee R, Palumbo MA, Fadale PD. Catastrophic cervical spine injuries in the collision sport athlete, part 1: epidemiology, functional anatomy, and diagnosis. Am J Sports Med. 2004; 32(4):1077–1087

[18] Banerjee R, Palumbo MA, Fadale PD. Catastrophic cervical spine injuries in the collision sport athlete, part 2: principles of emergency care. Am J Sports Med. 2004; 32(7):1760–1764

[19] Torlincasi A, Waseem M. Cervical injury. In: StatPearls. StatPearls Publishing; 2022

[20] Walters BC, Hadley MN, Hurlbert RJ, et al. American Association of Neurological Surgeons, Congress of Neurological Surgeons. Guidelines for the management of acute cervical spine and spinal cord injuries: 2013 update. Neurosurgery. 2013; 60 CN_suppl_1:82–91

[21] McCarthy J, Davis A. Diagnosis and management of vertebral compression fractures. Am Fam Physician. 2016; 94(1):44–50

[22] Park JI, King DR, Jonas RK, Phillips KB. An observational study of skier and snowboarder chairlift lap bar, helmet, and snow goggle usage. Proc Hum Factors Ergon Soc Annu Meet. 2022; 66(1):1330–1334

34 Combat Sports

Noah Lu, Max J. Kerensky, Andrew M. Hersh, Denis Routkevitch, Annie Pan, and Nicholas Theodore

Summary
Combat sports embody the essence of direct one-on-one athletic competition, where athletes adeptly capitalize on the vulnerabilities of the human body to propel themselves to victory. Ranging from unarmed techniques, including grappling, striking, and hybrid styles, to armed disciplines, such as fencing, combat sports capture the primal essence of athletic endeavor. This chapter focuses on the intended and unintended impacts of unarmed combat sports on the brain, spine, and nerves. It also delves into the examination of injuries incurred, along with the accompanying strategies for their prevention, mitigation, and treatment.

Keywords: combat, fighting, knock out, spinal cord injury, concussion, biomechanics, trauma, brain, chokes, spinal cord, boxing, wrestling, martial arts

34.1 Introduction

Combat sports encompass a broad category of modified and regulated one-on-one fighting. Widely recognized as one of the most expansive and ancient classes of sports, one-on-one combat comprises of diverse disciplines like boxing, wrestling, mixed martial arts, Taekwondo, Brazilian Jiu-Jitsu, and Judo among many others. These physical contact sports directly put one's skills and physical limitations to the test, although many combat sports, especially in the grappling domain such as wrestling, do not require the infliction of bodily damage to secure victory. Although combat sports like boxing are renowned for their highly regarded victories attained through severe physical damage, such as knockouts, it is important to note that accidental or incidental injuries can occur in any sport. In this discussion, we will examine injuries pertaining to the brain, spinal cord, and nerves, both through direct and indirect means (► Fig. 34.1). Additionally, we will shed light on typical injury examples, preventative measures, and emerging health trends within combat sports (► Fig. 34.2).

34.2 The Brain in Combat Sports

34.2.1 Common Brain Injury Forms in Combat Sports

Combat sports often lead to traumatic brain injury (TBI), which can result in significant health consequences including cognitive impairment. Individuals who are involved in combat sports are more susceptible to acute and chronic forms of TBI. Typically, acute TBI occurs as a result of direct head trauma. For example, a cerebral concussion, which is an acute TBI, constitutes the most commonly observed transient ailment in boxing.[1,2] The incidence of acute TBI rates in some professional boxing settings can even surpass 40%.[1] Conversely, chronic TBI can develop due to repetitive concussive and subconcussive head impacts, typically occurring later in a boxer's career after prolonged exposure to the sport. Symptoms of chronic TBI can include dysarthria, tremor, and cognitive deficits in executive function. The severe stage of chronic TBI, dementia pugilistica, manifests with cognitive dysfunction, including amnesia, executive frontal lobe dysfunction, and psychomotor retardation. However, unlike acute TBI, the prevalence of chronic TBI in modern-era boxing has not been as thoroughly investigated.[1]

34.2.2 Prevalent Brain Injuries and Return to Play Rules in Boxing

The distinctive biomechanical aspects inherent to boxing play a significant role in the specific characteristics and prevalence rates of neurological injuries associated with the sport. There are four primary punch categories in boxing: the jab, cross, hook, and uppercut, each distinguished by the method of force generation and the involvement of specific muscle groups. The objective in boxing is to deliver accurate punches on the opponent while employing defensive strategies to avoid counterattacks.[3] Considering that the majority of boxing injuries concentrate in the head and neck region, it comes as no surprise that boxers experience higher rates of neurological

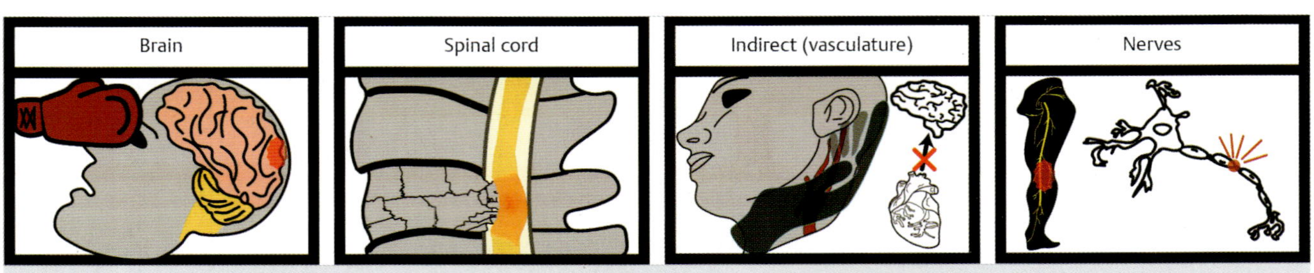

Fig. 34.1 Neural damage in combat sports. From punches and kicks to chokes and slams, the human body is pushed to the limits in combat sports. As a result, the brain, spinal cord, and nerves are at risk from both direct and indirect trauma.

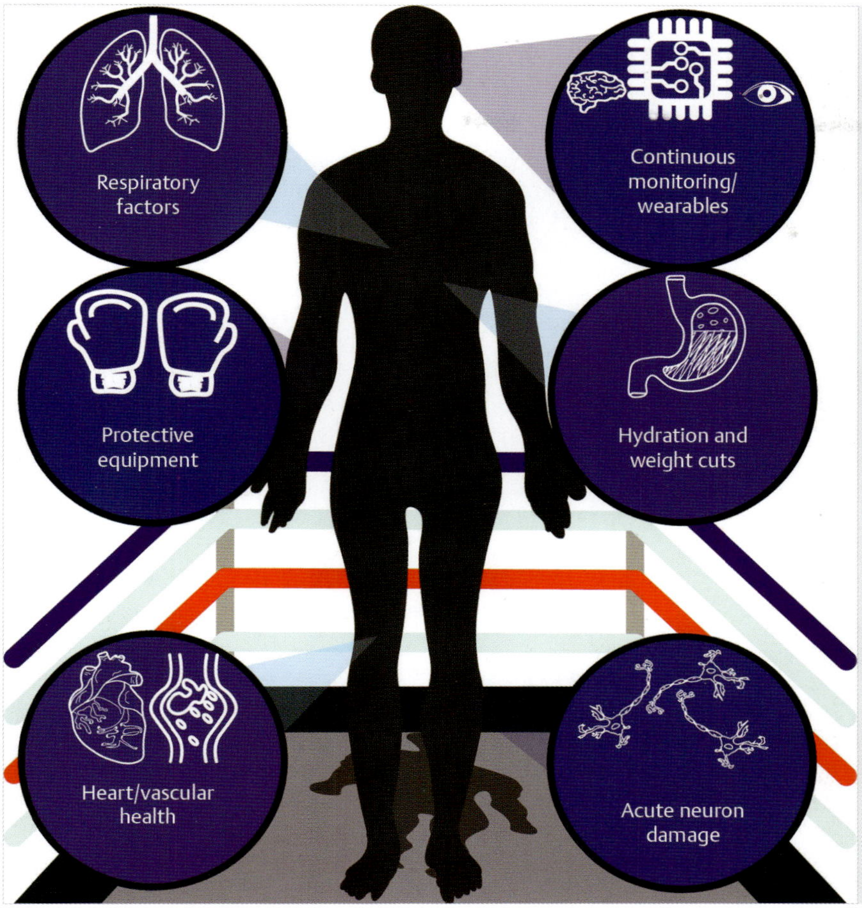

Fig. 34.2 Dynamic aspects of combat sports and human health. The damage that one may incur in combat sports is largely influenced by pre-competition factors. The rules, regulations, and monitoring protocols governing a particular sport play a crucial role in shaping its practices. Several influential parameters come into play, including acute weight cutting, equipment choices, and the combat environment, which can greatly impact the outcomes and potential for injuries.

injuries compared to their nonboxing counterparts. Similarly, in other combat sports, the head and neck region is either the most common injury site or the second most common injury site, following injuries to the lower extremities.[4] However, for boxing, it is important to note that the process of causing injury to the brain and its protective layers is complex due to the combined effects of a gloved fist's direct impact on the skull and the relative movement of the brain and skull in response to this impact.[2]

In boxing, concussion-related rest and inactivity recommendations vary by jurisdiction and competition level. However, the return to competition should align with the 2016 Berlin Consensus Statement on Concussion in Sport guidelines.[1,5] Following knockout or technical knockout, suspensions from contact/competition are mandated for varying durations (30–90 days or longer), with specific durations differing from state to state in the United States.[5] For acute brain injuries, it typically takes less than 35 days for uncomplicated concussions to recover. However, for individuals experiencing persistent headaches and other postconcussion symptoms, recovery often extends beyond 35 days.[2]

34.2.3 Prevalent Brain Injuries and Return to Play Rules in Judo

In Judo, choke techniques are employed to induce a player's submission before the player reaches a state of unconsciousness from a stranglehold. However, sometimes the player may experience a few involuntary jerking movements due to oxygen deprivation. If this occurs in adult judokas, the player is disqualified from further competition for the rest of the day due to safety concerns.[6] There is a possibility for the player to be assessed by a doctor who possesses expertise in choking techniques, and upon evaluation, the doctor may grant the player clearance to continue competing.[6] However, it is crucial for athletes who encounter oxygen deprivation during competition to take extra precautions. Cerebral hypoxia can result in various effects such as dizziness, disorientation, confusion, and loss of consciousness.[7] Additionally, prolonged or severe choking can result in more severe consequences, such as brain damage or sometimes even death.

34.3 The Spine in Combat Sports

34.3.1 Common Spine Injuries in Combat Sports

Spine injuries encompass various common forms, including cervical spine injury, lower back spine injury, and spinal cord injury (SCI). These injuries typically involve a combination of traction and compression forces, resulting in direct neural damage through fractured bone fragments, disk material, and ligaments as well as affecting both the central and peripheral nervous systems. This trauma leads to damaged blood vessels, disrupted axons, and broken neural-cell membranes. The reduction in blood flow disrupts and halts the transmission of nerve signals along axons, contributing to spinal shock.[8]

34.3.2 Prevalent Spine Injuries and Return to Play Rules in Wrestling

Cervical injuries incurred during wrestling are typically considered mild to moderate, with rupture being a rare occurrence. These injuries can arise from excessive mechanical stress. Lower back injuries commonly occur during takedowns, where wrestlers exert pressure on each other with a slightly extended lumbar spine. This combination of extension and twisting can lead to injury. Strains or sprains in the lower back can also happen when the spine is extended against resistance.[6] If the wrestler fully recovers and shows no symptoms within 1 to 2 minutes, the wrestler is allowed to resume the activity immediately. However, if there are any neurological abnormalities present after that time, the wrestler is not allowed to participate in the remainder of the competition.[9]

34.3.3 Prevalent Spine Injuries in Boxing

Although cervical spine injuries are less prevalent compared to TBIs in boxing, their consequences can be severe. Consequently, it is important to implement pre- and postparticipation screening of the cervical spine for all boxers.[10] For example, a report highlighted the case of a young male boxer with os odontoideum who experienced a transient SCI, raising concern that his condition may have increased his susceptibility to injury.

34.4 The Nerves in Combat Sports

34.4.1 Common Nerve Injuries in Combat Sports

In combat sports, peripheral nerve injuries are a recurrent phenomenon, typically arising from causes such as penetrating injury, crush, stretch, and ischemia.[11,12,13] After a peripheral nerve injury, the body initiates a series of actions to remove the damaged nerve fibers in a process known as Wallerian degeneration.[14] Once the damaged nerve fibers are removed, the healing process begins, with new nerve fibers growing to replace the old ones and reconnecting with their muscle and sensory receptors. The reaction to a peripheral nerve injury is not confined to the damage site but also engages cellular bodies located in the spinal cord and ganglia.[14]

34.4.2 Prevalent Nerve Injuries in Boxing

Although TBI and SCI are well-known risks in boxing, there are instances in boxing where peripheral nerve injuries can also occur. Although less frequent, spinal cord and peripheral nerve injuries can result in extended hospital stays, increased morbidity, and even mortality.[15]

Additionally, indirect optic neuropathy, or damage of the optic nerve, is often seen in high-impact sports such as boxing. The primary cause of indirect optic neuropathy is usually a blow to the brow or superior orbital rim that transmits force to the optic nerve canal, resulting in damage to the optic nerve. In cases of acute traumatic optic neuropathy, a distinct set of symptoms typically emerges, including vision loss, an afferent pupillary defect, and swelling of the optic nerve. A study conducted on boxers revealed that many of them exhibited optic nerve edema, which is believed to be closely associated with indirect traumatic optic neuropathy.[16]

34.4.3 Prevalent Nerve Injuries in Wrestling

Wrestling features a relatively high incidence of brachial plexus injuries compared to other activities. These injuries occur when holds are applied that force the opposing wrestler's head into extreme lateral flexion, as seen in full- or half-Nelson holds.[17] Another study indicates instances of catastrophic injuries most commonly associated with the defensive position during takedown maneuvers. These injuries led to outcomes such as quadriplegia, residual neurological deficits, paraplegia, and, in the most severe cases, even death.[18]

34.4.4 Nerve Injury Imaging and Clinical Care

The current surgical method for treating peripheral nerve injury involves timely repair of the damaged nerve through neurorrhaphy utilizing nylon sutures. In situations where the tension on the connection would be too great, nerve-cable autografts are employed to bridge the gap through grafting.[12] Alternatively, nonsurgical treatment options encompass a range of techniques, including electrical stimulation, magnetic stimulation, laser phototherapy, and the administration of nerve growth factors.[19] Ongoing research is focused on investigating pharmacologic agents, immune system modulators, and entubulation chambers to further enhance treatment outcomes.[12]

34.5 Preventative Measures and the Future Directions of Combat Sports

In light of the potential health consequences associated with combat sports, placing emphasis on preventive measures becomes imperative to safeguard athletes. For instance, boxing employs a range of preventive measures aimed at mitigating the risk of injuries and enhancing athlete safety. These measures include equipment regulations such as standardizing headgear, mouth guards, and glove weights, as well as the use of foot padding. Initially, headguards were mandated to reduce the risk of concussions, but in 2013, they were subsequently prohibited in amateur boxing. This controversial decision was made based on studies suggesting that headgear may increase the total number of hits to the head and removing it could potentially reduce the risk of concussions.[20] Conversely, the American Medical Association provides safety recommendations, such as the use of headgear, mouthguards, and increased glove size.[21]

Some advocate the use of appropriate ocular protective wear among individuals at high risk of injury, such as boxers, to prevent optic neuropathy.[22] Another precaution centers around the use of administrative controls, such as implementing new rules and scoring changes aimed at reducing head blows.[4]

Other preventive measures aimed at reducing injuries from combat sports focus on gear. In wrestling, high-quality gear such as wrestling shoes and kneepads likely provide assistance and protection. Additionally, it is also recommended to wear appropriately fitted headgear during both practice and competition. Similarly, in mixed martial arts, athletes must equip themselves with certain protective gear including a mouthguard, a cup to safeguard the groin area, and "grappling gloves" that leave the fingers and thumb uncovered.[6]

In the age of rapid advancements in wearable sensors and artificial intelligence, the monitoring of athletes can reach unprecedented levels. These technologies have the potential to track various aspects of a fighter's well-being, including the extent of injuries, the risk of further damage during fights, and the progression of chronic conditions. As one of the oldest and most primal sports, direct one-on-one combat necessitates extensive research into best practices and clinical care, as well as the adoption of new technologies, in order to minimize unnecessary injuries among combat athletes.

34.6 Clinical Pearls

- Combat sports place the central and peripheral nervous system at risk of serious injuries, with the governing regulations, monitoring protocols, equipment choices, and combat environment greatly influencing the potential for injuries and resulting outcomes.
- Professional boxing has a high proportion of injuries affecting the head and spine, including acute traumatic brain injury. Repeat impacts to the head can also cause lifelong dysfunction from chronic traumatic brain injury.
- Boxers, wrestlers, and other athletes exhibiting signs of neurological dysfunction should receive prompt attention to determine if the athlete requires further workup and should not return to play until symptoms resolve.

34.7 Disclosures

Noah Lu: None.
Max J. Kerensky: None.
Andrew M. Hersh: None.
Denis Routkevitch: None.
Annie Pan: None.
Nicholas Theodore: Royalties from Globus Medical. Stock Ownership in Globus Medical. Consultant for Globus Medical. On Scientific Advisory Board/Other Office for Globus Medical.

References

[1] Jordan BD. Brain injury in boxing. Clin Sports Med. 2009; 28(4):561–578, vi

[2] Ryan AJ. Intracranial injuries resulting from boxing. Clin Sports Med. 1998; 17(1):155–168

[3] Dinu D, Louis J. Biomechanical analysis of the cross, hook, and uppercut in junior vs. elite boxers: implications for training and talent identification. Front Sports Act Living. 2020; 2:598861

[4] Zazryn TR, McCrory PR, Cameron PA. Neurologic injuries in boxing and other combat sports. Neurol Clin. 2008; 26(1):257–270, xi

[5] Nalepa B, Alexander A, Schodrof S, Bernick C, Pardini J. Fighting to keep a sport safe: toward a structured and sport-specific return to play protocol. Phys Sportsmed. 2017; 45(2):145–150

[6] Jako P. Boxing. In: Wallace WA, Maffulli N, Wroble RR, Kordi R, eds. Combat Sports Medicine. Springer; 2009:193–213

[7] Dunn RJ, Sukhija K, Lopez RA. Strangulation Injuries. In: StatPearls. Treasure Island (FL): StatPearls Publishing; April 22, 2023

[8] McDonald JW, Sadowsky C. Spinal-cord injury. Lancet. 2002; 359(9304): 417–425

[9] Wroble RR. Wrestling. In: Wallace WA, Maffulli N, Wroble RR, Kordi R, eds. Combat Sports Medicine. Springer; 2009:215–245

[10] Place HM, Ecklund JM, Enzenauer RJ. Cervical spine injury in a boxer: should mandatory screening be instituted? J Spinal Disord. 1996; 9(1):64–67

[11] Toth C, McNeil S, Feasby T. Central nervous system injuries in sport and recreation: a systematic review. Sports Med. 2005; 35(8):685–715

[12] Lee SK, Wolfe SW. Peripheral nerve injury and repair. J Am Acad Orthop Surg. 2000; 8(4):243–252

[13] Campbell WW. Evaluation and management of peripheral nerve injury. Clin Neurophysiol. 2008; 119(9):1951–1965

[14] Burnett MG, Zager EL. Pathophysiology of peripheral nerve injury: a brief review. Neurosurg Focus. 2004; 16(5):E1

[15] Branston MM, Yee AH. Sports-related neurologic injuries: more than just concussion. Neurology. 2022; 98 S1:S9

[16] Corrales G, Curreri A. Eye trauma in boxing. Clin Sports Med. 2009; 28(4): 591–607, vi

[17] Toth C. Peripheral nerve injuries attributable to sport and recreation. Phys Med Rehabil Clin N Am. 2009; 20(1):77–100, viii

[18] Halloran L. Wrestling injuries. Orthop Nurs. 2008; 27(3):189–192, quiz 193–194

[19] Vijayavenkataraman S. Nerve guide conduits for peripheral nerve injury repair: a review on design, materials and fabrication methods. Acta Biomater. 2020; 106:54–69

[20] Mao Y, Zhao D, Li J, Fu W. Incidence rates and pathology types of boxing-specific injuries: a systematic review and meta-analysis of epidemiology studies in the 21st century. Orthop J Sports Med. 2023; 11(3): 23259671221127669

[21] Potter MR, Snyder AJ, Smith GA. Boxing injuries presenting to U.S. emergency departments, 1990–2008. Am J Prev Med. 2011; 40(4):462–467

[22] Jones NP. Eye injury in sport. Sports Med. 1989; 7(3):163–181

35 Ice Hockey

Victoria Bergstein, Carly Weber-Levine, and Nicholas Theodore

Summary

Ice hockey is a fast, often violent contact sport, and players are at high risk for neurological injury. Collisions with rink boards or body checks delivered by opposing players can cause traumatic brain injuries, which can be diagnosed with the Sport Concussion Assessment Tool. These high-impact collisions also put players at risk for cervical spine fracture and spinal cord injury, which can manifest as neck pain and weakness or sensory loss in the extremities. Immobilization and stabilization of these injuries are key to preventing further complications and can be accomplished with a cervical neck brace or by leaving the helmet in place. The three most common peripheral nerve injuries are to the cervical root, axillary nerve, and peroneal nerve. Cervical root injuries, commonly called "burners," and axillary nerve injuries frequently result from trauma to the shoulder or neck region. Peroneal nerve injuries can result from trauma to the knee region, or from chronic compression due to ill-fitting equipment. For all neurological injuries, the most important prevention strategies are implementing and enforcing safety rules to reduce the dangers of body checking. Understanding the symptoms, diagnoses, treatment, and prevention strategies is crucial for promoting the safety of ice hockey players.

Keywords: ice hockey, neurological injuries, concussion, spinal cord injuries, peripheral nerve injuries, sports medicine

35.1 Introduction

Ice hockey is a characteristically intense contact sport involving high velocities, quick accelerations, and violent collisions. By the nature of the sport, neurological injury in hockey is a major concern, and injuries to the brain, spine, and peripheral nerves are frequently reported. Most neurological injuries in hockey players are acute, caused by bodily impact from an opposing player or from the boards that surround the ice rink. However, repeated trauma or ill-fitting equipment can cause chronic neurologic injury. This chapter provides an overview of the most common neurological injuries observed in hockey players, common presentations of these injuries, and methods of treatment and prevention (▶ Table 35.1).

35.2 Brain

The two major mechanisms of brain injury in hockey players are: (1) colliding, being hit, or being body-checked by another player, and (2) being hit in the head by the puck. The former category, however, is much more common and results in more severe injuries.[9] Body checking is defined as a defensive player deliberately and forcefully using his or her body to separate an opposing player from the puck.[10] This can result in serious head injury when a player is checked from behind while the neck muscles are relaxed.[9,10] The most common brain injuries among hockey players are traumatic brain injury and concussion, and in severe head trauma, diffuse axonal injury and transient myelin disruption.[9,11,12]

35.2.1 Symptoms

The National Hockey League concussion guidelines mandate the immediate removal of a player with a suspected concussion from a game if the player displays certain signs, including lying motionless on the ice, motor incoordination/balance problems, blank or vacant look, or being slow to get up after a blow.

Table 35.1 Common neurological injuries in ice hockey players

Location	Cause	Presentation	Prevention
Brain			
TBI	Acute trauma	Headache, dizziness, nausea, neck pain, low energy or fatigue, blurred vision, and amnesia[1]	Helmets
Spine			
Cervical fracture	Acute trauma	Neck pain, stiffness, tenderness[2]	None
SCI	Acute trauma	Extremity weakness or numbness, painful dysesthesias or paresthesias, pain to palpation of the cervical region	Immediate immobilization of the spine following injury
Cervical cord neurapraxia	Acute trauma, spinal cord compression	Weakness and/or sensory loss in more than one extremity that normally resolves within 10 to 15 minutes[3,4]	None
Peripheral Nerve			
Upper trunk of brachial plexus	Acute trauma	Acute onset of burning pain or numbness radiating down to one extremity, transient weakness or paresthesia[5]	None
Axillary	Acute trauma, shoulder dislocation	Weakness of shoulder abduction and elevation, numbness and paresthesia throughout the superior lateral brachial cutaneous nerve distribution[6]	None
Peroneal	Acute trauma or chronic compression	Ankle pain, weakness of ankle dorsiflexors, ankle evertors, or toe flexors, numbness or paresthesia in the anterolateral leg, foot, and the webspace between the first two toes, foot drop[3,7,8]	Knee protective gear, wearing properly fitted ice skates

Abbreviations: SCI, spinal cord injury; TBI, traumatic brain injury.

The guidelines also include making direct contact with the ice as an indication.[13] Off-ice, the most common concussion symptoms include headache, dizziness, nausea, neck pain, fatigue, blurred vision, and amnesia.[1] These symptoms may take 24 to 48 hours to manifest.[13]

35.2.2 Diagnosis

The clinical assessment tool used to evaluate players with a suspected concussion is the Sport Concussion Assessment Tool Fifth Edition (SCAT5). Players take baseline tests at the beginning of the season in unimpaired states, allowing for comparison after head trauma.[13] SCAT5 includes symptom evaluation, immediate memory and delayed recall tasks, concentration tasks, a neurological screen, and a balance examination.[14] With the exception of the concentration tasks, every other evaluative component of SCAT5 has been shown to reliably identify concussed players.[14] Tissue damage from either focal or diffuse head injuries can be observed and diagnosed using computed tomography (CT) scans or magnetic resonance imaging (MRI) without contrast.[15] Myelin disruption resulting from diffuse axonal injury, a more severe complication, can be diagnosed using T2-weighted MRI.[12]

35.2.3 Treatment

Football players diagnosed with a concussion are not allowed to return to play or practice the same day, regardless of the severity of symptoms.[13] Players at all levels should undergo an initial 24 to 48 hours rest period, followed by a slow, progressive return to activity that does not aggravate any physical or cognitive symptoms.[13] It is recommended that all players seek consultation from a physician before being cleared to return to play.[13]

35.2.4 Prevention

The most important preventative measure in protecting hockey players from brain injury is implementing rules to reduce body checking. The Canadian Academy of Sport Medicine recommends that body checking be banned at the Peewee level (ages 12–13) due to the high incidence of injuries.[11] Proper use of helmets and mouthguards can also reduce the risk of concussion and TBIs. Mouthguards help absorb impact, distribute force across the mandible, and promote stability of the skull through increased neck muscle activity during teeth clenching.[15]

35.3 Spine

The violent and high-speed nature of ice hockey increases the risk of spinal cord injury (SCI). Cervical spine injury, including fractures and fracture-dislocations, comprises the majority of vertebral injuries in hockey players, with the most commonly affected vertebral level being C5–C6.[16] Teardrop cervical fractures secondary to a flexion-distraction injury, usually resulting from a push or check from behind, lead to a high risk of cervical SCI.[16,17] Impact with the boards accounts for nearly 70% of SCI recorded in hockey, owing to the axial compressive force imposed on the head and cervical vertebrae upon colliding with the strong, immovable boards.[16] The risk of catastrophic SCI resulting in permanent paralysis and severe neurological injury is greatly increased in ice hockey compared to other sports, even compared to other collision sports such as American football.[17] One study showed that three-quarters of hockey players who sustained an SCI during a game incurred a neurological deficit, with nearly one-third of these players becoming wheelchair-bound for life.[3,17]

35.3.1 Symptoms

Initial assessment following an acute injury depends on the athlete's level of consciousness. Unconscious athletes should be transported with spinal immobilization precautions and treated as if they have a cervical spine fracture until they regain consciousness or are cleared by imaging.[18] If the athlete is conscious, SCI may present with symptoms of extremity numbness, painful dysesthesias or paresthesias, weakness, or neck pain.[18] Neurologic deficits include paralysis of one or more extremities, gross weakness or numbness, or significant pain to palpation in the cervical region.[18] In relatively minor cases of spinal cord compression, hockey players have been shown to experience cervical cord neurapraxia, or transient quadriplegia.[3] These patients experience weakness and/or sensory loss in more than one extremity that normally resolves within 10 to 15 minutes, but can last up to 2 days.[4]

35.3.2 Diagnosis

Due to its lower cost and greater availability, X-ray imaging is the diagnostic method of choice for visualizing bony vertebral injuries.[2] The widely accepted standard for cervical spine X-ray imaging is to obtain the "3-view series," consisting of a lateral view from the base of the skull to the T1 vertebral body, an open-mouth odontoid view, and an anteroposterior view.[2] For high-risk patients, patients with neurological symptoms, or patients for whom the 3-view series cannot provide a sufficient assessment, CT scans are indicated.[2]

35.3.3 Treatment

It is crucial to stabilize the cervical spine to prevent further injury after the acute event. The player's helmet and shoulder pads should be left on in order to maintain the most neutral spinal alignment.[18] A cervical collar should be placed only if this can be accomplished without removing the helmet or shoulder pads, and athletes should be transferred to a rigid spine board.[18] For long-term management and return to play protocol, players with cervical spine fractures should wait 8 to 10 weeks for sufficient bony healing.[4] Athletes with any spinal injury should not return to the ice until they have painless, full range of motion and full muscle strength.[4]

35.3.4 Prevention

The most important method of prevention is implementing safety rules to protect players. An effective example is Hockey Canada's implementation of a rule prohibiting checking from behind in 1986, after which a notable reduction in SCIs was reported.[19] It is imperative to educate players, parents, coaches, team staff, and hockey officials about dangerous maneuvers. Efforts made on this front include stricter enforcement of checking rules, stricter penalties for infractions, and educational programs.[19] Equipment changes, such as installing more flexible boards around the rink, have been shown to reduce risk of spinal injury.[17] Of note, although helmets are important for protection against head and brain injury, they may unintentionally increase the risk of catastrophic SCI by increasing the burden on the cervical spine to decelerate the torso after a hit.[17]

35.4 Peripheral Nerves

Although injuries to the central nervous system are far more common in ice hockey, peripheral nerve injuries are not infrequent and warrant consideration. Peripheral nerve injuries in hockey are largely the result of trauma and subsequent nerve compression.[3] Although there have been reports of hockey-related peripheral nerve injuries throughout the body, the most common peripheral nerve injuries occur in the upper trunk of the brachial plexus, the axillary nerve, and the peroneal nerve.

35.4.1 Burners

A "burner" is the colloquial term for a traumatic injury to an upper cervical nerve root, specifically in the upper cord of the brachial plexus.[3] Burners are one of the most common neurologic injuries seen in athletes, and typically develop following trauma to the shoulder or neck region.[3] In hockey, common mechanisms include collisions with the boards and getting shoulder checked by opposing players.[3]

Symptoms

Burners are characterized by acute onset of burning pain or numbness radiating down one extremity in a nondermatomal distribution, sometimes accompanied by transient weakness, which usually resolves within minutes.[5] Upon physical examination after the acute impact, patients may shake their arm or hold it against their body to reduce discomfort.[5] In rare cases, shoulder depression and atrophy of the deltoid and supraspinatus muscles may occur.[5]

Diagnosis

At the time of injury, burners are diagnosed clinically.[5] If symptoms persist for longer than 3 weeks, an electromyograph (EMG) may be obtained to confirm the diagnosis, localize the lesion, and assess severity.[5]

Treatment

Burners should be carefully evaluated at the time of injury, and weekly reexamination is paramount to ensure the athlete is symptom-free before returning to play. Treatment includes addressing predisposing factors, improving strength, and restoring full range of motion through sport-specific physical therapy.[5]

Prevention

Burners can be prevented by improving protective equipment and enforcing rules that protect players from neck and shoulder trauma.[5]

35.4.2 Axillary Nerve

The axillary nerve is derived from the posterior cord of the brachial plexus and innervates the deltoid and teres minor muscles of the shoulder (▶ Fig. 35.1). The most common mechanisms of injury to the axillary nerve are anterior glenohumeral dislocation and a direct blow to the deltoid causing compression.[3] Because the nature of game of hockey predisposes players to extreme shoulder positions and forces, hockey players are at increased risk for acute or chronic overuse axillary nerve injury.[20]

Symptoms

Axillary nerve injury typically presents with weakness of shoulder abduction and elevation, as well as numbness and paresthesia throughout the superior lateral brachial cutaneous nerve distribution.[6] Because axillary nerve injuries commonly co-occur with shoulder dislocation, nervous symptoms can often be overshadowed by joint or bony injury, which highlights the importance of a thorough physical examination.[3]

Diagnosis

Axillary nerve lesions can be diagnosed by nerve conduction studies or EMG. However, electrophysiological tests should not be performed unless symptoms persist longer than 3 weeks, before which time electrical evidence of muscle denervation will not be detected.[6]

Treatment

Important aspects of axillary nerve injury rehabilitation include strengthening of the rotator cuff and deltoid muscles and restoration of full range of shoulder motion through passive and active movement.[6] It is also important that any associated dislocation, fracture, or ligamentous injury be appropriately treated with reduction and immobilization.[6] If symptoms persist longer

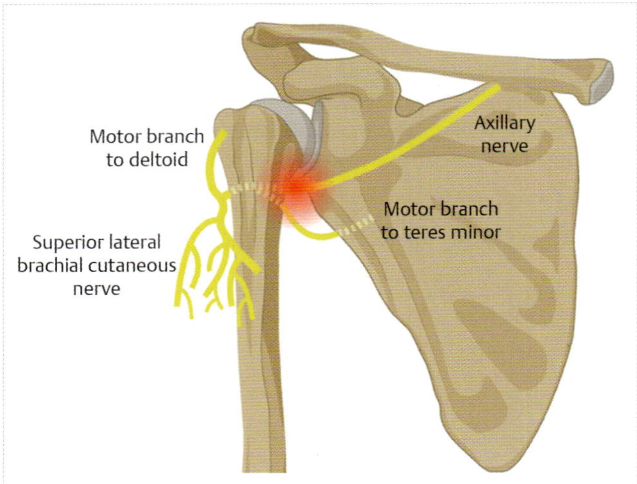

Fig. 35.1 The axillary nerve and its main motor and sensory branches. Anterior shoulder dislocation is a major culprit for axillary nerve injury in hockey players. (Created with BioRender.com.)

than 3 to 4 months, surgical exploration of the axillary nerve may be indicated.[6]

Prevention

As with burners, axillary nerve injuries can be avoided by implementing and following safety rules that limit shoulder checking, and by improving equipment, such as bolstering shoulder pads and making rink boards more flexible.[3,19]

35.4.3 Peroneal Nerve

The common peroneal nerve branches off the sciatic nerve, and itself gives rise to two main branches: the superficial peroneal nerve, which innervates muscles of the lateral compartment of the lower leg, and the deep peroneal nerve, which innervates muscles of the anterior compartment of the lower leg (▶ Fig. 35.2). The superficial peroneal nerve is susceptible to injury via compression at the fibular head, often by means of fracture or other trauma. Hockey players with ill-fitting ice skates have previously reported compression of the deep peroneal nerve, and there have been reports of laceration to the superficial peroneal nerve by the blade of another player's ice skate.[3,7]

Symptoms

Athletes with acute injuries to the peroneal nerve can experience numbness or paresthesia in the anterolateral leg, foot, and the webspace between the first two toes, as well as foot drop.[3,8] Ankle pain and weakness of the ankle dorsiflexors, ankle evertors, or toe extensors may also occur.[7] These symptoms generally resolve in minutes to days.[3]

Diagnosis

Physical examination is the primary method for peroneal nerve injury diagnosis, with expected findings of muscle weakness, sensory loss, or gait alterations.[8] Nerve conduction studies or EMG studies may also be used to strengthen diagnoses and determine prognoses.[8]

Treatment

Because most peroneal nerve injuries are self-limiting, most cases can be treated nonoperatively with bracing, symptom monitoring, and avoiding equipment or activities that induce pain or paresthesia.[8] If symptoms do not resolve, microsurgical decompression procedures can be performed under local anesthesia.[8]

Prevention

Wearing properly fitted ice skates is the best way to prevent deep peroneal nerve compression.[8] Injury to the common fibular nerve can be prevented by reducing risk of trauma to the fibular head through enhanced protective gear in the knee region.[8]

35.5 Conclusion

Given the high speeds and rough style of play in ice hockey, medical professionals should be aware of common hockey-related neurological injuries and how to treat them. The major concern comes from body checking, which results in injury from the blow itself, and from subsequent impact with the rink boards. Implementing rules against body checking has been shown to improve injury rates.[10,11] Helmets are pivotal for reducing brain injury; however,

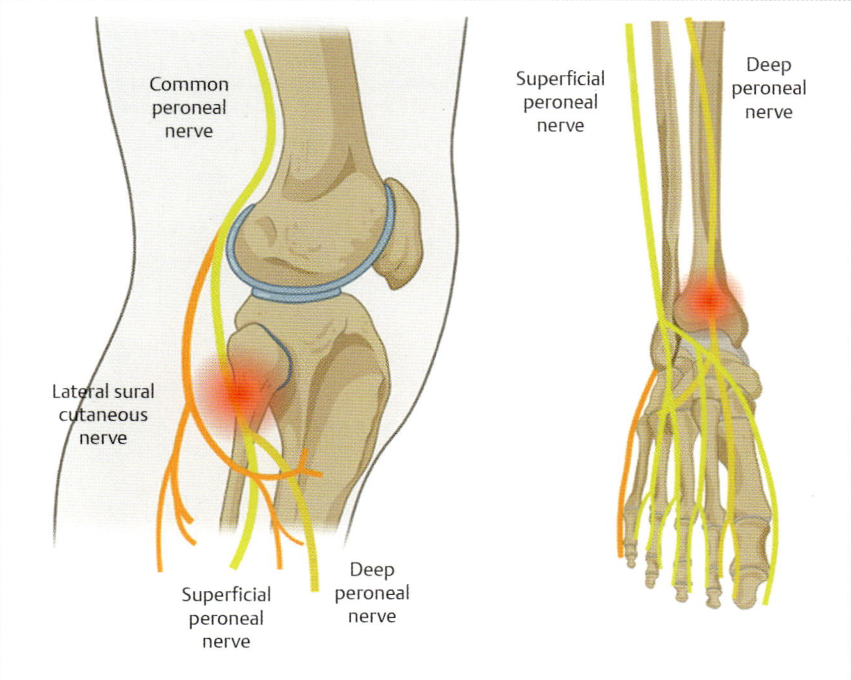

Fig. 35.2 The peroneal nerve and its main branches in the knee region and the foot region. Trauma to the fibular head can cause injury to the common or superficial peroneal nerve, and compression by ill-fitting ice skates can cause chronic injury to the deep peroneal nerve. (Created with BioRender.com.)

they can be unintentionally detrimental to players who sustain an SCI.[17] Neurological injuries in hockey are primarily acute, which results in injuries such as concussion, cervical spine injury, axillary nerve injury, or burners. Chronic injury, however, can develop from repeated head trauma or from peripheral nerve compression. Clinicians must make sure that players have restored full range of motion and have no pain before returning to play.

35.6 Clinical Pearls

- The most common mechanism of neurological injury in ice hockey is body checking into the boards that line the rink.
- Hockey players are at high risk for concussions, and the risk of catastrophic SCI is the highest of any contact sport.
- Peripheral nerve injuries are less common than central nervous system injuries, and they usually result from trauma.
- Helmets are crucial for protecting players from head or brain injuries, but can also introduce higher risk of catastrophic SCI.
- Because body checking is so ingrained into the game, the best ways to prevent the resulting neurological injuries are to implement and enforce safety rules, and improve player, coach, and parent education about the damage checking can cause.
- Treatment of neurological injuries in hockey mostly involves restoring painless, full range of motion through rest and gradual return to play.

35.7 Disclosures

Victoria Bergstein: None.
Carly Weber-Levine: None.
Nicholas Theodore: Royalties from Globus Medical. Stock Ownership in Globus Medical. Consultant for Globus Medical. On Scientific Advisory Board/Other Office for Globus Medical.

References

[1] Benson BW, Meeuwisse WH, Rizos J, Kang J, Burke CJ. A prospective study of concussions among National Hockey League players during regular season games: the NHL-NHLPA Concussion Program. CMAJ. 2011; 183(8): 905–911

[2] Saltzherr TP, Fung Kon Jin PHP, Beenen LFM, Vandertop WP, Goslings JC. Diagnostic imaging of cervical spine injuries following blunt trauma: a review of the literature and practical guideline. Injury. 2009; 40(8):795–800

[3] Wennberg RA, Cohen HB, Walker SR. Neurologic injuries in hockey. Neurol Clin. 2008; 26(1):243–255, xi

[4] Kepler CK, Vaccaro AR. Injuries and abnormalities of the cervical spine and return to play criteria. Clin Sports Med. 2012; 31(3):499–508

[5] Kuhlman GS, McKeag DB. The "burner": a common nerve injury in contact sports. Am Fam Physician. 1999; 60(7):2035–2040, 2042

[6] Perlmutter GS, Apruzzese W. Axillary nerve injuries in contact sports: recommendations for treatment and rehabilitation. Sports Med. 1998; 26 (5):351–361

[7] Hainline BW. Peripheral nerve injury in sports. Continuum (Minneap Minn). 2014; 20 6 Sports Neurology:1605–1628

[8] Fortier LM, Markel M, Thomas BG, Sherman WF, Thomas BH, Kaye AD. An update on peroneal nerve entrapment and neuropathy. Orthop Rev (Pavia). 2021; 13(2):24937

[9] Honey CR. Brain injury in ice hockey. Clin J Sport Med. 1998; 8(1):43–46

[10] Warsh JM, Constantin SA, Howard A, Macpherson A. A systematic review of the association between body checking and injury in youth ice hockey. Clin J Sport Med. 2009; 19(2):134–144

[11] Sullivan P. Sports MDs seek CMA support in bid to make hockey safer. CMAJ. 1990; 142(2):157–159

[12] Wright AD, Jarrett M, Vavasour I, et al. Myelin water fraction is transiently reduced after a single mild traumatic brain injury—a prospective cohort study in collegiate hockey players. PLoS One. 2016; 11(2):e0150215

[13] NHL concussion evaluation and management protocol for 2022–23 season. NHL.com. Accessed April 19, 2023 at: https://www.nhl.com/news/nhl-concussion-evaluation-and-management-protocol-for-2022-23-season/c-335002568

[14] Bruce JM, Thelen J, Meeuwisse W, et al. Use of the Sport Concussion Assessment Tool 5 (SCAT5) in professional hockey, part 2: which components differentiate concussed and non-concussed players? Br J Sports Med. 2020; 55(10):557–565

[15] Biasca N, Wirth SH, Maxwell WL, Simmen HP. Minor traumatic brain injury (mTBI) in ice hockey and other contact sports. Eur J Trauma. 2005; 31(2): 105–116

[16] Tator CH, Carson JD, Edmonds VE. Spinal injuries in ice hockey. Clin Sports Med. 1998; 17(1):183–194

[17] Self M, Mooney JH, Amburgy J, et al. Chasing the cup: a comprehensive review of spinal cord injuries in hockey. Cureus. 2022; 14(4):e24314

[18] Bailes JE, Petschauer M, Guskiewicz KM, Marano G. Management of cervical spine injuries in athletes. J Athl Train. 2007; 42(1):126–134

[19] Tator CH, Provvidenza C, Cassidy JD. Update and overview of spinal injuries in Canadian ice hockey, 1943 to 2011: the continuing need for injury prevention and education. Clin J Sport Med. 2016; 26(3):232–238

[20] Colak T, Bamaç B, Alemdar M, et al. Nerve conduction studies of the axillary, musculocutaneous and radial nerves in elite ice hockey players. J Sports Med Phys Fitness. 2009; 49(2):224–231

36 Weightlifting

Vikas Vattipally, A. Daniel Davidar, Kimberly Ashayeri, and Nicholas Theodore

Summary

Weightlifting is a common recreational and competitive sport that puts significant stress, load, and potential shearing forces on the spine and joints. Although vertebral fractures, spinal cord pathologies, and peripheral nerve injuries are rare in weightlifting, they can have serious consequences due to the large forces athletes' bodies must withstand. Weightlifters should be diligent about learning and maintaining proper form while performing movements, and providers should recognize the injuries that can occur during this sport. In this chapter, we will discuss an overview of the effects of weightlifting on neurological structures. We will also address the physiology of neurological injuries in weightlifting, including treatments, prevention, and future directions.

Keywords: weightlifting, back pain, return to play, spine, peripheral nerve

36.1 Introduction

Weightlifting encompasses a vast range of musculoskeletal movements against the resistance of a fixed weight to build muscle mass and strength. With an increasing presence in recreational and professional sports, weightlifting has steadily increased in popularity. It has further been propelled by prominent events such as the Olympics, Strongmen competitions, and various bodybuilding tournaments. Weightlifting can be broadly classified into powerlifting and Olympic weightlifting. Powerlifting consists of the "squat," "deadlift," and "bench press" movements, while Olympic weightlifting includes the "snatch" and "clean and jerk" movements.[1,2] Additionally, other sports, such as CrossFit, involve a combination of weightlifting, gymnastics, and aerobic exercises to build muscle, with a vast majority of CrossFit injuries caused by these movements.[3,4] Weightlifting movements place a large amount of stress, load, and potential shearing forces on the spine and joints, which have the potential to cause acute and chronic injuries.[5,6,7] In this chapter, we will discuss an overview of the effects of weightlifting on neurological structures. We will also address the physiology of neurological injuries in weightlifting, including treatments, prevention, and future directions (▶ Fig. 36.1).

36.2 Pathophysiology of Weightlifting Injuries

36.2.1 Athlete Baseline Factors

In the following section, we will discuss athlete characteristics that may contribute to the risk of weightlifting-associated injury.

Age

Weightlifting is performed by individuals across different age groups, with youth divisions in some national competitions including athletes as young as 13 years old.[8] Although some believe that lifting weights can lead to abnormalities in growth plates and height, there has been no substantial literature supporting this claim.[9] The relationship between weightlifting, age, and neurological injuries remains understudied, but age has been shown to play a role in other weightlifting injury types. Younger weightlifting athletes may be at higher risk of accidental injury, injury due to improper technique, or injury due to insufficient supervision.[10] One study of emergency department visits after weightlifting injuries found that the risk of "accidental" injuries, such as dropping weights on a body part, was increased in younger age groups, while the inverse was true for weightlifting-related stress and strain injuries.[11] However, increased age was found to be a risk factor for CrossFit injuries, potentially due to an increased need for mobility that older patients may struggle with.[4,12]

Sex

Males and females have been shown to experience different rates of injury from weightlifting. One study found the overall incidence of cervical neck sprains to be higher in males compared to females, though weightlifting was the third-highest cause of neck sprains in males and the primary cause in females.[13] In another study of traumatic lumbar spine injuries, weightlifting was the third overall sporting cause, but these weightlifting injuries comprised a larger proportion of injuries in males than in females.[14] Potential sources of these differences include the differential participation in weightlifting by sex and an inclination for males to lift heavier weights than women, predisposing them to greater injury.

Performance-Enhancing Drugs

Several performance-enhancing drugs alter physiology to enable a higher output during weight training. Although some have been proven to increase muscle bulk, others, such as recombinant growth hormone, provide insufficient benefits to outweigh the adverse effects that can include fatigue, arthralgia, or acromegaly.[15,16] Certain studies demonstrate that growth hormone supplementation has no functional strength improvements,[17,18] and others note a predisposition to develop carpal tunnel syndrome and de Quervain's tenosynovitis, potentially due to increased peripheral edema.[15,16,19]

36.2.2 Physiological Forces

Intra-abdominal Pressure on the Spine

Weightlifting in excess of 2.5 kg (5.5 lb) can cause a significant increase in intra-abdominal pressure.[20] Studies have shown that increased intra-abdominal pressure leads to increased intradiskal pressure within the vertebral column.[21,22] As a result, as individuals lift increasingly more weight, they increase their risk of disk herniation.[23] Other studies, however, have postulated that increased intra-abdominal pressure counters pressure on the spine, preventing injury.[21] In one rare case, pneumorrachis, which is the presence of gas within the spinal canal, was reported to develop

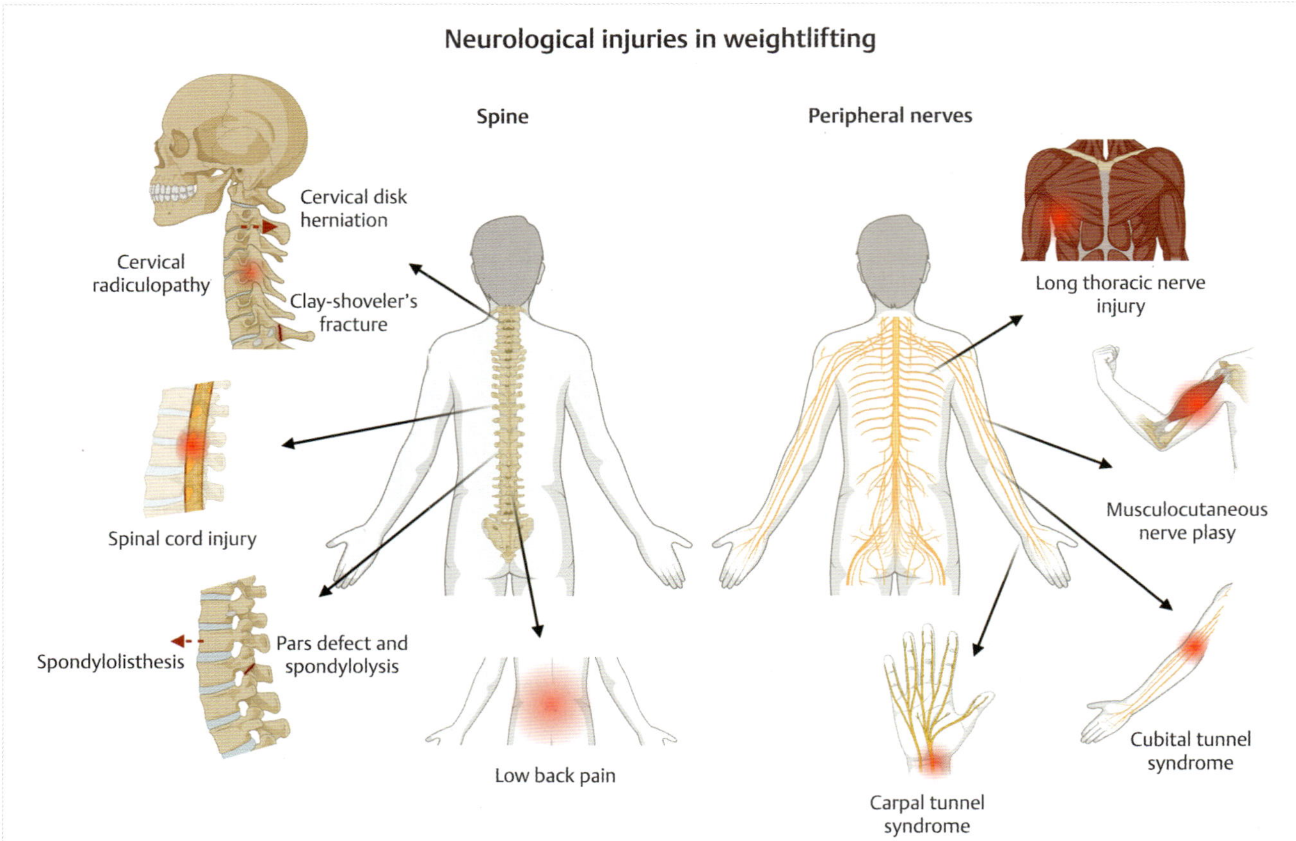

Fig. 36.1 Neurological injuries that can occur in weightlifting. Injuries to the spine include cervical disk herniation, cervical spinous process fracture ("clay-shoveler's fracture"), cervical radiculopathy, spinal cord injury, pars interarticularis defects that can progress to spondylolysis or spondylolisthesis, and low back pain. Peripheral nerves may be affected from weightlifting as in carpal tunnel syndrome (median nerve), cubital tunnel syndrome (ulnar nerve), musculocutaneous nerve palsy, and long thoracic nerve injury. (Created with BioRender.com.)

extending from the skull base to the thoracolumbar junction and accompanied by axio-atlanto-occipital hyperpneumatization, because of repeated Valsalva maneuvers during weightlifting exercises.[24]

Pressure Mitigation

Weightlifters performing the deadlift movement can be encouraged to employ the "sumo stance," which utilizes a wider stance and offloads pressure on lumbar joints.[7] A supportive belt for weightlifting may help stabilize the lumbar spine by increasing intrabdominal and erector spinae pressure.[25,26] Nevertheless, it is important to note that weight belts have previously been associated with a higher rate of lumbar spine injury among competitive and elite powerlifters, which is hypothesized to be because of nonphysiological loading forces placed on the lower back.[27]

36.2.3 Onset of Injury

Acute Injuries

The etiology of acute weightlifting injuries often involves improper technique, repetitive stress leading to an acute event, or equipment-related malfunctions. In strength training exercises, 46% of acute injuries were a strain or sprain, with improper dropping of weights being a predominant mechanism of injury.[28] Moreover, free weight exercises accounted for a large amount of these injuries. Increased attention has also been brought to acute equipment-related injuries as athletes or bystanders have suffered paralysis or even death in certain instances.[29]

Chronic Injuries

Repetitive weightlifting movements render the individual susceptible to stress fractures, especially at locations of repetitive loads.[30] Chronic injuries were common due to the now-discontinued "clean and press" Olympic weightlifting event, in which extreme lordosis led to significant stress on the lumbar spine.[31] Repetitive squatting has also been suggested to cause osteoarthritis of the knee, with one cohort study of former top-level athletes across sports finding former weightlifters to have a higher incidence of osteoarthritis, especially among those with a higher body mass index (BMI).[32]

36.3 Common Injuries Caused by Weightlifting

36.3.1 Spine

As the spine serves to stabilize the body and bears much of the mechanical stress during sports activities, the significant forces experienced during weightlifting can create susceptibility to injury.

Lumbar Spine

Low back pain is prevalent among athletes, with up to 30% experiencing this symptom at some point during their career.[33,34] This holds true among weightlifting athletes, with low back pain being commonly reported.[35,36] The use of heavy weights and improper form place excessive strain on the muscles and joints of the lower back, further predisposing weightlifters to low back pain.[37] Abnormal radiographic lumbar spine findings, such as disk degeneration or extrusion, have been found in both long-term weightlifters as well as in small prospective cohorts of young weightlifters.[38,39]

The pars interarticularis is the narrow isthmus between the superior and inferior articulating processes of vertebral bodies. Pars defects have been reported in upwards of 20% of weightlifters.[40] Repetitive stress to the pars interarticularis, such as repetitive hyperextension of the lower back in weightlifting, is hypothesized to cause radiologically occult injuries that do not breach the bony cortex.[41,42] This may progress to spondylolysis, meaning a stress fracture in the pars, which can further develop into spondylolisthesis, indicated by displacement of a vertebral body in relation to an adjacent one.[43] Mechanical stress is postulated to be a causal factor of spondylolysis due to its absence in nonambulatory individuals and progression from unilateral to bilateral spondylolysis with age in ambulatory individuals.[44,45]

Evaluation of weightlifting-related low back pain is dependent on each athlete's individual history, with a thorough history and physical examination warranted for each patient. Management includes rest, physical therapy, and anti-inflammatory medications. It is also important that the patient be educated on proper weightlifting techniques to prevent further injury.[36] Evaluation of pars defects can be performed via plain radiography or computed tomography (CT) of the suspected area. Among athletes, nonoperative management, which includes physical therapy, lumbosacral orthosis, and activity modification, is often effective. Operative intervention is recommended for patients who are refractory to nonoperative treatment, those who progress to spondylolisthesis, or those who present with neurological deficits.[46]

Cervical Spine

Cervical injuries occurring during weightlifting include fractures, arthrosis, disk herniation, and spondylolisthesis. In a cross-sectional study of powerlifters, it was found that approximately one-fourth of athletes have sustained a cervical spine injury.[27]

Avulsion of the cervical spinous process, commonly known as clay-shoveler's fracture, can occur during forceful flexion of the cervical spine or excessive contraction of the trapezius and rhomboid muscles while weightlifting.[47] The most common location for this fracture is at the C7 vertebra, but fractures at other levels have also been reported.[48,49] Cervical vertebrae fractures can also occur when resting heavy weights on the neck or shoulders.[49] One large study indicated a possible association between the use of free weights and cervical disk herniation.[50] Weightlifting may also exacerbate pre-existing degenerative cervical changes, resulting in radiculopathy, as was reported in a case series of three athletes.[51]

For structural injuries of the cervical spine, radiographs are indicated for initial evaluation followed by CT or magnetic resonance imaging (MRI) if findings are inconclusive and symptoms persist. Management may include anti-inflammatory medications, activity modification, and a cervical collar.[51,52]

Spinal Cord

Sports-related traumatic spinal cord injuries account for 8.7% of all traumatic spinal cord injuries.[47] Although exceedingly rare, some spinal cord injuries have been reported in association with weightlifting throughout the literature. Spinal epidural hematomas which result in neurological symptoms and require surgical intervention have been associated with intense weightlifting.[53] One patient was found to have an infarction of the conus medullaris after repeated lumbar hyperextension exercises, and another athlete presented with spontaneous tetraplegia after weight training due to a posterior disk herniation impinging the spinal canal.[54,55] Finally, one patient was noted to develop syringomyelia that expanded over time in association with neck extensor exercises.[56]

Typically, MRI is used for evaluation and operative planning in the case of spinal cord pathologies. Management should be tailored specifically for each patient's injury.

36.3.2 Peripheral Nerve

Carpal Tunnel Syndrome

Carpal tunnel syndrome is an entrapment of the median nerve, which can result from repetitive movements of the arm and wrist muscles and can result in pain, numbness, and paresthesia, especially of the first three digits.[57,58] Although lifting weights is a rare cause of carpal tunnel syndrome, the initial assessment includes Phalen's maneuver and nerve conduction studies.[59,60] One study indicated that the degree of motor dysfunction was associated with the duration of weight training.[60] Management involves activity modification, splinting, and carpal tunnel release surgery if other treatments fail.[59]

Cubital Tunnel Syndrome

Cubital tunnel syndrome involves subluxation of the ulnar nerve at the elbow joint, which can result in pain, numbness, and paresthesia along the medial forearm and fourth to fifth digits.[61] One study found that the degree of ulnar nerve luxation is related to hypertrophy of the triceps muscle, which was increased in amateur bodybuilders as compared to control patients.[62] In a case report, one patient was reported to experience cubital tunnel syndrome after a powerlifting-related triceps tendon rupture, which eventually necessitated surgical intervention.[63]

Musculocutaneous Nerve

Musculocutaneous nerve palsy is a rare syndrome seen in weightlifters that is characterized by weakness of the elbow flexors due to biceps brachii and brachialis weakness and dysesthesias of the lateral forearm.[64,65,66] It primarily involves the dominant arm and resolves with exercise modification or decreased exercise intensity and rest.

Long Thoracic Nerve

The long thoracic nerve arises from the C5–C7 nerve roots and innervates the serratus anterior muscle. Weightlifting injuries to the long thoracic nerve have been associated with repetitive performance of overhead exercises.[67] Patients present with weakness of the affected arm for pushing motions and complete absence of contraction of the serratus anterior on the affected side.[68] Restriction of overhead arm movements is also possible. Management involves physical therapy or restrengthening programs.[67]

36.4 Conclusion

Weightlifting is a common recreational and competitive activity athletes of all ages participate in to improve their strength and overall fitness. It is, therefore, important for athletes and care providers to recognize predisposing factors, clinical signs, and optimal treatment strategies for common injuries to the spine or peripheral nerves that can arise from this sport. Low back pain is particularly frequent among these athletes and can be exacerbated by improper form or overuse. Although vertebral fractures and spinal cord pathologies are rare, they can have serious consequences if athletes continue to lift weights despite their injury. Injuries to peripheral nerves may also arise or be exacerbated by lifting weights, and typically present with weakness in the corresponding muscles. All athletes interested in weightlifting, either on a recreational or competitive basis, should be diligent about learning and maintaining proper form while performing movements, and should always seek medical attention if they suspect a neurological injury.

36.5 Clinical Pearls

- Weightlifting is a popular hobby and competitive sport and involves large amounts of stress on the muscles and joints of the body.
- Male weightlifters and younger athletes may be more susceptible to weightlifting injuries.
- Acute injuries are commonly attributable to improper weightlifting form, while chronic injuries can occur due to repetitive stress on a joint over time.
- Low back pain is common among weightlifters and can be exacerbated by heavier weights or poor technique.
- Spinal pathologies such as vertebral fractures, disk herniations, or spinal cord injuries are rare but require medical evaluation to ensure further injury does not occur.
- Repetitive movements and muscle hypertrophy can contribute to carpal tunnel syndrome and cubital tunnel syndrome, respectively.
- Providers should emphasize proper form and technique to minimize the risk of acute weightlifting injuries and prevent the development of chronic injuries.
- Early evaluation and intervention are important for suspected weightlifting injuries as most are treatable with activity modification.

36.6 Disclosures

Vikas Vattipally: None.
A. Daniel Davidar
Kimberly Ashayeri
Nicholas Theodore: Royalties from Globus Medical. Stock Ownership in Globus Medical. Consultant for Globus Medical. On Scientific Advisory Board/Other Office for Globus Medical.

References

[1] International Weightlifting Federation. International Weightlifting Federation. Accessed January 5, 2024 at: https://beta.iwf.sport
[2] International Powerlifting Federation. International Powerlifting Federation. Accessed January 5, 2024 at: https://powerlifting.sport
[3] Meyer J, Morrison J, Zuniga J. The benefits and risks of CrossFit: a systematic review. Workplace Health Saf. 2017; 65(12):612–618
[4] Ángel Rodríguez M, García-Calleja P, Terrados N, Crespo I, Del Valle M, Olmedillas H. Injury in CrossFit®: a systematic review of epidemiology and risk factors. Phys Sportsmed. 2022; 50(1):3–10
[5] Brown EW, Abani K. Kinematics and kinetics of the dead lift in adolescent power lifters. Med Sci Sports Exerc. 1985; 17(5):554–566
[6] Cholewicki J, McGill SM. Lumbar posterior ligament involvement during extremely heavy lifts estimated from fluoroscopic measurements. J Biomech. 1992; 25(1):17–28
[7] Cholewicki J, McGill SM, Norman RW. Lumbar spine loads during the lifting of extremely heavy weights. Med Sci Sports Exerc. 1991; 23(10):1179–1186
[8] Huebner M, Perperoglou A. Performance development from youth to senior and age of peak performance in Olympic weightlifting. Front Physiol. 2019; 10:1121
[9] American Academy of Pediatrics. Care of the Young Athlete Patient Education Handouts: Strength Training; 2011. https://www.aap.org/globalassets/publications/coya/strength_training_final_secured.1.0.pdf
[10] Faigenbaum AD, Myer GD. Resistance training among young athletes: safety, efficacy and injury prevention effects. Br J Sports Med. 2010; 44(1):56–63
[11] Myer GD, Quatman CE, Khoury J, Wall EJ, Hewett TE. Youth versus adult "weightlifting" injuries presenting to United States emergency rooms: accidental versus nonaccidental injury mechanisms. J Strength Cond Res. 2009; 23(7):2054–2060
[12] Everhart JS, Kirven JC, France TJ, Hidden K, Vasileff WK. Independent risk factors for recurrent or multiple new injuries in CrossFit athletes. J Sports Med Phys Fitness. 2020; 60(11):1470–1476
[13] DePasse JM, Durand W, Palumbo MA, Daniels AH. Sex- and sport-specific epidemiology of cervical spine injuries sustained during sporting activities. World Neurosurg. 2019; 122:e540–e545
[14] Cheng R, Kahan JB, Li D, Schneble CA, Gardner EC. Sex- and sports-specific epidemiology of traumatic lumbar spine injuries sustained during sporting activities: male snowboarders and female horseback riders at greatest risk. Arthrosc Sports Med Rehabil. 2021; 3(2):e515–e520
[15] Warrier AA, Azua EN, Kasson LB, et al. Performance-enhancing drugs in healthy athletes: an umbrella review of systematic reviews and meta-analyses. Sports Health. 2023:19417381231197389
[16] Siebert DM, Rao AL. The use and abuse of human growth hormone in sports. Sports Health. 2018; 10(5):419–426
[17] Tavares ABW, Micmacher E, Biesek S, et al. Effects of growth hormone administration on muscle strength in men over 50 years old. Int J Endocrinol. 2013; 2013:942030
[18] Macintyre JG. Growth hormone and athletes. Sports Med. 1987; 4(2): 129–142
[19] Pagonis T, Ditsios K, Givissis P, Pagonis A, Christodoulou A. Abuse of growth hormone increases the risk of persistent de Quervain tenosynovitis. Am J Sports Med. 2009; 37(11):2228–2233
[20] Gerten KA, Richter HE, Wheeler TL, II, et al. Intraabdominal pressure changes associated with lifting: implications for postoperative activity restrictions. Am J Obstet Gynecol. 2008; 198(3):306.e1–306.e5
[21] Bartelink DL. The role of abdominal pressure in relieving the pressure on the lumbar intervertebral discs. J Bone Joint Surg Br. 1957; 39-B(4):718–725
[22] Nachemson AL, Andersson BJ, Schultz AB. Valsalva maneuver biomechanics. Effects on lumbar trunk loads of elevated intraabdominal pressures. Spine. 1986; 11(5):476–479

[23] Noguchi M, Gooyers CE, Karakolis T, Noguchi K, Callaghan JP. Is intervertebral disc pressure linked to herniation?: An in-vitro study using a porcine model. J Biomech. 2016; 49(9):1824–1830

[24] Germino JC, Medverd JR, Nguyen VT, Favinger JL, Marder CP. Craniocervical hyperpneumatization with concurrent pneumorrhachis, pneumomediastinum, and subcutaneous emphysema in a weightlifter. Spine J. 2013; 13(10):e47–e53

[25] Harman EA, Rosenstein RM, Frykman PN, Nigro GA. Effects of a belt on intra-abdominal pressure during weight lifting. Med Sci Sports Exerc. 1989; 21 (2):186–190

[26] Miyamoto K, Iinuma N, Maeda M, Wada E, Shimizu K. Effects of abdominal belts on intra-abdominal pressure, intra-muscular pressure in the erector spinae muscles and myoelectrical activities of trunk muscles. Clin Biomech (Bristol, Avon). 1999; 14(2):79–87

[27] Siewe J, Rudat J, Röllinghoff M, Schlegel UJ, Eysel P, Michael JWP. Injuries and overuse syndromes in powerlifting. Int J Sports Med. 2011; 32(9):703–711

[28] Kerr ZY, Collins CL, Comstock RD. Epidemiology of weight training-related injuries presenting to United States emergency departments, 1990 to 2007. Am J Sports Med. 2010; 38(4):765–771

[29] George DH, Stakiw K, Wright CJ. Fatal accident with weight-lifting equipment: implications for safety standards. CMAJ. 1989; 140(8):925–926

[30] Lavallee ME, Balam T. An overview of strength training injuries: acute and chronic. Curr Sports Med Rep. 2010; 9(5):307–313

[31] Calhoon G, Fry AC. Injury rates and profiles of elite competitive weightlifters. J Athl Train. 1999; 34(3):232–238

[32] Hartmann H, Wirth K, Klusemann M. Analysis of the load on the knee joint and vertebral column with changes in squatting depth and weight load. Sports Med. 2013; 43(10):993–1008

[33] Dreisinger TE, Nelson B. Management of back pain in athletes. Sports Med. 1996; 21(4):313–320

[34] De Luigi AJ. Low back pain in the adolescent athlete. Phys Med Rehabil Clin N Am. 2014; 25(4):763–788

[35] Aasa U, Svartholm I, Andersson F, Berglund L. Injuries among weightlifters and powerlifters: a systematic review. Br J Sports Med. 2017; 51(4): 211–219

[36] Ross R, Han J, Slover J. Chronic lower back pain in weight lifters: epidemiology, evaluation, and management. JBJS Rev. 2023; 11(6)

[37] Fares MY, Fares J, Salhab HA, Khachfe HH, Bdeir A, Fares Y. Low back pain among weightlifting adolescents and young adults. Cureus. 2020; 12(7): e9127

[38] Yoshimizu R, Nakase J, Yoshioka K, et al. Incidence and temporal changes in lumbar degeneration and low back pain in child and adolescent weightlifters: a prospective 5-year cohort study. PLoS One. 2022; 17(6):e0270046

[39] Shimozaki K, Nakase J, Yoshioka K, et al. Incidence rates and characteristics of abnormal lumbar findings and low back pain in child and adolescent weightlifter: a prospective three-year cohort study. PLoS One. 2018; 13(10): e0206125

[40] Tawfik S, Phan K, Mobbs RJ, Rao PJ. The incidence of pars interarticularis defects in athletes. Global Spine J. 2020; 10(1):89–101

[41] Hollenberg GM, Beattie PF, Meyers SP, Weinberg EP, Adams MJ. Stress reactions of the lumbar pars interarticularis: the development of a new MRI classification system. Spine. 2002; 27(2):181–186

[42] Mohile NV, Kuczmarski AS, Lee D, Warburton C, Rakoczy K, Butler AJ. Spondylolysis and isthmic spondylolisthesis: a guide to diagnosis and management. J Am Board Fam Med. 2022; 35(6):1204–1216

[43] McDonald BT, Hanna A, Lucas JA. Spondylolysis. In: StatPearls [Internet]. Treasure Island, FL: StatPearls Publishing; 2023

[44] Rosenberg NJ, Bargar WL, Friedman B. The incidence of spondylolysis and spondylolisthesis in nonambulatory patients. Spine. 1981; 6(1):35–38

[45] Beutler WJ, Fredrickson BE, Murtland A, Sweeney CA, Grant WD, Baker D. The natural history of spondylolysis and spondylolisthesis: 45-year follow-up evaluation. Spine. 2003; 28(10):1027–1035, discussion 1035

[46] Blanda J, Bethem D, Moats W, Lew M. Defects of pars interarticularis in athletes: a protocol for nonoperative treatment. J Spinal Disord. 1993; 6(5): 406–411

[47] Boden BP, Jarvis CG. Spinal injuries in sports. Neurol Clin. 2008; 26(1): 63–78, viii

[48] Herrick RT. Clay-shoveler's fracture in power-lifting. A case report. Am J Sports Med. 1981; 9(1):29–30

[49] Watson DJ, Dolbeer JA. C6 spinous process fracture in a young adult. J Orthop Sports Phys Ther. 2017; 47(9):692–692

[50] Mundt DJ, Kelsey JL, Golden AL, et al. The Northeast Collaborative Group on Low Back Pain. An epidemiologic study of sports and weight lifting as possible risk factors for herniated lumbar and cervical discs. Am J Sports Med. 1993; 21(6):854–860

[51] Jordan BD, Istrico R, Zimmerman RD, Tsairis P, Warren RF. Acute cervical radiculopathy in weight lifters. Phys Sportsmed. 1990; 18(1):73–76

[52] Posthuma de Boer J, van Wulfften Palthe AFY, Stadhouder A, Bloemers FW. The clay shoveler's fracture: a case report and review of the literature. J Emerg Med. 2016; 51(3):292–297

[53] Anghelescu A, Rasina A. Acute spontaneous thoracic epidural hematoma, triggered by weight-lifting training, in a retired sportsman: case report and literature review. Spinal Cord Ser Cases. 2017; 3:17090

[54] Cipriano K, Mansfield JT, Batal H, Gosai E. Nontraumatic acute hyperextension myelopathy associated with weightlifting. Am J Phys Med Rehabil. 2021; 100(8):e113–e115

[55] Clewer G, Carmont M, Jaffray D. Spontaneous tetraplegia during weight training. Br J Sports Med. 2006; 40(12):1011–1012

[56] Balmaseda MT, Jr, Wunder JA, Gordon C, Cannell CD. Posttraumatic syringomyelia associated with heavy weightlifting exercises: case report. Arch Phys Med Rehabil. 1988; 69(11):970–972

[57] Katz RT. Carpal tunnel syndrome: a practical review. Am Fam Physician. 1994; 49(6):1371–1379, 1385–1386

[58] Sevy JO, Sina RE, Varacallo M. Carpal Tunnel Syndrome. In: StatPearls [Internet]. Treasure Island, FL: StatPearls Publishing; 2023

[59] Steyers CM, Schelkun PH. Practical management of carpal tunnel syndrome. Phys Sportsmed. 1995; 23(1):83–88

[60] Mauer UM, Lotspeich E, Klein HJ, Rath SA. [Body building—effect on neural conduction velocity of the median nerve in the carpal tunnel]. Z Orthop Ihre Grenzgeb. 1991; 129(4):319–321

[61] Chauhan M, Anand P, Das JM. Cubital Tunnel Syndrome. In: StatPearls [Internet]. Treasure Island, FL: StatPearls Publishing; 2023

[62] Michael AE, Young P. Is triceps hypertrophy associated with ulnar nerve luxation? Muscle Nerve. 2018; 58(4):523–527

[63] Herrick RT, Herrick S. Ruptured triceps in a powerlifter presenting as cubital tunnel syndrome. A case report. Am J Sports Med. 1987; 15(5):514–516

[64] Matz SO, Nibbelink G. Bilateral musculocutaneous nerve palsy from strength training. Phys Sportsmed. 2004; 32(3):18–20

[65] Braddom RL, Wolfe C. Musculocutaneous nerve injury after heavy exercise. Arch Phys Med Rehabil. 1978; 59(6):290–293

[66] Lorei MP, Hershman EB. Peripheral nerve injuries in athletes. Treatment and prevention. Sports Med. 1993; 16(2):130–147

[67] Berthold JB, Burg TM, Nussbaum RP. Long thoracic nerve injury caused by overhead weight lifting leading to scapular dyskinesis and medial scapular winging. J Am Osteopath Assoc. 2017; 117(2):133–137

[68] Stanish WD, Lamb H. Isolated paralysis of the serratus anterior muscle: a weight training injury. Case report. Am J Sports Med. 1978; 6(6):385–386

37 Rugby

Nicholas D. Cassimatis, Andrew K. Chan, and John Knightly

Summary

Rugby delves into the captivating world of one of the most physically demanding and strategically complex sports, originating in the 19th century in England and known for its blend of speed, power, and team play. Highlighting the nuances between different elements of rugby, the chapter meticulously explores the continuous and full-contact nature of the game, the roles and risks associated with various positions, and the evolution of medical awareness and neurological injury management protocols. Through a focus on the increasing concerns around neurotrauma, such as concussions and their long-term effects, this chapter sheds light on the significant measures taken to enhance player safety without compromising the sport's integrity. This chapter is a must-read for those interested in the intersection of sports, health, and safety protocols, offering deep insights into the challenges and changes shaping modern rugby.

Keywords: concussion/prevention and control in rugby, sports medicine/methods in rugby, rugby-related athletic injuries, spinal injuries in rugby, chronic traumatic encephalopathy/epidemiology, risk management/methods in rugby neurotrauma, health policy/legislation and jurisprudence (rugby safety), physical endurance/physiology (rugby athletes), emergency medical services/standards (rugby-related neurotrauma)

37.1 Rugby Basics

Rugby, a highly physical and tactically complex sport, requires a blend of speed, power, and strategic team play. It originated in the 19th century in England and has since spread globally, having two primary forms: Rugby Union and Rugby League, each with its own variations of rules and team sizes. The game is characterized by its continuous nature, with play only stopping for infractions, injuries, or point scores. Rugby is a full-contact sport often leading to a broad spectrum of injuries with which medical professionals need to be familiar.

Rugby consists of two 40-minute halves where teams score points by grounding the ball in the opposition's in-goal area (a try), which is worth five points. Following a try, the scoring team has an opportunity to kick a conversion for an additional two points. Teams can also score through penalty kicks or drop goals, each worth three points. Rugby Union is played by two teams of 15 players each, whereas Rugby League typically has 13-player teams. The play is continuous, and athletes can pass the ball laterally or backward, but not forward, while trying to run forward and dodge defenders. Tackling is an essential part of rugby, but players can only tackle the ball carrier and must do so below the shoulders. Blocking is not allowed, and in most instances, the player carrying the ball attempts to pass the ball before being tackled. Tackling in rugby focuses more on wrapping and dragging opponents to the ground, and players do not wear protective gear. In comparison, tackling in American football is typically more high-impact, involving direct, forceful collisions with players wearing substantial protective equipment.

Rugby positions, typically divided into "forwards" and "backs," each have distinct roles. Forwards, consisting of eight players in Rugby Union (six in Rugby League), engage in physical battles for possession and territory in events called "scrums" and "line-outs." They are generally larger and stronger, often leading to injuries associated with high-impact collisions.[1] The backs are generally quicker and more agile, using speed, skill, and strategy to outmaneuver the opposition. They are more prone to injuries related to high-speed running, such as hamstring strains.[1] Understanding these positions and the typical injuries associated with each is crucial for medical professionals dealing with rugby players.

The physically demanding nature of rugby, coupled with the sport's various plays and positions, contributes to a wide array of potential injuries.

37.2 Historical Numbers

Rugby, among other contact sports, has a long history of neurotrauma. This is manifested as sports-related concussions (SRCs) and mild traumatic brain injuries (TBIs), more severe TBI, injuries to the spine, or peripheral nerve injuries. The awareness and understanding of these injuries in rugby have significantly evolved over time, reflecting both developments in medical science and shifts in societal attitudes toward player safety. In the early days of the sport, there was little recognition of the long-term effects of repetitive head trauma, with players often continuing to play after suffering a head injury.[2] Reports of neurotrauma were scant due to underreporting and lack of comprehensive medical surveillance.[2]

Starting from the late 20th century, researchers began to better understand the dangers of neurotrauma and chronic traumatic encephalopathy (CTE). Consequently, attitudes toward neurotrauma in rugby started to shift. Evidence from the 1990s onwards indicated an increasing trend in the reported incidence of concussions in the sport.[3] This was attributed not only to the increasing physicality and professionalization of the game but also to improvements in medical awareness and SRC management protocols. In the Annual England Professional Rugby Injury Surveillance Project of 2019–2020, SRC was the most commonly reported match injury, with an incidence of nearly 20 SRCs per 1,000 hours of match play.[3] The Surveillance Project also highlighted that SRCs resulted in 16 days missed per match on average.[3] Although the incidence of overall injury has been relatively stable since surveillance began in 2002, injury severity, measured by days missed due to injury, has increased. Furthermore, the incidence of concussions has also increased.

Over the years, highly publicized cases of contact sport players suffering from long-term neurological complications, including early-onset dementia, further galvanized attention toward the issue.[2,4,5,6,7] Due to the growing recognition of the potential life-altering effects of neurotrauma, rugby's governing bodies have introduced stricter regulations and management protocols around head and spine injuries.[8,9,10] There is increased emphasis on prevention, including safer tackling techniques, rules enforcement (such as sanctioning illegal tackles), and new assessment protocols for suspected neurotrauma with mandatory rest periods following suspected SRCs. Simultaneously, technological advancements have enabled better on-field diagnosis and post-game review of potential neurotraumatic events.[3,11,12] Although these measures have increased the reported instances of neurotrauma in the short term due to improved detection, they represent a crucial step toward reducing the long-term incidence and severity of these injuries in rugby.

37.3 Plays Likely to Cause Neurotrauma

Neurotrauma in rugby can occur in a variety of play situations, with some presenting a higher risk than others due to the nature of the contact and forces involved. Some of the most common high-energy rugby plays, and their basic definitions are as follows:

- **Tackle:** A method of halting the progress of an opponent carrying the ball by bringing them to the ground. The tackler must wrap his or her arms around the ball carrier, typically targeting below the shoulders and above the knees, and use the momentum to bring the opponent down. Once a player is successfully tackled, the tackler must release the ball, allowing for a contest for possession.
- **Maul:** When a ball carrier is held up by one or more opponents, and one or more of the ball carrier's teammates bind on the ball carrier.
- **Ruck:** Structure formed following a tackle, when at least one player from each team is in contact, on their feet, over the ball (▶ Fig. 37.1).
- **Scrum:** A method of restarting play that involves players packing closely together with their heads down and attempting to gain possession of the ball. It consists of eight players from each team, bound together in three rows, pushing against the opposing team's similar formation, with the ball thrown into the gap between the two teams (▶ Fig. 37.2).

Among the riskiest maneuvers, tackling accounts for the majority of injuries due to the high-speed, high-impact collisions.[3] Misdirected tackles, in particular, can result in shoulder, neck, and head injuries, including concussions.[13] The England Professional Rugby Injury Surveillance Project of 2019–2020 found that 52% of all match injuries were attributed to tackles, with ball carriers and tacklers each accounting for half of the total percentage.[3] This same investigation also found that the most common injury resulting from a tackle was an SRC, which made up 39% of all injuries to the tackler and 17% of the ball carrier. In this 2019–2020 season, it was found that 19% of reported SRCs occurred during training, and 17% of players sustained at least one match SRC with 4% sustaining more than one match SRC.[3] High or illegal tackles, where the tackler's head contacts another player's head or neck, or tackles where the tackler is upright rather than crouched, are particularly associated with a higher risk of SRC.[14] A 2015 systematic review of rugby league SRCs found these injuries account for nearly 29% of all injuries resulting from illegal play, while only accounting for 9% of injury in legal play.[14]

Scrummages (or "scrums") are unique to rugby and involve a head-on competition between two teams' forward players, often leading to injuries. Although rules have been modified over the years to reduce risk, scrums are still a common source of spinal injuries due to extreme pressure and unusual loading on the neck and spine.[9,13,15]

Peripheral nerve injuries can occur during direct contact, such as a tackle or collision, but they also frequently result from the compression forces involved in scrummaging, potentially leading to conditions like "burners" or "stingers."[16]

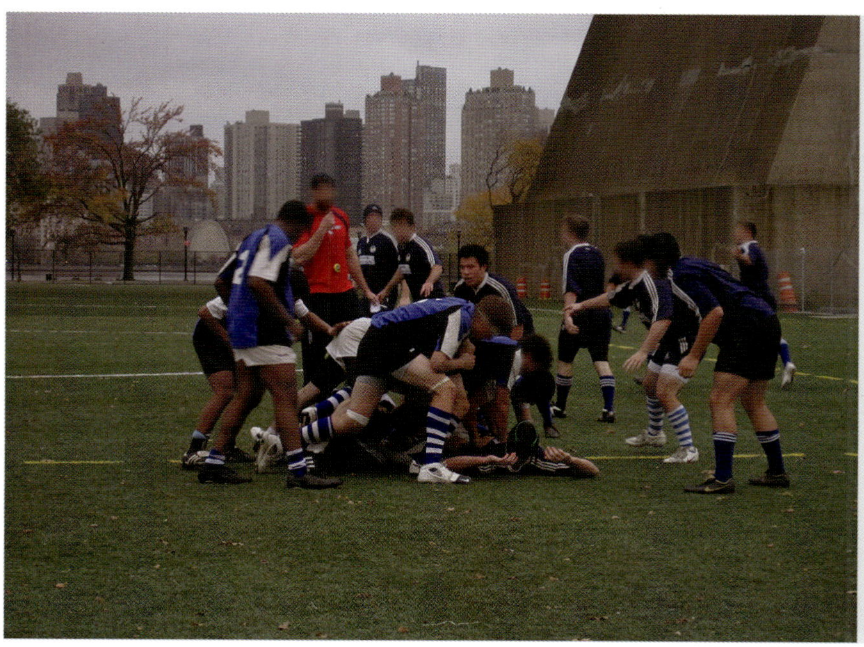

Fig. 37.1 Rugby ruck. (Image courtesy of Dr. Andrew K. Chan.)

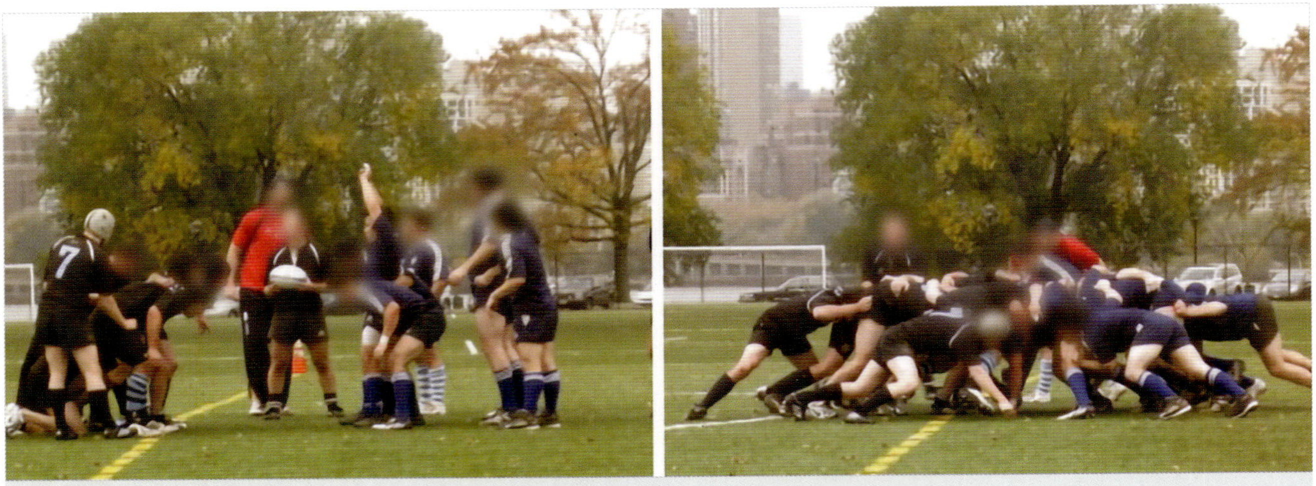

Fig. 37.2 Rugby scrum line-up on left, and active scrum on right. (Images courtesy of Dr. Andrew K. Chan.)

These are injuries to the brachial plexus causing temporary, intense burning or stinging pain shooting down the arm. Neurological finger injuries in rugby are also common and can include ulnar nerve injuries, which result in a claw hand, or median nerve injuries leading to conditions like ape hand or carpal tunnel syndrome.

37.4 Most Neurotrauma by Position

In rugby, the forwards, numbered 1 to 8, are typically the larger and stronger players responsible for winning possession of the ball through scrums, lineouts, rucks, or mauls. The forwards are generally involved in physical aspects of the game requiring close contact situations. They are often more exposed to high-impact collisions and, consequently, have a higher propensity for injuries such as SRC, shoulder dislocations, and spinal injuries.[1,17]

The backs, numbered 9 to 15, are usually smaller, quicker, and more agile than the forwards. Their roles often involve exploiting space on the field, running with the ball, passing, kicking, and scoring tries. The backs are more likely to be involved in high-speed collisions, often when being tackled while running at pace, increasing their risk for SRCs. They are also more prone to ligament and joint injuries, such as ankle sprains and knee ligament injuries.[1,17]

Studies have found that forwards experience approximately double the rate of injuries to the head, neck, and peripheral nervous system.[1,17] The majority of injuries to forwards primarily stemmed from the ruck and maul aspects of the game, whereas the most common cause of injuries to backs resulted from being tackled.[2] The hooker, who plays a crucial role in the scrum and lineouts, and the outside center, responsible for creating opportunities in open play and defending against the opposition's attacks, represented the playing positions most susceptible to injury.[2] However, it is important to note that other studies have found no significant differences in injury rates or severity between the broad positions.[18]

37.5 Rule Changes

Rugby governing bodies have made several rule changes and implemented measures over the years to enhance player safety and reduce the risk of neurotrauma. This reflects a growing recognition of the potential long-term effects of SRCs and other head injuries.

One of the most significant changes is the High Tackle Sanction Framework, introduced to reduce the risk of head injuries by changing player behavior.[19] This rule prioritizes the sanctioning of high tackles, which are more likely to result in head injuries. The framework provides clear definitions and guidelines for determining whether a high tackle warrants a penalty, a yellow card (temporary removal from the game), or a red card (permanent removal from the game).

Another important change has been the introduction of the Head Injury Assessment (HIA) protocol.[20] This allows for a player suspected of having an SRC to be temporarily replaced while a medical assessment is conducted off-field. If an SRC is diagnosed, the athlete is not allowed to return to the game. This ensures that players are not pressured to continue playing when an SRC is suspected, reducing the risk of further injury.

The sport has also revised the laws around scrummaging to reduce the force of impact upon engagement, thus reducing the risk of neck and spinal injuries.[9,21] In 2007, the International Rugby Board implemented a new law for scrum engagement. Changes include alterations to the engagement sequence and the requirement for front-row players to be bound before the scrum engagement. The aim was to reduce impact force and scrum collapses, a frequent cause of head and neck injuries.

Moreover, in youth rugby, there are rules to limit or eliminate certain elements of the adult game that are associated with a higher risk of injury. For instance, some youth leagues do not allow full-contact tackles or introduce scrums and tackles gradually as players get older and more experienced.

Collectively, the combination of rule changes and enforcement, along with improvements in coaching and player awareness, aims to make the game safer without fundamentally altering its nature of strength and athleticism. They represent a recognition by all parties (organizations, fans, and the players themselves) of the paramount importance of player safety, and particularly brain health, in the long-term success of rugby.

37.6 Clinical Pearls

- Proper tackling techniques and adherence to the High Tackle Sanction Framework are crucial in reducing the incidence of concussions and other head injuries in rugby.
- The Head Injury Assessment (HIA) protocol is a critical tool for the immediate evaluation of players suspected of sustaining a sports-related concussion, ensuring timely and appropriate medical intervention.
- Modifications in scrum engagement laws aim to decrease the risk of neck and spinal injuries by reducing the force of impact upon engagement.
- Early recognition and management of neurotrauma, including concussions, are imperative for preventing long-term neurological complications in rugby players.

References

[1] Evans SL, Davis OE, Jones ES, Hardy J, Owen JA. Match and training injury risk in semi-professional rugby union: a four-year study. J Sci Med Sport. 2022; 25(5):379–384

[2] Symons GF, Clough M, Fielding J, et al. The neurological consequences of engaging in Australian collision sports. J Neurotrauma. 2020; 37(5):792–809

[3] Kemp S, Starling L, Anstiss T, et al. England Professional Rugby Injury Surveillance Project: Season Report 2019-20. 2021

[4] Brooks JH, Fuller CW, Kemp SP, Reddin DB. Epidemiology of injuries in English professional rugby union: part 1 match injuries. Br J Sports Med. 2005; 39(10):757–766

[5] Adams JW, Alvarez VE, Mez J, et al. Lewy body pathology and chronic traumatic encephalopathy associated with contact sports. J Neuropathol Exp Neurol. 2018; 77(9):757–768

[6] Kenney K, Iacono D, Edlow BL, et al. Dementia after moderate-severe traumatic brain injury: coexistence of multiple proteinopathies. J Neuropathol Exp Neurol. 2018; 77(1):50–63

[7] Ling H, Morris HR, Neal JW, et al. Mixed pathologies including chronic traumatic encephalopathy account for dementia in retired association football (soccer) players. Acta Neuropathol. 2017; 133(3):337–352

[8] Raftery M, Tucker R, Falvey ÉC. Getting tough on concussion: how welfare-driven law change may improve player safety—a Rugby Union experience. Br J Sports Med. 2020; 55(10):527–529

[9] Gianotti S, Hume PA, Hopkins WG, Harawira J, Truman R. Interim evaluation of the effect of a new scrum law on neck and back injuries in rugby union. Br J Sports Med. 2008; 42(6):427–430

[10] Stokes KA, Locke D, Roberts S, et al. Does reducing the height of the tackle through law change in elite men's rugby union (The Championship, England) reduce the incidence of concussion? A controlled study in 126 games. Br J Sports Med. 2021; 55(4):220–225

[11] Echemendia RJ, Meeuwisse W, McCrory P, et al. The Sport Concussion Assessment Tool 5th Edition (SCAT5): background and rationale. Br J Sports Med. 2017; 51(11):848–850

[12] Echemendia RJ, Ahmed OH, Bailey CM, et al. The Concussion Recognition Tool 6 (CRT6). Br J Sports Med. 2023; 57(11):692–694

[13] Quarrie KL, Cantu RC, Chalmers DJ. Rugby union injuries to the cervical spine and spinal cord. Sports Med. 2002; 32(10):633–653

[14] Gardner A, Iverson GL, Levi CR, et al. A systematic review of concussion in rugby league. Br J Sports Med. 2015; 49(8):495–498

[15] Silver JR. Injuries of the spine sustained in rugby. Br Med J (Clin Res Ed). 1984; 288(6410):37–43

[16] Bowles DR, Canseco JA, Alexander TD, Schroeder GD, Hecht AC, Vaccaro AR. The prevalence and management of stingers in college and professional collision athletes. Curr Rev Musculoskelet Med. 2020; 13(6): 651–662

[17] Gissane C, Jennings DC, Cumine AJ, Stephenson SE, White JA. Differences in the incidence of injury between rugby league forwards and backs. Aust J Sci Med Sport. 1997; 29(4):91–94

[18] Whitehouse T, Orr R, Fitzgerald E, Harries S, McLellan CP. The epidemiology of injuries in Australian Professional Rugby Union 2014 Super Rugby Competition. Orthop J Sports Med. 2016; 4(3):2325967116634075

[19] Worldrugby.org. Laws of the game: World Rugby Laws. Laws of the Game | World Rugby Laws. Accessed June 23, 2023 at: https://www.world.rugby/the-game/laws/home

[20] Worldrugby.org Laws of the Game: World Rugby Laws. Accessed June 23, 2023 at https://www.world.rugby/the-game/laws/home

[21] Fuller C W, Raftery M, Readhead C, Targett SGR, Molloy MG. Impact of the International Rugby Board's experimental law variations on the incidence and nature of match injuries in southern hemisphere professional rugby union. S Afr Med J. 2009; 99(4):232–237

38 Aquatic Sports

Kelly Jiang and Nicholas Theodore

Summary

Aquatic sports can lead to severe neurological injuries as a result of high-force mechanisms of watercrafts and sporting equipment, marine organism exposure, prolonged time to treatment, and the potential for drowning and developing hypothermia. Injury patterns depend on the sport and can include high cervical spine injuries from diving into shallow water, traumatic brain injury from ejection off watercrafts, decompression sickness from scuba diving, or more minor traumatic injuries to the brain and spine from surfing. Spinal immobilization is critical to reduce the severity of injury during patient extrication. In drowning victims, airway management should be prioritized.

Keywords: water sports, surfing, diving, swimming, watercrafts

38.1 Introduction

Aquatic sports represent a less common but often severe cause of injuries to the central nervous system (CNS) compared to other athletic activities. They account for only 3.5% of sports-related traumatic brain injuries (TBIs), but nonetheless are associated with significantly longer hospital admissions, increased medical complications, and higher mortality.[1] Compared to athletic injuries that occur on land, aquatic injuries are proportionally more likely to involve the spinal column and cause spinal cord injury (SCI).[2] The severity of water-related injuries relates to the unique set of risk factors experienced by athletes, including high-force mechanisms of watercrafts and sporting equipment, marine organism exposure, prolonged time to treatment due to difficult patient extrications, and susceptibility to drowning and hypothermia.[3] Injuries during water activities are most commonly sustained by young males and associated with reckless behavior, lack of experience with the sport, intoxication, or incapacitating disorders such as epilepsy.[4,5] Water sports injuries also follow seasonal and geographic patterns, with more injuries occurring during summer months and in coastal areas.[6] However, water sports are a heterogeneous entity which vary greatly in speed, body positioning, and the likelihood of impact with the floor, equipment, or other people. Consequently, CNS injuries differ by the activity performed and can be broadly categorized as traumatic, submersion, or decompression injuries (▶ Table 38.1; ▶ Fig. 38.1).

38.2 Mechanisms of CNS Injuries in Common Aquatic Sports

38.2.1 Diving

Diving is the leading cause of recreation-related quadriplegia.[7] Diving injuries commonly affect the cervical spine due to head-first jumps into shallow water or water of unknown depth, resulting in impact with the floor of the body of water. Injuries arising from head strikes are usually the result of significant axial force on the flexed or hyperextended cervical spine. High speeds associated with diving and full bodyweight loading onto the axial skeleton in the inverted position often causes fractures or dislocations at the C5–C7 levels that may injure the spinal cord.[7] Cervical spine injuries sustained during diving can be severe, often causing permanent neurologic disability with minimal improvement over time.[7]

38.2.2 Personal Watercraft Riding

Personal watercrafts (PWCs) are motorized boats such as jet skis or wave runners upon which riders sit or stand. PWCs are powered by jet propulsion and can reach speeds up to 70 miles per hour. Despite being able to travel at the same speeds as motor vehicles traversing a highway, PWCs can be operated without a license and even by children as young as 12 years old in some states. Unfortunately, injuries while riding PWCs can be severe. Traumatic brain and spine injuries can occur from direct collision with a stationary object or another vehicle, ejection off the watercraft, axial loading, straddling of handlebars, or falling into the stream of the hydrostatic jet.[8,9] Spine injuries most commonly involve fractures in the thoracic and lumbar regions. Although most injuries occur in young men, epidemiological studies have shown that females have greater risk of mortality

Table 38.1 Neurological injuries associated with aquatic sports and their presentations, diagnoses, and treatments

Neurological injury	Sport	Presentation	Diagnosis	Treatment
Spinal cord injury	Diving, watercraft riding, wave-related activities	Neck pain, paralysis, numbness, dyspnea	CT	Skull traction for cervical injury, decompressive laminectomy
Traumatic brain injury	Surfing, diving, watercraft riding	Loss of consciousness, headache, vomiting, nausea, seizure, pupil dilation, slurred speech	CT	Oxygen, intravenous fluids, decompressive craniectomy for surgical emergencies, cognitive and physical rest for mild cases
Decompression illness	Scuba diving	Joint pain, headache, paresthesia, numbness, livedo reticularis rash, stroke symptoms, ataxia, seizure	Clinical examination	Hyperbaric oxygen, intravenous fluids
Myelopathy	Surfing, swimming	Paraparesis, urinary retention, hyperesthesia	MRI	Physical therapy, spinal decompression surgery

Abbreviations: CT, computed tomography; MRI, magnetic resonance imaging.

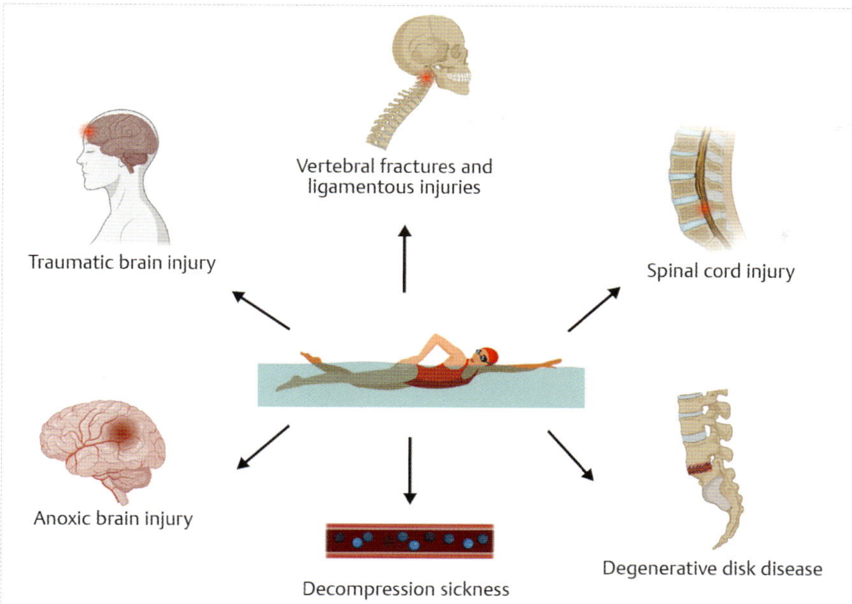

Fig. 38.1 Mechanisms of axial loading causing traumatic cervical spine injuries in aquatic sports. (Created with BioRender.com.)

and severe systemic injuries.[8] Riding PWCs can be especially dangerous for children, with 42% of pediatric injuries from PWCs requiring admission to the intensive care unit and unfortunately causing disability.[10]

38.2.3 Scuba Diving

There are over three million scuba divers in the United States.[11] The sport has increased in popularity in recent years, along with improvements in diving equipment and training regimens. Injuries are relatively uncommon owing to widespread access to professional dive guides and devices that improve navigation ability such as modern diving computers. Decompression sickness and arterial gas embolisms are collectively referred to as decompression illness, and colloquially known as "the bends." Decompression illness occurs when divers rapidly ascend to the surface of the water and inert gas bubbles dissolved in the tissues release into the bloodstream. Bubble embolization can obstruct venous drainage or arterial flow in the brain and spinal cord, resulting in infarction, tissue death, and subsequent neurological deficits.[12] In 2014, approximately 500 divers suffered from decompression sickness and required evacuation to a hyperbaric chamber facility for specialized treatment.[11] Despite treatment morbidity is high, with nearly a third of patients suffering long-term neurological symptoms.[13]

38.2.4 Surfing

Surfing has also gained popularity over the last few decades, and consequently, the number of CNS injuries sustained during the sport have also increased.[14] Most surfing injuries are relatively minor and are caused by the athlete striking a surfboard, another surfer, or the ocean floor.[15] However, injuries can become especially severe during wipeouts, referring to a fall off the board from high wave forces, and in dangerous weather conditions. Injuries to the head and neck, including TBI, account for up to 37% of all surfing injuries.[16]

Surfer's myelopathy, an atraumatic SCI causing symptoms of paraparesis, urinary retention, and hyperesthesia, is a rare but significant form of injury that can result from surfing.[17] This form of injury most frequently occurs in first-time surfers and is caused by abnormal posturing or prolonged hyperextension, which is believed to cause ischemia to the spinal arteries. Most patients completely recover, but some remain paraplegic.[18]

38.2.5 Swimming

Swimming features low-impact forces and is recommended as a rehabilitation activity for people recovering from injuries including incomplete SCI.[19] When swimming pool rules are followed, the risk of severe neurological injury is low as collisions between athletes, equipment, or the pool floor are rare and usually occur at low velocity. The most common swimming injuries are therefore typically due to overuse and degeneration in long-term swimmers. Hyperextension of the back is commonly required for proper swim strokes, and chronic hyperextension can result in degenerative disk disease and spondylosis.[20]

38.2.6 Wave-Related Activities

Shallow water beaches are sites of casual recreation for people of all ages and abilities who may be inexperienced in the ocean and who may not understand the danger of waves. Unlike other aquatic sports, injuries from wave-related recreation often occur to people who do not participate in high-risk athletic activities. These injuries are typically seen in older individuals with preexisting degenerative spine conditions such as spinal stenosis or spondylosis which can predispose to spinal injury.[21] Injuries usually result from the patient striking against an oncoming wave or the ocean floor while tumbling in waves. There is a wide range of severity of wave-related traumas, with age and wave height associated with greater injury severities.[22] Cervical injuries including fractures and dislocations are the most commonly reported neurological traumatic injuries. Permanent neurological injury is present in an estimated 65% of patients with these cervical injuries, with permanent quadriplegia affecting nearly 13%.[23]

38.3 Diagnosis and Treatment of Aquatic Injuries

38.3.1 Traumatic Spine Injuries

Traumatic injuries during water sports pose significant additional risk due to difficulty with patient extrication. Improper manipulation of the patient during extrication, transport, or handling causes a substantial amount of SCI.[24,25] Recognition of potential spinal trauma and immobilization of the spine prior to removal from the water is crucial to prevent further injury. Spinal immobilization should be considered when there is significant trauma, altered mental status, loss of consciousness, back pain, numbness or weakness, or a significant distracting injury.[25] Immediate threats to airway, breathing, and circulation should be addressed in accordance with Advanced Trauma and Life Support protocols.

When the victim is found in the water, manual stabilization techniques such as the extended arm head splint should be applied. In this maneuver, the rescuer positions both the arms of the victim above the head and against the ears. The rescuer can then maintain this head splint by holding the two arms of the victim together with one hand while swimming to shore. Several other methods like the vice-grip and body hug have also been described.[26] Once removed from the water, the victim should be secured to a backboard with a cervical collar and blocks as soon as feasible with as little spinal motion as possible.

Patients with SCI can be subject to acute, life-threatening cardiovascular and respiratory complications which should be managed immediately.[27] Once the patient has been stabilized at the hospital, clinicians should obtain a computed tomography (CT) scan and perform a thorough neurological examination. The decision for surgical management should be made as soon as possible as early intervention is associated with improved neurological recovery and reduced morbidity.[27] When there is significant cord compression, neurological deficits, or vertebral instability, a decompressive laminectomy should be performed with traction considered in cervical spine injuries.[27]

38.3.2 Traumatic Brain Injuries

Prior to admitting a patient with TBI to the hospital, the most important priority is the prevention of secondary brain injury caused by hypoxia and hypotension.[28] When severe TBI is suspected, patients should be rapidly transferred to definitive care with basic airway strategies, oxygenation, and fluid resuscitation using isotonic crystalloids. At the hospital, patients should be initially managed using the Advanced Trauma Life Support algorithm prioritizing airway, breathing, and circulation. Neurological assessment using the Glasgow Coma Score and pupillary examination should be performed every 1 to 2 hours to determine injury severity as rapid deterioration is possible.[28] Patients with reduced level of consciousness, suspected skull fracture, multiple episodes of vomiting, or dangerous mechanisms of injury should receive CT imaging immediately.[29] CT scans can identify large epidural and subdural hematomas, intracerebral hemorrhage, and dural penetrating injuries which are life-threatening neurosurgical emergencies that should be treated with decompressive craniectomy.[28] Fortunately, most cases of water sport related TBI are mild and do not require surgical or inpatient management. Cognitive and physical rest is recommended when an athlete sustains a mild TBI, with gradually increasing levels of activity until full recovery.[29]

38.3.3 Submersion Injuries

Unlike land sports, aquatic sports have a risk of drowning. In the United States, 11 fatal drownings are estimated to occur each day.[30] The competitive nature of sports may lead individuals to misjudge their capability to navigate the water, engage in dangerous behaviors, or become subject to injury preventing the person from staying afloat. Hypoxic-ischemic brain damage following cardiac arrest occurs within the first few minutes of submersion. Of patients who sustain injury in a drowning incidence, around 16% will die from anoxic brain injury.[31] Primary management of the cardiac arrest is critical to prevent further neurological impairment. Drowning victims should be placed supine and evaluated for responsiveness and breathing. When resuscitation is necessary, airway management should be prioritized before compressions as the cardiac arrest is usually from hypoxia. Unfortunately, submersion injuries often cause permanent long-term neurological dysfunction.[32]

38.3.4 Decompression Injuries

Decompression illness is not limited to scuba divers and can occur beginning at depths of about 20 feet. Decompression illness often presents immediately after surfacing from a dive. Over half of the patients show symptoms within 10 minutes of surfacing, and nearly all present within 4 hours.[33] The diagnosis of decompression illness is clinical, so careful neurological examination is critical. Any divers with symptoms arising after surfacing should be thoroughly assessed. Neurological symptoms may initially appear mild, and the diver may not be aware of the deficits. Symptoms can range from fatigue and joint pain to altered consciousness, ataxia, and seizure. In 85% of cases, pain, constitutional symptoms, numbness, paresthesias, and rash are the initial symptoms.[12] Divers with suspected decompression illness should be given 100% oxygen and intravenous fluids while placed horizontally.[12] Oxygen administration flushes out the inert gases and can attenuate damage caused by tissue hypoxia. In severe cases, recompression therapy in a hyperbaric chamber should be considered. When oxygen is administered during recompression, bubble volumes decrease, improving oxygenation in affected tissues.[12] Approximately half of the patients with decompression illness affecting the spinal cord will make a full recovery with no residual symptoms following recompression therapy.[12] Due to the severity of decompression illness and the possibility of recurrence, clinicians should maintain a high index of suspicion in any patient with a recent history of diving.

38.4 Conclusion

CNS injuries in aquatic sports are uncommon but can cause severe and permanent neurological deficits. Aquatic sports can involve high-risk maneuvers, often with overconfident partakers who may be unaware of the hazards. Prevention efforts should focus on public health education discouraging dangerous behaviors such as diving in waters of unknown depths, participating in aquatic activities while intoxicated, and unsupervised operation of personal watercrafts.

38.5 Clinical Pearls

- Aquatic sports can lead to severe neurological injuries as a result of high-force mechanisms of watercrafts and sporting equipment, marine organism exposure, prolonged time to treatment, and the potential for drowning and developing hypothermia.
- Diving is the leading cause of quadriplegia due to head-first jumps into shallow water or water of unknown depth.
- Personal watercrafts, such as jet skis or wave runners, can lead to traumatic brain and spine injuries as a result of direct collision, ejection off the watercraft, axial loading, straddling of handlebars, or falling into the stream of the hydrostatic jet.
- Scuba divers who ascend too quickly can develop decompression illness, also known as "the bends," and should be treated with 100% oxygen and intravenous fluids.
- Surfers can develop injuries to the head and neck most commonly from wipeouts into high-speed waves.
- Spinal immobilization is critical to reduce the severity of injury during patient extrication.
- In drowning victims, airway management should be prioritized before compressions as cardiac arrest is typically due to hypoxia.

38.6 Disclosures

Kelly Jiang: None.
Nicholas Theodore: Royalties from Globus Medical. Stock Ownership in Globus Medical. Consultant for Globus Medical. On Scientific Advisory Board/Other Office for Globus Medical.

References

[1] Winkler EA, Yue JK, Burke JF, et al. Adult sports-related traumatic brain injury in United States trauma centers. Neurosurg Focus. 2016; 40(4):E4

[2] Kane I, Ong A, Radcliff KE, Austin LS, Maltenfort M, Tjoumakaris F. Epidemiology of aquatic and recreational water sport injuries: a case-control analysis. Orthopedics. 2015; 38(9):e813–e818

[3] Ehrhardt JD, Jr, Newsome K, Das S, McKenney M, Elkbuli A. Evaluation and management of watercraft-related injuries for acute care surgeons: towards improving care and implementing effective public health prevention policies. Ann Surg Open. 2022; 3(1):e149

[4] Bell GS, Gaitatzis A, Bell CL, Johnson AL, Sander JW. Drowning in people with epilepsy: how great is the risk? Neurology. 2008; 71(8):578–582

[5] Chalmers D, Morrison L. Epidemiology of non-submersion injuries in aquatic sporting and recreational activities. Sports Med. 2003; 33(10):745–770

[6] Karantanas AH. Common injuries in water sports. In: Karantanas AH, ed. Sports Injuries in Children and Adolescents. Springer; 2010:289–317

[7] Korres DS, Benetos IS, Themistocleous GS, Mavrogenis AF, Nikolakakos L, Liantis PT. Diving injuries of the cervical spine in amateur divers. Spine J. 2006; 6(1):44–49

[8] Donnally CJ, III, Metser G, Roth ES, Moo Young JP, Rush AJ, III, Al Maaieh MA. Spine trauma from personal watercraft usage. Spine. 2018; 43(17): E1033–E1039

[9] Shin SH, Johnson BP, Mentzer CJ, et al. Personal watercraft related injuries—16-year experience from a level I trauma center. Am Surg. 2017; 83(12): e485–e487

[10] Rubin LE, Stein PB, DiScala C, Grottkau BE. Pediatric trauma caused by personal watercraft: a ten-year retrospective. J Pediatr Surg. 2003; 38(10): 1525–1529

[11] Buzzacott P, Schiller D, Crain J, Denoble PJ. Epidemiology of morbidity and mortality in US and Canadian recreational scuba diving. Public Health. 2018; 155:62–68

[12] Vann RD, Butler FK, Mitchell SJ, Moon RE. Decompression illness. Lancet. 2011; 377(9760):153–164

[13] Gempp E, Blatteau JE. Risk factors and treatment outcome in scuba divers with spinal cord decompression sickness. J Crit Care. 2010; 25(2):236–242

[14] Kozminski BU, Ahmed N, Cautela FS, et al. Surfing-related head injuries presenting to United States emergency departments. J Orthop. 2019; 19: 184–188

[15] Taylor DMD, Bennett D, Carter M, Garewal D, Finch CF. Acute injury and chronic disability resulting from surfboard riding. J Sci Med Sport. 2004; 7 (4):429–437

[16] Nathanson A, Haynes P, Galanis D. Surfing injuries. Am J Emerg Med. 2002; 20(3):155–160

[17] Swinney C, Flick D, Cheng M. Atraumatic spinal cord injury in the novice surfer: a comprehensive review and update. Hawaii J Med Public Health. 2017; 76(2):43–47

[18] Thompson TP, Pearce J, Chang G, Madamba J. Surfer's myelopathy. Spine. 2004; 29(16):E353–E356

[19] Loy K, Bareyre FM. Rehabilitation following spinal cord injury: how animal models can help our understanding of exercise-induced neuroplasticity. Neural Regen Res. 2019; 14(3):405–412

[20] Wanivenhaus F, Fox AJS, Chaudhury S, Rodeo SA. Epidemiology of injuries and prevention strategies in competitive swimmers. Sports Health. 2012; 4 (3):246–251

[21] Chang SKY, Tominaga GT, Wong JH, Weldon EJ, Kaan KT. Risk factors for water sports-related cervical spine injuries. J Trauma. 2006; 60(5): 1041–1046

[22] Lurie T, Berman E, Hassan S, et al. Early predictors of near-shore spinal injuries among emergency department patients. J Emerg Med. 2021; 60(1):17–24

[23] Griepp DW, De la Garza Ramos R, Lee J, et al. Beach breaking waves and related cervical spine injuries: a level one trauma center experience and systematic review. World Neurosurg. 2022; 160:e471–e480

[24] Green BA, Gabrielsen MA, Hall WJ, O'Heir J. Analysis of swimming pool accidents resulting in spinal cord injury. Paraplegia. 1980; 18(2):94–100

[25] Theodore N, Hadley MN, Aarabi B, et al. Prehospital cervical spinal immobilization after trauma. Neurosurgery. 2013; 72 Suppl 2:22–34

[26] Wernicki P, Szpilman D. Immobilization and extraction of spinal injuries. In: Bierens J, ed. Drowning. Springer;2014:621–628

[27] Sandean D. Management of acute spinal cord injury: a summary of the evidence pertaining to the acute management, operative and non-operative management. World J Orthop. 2020; 11(12):573–583

[28] Vella MA, Crandall ML, Patel MB. Acute management of traumatic brain injury. Surg Clin North Am. 2017; 97(5):1015–1030

[29] Silverberg ND, Iaccarino MA, Panenka WJ, et al. American Congress of Rehabilitation Medicine Brain Injury Interdisciplinary Special Interest Group Mild TBI Task Force. Management of concussion and mild traumatic brain injury: a synthesis of practice guidelines. Arch Phys Med Rehabil. 2020; 101 (2):382–393

[30] CDC WONDER. Accessed February 3, 2023 at: https://wonder.cdc.gov/

[31] Hwang V, Shofer FS, Durbin DR, Baren JM. Prevalence of traumatic injuries in drowning and near drowning in children and adolescents. Arch Pediatr Adolesc Med. 2003; 157(1):50–53

[32] Suominen PK, Sutinen N, Valle S, Olkkola KT, Lönnqvist T. Neurocognitive long term follow-up study on drowned children. Resuscitation. 2014; 85(8): 1059–1064

[33] Howle LE, Weber PW, Hada EA, Vann RD, Denoble PJ. The probability and severity of decompression sickness. PLoS One. 2017; 12(3):e0172665

39 The Future of Traumatic Brain Injury

Meghana Bhimreddy, Andrew M. Hersh, and Nicholas Theodore

Summary
Traumatic brain injury (TBI) is a significant public health burden with lifelong effects, prompting the development of tools and devices that can enhance our diagnostic accuracy and provide more effective management options that improve patient outcomes. These tools range from imaging and biological markers to innovative devices utilizing eye-tracking, pupillometry, virtual reality, and more. Greater application and development of these resources will pave the way for more personalized and targeted interventions that optimize patient care and recovery in the future.

Keywords: traumatic brain injury, biomarkers, pupillometry

39.1 Overview

Traumatic brain injury (TBI) is responsible for more than 69 million disability-adjusted life years (DALYs) lost annually.[1] As the proportion of patients living with neurological deficits continues to rise, the development of advanced tools for assessment and workup is an active area of research. New technologies are being designed and implemented to improve the accuracy, reliability, and sensitivity of TBI grading and management, including the use of imaging biomarkers, blood and saliva biomarkers, pupillometry, and eye tracking. This chapter will delve into greater detail on these tools.

39.2 Imaging Biomarkers

Computed tomography (CT) and magnetic resonance imaging (MRI) scans are routinely used for the workup of TBI and to assist in treatment planning and monitoring. CT scans can help identify fractures, foreign objects, hemorrhage, and edema, while MRI provides a sharper view of the soft tissue anatomy and can identify microhemorrhages that are otherwise absent on CT. Several neuroimaging techniques for biomarkers are under investigation for their potential in diagnosis and evaluation of injury progression, including various MRI techniques, positron emission tomography (PET), and electroencephalography (EEG).

One of these MRI tools is diffusion tensor imaging (DTI), which is capable of visualizing the organization and integrity of white matter tracks in the brain.[2] DTI offers several helpful measurements, such as fractional anisotropy (FA), which quantifies the coherence and directionality of water diffusion within white matter tracts. The FA magnitude varies over the acute-to-subacute phases of TBI and can be correlated with neurological recovery. Higher FA values in the splenium of the corpus callosum during the acute and subacute phases of injury are correlated with improved outcomes; however, higher FA in the genu of the corpus callosum has been associated with inferior outcomes.[3] The variability in FA values over time has complicated studies examining the predictability and clinical utility of DTI and imaging biomarkers for TBI, leading some to consider it unreliable. However, by studying precisely how these values change over time, a correlation can be drawn between the FA values at any given timepoint after injury and the predicted neurological recovery. Other DTI measurements, such as mean diffusivity, axial diffusivity, and radial diffusivity, also show potential as markers for tissue microstructure alterations, such as edema and myelin damage.[4]

Additionally, dynamic contrast-enhanced imaging, which provides information on the hemodynamic and vascular characteristics of tissue, can detect perfusion deficits in specific locations of the brain in patients with a history of TBI. These scattered deficits show a significant correlation to measures of memory, reaction time, and self-reported symptoms of stress.[5] As a result, these markers may have prognostic value for the long-term recovery of TBI. Similarly, cerebrovascular reactivity imaging, which assesses the ability of intracranial blood vessels to dilate and constrict in response to changes in blood flow and metabolic demands, is emerging as an additional imaging tool for classifying TBI. Lower values of the cerebrovascular reactivity index, which represents the relative vasodilatory capacity of the brain, are associated with worse outcomes and more severe TBI.[6]

PET generates three-dimensional images of the distribution and concentration of a radioactive tracer in the body and is widely used for workup of cancer by detecting increased metabolic activity at the site of cancer tissue. PET scans can provide insight on cerebral blood flow, cerebral metabolism, neurodegenerative processes, and neuroinflammation. PET scans show significant differences in glucose metabolism in the thalamus, brain stem, and cerebellum of patients with TBI based on the level of consciousness at the time of the test.[7] PET imaging with ^{11}C-PBB3, a radiotracer for tau aggregates, revealed an association between increased tau deposits and late-onset neuropsychiatric outcomes in patients with chronic TBI. These individuals demonstrated a close correlation between ^{11}C-PBB3 binding capacity in the white matter and post-traumatic psychosis, suggesting a role for tau as a marker for long-term psychiatric outcomes post TBI.[8]

EEG has had some commercial success for patients with TBI, including the BrainScope One system, an FDA-approved medical tool consisting of a handheld device and a disposable headset with integrated EEG sensors. The system utilizes signal processing algorithms and machine learning techniques to analyze EEG signals and other physiological data collected from the patient. The machine compares this data to a reference database and provides an assessment of the patient's brain activity, as well as an objective measure of the likelihood of the presence of intracranial bleeding. For a healthcare provider, this data can be useful in the triage and management of TBI patients.[9]

Although these imaging approaches are promising, further studies are needed to determine their sensitivity for identifying TBI. In addition, some tools have been predominantly limited to research settings and necessitate further refinement before widespread clinical applicability or device innovation can be achieved.

39.3 Blood and Saliva Biomarkers

Blood and saliva-based biomarkers are also emerging as important tools for TBI diagnosis and management. Notably, the

FDA has approved the use of glial fibrillary acidic protein (GFAP) and ubiquitin C-terminal hydrolase (UCH-L1) for the detection of intracranial lesions after mild to moderate TBI.[10] In addition to these markers, neurofilament light chain protein (NF-L), tau, and S100B have been extensively studied for their role in aiding the diagnosis, prognosis, and monitoring of brain injury.[11] GFAP is an intermediate filament protein found predominantly in astrocytes. Studies indicate that GFAP is superior to other established markers in differentiating between TBI patients with head CT abnormalities and those with normal CT scans. Higher levels of GFAP are correlated with the severity of TBI, as well as the level of care needed for treatment.[12] Similarly, neuron-specific enolase is an enzyme primarily found in neurons that exhibits increased serum levels with greater severity of injury.[13] Furthermore, S100B, a calcium-binding protein found mostly in astrocytes, can be used to determine the presence of secondary injury in TBI patients, as well as predict long-term outcomes.[14]

Blood and saliva biomarkers also include hormones, miRNA species, and extracellular vesicles.[15] Some miRNA species, such as miR-320c-1, miR-133a-5p, miR-769–5p, let-7a-3p, and miR-1307–3p, can be used to classify the level of concussion. These markers show a strong correlation to the reaction time component of the ImPACT concussion assessment tool.[16] Other miRNA species are associated with the number of head impacts during football practice and the number of previous concussions in a patient, suggesting that miRNA expression may have substantial utility and accuracy in predicting TBI severity and outcomes.[17]

The medical technology sector is developing handheld, portable devices that can measure the levels of biomarkers in the blood or saliva to aid physicians in their diagnostic and management decisions. The i-STAT Alinity platform's TBI Plasma test was the first to receive FDA clearance for its ability to rapidly measure and display the levels of GFAP and UCH-L1 in the blood.[18] Despite these advancements, there are a number of confounding variables that influence biomarker expression, thereby limiting their utility in the clinical space. For instance, there is no standard as to the optimal sampling time. Furthermore, blood biomarkers show success in predicting outcomes for mild TBI but decrease in utility for more complex cases involving multiple concussive episodes. In addition, there is a lack of demographic diversity among studies on the newer biomarkers, resulting in decreased generalization to the entire TBI cohort.[19]

39.4 Pupillometry/Eye Tracking

Quantitative pupillometry, which involves the measurement and analysis of pupillary responses, has shown promise as an affordable, noninvasive tool for diagnosing, classifying, and predicting outcomes in TBI. Modern pupillometers are quite sophisticated and have the capacity to store data regarding pupil size, constriction velocity, dilation velocity, latency, redilation time, and pupillary escape.[20] These variables are typically combined using the neurological pupil index (NPi), a metric developed by NeurOptics to quantify pupillary reactivity and provide an objective measure of the pupillary light reflex.[21] A higher NPi value indicates a more intact and healthier pupillary response, while a lower value suggests impaired pupillary function. The application of pupillometry to TBI has great promise, with studies correlating decreased pupillary constriction, dilation velocity, and NPi with TBI severity.[20] Pupillometry can also be used to monitor recovery from TBI. Studies conducted on post-TBI military personnel found longer constriction latency and slower constriction and dilation velocities.[22]

Eye-tracking technology is another noninvasive tool with significant developments in modern TBI diagnosis and management. The FDA has approved devices that conduct rapid eye-tracking assessments, including visual tracking tasks or stimulus recognition tasks. NeuroSync, which received FDA clearance in 2021, uses virtual reality and artificial intelligence to combine 60-second eye-tracking assessments and neurocognitive assessments with physician-provided patient symptoms and medical history to provide an individualized report on the severity and type of deficit caused by TBI.[23] RightEye's Brain Health EyeQ system is another tool that can help diagnose moderate-to-severe TBI by measuring vertical smooth pursuit. The system tracks participants' eye movements as they follow a white dot that moves up and down the screen. Alterations from this path are associated with severity of injury.[24]

39.5 Sports-Specific Tools

Several tools are actively being developed and utilized in the athletic realm for TBI diagnosis and management. Video analysis is increasingly used to not only determine extent of injury, but also reveal trends in TBI occurrence. A review of video footage of concussions from 2015 to 2017 in the National Football League (NFL) revealed that cornerbacks were at highest risk of brain injury. The investigation also determined that tackling was more likely to result in a concussive episode compared to other contact interactions. Furthermore, a rising trend was noted in the number of helmet-to-ground impacts, revealing an area for future investment and improvement.[25]

In addition, the NFL launched a mouthguard sensor program in 2019 as part of a commitment to promoting the health and safety of players. These devices measure the magnitude and direction of linear and rotational severity and acceleration.[26] Innovations in helmet design are also being made in an effort to decrease the likelihood of concussive episodes. Guardian Cap and Defend Your Head ProTech Helmet Cap are two add-on caps to traditional football helmets. These two pieces of supplementary equipment are currently being tested by the NFL in simulated impacts. Guardian Cap and Defend Your Head ProTech Helmet Cap show potential for minimizing injury, with a 9 and 5% reduction in force impact, respectively.[27]

39.6 Conclusion

Over the past decade, numerous innovations have been made surrounding the diagnosis, management, and prevention of TBI. Both imaging and blood/saliva biomarkers have seen increased interest and commercial success. The enhanced capabilities of virtual reality, machine learning, and artificial intelligence have

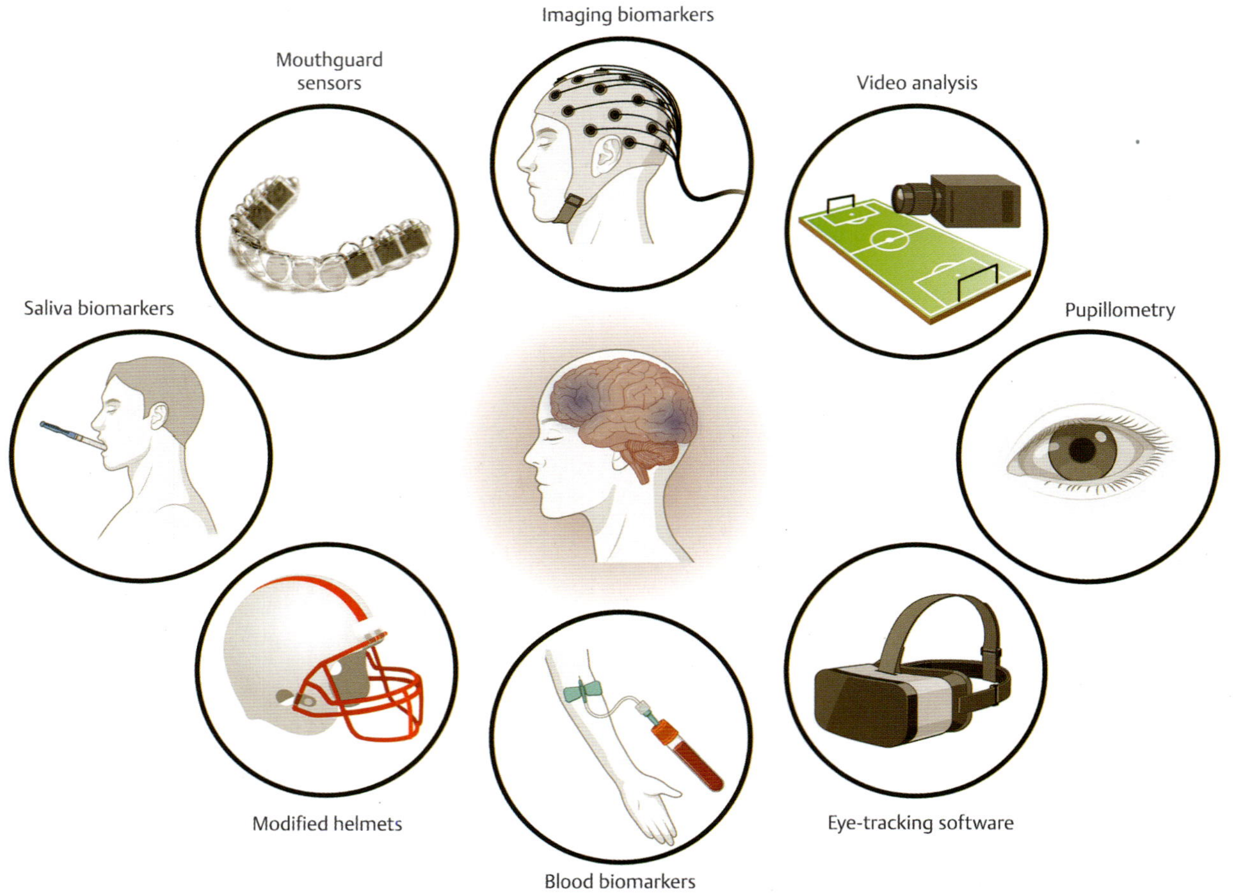

Fig. 39.1 Current areas of innovation for traumatic brain injury (TBI) diagnosis, tracking, management, and prevention. (Created with BioRender.com)

supported the development of pupillometry, eye-tracking, and video analysis software. Due to increased public awareness surrounding the effects of TBI in sports-related settings, athletic organizations are also investing heavily in the creation of new metrics and sensors that can help characterize concussive episodes. Due to the complexity of TBI, the optimal tools will likely involve a combination of the aforementioned components (▶ Fig. 39.1). Continued research in these areas holds promise for advancing our understanding of TBI, improving diagnostics, and optimizing treatment and prevention strategies.

39.7 Clinical Pearls

- Emerging technologies, such as imaging biomarkers, blood and saliva biomarkers, pupillometry, and eye tracking, can enhance the precision, dependability, and sensitivity of TBI grading and management.
- FA values, which can be obtained from DTI during acute-to-subacute phases of TBI, appear to be correlated to neurological recovery.
- Dynamic contrast-enhanced imaging and cerebrovascular reactivity imaging provide valuable insight into perfusion deficits and vascular reactivity after TBI, with prognostic implications for long-term recovery.
- PET scans can suggest level of consciousness and long-term psychiatric outcomes after TBI based on detection of glucose metabolism and tau aggregates, respectively.
- Higher serum levels of GFAP, neuron-specific enolase, and S100B are correlated with greater severity of TBI.
- miRNA species can classify both previous and current concussion severity.
- Development of handheld devices to measure biomarkers is currently in progress and can be useful for rapid diagnostic and management decisions during triage.
- Quantitative pupillometry can record pupil size, constriction velocity, dilation velocity, latency, redilation time, and pupillary escape to track TBI recovery over time.
- Sports organizations, such as the NFL, are using video analysis and mouthguard sensors to proactively decrease occurrence and severity of TBI among players.

39.8 Disclosures

Meghana Bhimreddy: None.
Andrew M. Hersh: None.
Nicholas Theodore: Royalties from Globus Medical. Stock Ownership in Globus Medical. Consultant for Globus Medical. On Scientific Advisory Board/Other Office for Globus Medical.

References

[1] Dewan MC, Rattani A, Gupta S, et al. Estimating the global incidence of traumatic brain injury. J Neurosurg. 2018; 130(4):1080–1097

[2] Douglas DB, Iv M, Douglas PK, et al. Diffusion tensor imaging of TBI: potentials and challenges. Top Magn Reson Imaging. 2015; 24(5): 241–251

[3] Edlow BL, Copen WA, Izzy S, et al. Diffusion tensor imaging in acute-to-subacute traumatic brain injury: a longitudinal analysis. BMC Neurol. 2016; 16:2

[4] Winklewski PJ, Sabisz A, Naumczyk P, Jodzio K, Szurowska E, Szarmach A. Understanding the physiopathology behind axial and radial diffusivity changes—what do we know? Front Neurol. 2018; 9:92

[5] Liu W, Wang B, Wolfowitz R, et al. Perfusion deficits in patients with mild traumatic brain injury characterized by dynamic susceptibility contrast MRI. NMR Biomed. 2013; 26(6):651–663

[6] Zeiler FA, Ercole A, Czosnyka M, et al. Continuous cerebrovascular reactivity monitoring in moderate/severe traumatic brain injury: a narrative review of advances in neurocritical care. Br J Anaesth. 2020: S0007–0912(19)30966–3

[7] Hattori N, Huang SC, Wu HM, et al. Correlation of regional metabolic rates of glucose with Glasgow coma scale after traumatic brain injury. J Nucl Med. 2003; 44(11):1709–1716

[8] Takahata K, Kimura Y, Sahara N, et al. PET-detectable tau pathology correlates with long-term neuropsychiatric outcomes in patients with traumatic brain injury. Brain. 2019; 142(10):3265–3279

[9] Science & Technology. BrainScope. Accessed May 11, 2023 at: https://www.brainscope.com/sciencetechnology

[10] Anderson TN, Hwang J, Munar M, et al. Blood-based biomarkers for prediction of intracranial hemorrhage and outcome in patients with moderate or severe traumatic brain injury. J Trauma Acute Care Surg. 2020; 89(1):80–86

[11] Shahim P, Zetterberg H. Neurochemical markers of traumatic brain injury: relevance to acute diagnostics, disease monitoring, and neuropsychiatric outcome prediction. Biol Psychiatry. 2022; 91(5):405–412

[12] Abdelhak A, Foschi M, Abu-Rumeileh S, et al. Blood GFAP as an emerging biomarker in brain and spinal cord disorders. Nat Rev Neurol. 2022; 18(3): 158–172

[13] Giacoppo S, Bramanti P, Barresi M, et al. Predictive biomarkers of recovery in traumatic brain injury. Neurocrit Care. 2012; 16(3):470–477

[14] Raabe A, Kopetsch O, Woszczyk A, et al. S-100B protein as a serum marker of secondary neurological complications in neurocritical care patients. Neurol Res. 2004; 26(4):440–445

[15] Porteny J, Tovar E, Lin S, Anwar A, Osier N. Salivary biomarkers as indicators of TBI diagnosis and prognosis: a systematic review. Mol Diagn Ther. 2022; 26(2):169–187

[16] Di Pietro V, Porto E, Ragusa M, et al. Salivary microRNAs: diagnostic markers of mild traumatic brain injury in contact-sport. Front Mol Neurosci. 2018; 11:290

[17] Hicks SD, Onks C, Kim RY, et al. Refinement of saliva microRNA biomarkers for sports-related concussion. J Sport Health Sci. 2023; 12(3):369–378

[18] Korley FK, Jain S, Sun X, et al. TRACK-TBI Study Investigators. Prognostic value of day-of-injury plasma GFAP and UCH-L1 concentrations for predicting functional recovery after traumatic brain injury in patients from the US TRACK-TBI cohort: an observational cohort study. Lancet Neurol. 2022; 21(9): 803–813

[19] Hier DB, Obafemi-Ajayi T, Thimgan MS, et al. Blood biomarkers for mild traumatic brain injury: a selective review of unresolved issues. Biomark Res. 2021; 9(1):70

[20] Boulter JH, Shields MM, Meister MR, Murtha G, Curry BP, Dengler BA. The expanding role of quantitative pupillometry in the evaluation and management of traumatic brain injury. Front Neurol. 2021; 12:685313

[21] Chen JW, Vakil-Gilani K, Williamson KL, Cecil S. Infrared pupillometry, the Neurological Pupil index and unilateral pupillary dilation after traumatic brain injury: implications for treatment paradigms. Springerplus. 2014; 3:548

[22] Capo-Aponte J, Urosevich T, Walsh D, Temme L, Tarbett A. Pupillary light reflex as an objective biomarker for early identification of blast-induced mTBI. J Spine. 2013; S4:1–4

[23] Product. NeuroSync. December 12, 2022. Accessed May 11, 2023 at: https://www.neurosync.health/product/

[24] Carter G. RightEye introduces functional vision EyeQ-the first automated test designed to measure dynamic vision skills that impact quality of life. RightEye, LLC. January 4, 2023. Accessed May 11, 2023 at: https://righteye.com/righteye-introduces-functional-vision-eyeq-the-first-automated-test-designed-to-measure-dynamic-vision-skills-that-impact-quality-of-life/

[25] Lessley DJ, Kent RW, Funk JR, et al. Video analysis of reported concussion events in the National Football League during the 2015–2016 and 2016–2017 seasons. Am J Sports Med. 2018; 46(14):3502–3510

[26] NFL. NFL expands partnership to eight research universities to measure on-field head impacts using novel mouthguard sensors. NFL.com. February 28, 2023. Accessed May 11, 2023 at: https://www.nfl.com/playerhealthandsafety/equipment-and-innovation/equipment-testing/nfl-expands-partnership-to-eight-research-universities-to-measure-on-field-head-

[27] Newton D. Guardian caps: are the soft-shelled football helmet covers effective at limiting head injuries? ESPN. Accessed May 11, 2023 at: https://www.espn.com/nfl/story/_/id/32140546/guardian-caps-soft-shelled-football-helmet-covers-effective-limiting-head-injuries

40 Concussions in the National Football League: Using Data to Improve Game Safety

Christina Mack, Scott L. Zuckerman, Erin B. Wasserman, Mackenzie M. Herzog, Gary S. Solomon, Soren Jonzzon, Patricia Roby, and Allen Sills

Summary
Throughout the last decade, the National Football League (NFL) has implemented significant changes to improve head injury and sports-related concussion (SRC) safety through all facets of the league. The data-driven approach to SRC management that includes robust diagnosis and detection programs, rigorous return to play protocols, and rules changes are all aimed toward making the game safer. The objectives of this chapter are to: (1) report the process of building the NFL's concussion data source, (2) describe the injury data collected through the NFL's concussion protocol, and (3) explain how the data are used to implement injury reduction initiatives. Through the utilization of the data, research, and technology, the NFL has enhanced safety with over 50 rules changes while preserving key elements of game play. Through the detailed data collection, the knowledge of SRC has increased while the rates of concussion have decreased. Player safety has been and will continue to be a priority and an ever-evolving point of emphasis to protect all NFL athletes.

Keywords: concussion, injury reduction, American football/National Football League, data linkage/integrated evidence hubs, evidence-based medicine, agile analytics

40.1 Introduction

The National Football League (NFL) represents the pinnacle of American football and is the most watched sport in the United States (US).[1] When it comes to player health and safety, the NFL takes a comprehensive and evidence-based approach. The strategies utilized to enhance player health and safety include standardized data collection and linkage, collaboration with focused epidemiologic, medical, and engineering experts to test products and analyze data, and communication across the NFL to discuss findings and enact interventions. Evidence generated from robust, NFL-wide data collection is reviewed and discussed by medical experts as well as decision-makers across football operations, the NFL Players Association, the NFL Competition Committee, and club leadership to identify channels through which to make the game safer and inform decisions to improve player health and safety. This continuous evaluation and data-driven approach is central to strategic planning to further game safety.

Player health and safety programs are evidence-driven and directed toward all injuries that impact NFL athletes with priority given to those injuries that have a high measurable burden (i.e., frequently occurring and/or resulting in a large number of days missed from football participation). For this reason, sports-related concussion (SRC) is a longstanding and high priority focus of NFL injury detection, prevention, and management efforts.[2,3] The programs in place have been critical to increasing the safety of the game for NFL athletes and are shared with all other levels of play to improve safety for football players of all ages. The NFL's approach to SRC management includes prevention, detection, diagnosis, and return to football participation. All protocols, interventions, and programs are subject to annual evaluation for quality and effectiveness and to inform further opportunities to prevent injuries based on the data collected.

The current chapter summarizes the NFL's data-driven approach to SRC management including implementing robust diagnosis and detection programs, defining and applying return to play protocols, and policy and rule changes aimed at making the game safer. Our objectives in this chapter are to: (1) report the process of building the NFL's concussion data source, (2) describe the injury data collected through the NFL Head, Neck and Spine Committee's Concussion Diagnosis and Management Protocol ("Concussion Protocol"), and (3) explain how the data are used to implement injury reduction initiatives.

40.2 Building the Data Source

40.2.1 The NFL Injury Analytics Database

The NFL has dedicated significant time and resources to the collection and analysis of injury data, along with contextual information about the players and their injuries. These efforts were enhanced in 2011 with the creation of an evidence hub and analytic program.[4] The backbone of the data collection system is an audited electronic medical record (EMR) system, which collects all workplace injuries that impact NFL players, regardless of whether the injury resulted in missed time. NFL team athletic trainers and physicians report medical data into the EMR, which then provides a foundation for a large, linked evidence platform. Real-time quality checks and linkage with other sources occur consistently throughout the season. These other sources include all game day SRC evaluation reports submitted in real time by health professionals present at each game on the sidelines and in the booth, video evaluation of each play in which a game day concussion occurs, equipment and field surface information, and documentation of return to participation through an external concussion management application (C3Logix). These data may be analyzed alongside NFL game statistics, player participation data, and player tracking data ascertained through certain wearable tracking devices to provide a comprehensive view of the injury. Combined with the data extracted from the NFL player EMR, these data form the concussion-related portion of the NFL Injury Analytics Database (▶ Fig. 40.1).

40.2.2 Medical Data Optimization

Data optimization includes two major advances, namely, the use of the player EMR and in-season auditing of data, as described above. An independent group of epidemiologists provide daily, in-season audits of both the EMR and concussion management data captured within C3Logix to ensure completeness of the data

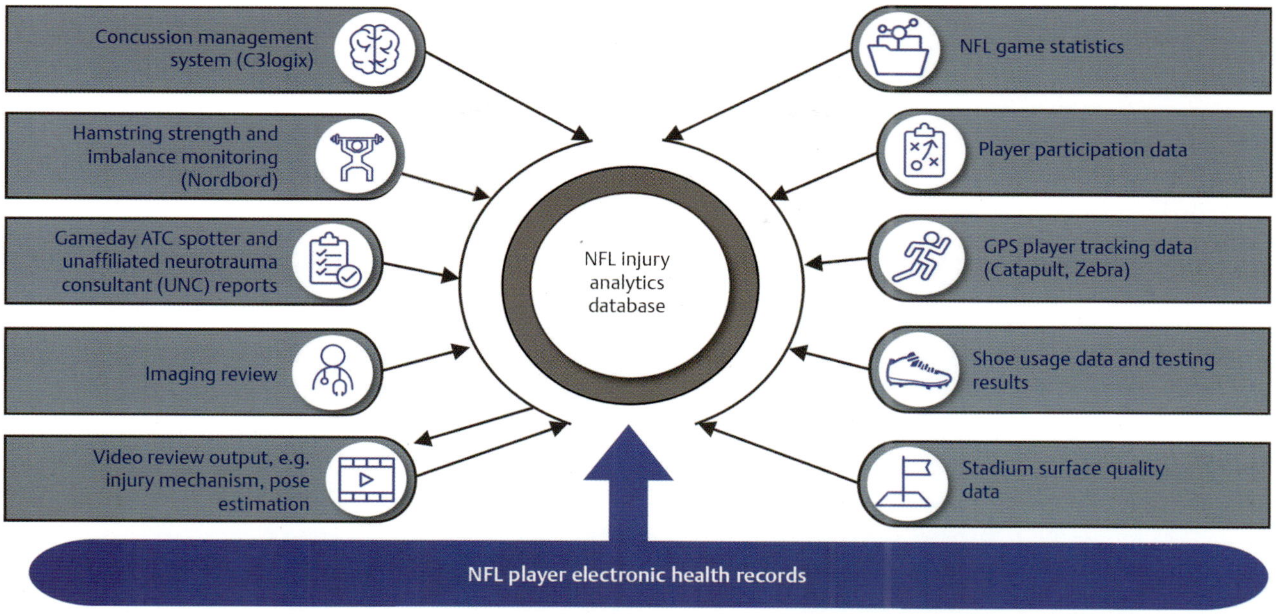

Fig. 40.1 The National Football League (NFL) Injury Analytics Database is built on an electronic medical record foundation with linkage to real-time data entry from several sources of each game. ATC, certified athletic trainer. (Source: Figure modified from Dreyer NA, et al. *Sports Health*. 2019;11(5):440–445, with permission from Sage Journals.)

entered. Additionally, all data sources are compared against each other to detect any inconsistencies. Comparison between data sources improves documentation of concussion diagnoses and associated information by providing a continuous feedback loop to medical staff who are caring for players. Missing data are noted and audited in real time to avoid memory decay by the medical staff inputting the information. These high-quality, trusted, well-described, and often-used evidence sources drive the use of these data for decision-making across operational bodies, the Competition Committee, and club leadership.

Medical staff entering data in the EMR are trained at least annually on data entry, and the data submitted are regularly audited for data quality, discrepancies, and completeness. Medical staff also receive reference guidance documents for data entry in key areas or confusing workflows within the EMR. These practices provide standardized definitions and improve consistency in data entry across the 32 NFL clubs. Media reports on injuries are assessed by trained reviewers with a background in epidemiology and compared with EMR-based reports to ensure completeness, although medical staff assessment of the injury is the source of truth over media reports, which are used to identify potential missed reports. Data issues are queried in near real time by trained analytic staff, and continual feedback and training are provided on standardized reporting procedures and data quality.

40.2.3 Team Behind the Team

Good data quality requires consistent and reliable reporting from qualified sources. The data source is only as good as the information entered into it, and accurate, complete data comes from experienced medical professionals. Without accurate injury data, the ability to analyze concussion trends and design efforts to improve safety would be compromised.[4,5,6] At each NFL game, at least 30 gameday medical staff are present (▶ Fig. 40.2). One type of medical personnel critical to acute concussion evaluation is the unaffiliated neurotrauma consultant (UNC), an independent clinician who works alongside the team physician to perform an acute assessment for a potential concussion, with the team physician responsible for the final decision.[7] Additionally, each team may have other specialists including certified athletic trainers (ATs), primary care physicians, orthopedists, and chiropractors. The stadium team consists of an additional UNC and two AT spotters located in an elevated stadium booth, a radiology technician, an ophthalmologist, two paramedics, one dentist, one emergency response physician, and one airway management physician.[8]

40.3 Concussion Detection, Diagnosis, and Return to Participation

Following a concussion, early diagnosis and proper management have` been shown to improve clinical outcomes.[9] Moreover, concussions often rely on an athlete communicating his/her own symptoms, and even then, diagnosis can prove challenging, especially on a busy sideline.[10] As such, the NFL and NFL Players Association (NFLPA) have implemented several sequential measures over the last decade to enhance SRC detection, diagnosis, and reporting on game days, which are summarized in the following (▶ Table 40.1). Additionally, we herein summarize acute assessment involved in making the concussion diagnosis and the return to participation (RTP) process.

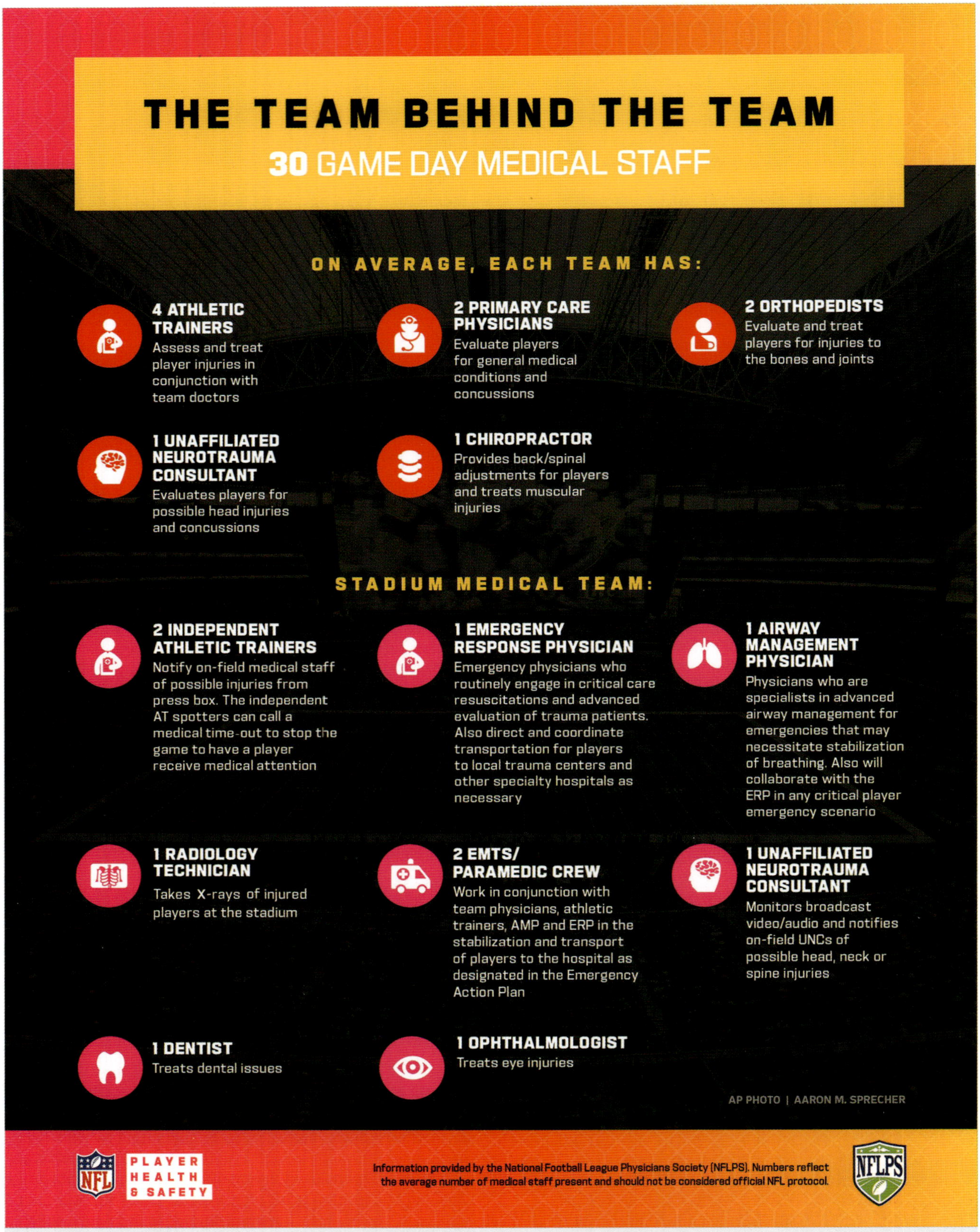
THE TEAM BEHIND THE TEAM
30 GAME DAY MEDICAL STAFF
ON AVERAGE, EACH TEAM HAS:
4 ATHLETIC TRAINERS
Assess and treat player injuries in conjunction with team doctors
2 PRIMARY CARE PHYSICIANS
Evaluate players for general medical conditions and concussions
2 ORTHOPEDISTS
Evaluate and treat players for injuries to the bones and joints
1 UNAFFILIATED NEUROTRAUMA CONSULTANT
Evaluates players for possible head injuries and concussions
1 CHIROPRACTOR
Provides back/spinal adjustments for players and treats muscular injuries
STADIUM MEDICAL TEAM:
2 INDEPENDENT ATHLETIC TRAINERS
Notify on-field medical staff of possible injuries from press box. The independent AT spotters can call a medical time-out to stop the game to have a player receive medical attention
1 EMERGENCY RESPONSE PHYSICIAN
Emergency physicians who routinely engage in critical care resuscitations and advanced evaluation of trauma patients. Also direct and coordinate transportation for players to local trauma centers and other specialty hospitals as necessary
1 AIRWAY MANAGEMENT PHYSICIAN
Physicians who are specialists in advanced airway management for emergencies that may necessitate stabilization of breathing. Also will collaborate with the ERP in any critical player emergency scenario
1 RADIOLOGY TECHNICIAN
Takes X-rays of injured players at the stadium
2 EMTS/ PARAMEDIC CREW
Work in conjunction with team physicians, athletic trainers, AMP and ERP in the stabilization and transport of players to the hospital as designated in the Emergency Action Plan
1 UNAFFILIATED NEUROTRAUMA CONSULTANT
Monitors broadcast video/audio and notifies on-field UNCs of possible head, neck or spine injuries
1 DENTIST
Treats dental issues
1 OPHTHALMOLOGIST
Treats eye injuries
AP PHOTO | AARON M. SPRECHER
NFL
PLAYER HEALTH & SAFETY
Information provided by the National Football League Physicians Society (NFLPS). Numbers reflect the average number of medical staff present and should not be considered official NFL protocol.
NFLPS

Fig. 40.2 All medical personnel present at each National Football League (NFL) game. AMP, airway management physician; EMTS, emergency medical technicians; ERP, emergency response physician; UNCs, unaffiliated neurotrauma consultants. (Reproduced from The National Football League and the National Football League Players Association.)

Table 40.1 Measures to increase concussion detection

Program
Certified Athletic Trainer (AT) Spotter Program
Unaffiliated Neurotrauma Consultant (UNC) Program
Pregame "60-Minute Meeting"
Gameday Technology and Injury Video Review System (IVRS)
Medical Tents
Player Education

40.3.1 Athletic Trainer (AT) Spotter Program

The AT Spotter Program was initiated as a pilot venture in 2011 and was launched formally in 2012.[11] All AT spotters undergo annual training and receive regular online video education related to signs of injury identification and the decision-making processes involved in calling a medical time-out. The AT spotters are independent from any NFL team. Each AT spotter is an experienced sports medicine provider, with a minimum of 10 years of athletic training experience and a requirement of clinical experience at the collegiate or professional level. The primary duty of the AT spotter is to alert the officials and/or sideline medical staff about players on the field who may need medical evaluation for potentially concussive injuries, but go undetected.[11] At each game, two AT spotters monitor the field of play as well as video during the game via the Injury Video Replay System (IVRS), which includes nine camera angles *(see the section "Gameday Technology and Injury Video Review System (IVRS)" for more on the IVRS)*, to serve as an extra sets of eyes to detect potential concussions. In case a player sustains an impact and appears to need medical attention, but is not removed from the game for evaluation, the AT spotter may call a game official to initiate a "medical time-out." At that time, the medical staff will evaluate the player using the previously described assessments. AT spotters are the only individuals with the authority to call a medical time-out. AT spotters document all potential injuries they observe, tag them to a corresponding play on video to be reviewed after the game, and note whether the evaluation resulted in a concussion diagnosis. Moreover, AT spotters also identify head impacts that do not result in injurious behavior and work with the IVRS technicians to tag these within the videos. During each game, AT spotters communicate regularly with head team athletic trainers and medical staff via radio.

From 2015 to 2017, as many as 680 head or neck injuries were flagged by the AT spotter program, representing about 30% of all tagged injuries and an average of two per game. Although most of these flags did not result in a diagnosis of concussion, they facilitated evaluation and communication with the sideline medical team.[11] In 2023, there were 33 total medical time-outs called by an AT spotter during the 2023 season, which was almost double the previous season.

40.3.2 Unaffiliated Neurotrauma Consultant (UNC) Program

The UNC program began in 2013, after a 2012 pilot, as a joint venture between the medical leadership of the NFL Head, Neck and Spine (HNS) Committee and the NFLPA.[12] Each UNC is an independent physician board certified in neurology, neurologic surgery, emergency medicine, or physical medicine and rehabilitation, or a sports medicine primary care physician. All are approved by the HNS Committee, the NFL, and the NFLPA, and undergo yearly trainings on the Concussion Protocol and game day processes, the prior season's concussion data, the pregame medical meeting, use of the sideline tent, locker room evaluations, the video review process, and game day communications. The program began with one UNC at each game and increased to two field UNCs (one on each sideline), and then, based on data showing the effectiveness of the program, added a third UNC to the booth. Field UNCs serve as independent experts available to assist each team's medical staff in identifying injury behavior and evaluating for concussion, pursuant to the Concussion Protocol. The field UNCs are present for all evaluations of potential concussions and stingers that occur during the game and assist with identifying mechanisms and signs of injury. The booth UNC assists AT spotters in identification of injury behavior through video review of the IVRS. Each UNC has access to video review both on the sideline and in the booth.

Each UNC submits a report following each game that includes all concussion evaluation activities that occurred in the game. These reports are used throughout the season to monitor game day concussion protocols, as well as at the end of the season for program evaluation and identification of any needed protocol additions or modifications. In 2016 and 2017, UNCs submitted an average of 1.9 evaluations per game with high sensitivity (93–97%) and specificity (81–88%) for concussion diagnosis among players who were evaluated.[12] Although not published in peer-reviewed manuscript form, a 2023 NFL press release reported that the average rate of evaluations per game was 1.6.[13] The NFL and NFLPA review the UNC program each year from the perspective of program evaluation and improvement.

40.3.3 Pregame "60-Minute Meeting"

To ensure that the Emergency Action Plan (EAP) is well understood by all stakeholders, the pregame "60-minute meeting" is performed 1 hour prior to game start and is led by the officials with all team- and stadium-based medical staff in attendance. The head home team physician reviews the aforementioned EAP, which includes all emergency procedures, medical equipment, ambulance location, airway management plan, and location of the designated Level I trauma center. The officiating team also meets the medical personnel on each sideline and encourages all health care providers present to speak up if there is concern for a player. The pregame medical meeting is analogous to the presurgical "time-out," which has been adopted worldwide to ensure clear expectations and open communication of the subsequent surgical procedure.[14] Just as in an operating room, the 60-minute meeting ensures that all appropriate channels for critical safety information are known by all medical personnel in the event of a potentially serious injury that would require enacting the EAP (e.g., cardiac arrest, severe spinal injury). It also provides a key benefit of ensuring visual identification of medical providers who may need to enter the field during the game.

40.3.4 Gameday Technology and Injury Video Review System (IVRS)

As alluded to in the AT spotter section, IVRS technology is present on the sidelines and in the booth. It allows for easy and quick review of each play by medical personnel. Implemented in 2012, the IVRS helps medical staff to review the mechanism of an injury to better understand the impacts that took place. Recently, the IVRS was expanded to include the HawkEye system, which uses many different stadium-based camera angles. Although this includes the live television video feed, the comprehensive set of views is independent of the broadcast feed. The AT spotters and UNCs have full access to the IVRS, which includes the ability to rewind, slow down, and zoom in to certain plays. Additionally, the IVRS helps to observe player behavior following a potential injury, which can guide evaluation, diagnosis, and management for head injuries.[15] Importantly, to maintain focus on the game and not get slowed down by the technology, each medical provider has several IVRS technicians available to help expedite review. Moreover, video review of the injury is now a mandatory part of the concussion evaluation to aid in detection of post-impact behaviors that may be obscured by other players or sideline personnel in real time. In addition to the IVRS, two-way radios are used as a mechanism for all medical providers to communicate during the game in an organized fashion.

40.3.5 Medical Tents

In 2017, the NFL implemented blue medical examination tents that can help medical staff immediately evaluate players in private and with fewer distractions, with a focus on concussion evaluation (▶ Fig. 40.3). All sideline concussion evaluations must be conducted in the tent. The NFL sideline is often a busy and hectic place. Taking the time to talk to a player, elicit potential symptoms, and administer a concussion examination is more effective in a controlled environment. This patient-centric approach embraces patient privacy as well, which may allow the athlete to be more forthright with symptoms. Additionally, other medical evaluations may be made in the tent, such as musculoskeletal injuries.

40.3.6 Player Education

The Concussion Protocol mandates that players receive concussion education annually.[16] This includes a description of the signs and symptoms of concussion, the Concussion Protocol, the medical providers involved in the protocol, and the importance of reporting any indications of concussion, including signs observed in other players. A growing and meaningful proportion of sideline evaluations are prompted in part or in full by self-reporting by the player, reflecting a culture change in football and sports overall.

40.3.7 Concussion Assessment

A detailed description of the Concussion Game Day Checklist can be found in ▶ Fig. 40.4. A player can be removed for an evaluation following specific triggers: (1) the player receives an impact to the head followed by injury behavior, signs, or symptoms; (2) the player reports symptoms or has signs of a concussion or stinger; or (3) an evaluation is triggered by any of the following people: team AT, booth AT, team physician, NFL official, coach, teammate, or UNC. In such a case, the player is then removed from the play and taken to the tent. The team physician and UNC review the video on the IVRS, and concomitantly, the booth UNC and AT spotters also review the video for any "No-Go" signs. "No-Go" signs trigger immediate removal from participation, even if the player's examination is normal, and the player is diagnosed with a concussion and enters the Concussion Protocol. These "No-Go" signs are loss of consciousness (including impact seizure and/or "fencing posture"), ataxia

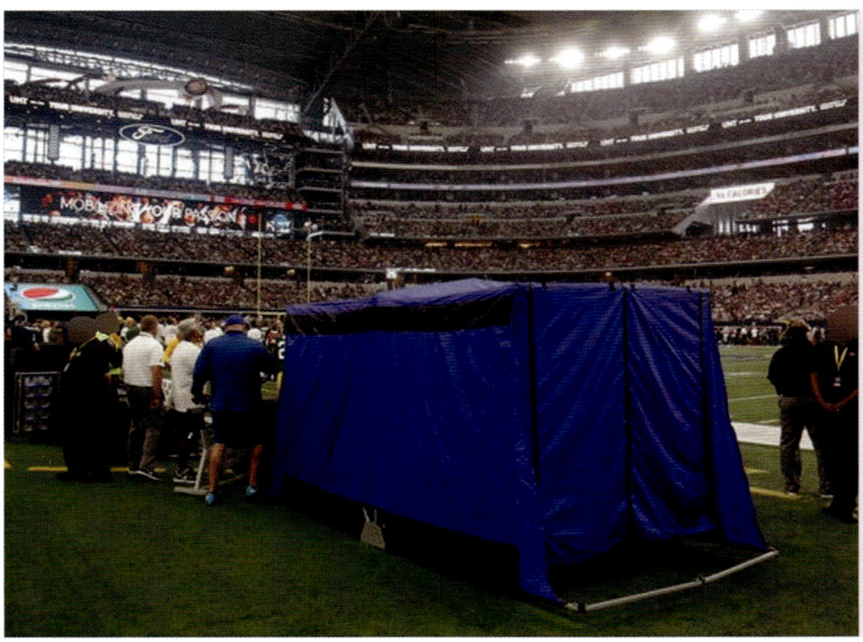

Fig. 40.3 Sideline medical evaluation tent. (Reproduced from The National Football League and the National Football League Players Association.)

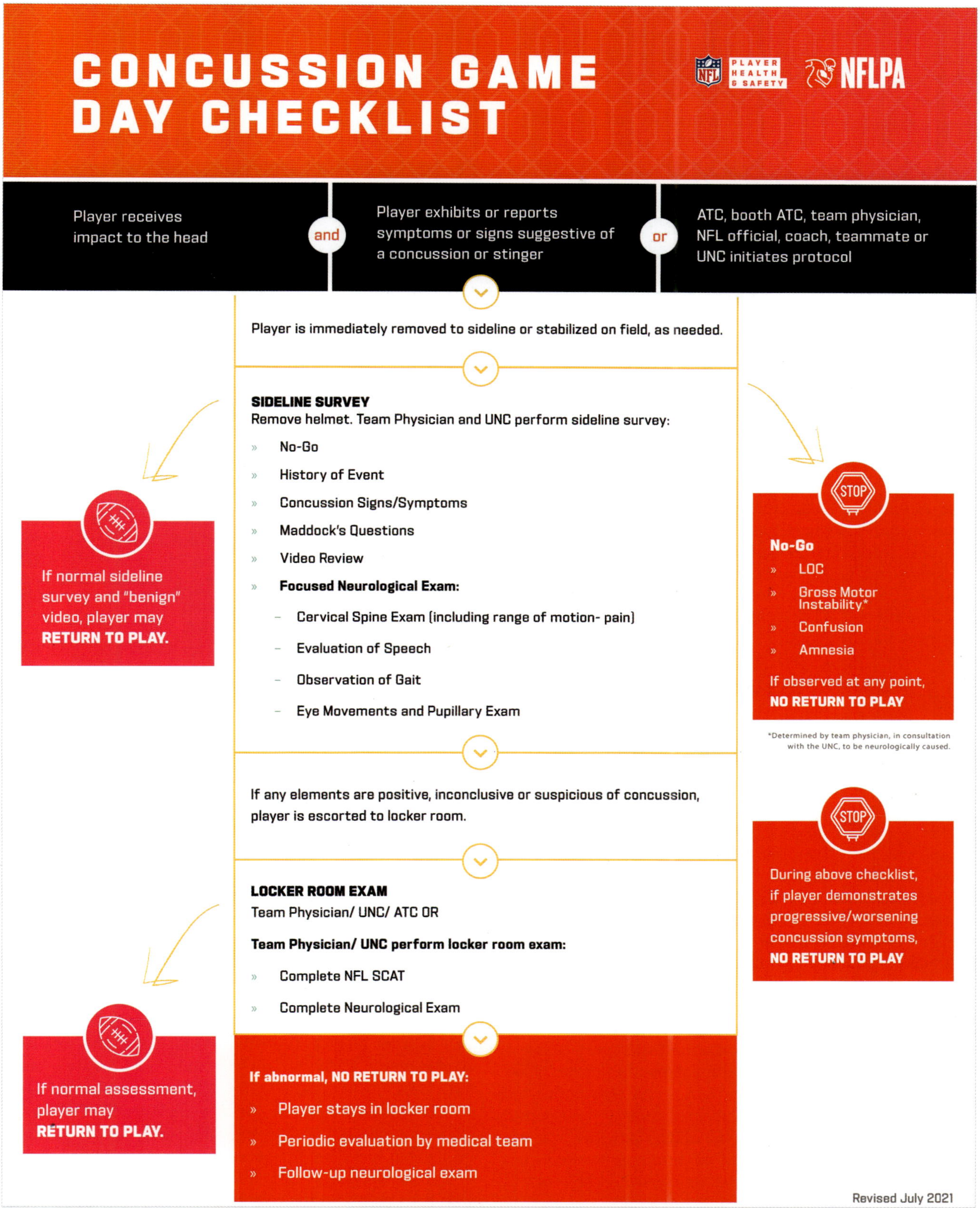

Fig. 40.4 National Football League (NFL) Concussion Game Day Checklist. ATC, certified athletic trainer; NFL SCAT, NFL Sports Concussion Assessment Test; LOC, loss of consciousness; UNC, unaffiliated neurotrauma consultant. (Reproduced from The National Football League and the National Football League Players Association.)

(abnormality of balance/stability, motor coordination, or dysfunctional speech), confusion, or amnesia. If the "No-Go" criteria are not present, the Sideline Survey begins. The Sideline Survey is performed by the designated team physician and UNC together and includes history of the event, assessment of any signs/symptoms, and Maddock's questions, which consist of the following: What venue are we at? What quarter is it? Who scored last? Who did you play last week? Did your team win the last game? A focused neurological examination is then performed, which includes a cervical spine examination, speech evaluation, gait observation, and extraocular and pupillary examination, as well as video review of the injury. If there is any concern for potential concussion, the player is escorted to the locker room for completion of the NFL Sports Concussion Assessment Test (SCAT) and the full neurologic examination by both the designated team physician and UNC. The UNC and team physician must reach a unanimous decision to clear the player; otherwise, the player will be held out. At the conclusion of each game, the UNC completes a full report that includes information on every evaluation, regardless of concussion diagnosis. Importantly, if a player is diagnosed with a concussion, the player stays in the locker room, and the medical team must continually evaluate the player with questions and serial neurologic examinations. All athletes assessed for concussion on game day (including those cleared) are reassessed the following day. This represents an attempt to capture athletes whose symptoms and/or signs present in a delayed fashion. The data from the UNC program is reviewed continually in-season as well as at the end of the season to identify any areas of needed training or improvement.

40.3.8 Return to Participation

After a diagnosis has been made, the player is removed from play and enters the Return-to-Participation (RTP) Protocol. The Protocol consists of five phases of progressively rigorous activity to assess presence or recurrence of concussion symptoms (▸ Fig. 40.5). Phase 1, symptom limited activity, involves participation in activities of daily living and light exercise. Phase 2, aerobic exercise, allows the athlete to utilize exercise equipment including treadmills and stationary bikes. Phase 3, football-specific exercise, allows the athlete to take part in noncontact sport-specific exercises limited to 30 minutes. The athlete should undergo neurocognitive testing overseen by the club neuropsychology consultant no earlier than the completion of Phase 2 and no later than the end of Phase 4 and is not permitted to participate in any contact activities until determined to be at neurocognitive baseline, or that any continued deficits are determined to have a nonconcussion cause. Phase 4, club-based noncontact training drills, allows the athlete to participate in all aspects of practice/training but does not permit contact with objects or other athletes. Phase 5, full football activity/clearance, is a return to full contact activities. If at any point during any of the phases of the protocol the athlete has recurrence or new symptoms, the athlete should be removed from that tier of activity and re-evaluated from a symptom and concussion burden perspective. Players spend a median time from concussion to return to participation of 9 days.[7]

Once a player progresses through Phase 5 without recurrence of signs and symptoms and neurocognitive testing is back to baseline, the team physician may fully clear the player to return to full participation. The player is also evaluated by an independent neurological consultant (INC) who is board certified in neurology, neurological surgery, emergency medicine, or physical medicine and rehabilitation, or is a certified sports medicine physician. All relevant tests and documentation of symptoms throughout the RTP protocol are shared with the INC, and the INC must confirm the team physician's decision for the player to return; only at that time, the athlete may then return to play.

40.4 Data-Driven Injury Prevention

Through the above-mentioned data collection measures, concussion detection efforts, and data optimization strategies, the NFL has established a strong research and program evaluation infrastructure for concussive injury. From this foundation, several scientific reports have summarized relevant concussion data to identify interventions and contribute to the body of evidence related to SRC. A total of 26 peer-reviewed manuscripts detailing the NFL's concussion policies, medical personnel, and head injury safety measures are summarized in ▸ Table 40.2. One key published peer-reviewed manuscript was the publication of the official Concussion Protocol.[17] Using data from the NFL Injury Analytics Database linked with biomedical engineering data, such as helmet testing and video review, the NFL has changed the game in a multitude of ways to improve player safety and reduce the number of concussions. Efforts have been focused on improving helmet technology, decreasing the forces of each head impact, reducing the number of head impacts, and changing play rules to mitigate the frequency of severe head impact. A timeline and summary of all key reporting measures and rules changes are shown in ▸ Fig. 40.6.

40.4.1 Equipment-Related Changes

Helmet Safety

Each year the NFL and the NFLPA publish helmet laboratory testing performance results, an initiative led by appointed biomechanical experts from each organization (▸ Fig. 40.7).[38] Each helmet model worn by NFL players is listed in order of its performance in laboratory testing, with rankings based on the ability of the helmet to reduce head impact severity.[38] Performance is most often evaluated based on linear and rotational accelerations.[27] Each year, the NFL and NFLPA release a document outlining permissible helmets by brand and model based on laboratory performance. Helmets highlighted in green are top performing and recommended for use by the NFL. Helmets highlighted in red are the poorest performing and are prohibited. For newly prohibited helmets (red), new players and those who have not worn the helmets in the previous year are not permitted to use these helmets. All players are required to discontinue use of a prohibited helmet 1 year after it becomes prohibited.[39] Data has shown strong correlation of lab testing to on field injury rates for each helmet.[26]

RETURN-TO-PARTICIPATION PROTOCOL

NFL NFLPA

PHASE 1

SYMPTOM LIMITED ACTIVITY

The player is prescribed rest, limiting or, if necessary, avoiding activities (both physical and cognitive) which increase or aggravate symptoms. Under athletic training staff supervision, limited stretching and balance training can be introduced, progressing to light aerobic exercise, all as tolerated.

PHASE 2

AEROBIC EXERCISE

Under direct oversight of the team's medical staff, the player should begin graduated cardiovascular exercise and may also engage in dynamic stretching and balance training. Neurocognitive and balance testing can be administered after completion of Phase Two and the results should be interpreted as back to baseline.

PHASE 3

FOOTBALL-SPECIFIC EXERCISE

The player continues with supervised cardiovascular exercises that are increased and may mimic sport-specific activities, and supervised strength training is introduced. The player is allowed to practice with the team in sport-specific exercise for 30 minutes or less with ongoing and careful monitoring.

PHASE 4

CLUB-BASED NONCONTACT TRAINING DRILLS

The player continues cardiovascular, strength and balance training, team-based sports-specific exercise, and participates in noncontact football activities (e.g. throwing, catching, running, and other position-specific activities). Neurocognitive and balance testing should be completed no later than the end of Phase Four with the results interpreted as back to baseline.

PHASE 5

FULL FOOTBALL ACTIVITY / CLEARANCE

Upon clearance by the Club physician for full football activity involving contact, the player must be examined by the Independent Neurological Consultant (INC) assigned to the Club. If the INC concurs with the Club physician that the player's concussion has resolved, the player may participate in the Club's next practice or game.

Revised July 2020

Fig. 40.5 National Football League (NFL) Return-to-Participation Protocol. (Reproduced from The National Football League and the National Football League Players Association.)

Table 40.2 Summary of peer-reviewed scientific research about head injury safety, head impacts, and concussion in the NFL

Study	Year	Title	Key takeaway
Lessley et al[18]	2018	Video analysis of reported concussion events in the National Football League during the 2015–2016 and 2016–2017 seasons	• This study evaluated all concussions from 2015 to 2017 in the NFL by video review and found cornerbacks had highest number of concussions • Concussions most commonly occurred on passing plays often involving tackling and impact to the side of head, which was inconsistent with patterns in previous seasons
Gabler et al[19]	2018	Development of a metric for predicting brain strain responses using head kinematics	• This study successfully aimed to develop a new brain injury metric, Universal Brain Injury Criterion (UBrIC), to improve impact modeling with a goal of implementation within the domain of helmet design
Ellenbogen et al[17]	2018	National Football League Head, Neck and Spine Committee's Concussion Diagnosis and Management Protocol: 2017–18 season	• This paper established the updated NFL Head, Neck, and Spine Committee's recommendations regarding concussion management based on the evolving literature • Management protocol, diagnosis of concussion, and implementation are thoroughly outlined using known literature at that time
Joodaki et al[20]	2019	Relative motion between the helmet and the head in football impact test	• This study aimed to compare head and helmet motion in football impacts using an impact model • Linear acceleration and angular velocity were significantly different between the helmet and the head suggesting that evaluating only helmet impact forces is insufficient for accurate understanding of forces to the head
Sanchez et al[21]	2019	A reanalysis of football impact reconstructions for head kinematics and finite element modeling	• Evaluation of accelerometer consistency and error evolved over time, which suggested interpretation of prior data may have been flawed • This study applied these new techniques to previously evaluated data and found a significant change in the forces seen in these impacts suggesting prior study conclusions should be re-evaluated based on this new information
Mack et al[11]	2019	Engaging athletic trainers in concussion detection: overview of the National Football League ATC Spotter Program, 2011–2017	• This paper discusses the growth and evolution of the certified athletic trainer spotter program from its inception to the 2017 current state including increased numbers of spotters, as well as placement of injury review systems on field
Funk et al[22]	2020	Laboratory reconstructions of concussive helmet-to-helmet impacts in the National Football League	• This study compared 17 concussive events and video-determined forces with modeled simulation data • Detailed video evaluation, physical surrogate determination, and iterative testing were necessary to optimize error to less than half of the effect size
Bailey et al[23]	2020	Characterization of concussive events in professional American football using videogrammetry	• Use of high-speed cameras and laser scanning allowed for calculation of change in velocity of helmets during impact • Results found helmet-to-ground impacts to have highest change in translational velocity which provides useful information for helmet design
Kent et al[24]	2020	The biomechanics of concussive helmet-to-ground impacts in the National Football League	• This study looked to assess the characteristics of 16 concussion generating impacts • The average impact velocity was found to be 8.3 m/s with an average angle of nearly 45 degrees • The study also assessed head motion relative to helmet motion and found significant decoupling resulting in greater force to the head than helmet over a short impact window of 15 to 30 milliseconds
Lessley et al[25]	2020	Position-specific circumstances of concussions in the NFL: Toward the development of position-specific helmets	• A total of 647 concussions over the course of four seasons were evaluated showing that certain impact characteristics are prevalent among all positions while some types of impacts are disproportionately common in specific positions which may lead to benefit of position-specific helmet design
Bailey et al[26]	2020	Comparison of laboratory and on-field performance of American football helmets	• Modeled impacts were generated within the laboratory setting and a helmet performance score was created which positively correlated with the rate of concussion seen among athletes • These findings suggest that helmets could be evaluated for safety in the laboratory and allow for determination of inferior helmet designs that needed to be prohibited to protect the athlete
Bailey et al[27]	2020	Development and evaluation of a test method for assessing the performance of American football helmets	• This study developed a model to test for helmet performance and performed tests at two locations to assess inter-lab variability • They found the inter-lab results to have a variability of 1.1% and found there was as much as a 33% difference in the performance of the best and worst helmets
Kent et al[28]	2020	Surface contact features, impact obliquity, and preimpact rotational motion in concussive helmet-to-ground impacts: assessment via a new impact test device	• This study aimed to create a model to evaluate head to ground impacts since they are a common driver of concussions • The study creates a model that takes into account oblique impact velocity, compliance of the surface, friction of the surface, head loading, and rotational velocity during ground contact to optimize helmet evaluation

(Continued)

Table 40.2 (*Continued*) Summary of peer-reviewed scientific research about head injury safety, head impacts, and concussion in the NFL

Study	Year	Title	Key takeaway
Bailey et al[29]	2020	Validation of a videogrammetry technique for analysing American football helmet kinematics	• This study evaluated modeled concussion impacts and reviewed video footage from high-speed recording typically available from broadcasting to validate its use for impact evaluation • Results showed that high-speed footage is capable of accurately evaluating the forces of impact, but low frame rate was only able to assess preimpact characteristics accurately
Gabler et al[30]	2020	On-field performance of an instrumented mouthguard for detecting head impacts in American football	• This study evaluated the precision of instrumented mouthguards in detecting head strikes after initial data was modeled to account for spurious activity • The instrumented mouthguard using the model was able to achieve 98.3% precision and 81.6% recall
Mack et al[12]	2020	Enhancing concussion management in the National Football League: evolution and initial results of the unaffiliated neurotrauma consultants program, 2012–2017	• This paper discusses the evolving role of unaffiliated neurotrauma consultants in the National Football League • The paper also discusses the increase in compliance, average evaluations per game (1.9), and establishes high sensitivity (93.4–97.4%) and specificity (81.0–88.3%)
Zuckerman et al[31]	2020	Concussions in the National Football League: the evolution of video review for assessing the frequency and reliability of visible signs	• This paper looked at visible signs of athlete injury including lack of coordination, slow to get up, seizure, and facial injury • With expert raters, total percentage agreement in evaluation of visible signs was 83 to 100%
Elbin et al[32]	2020	Sensitivity and specificity of on-field visible signs of concussion in the National Football League	• This study defined the percentage of concussion events with visible signs of concussion • Most commonly seen was the athlete being slow to get up (65.9%) with blank/vacant look and seizure being the most specific (100%) • The study also showed that visible signs of concussion alone were not sufficient for diagnosis of concussion but served a valuable function in comprehensive athlete evaluation
Bailey et al[33]	2021	Laboratory evaluation of shell add-on products for American football helmets for professional linemen	• This study looked at externally worn helmet shell add-on products and found that they decreased the force that a helmet received in linear impact but worsened helmet characteristics in some scenarios • Additionally, they found no significant difference in the predicted effect on neck injury
Gabler et al[34]	2021	Development of a low-power instrumented mouthpiece for directly measuring head acceleration in American football	• This study successfully aimed to develop an instrumented mouthpiece that allowed for measurement rather than calculation of linear and angular acceleration of the head • Additionally, they aimed to decrease power usage and size of mouthguard while maintaining accuracy
Mack et al[3]	2021	Epidemiology of concussion in the National Football League, 2015–2019	• This study evaluated the rates and trends of concussions from 2015 to 2019 • The study found a downtrend in the number of concussions from 231 concussions per year to 177 concussions per year during the study window • The study compares game versus practice concussion rates as well as position-specific concussion frequency
Park et al[35]	2022	Head shape analysis of National Football League players	• The goal of this study was to better characterize the shape of football players' heads to optimize helmet sizing • A three-dimensional scan was performed showing that variation was mostly related to sagittal plane height and length as well as prominent shape and size of back of the head
Cools et al[36]	2022	Same-year repeat concussions in the National Football League: trends from 2015 through 2019	• This study evaluated the likelihood of athletes having a same-year concussion and found the rate to be 0.38 to 0.69% per season • The likelihood of an athlete sustaining a second concussion was similar to what is seen in first concussion events but were noted to have longer return to play after the second concussion
Mack et al[37]	2022	Return to full participation following concussion in the National Football League, 2015 through 2020	• Among National Football League players who suffered a concussion from 2015 to 2020, the median time to return to play was 9 days • About 38% of athletes who sustained a concussion in a Sunday game were able to participate in a game the following week while the majority were not
Jacobi et al[16]	2023	The National Football League Concussion Protocol: a review	• This article reviews the current state of the National Football League concussion protocol • Aspects of the protocol discussed include education, baseline testing, surveillance, concussion evaluation, and return to play recommendations
Inclan et al[6]	2023	Validity of research based on publicly obtained data in sports medicine: a quantitative assessment of concussions in the National Football League	• This study evaluated the accuracy of publicly obtained data on concussions compared with National Football League databases • The study showed that approximately 70% of concussions are documented in the public data with a wide range between various studies • Difference was also noted in the position-specific reported rates of concussion between the two groups

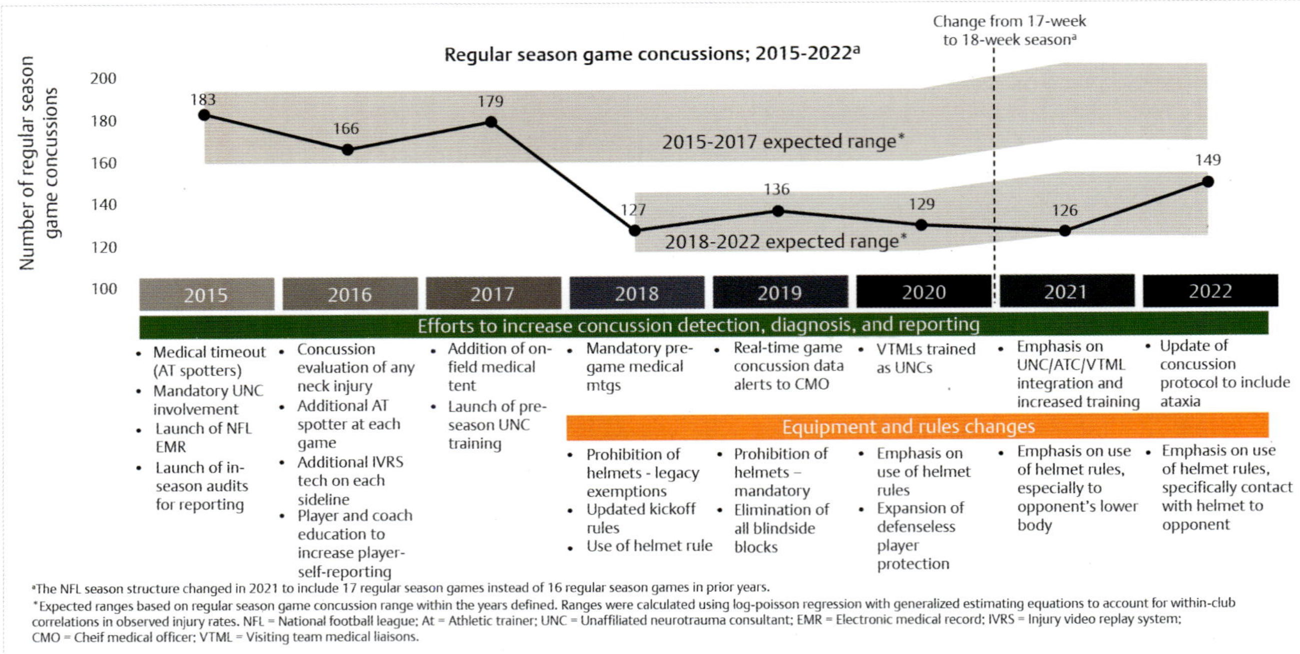

Fig. 40.6 Comprehensive review of decreased concussion counts, efforts to increase concussion detection, and key rule changes. ATC, certified athletic trainer; CMO; IVRS, Injury Video Replay System; mtgs; NFL EMR, National Football League electronic medical record; UNC, unaffiliated neurotrauma consultant; VTMLs, visiting team medical liaisons. (Source: Used with permission from Mack CD, et al. *Sports Health.* Sage Publications: 2021;13(5):423–430)

Guardian Cap

The Guardian Cap is an add-on device worn over the football helmet that has been shown to reduce the magnitude of head impacts. For the 2022 preseason, the NFL required Guardian Cap use among all offensive and defensive linemen, tight ends, and linebackers in practices from the start of the training camp contact period through the second preseason game.[40] The Guardian Cap has been available for several years, and although the first iteration was not as successful in reducing head impact severity,[41] there is laboratory evidence that the second version reduced the linear and rotational accelerations of some impacts.[42] The theory behind the Guardian Cap is that an external pad increases the thickness of the overall padding system, which can absorb additional force and subsequently reduce the amount of force that is transmitted to the head and brain.[42] A recent study published by NFL- and NFLPA-affiliated biomechanical engineers revealed that, in laboratory tests, the NFL version of the Guardian Cap resulted in a 10% reduction in severity of impact, and an estimated 20% reduction in dummy-to-dummy testing with both helmets wearing the Guardian Cap.[33] Although the primary purpose of the Guardian Cap is to reduce the severity of head impacts, there was a 52% decrease in preseason practice concussions among players in Guardian Cap–mandated positions (offensive line, tight end, defensive line, and linebackers) in the first year of the mandate.[13] Due to positive feedback and a 52% decrease in 2022 concussions among Guardian Cap–mandated positions, the NFL expanded the mandate in 2023 to require Guardian Cap use among running backs and for all preseason and regular season contact practices.

Position-Specific Helmets

Over the past two seasons, position-specific helmets have been introduced. Based on studies conducted by NFL and NFLPA engineers, data from epidemiologic investigations, as well as funding from the NFL to innovate helmet technology, helmet manufacturers have developed helmets specifically designed for both linemen and quarterbacks.[25,39,43] Data show that over half of all quarterback concussions occur due to helmet-to-ground contact, and a large proportion occur when the back of the head hits the ground.[39] Therefore, new quarterback helmets have additional padding in the occipital area to reduce the head-to-ground impacts. In addition, the top-ranked helmets in the NFL's 2023 helmet rankings include offensive and defensive lineman (OL/DL) helmets that protect common points of contact for linemen, including the front and upper sides. Although historically the side of the helmet has been one of the least padded areas of the entire helmet, the OL/DL helmets have bumpers in these locations which are intended to absorb higher head impacts and mitigate the forces of these side-to-side head impacts.[44]

40.4.2 Changes to Game Play

A key change within the NFL is the increased ability for player health and safety data to generate informative evidence that is used by the NFL Competition Committee to create and modify rules that make the game safer. Over 50 rules have been added or changed based on an evidence-driven approach since 2002 with 22 coming in the last decade.[45] Here, we highlight four that are focused on concussion reduction.

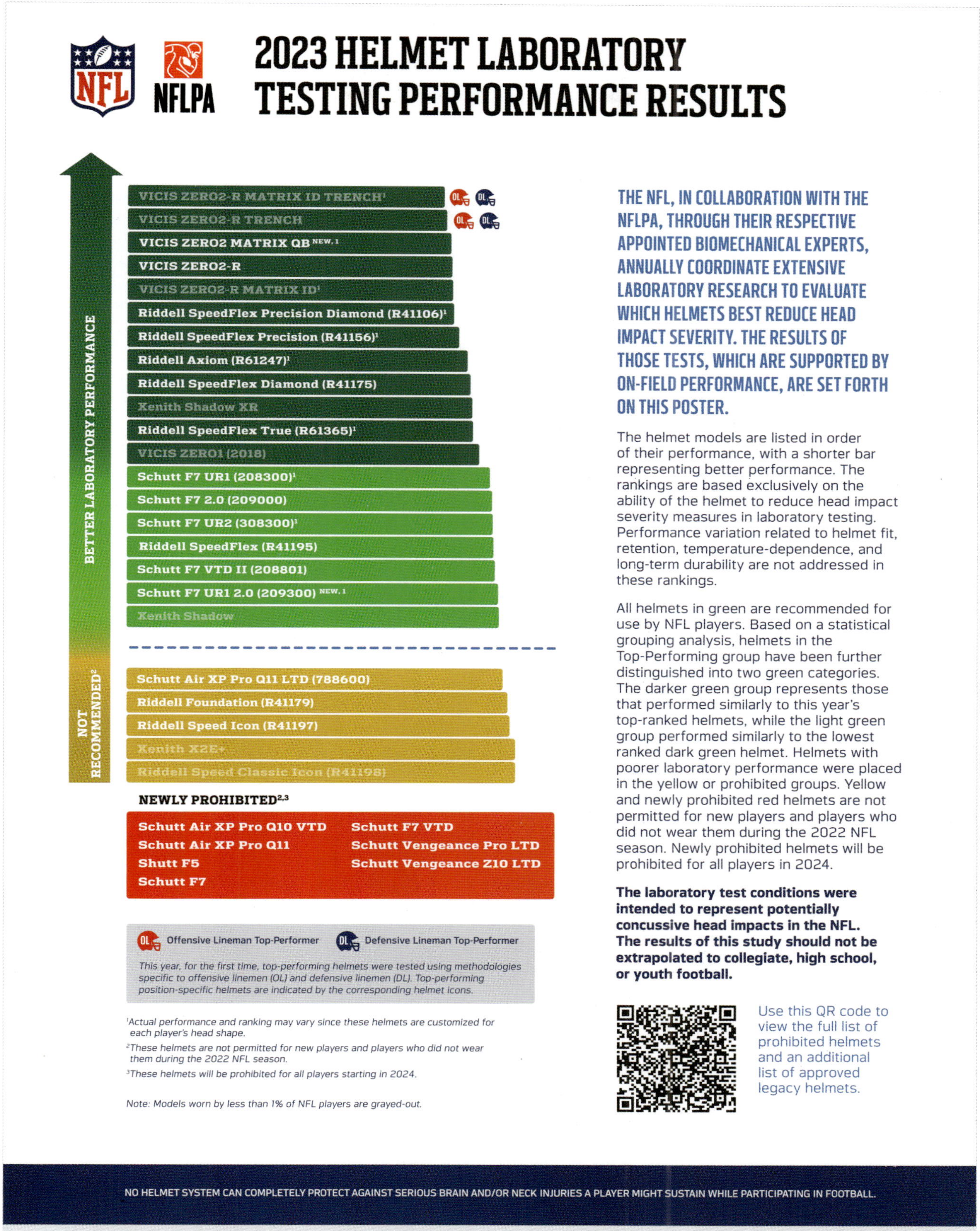

Fig. 40.7 Helmet laboratory testing performance results from 2023. (Reproduced from The National Football League and the National Football League Players Association.)

Updated Kickoff Rules

In a single season, approximately 2,700 NFL plays are kickoffs, where a team cedes possession after a scoring play, or a half is started by kicking deep from one side of the field to the other. Data showed that the combination of space and speed between the two teams on kickoff plays led to high rates of concussion compared to rushing and passing plays.[46] Several iterations of kickoff rules have been implemented with the intent to reduce injuries in the kickoff play. As one example, in 2009, the "wedge" style of block by the return team, where multiple players would align next to one another to form a shield, was eliminated.[45] In 2016, the NFL moved up the starting point from where the ball was kicked, thereby decreasing the distance from kickoff point to the endzone and increasing the probability of a touchback.[45] The offense's starting point also moved from the 20- to the 25-yard line, further incentivizing teams to refrain from returning a kickoff.[45]

With concussion rates per kickoff return still elevated in 2018, the league changed permissible formations on kickoff plays, including (i) where players can align at the start of the play and (ii) where players on the receiving team can block opponents. In May of 2023, the NFL further refined the kickoff play. Beginning in the 2023 season, if a player calls for a fair catch behind the 25-yard line, the ball will be placed at the 25-yard line. Given the risk for concussion with multiple special team players charging at full speed over a long distance, these kickoff rule changes have helped mitigate the frequency of high-energy head impacts leading to concussions.[46]

Use-of-Helmet Rule

The aligning of the head, neck, and thoracic spine creates a high force vector. Of note, this vector is created when tacklers lead with their helmet to make contact with another player's helmet.[46] Due to the lab and on-field evidence illustrating the high risk of this style of play, the NFL initiated the use-of-helmet rule in 2018. This rule made it a foul for players to deliberately lower their head to initiate contact with their helmet against the opponent, which would result in loss of yards and/or discipline to the offending player.[47] In 2022, the word "initiate" was replaced with "make forcible contact" (if players lower their head and make forcible contact with their helmet against the opponent). This subtle change was meant to only capture behavior that evidenced a player's specific intent to make contact with the helmets against another player.[48] In 2023, the NFL built on the rule to make it a foul for a player to use the helmet to butt, spear, ram, or make forcible contact to an opponent's head or neck area.

Elimination of Blindside Blocks

In 2019, the NFL banned "blindside blocks," defined as when "the blocker is moving toward his own endline and approaches the opponent from behind or from the side, and the initial force of the contact by the blocker's helmet, forearm, or shoulder is to the head or neck area of an opponent."[45] These blocks were noted to account for approximately one-third of concussions on punt returns.[49] When players are not aware of an oncoming hit and cannot brace their neck to protect against a head impact, high rates of rotational acceleration can occur bringing an increased risk of concussion.[50]

Defenseless Player Rules

Over the past decade, there have been several modifications and expansions to the "defenseless player" rule. The first iteration, initiated in 2009, made the "blindside block" illegal, i.e., hitting a defenseless receiver if the initial force of the contact by the defender is to the head or neck area of the receiver.[45] In 2011, the rule was further refined to provide that receivers who had completed a catch are considered "defenseless" until they have had time to protect themselves or have clearly become a runner.[51] The list of defenseless players was also expanded to include a kicker/punter during the kick or during the return and a quarterback at any time after a change of possession. In 2013, further expansion included long snappers during field goals and the point after touchdown attempts. The list was later expanded to include a receiver when a pass was not caught or there was an interception.

40.5 Conclusions

The NFL's approach to head injury data collection and evidence-based concussion reduction initiatives shows that player health and safety data collection is an ever-evolving practice. Established programs are continually evaluated, as evidenced by the expansion of the AT spotter and UNC programs as new data emerge and new clinical guidelines are developed. New areas of focus are constantly arising. The NFL will continue to advance studies that will aim to better inform individual concussion management and assist in modifying playing style to reduce the number and severity of head impacts.

In addition to internal research efforts, the NFL has also funded external efforts to empirically investigate the nature of head impacts associated with SRC. The NFL has contributed hundreds of millions of dollars to medical research and education involving all aspects of player health and safety, including funding to the Head Health Initiative and to independent university-sponsored research.[20]

Although these data and safety changes are taking place at the highest level of American football, we would be remiss not to mention the potential trickle-down effect that NFL player safety changes can have on lower levels of football play. There are over 3 million high school and youth football players in the US.[52] The evidence-driven programs at the NFL level as well as the scientific findings around concussions hold applicability to safety efforts at lower levels of play, and dissemination of this information can contribute broadly to enhanced safety across collision sports. This is critical as studies continue to show the positive impact that participation in team sports has on young athletes.[53,54,55,56,57]

Participation in any sport incurs a risk of injury. However, robust data collection and methodologically sound research can lead to insights that drive evidence-based strategies that reduce injuries. This knowledge can be applied to the NFL but may also provide insights that influence all levels of football.

40.6 Clinical Pearls

- High-quality data can be leveraged to identify areas of focus and drive effectiveness in athletic safety programs and injury reduction efforts.
- The NFL has built robust, data-driven SRC diagnosis and detection programs with components that can be applied to other settings in sports.
- Evidence-based programs, rule changes, and equipment improvements have led to an overall reduction in SRC in the NFL.

40.7 Conflicts of Interest and Source of Funding

Drs. Mack, Wasserman, Herzog, and Roby are full-time employees for IQVIA which is in a paid consultancy with sports organizations including the NFL. Dr. Zuckerman reports being an unaffiliated neurotrauma consultant for the NFL and a member of the NFL Head, Neck and Spine Committee. Dr. Solomon is a paid consultant of the NFL and Dr. Sills is a full-time NFL employee.

References

[1] Statistics and Data: Most popular sports in the United States. Statisticsanddata.org. 2022. Accessed at: https://statisticsanddata.org/data/most-popular-sports-in-the-united-states/

[2] Mack CD, Kent RW, Coughlin MJ, et al. Incidence of lower extremity injury in the National Football League: 2015 to 2018. Am J Sports Med. 2020; 48 (9):2287–2294

[3] Mack CD, Solomon G, Covassin T, Theodore N, Cárdenas J, Sills A. Epidemiology of concussion in the National Football League, 2015–2019. Sports Health. 2021; 13(5):423–430

[4] Dreyer NA, Mack CD, Anderson RB, Wojtys EM, Hershman EB, Sills A. Lessons on data collection and curation from the NFL Injury Surveillance Program. Sports Health. 2019; 11(5):440–445

[5] Inclan PM, Chang PS, Mack CD, et al. Validity of research based on public data in sports medicine: a quantitative assessment of anterior cruciate ligament injuries in the National Football League. Am J Sports Med. 2022; 50 (6):1717–1726

[6] Inclan PM, Kuhn AW, Chang PS, et al. Validity of research based on publicly obtained data in sports medicine: a quantitative assessment of concussions in the National Football League. Sports Health. 2023; 15(4):527–536

[7] NFL Head, Neck and Spine Committee's Concussion Diagnosis and Management Protocol. Published October 8, 2022. Accessed at: https://static.www.nfl.com/image/upload/v1665264248/league/moexjmdzy2kvjtqsdpbx.pdf

[8] NFL Presents: Emergency Preparedness in Sports (VIDEO). Published February 2, 2023. Accessed at: https://www.nfl.com/playerhealthandsafety/health-and-wellness/player-care/nfl-presents-emergency-preparedness-in-sports-webinar

[9] Ochiai H, Abe T. Clinical features and early detection of sport-related concussion. Acute Med Surg. 2018; 6(1):49–53

[10] Register-Mihalik JK, Guskiewicz KM, McLeod TC, Linnan LA, Mueller FO, Marshall SW. Knowledge, attitude, and concussion-reporting behaviors among high school athletes: a preliminary study. J Athl Train. 2013; 48(5): 645–653

[11] Mack C, Myers E, Barnes R, Solomon G, Sills A. Engaging athletic trainers in concussion detection: overview of the National Football League ATC Spotter Program, 2011–2017. J Athl Train. 2019; 54(8):852–857

[12] Mack C, Sendor RR, Solomon G, et al. Enhancing concussion management in the National Football League: evolution and initial results of the Unaffiliated Neurotrauma Consultants program, 2012–2017. Neurosurgery. 2020; 87(2): 312–319

[13] Transcript: End-of-Season Health & Safety Briefing, February 3, 2023. Published February 3, 2023. Accessed at: https://www.nfl.com/playerhealthandsafety/resources/press-releases/transcript-end-of-season-health-safety-briefing-february-3-2023

[14] Haugen AS, Sevdalis N, Søfteland E. Impact of the World Health Organization surgical safety checklist on patient safety. Anesthesiology. 2019; 131(2): 420–425

[15] A 21st Century Sideline. Published November 23, 2016. Accessed at: https://www.nfl.com/playerhealthandsafety/health-and-wellness/player-care/a-21st-century-sideline#:~:text=This%20Injury%20Video%20Review%20System%20%28IVRS%29%2C%20implemented%20in,staffs%20to%20communicate%20with%20the%20booth%20ATC%20spotters

[16] Jacobi J, Wasserman EB, Mack CD, et al. The National Football League Concussion Protocol: a review. HSS J. 2023; 19(3):269–276

[17] Ellenbogen RG, Batjer H, Cardenas J, et al. National Football League Head, Neck and Spine Committee's Concussion Diagnosis and Management Protocol: 2017–18 season. Br J Sports Med. 2018; 52(14):894–902

[18] Lessley DJ, Kent RW, Funk JR, et al. Video analysis of reported concussion events in the National Football League during the 2015–2016 and 2016–2017 seasons. Am J Sports Med. 2018; 46(14):3502–3510

[19] Gabler LF, Crandall JR, Panzer MB. Development of a metric for predicting brain strain responses using head kinematics. Ann Biomed Eng. 2018; 46(7): 972–985

[20] Joodaki H, Bailey A, Lessley D, Funk J, Sherwood C, Crandall J. Relative motion between the helmet and the head in football impact test. J Biomech Eng. 2019; 141(8):081006

[21] Sanchez EJ, Gabler LF, Good AB, Funk JR, Crandall JR, Panzer MB. A reanalysis of football impact reconstructions for head kinematics and finite element modeling. Clin Biomech (Bristol, Avon). 2019; 64:82–89

[22] Funk JR, Jadischke R, Bailey A, et al. Laboratory reconstructions of concussive helmet-to-helmet impacts in the National Football League. Ann Biomed Eng. 2020; 48(11):2652–2666

[23] Bailey AM, Sherwood CP, Funk JR, et al. Characterization of concussive events in professional American football using videogrammetry. Ann Biomed Eng. 2020; 48(11):2678–2690

[24] Kent R, Forman J, Bailey AM, et al. The biomechanics of concussive helmet-to-ground impacts in the National Football League. J Biomech. 2020; 99: 109551

[25] Lessley DJ, Kent RW, Cormier JM, et al. Position-specific circumstances of concussions in the NFL: toward the development of position-specific helmets. Ann Biomed Eng. 2020; 48(11):2542–2554

[26] Bailey AM, McMurry TL, Cormier JM, et al. Comparison of laboratory and on-field performance of American football helmets. Ann Biomed Eng. 2020; 48 (11):2531–2541

[27] Bailey AM, Sanchez EJ, Park G, et al. Development and evaluation of a test method for assessing the performance of American football helmets. Ann Biomed Eng. 2020; 48(11):2566–2579

[28] Kent R, Forman J, Bailey A, et al. Surface contact features, impact obliquity, and preimpact rotational motion in concussive helmet-to-ground impacts: assessment via a new impact test device. Ann Biomed Eng. 2020; 48(11): 2639–2651

[29] Bailey A, Funk J, Lessley D, et al. Validation of a videogrammetry technique for analysing American football helmet kinematics. Sports Biomech. 2020; 19(5):678–700

[30] Gabler LF, Huddleston SH, Dau NZ, et al. On-field performance of an instrumented mouthguard for detecting head impacts in American football. Ann Biomed Eng. 2020; 48(11):2599–2612

[31] Zuckerman SL, Elbin RJ, Sills AK, et al. Concussions in the National Football League: the evolution of video review for assessing the frequency and reliability of visible signs. Phys Sportsmed. 2020; 48(4):424–429

[32] Elbin RJ, Zuckerman SL, Sills AK, Crandall JR, Lessley DJ, Solomon GS. Sensitivity and specificity of on-field visible signs of concussion in the National Football League. Neurosurgery. 2020; 87(3):530–537

[33] Bailey AM, Funk JR, Crandall JR, Myers BS, Arbogast KB. Laboratory evaluation of shell add-on products for American football helmets for professional linemen. Ann Biomed Eng. 2021; 49(10):2747–2759

[34] Gabler LF, Dau NZ, Park G, Miles A, Arbogast KB, Crandall JR. Development of a low-power instrumented mouthpiece for directly measuring head acceleration in American football. Ann Biomed Eng. 2021; 49(10):2760–2776

[35] Park G, Gabler LF, Bailey AM, et al. Head shape analysis of National Football League players. Proc Inst Mech Eng Part P J Sports Eng Technol. 2022; 236 (4):334–340

[36] Cools M, Zuckerman SL, Herzog M, et al. Same-year repeat concussions in the National Football League: trends from 2015 through 2019. World Neurosurg. 2022; 161:e441–e447

[37] Mack CD, Herzog MM, Solomon G, et al. Return to full participation following concussion in the National Football League, 2015 through 2020. Clin J Sport Med. 2022; 32(6):e605–e613

[38] Helmet Laboratory Testing Performance Results. Published April 13, 2023. Accessed at: https://www.nfl.com/playerhealthandsafety/equipment-and-innovation/equipment-testing/helmet-laboratory-testing-performance-results

[39] NFL Enters Next Era of Helmet Safety with Quarterback-Specific Helmet. Published April 13, 2023. Accessed at: https://operations.nfl.com/updates/the-game/nfl-enters-next-era-of-helmet-safety-with-quarterback-specific-helmet/

[40] Guardian Cap Debuts at Training Camps around the NFL. Published July 29, 2022. Accessed at: https://operations.nfl.com/updates/the-game/guardian-cap-debuts-at-training-camps-around-the-nfl/

[41] Quigley KG, Hopfe D, Taylor MR, et al. Preliminary examination of Guardian Cap head impact data using instrumented mouthguards. ArXiv. 2023. Preprint

[42] Breedlove KM, Breedlove E, Nauman E, Bowman TG, Lininger MR. The ability of an aftermarket helmet add-on device to reduce impact-force accelerations during drop tests. J Athl Train. 2017; 52(9):802–808

[43] Nathanson JT, Connolly JG, Yuk F, et al. Concussion incidence in professional football: position-specific analysis with use of a novel metric. Orthop J Sports Med. 2016; 4(1):2325967115622621

[44] Rapp T. NFL, NFLPA Approve Position-Specific Helmets for OL, DL; Features Safety Bumpers. Published April 21, 2021. Accessed at: https://bleacherreport.com/articles/2940595-nfl-nflpa-approve-position-specific-helmets-for-ol-dl-features-safety-bumpers

[45] NFL Health and Safety Related Rules Changes Since 2002: A Constant Evolution. Published September 26, 2019. Accessed at: https://www.nfl.com/playerhealthandsafety/equipment-and-innovation/rules-changes/nfl-health-and-safety-related-rules-changes-since-2002#:~:text=Defenseless%20player%20protections%20are%20expanded,on%20the%20line%20of%20scrimmage

[46] Pellman EJ, Powell JW, Viano DC, Casson IR, Tucker AM, Feuer H, et al. Concussion in professional football: epidemiological features of game injuries and review of the literature–part 3. Neurosurgery. 2004; 54(1):81–94; discussion -6

[47] Health and Safety Related Changes for the 2018 Season. Published August 1, 2018. Accessed at: https://www.nfl.com/playerhealthandsafety/equipment-and-innovation/rules-changes/health-and-safety-related-changes-for-the-2018-season

[48] NFL Video Rulebook. Use of the Helmet. Accessed at: https://operations.nfl.com/the-rules/nfl-video-rulebook/use-of-the-helmet/#:~:text=Rule%20Summary%20View%20Official%20Rule&text=It%20is%20a%20foul%20if,The%20player%20may%20be%20disqualified

[49] Teope H. League owners vote to eliminate blindside blocks. Updated March 26, 2019. Accessed at: https://www.nfl.com/news/league-owners-vote-to-eliminate-blindside-blocks-0ap3000001024314

[50] Zuckerman SL, Totten DJ, Rubel KE, Kuhn AW, Yengo-Kahn AM, Solomon GS. Mechanisms of injury as a diagnostic predictor of sport-related concussion severity in football, basketball, and soccer: results from a regional concussion registry. Neurosurgery. 2016; 63 Suppl 1:102–112

[51] NFL Video Rulebook. Defenseless Player. Accessed at: https://operations.nfl.com/the-rules/nfl-video-rulebook/defenseless-player/

[52] Farrey T. Youth football participation increases in 2015; teen involvement down, data shows. Published April 15, 2016. Accessed at: https://www.espn.com/espn/otl/story/_/id/15210245/slight-one-year-increase-number-youth-playing-football-data-shows

[53] Zuckerman SL, Tang AR, Richard KE, et al. The behavioral, psychological, and social impacts of team sports: a systematic review and meta-analysis. Phys Sportsmed. 2021; 49(3):246–261

[54] Andersen MH, Ottesen L, Thing LF. The social and psychological health outcomes of team sport participation in adults: an integrative review of research. Scand J Public Health. 2019; 47(8):832–850

[55] Harrison PA, Narayan G. Differences in behavior, psychological factors, and environmental factors associated with participation in school sports and other activities in adolescence. J Sch Health. 2003; 73(3):113–120

[56] Eime RM, Young JA, Harvey JT, Charity MJ, Payne WR. A systematic review of the psychological and social benefits of participation in sport for children and adolescents: informing development of a conceptual model of health through sport. Int J Behav Nutr Phys Act. 2013; 10:98

[57] Zuckerman SL, Yengo-Kahn AM, Brett BL, Kuhn AW, Wolfson DI, Kerr ZY. Benefits of team sport participation versus concerns of chronic traumatic encephalopathy: prioritizing the health of our youth. Concussion. 2020; 5(2):CNC75

Index

Note: Page numbers set **bold** or *italic* indicate headings or figures, respectively.

A

B

C

D

E

F

G

H

I

J

K

L

Q

R

S

T

U

V

W

X